Comprehensive Management of Spine Trauma

Comprehensive Management of Spine Trauma

Daniel A. Capen, M.D.
Associate Clinical Professor
Neurotrauma Service
USC-Rancho Los Amigos Medical Center
Downey, California

Willi Haye, RN
H-D Medical Projects
Santa Fe, New Mexico

with 430 *illustrations*

Mosby

St. Louis Baltimore Boston Carlsbad Chicago Minneapolis New York Philadelphia Portland
London Milan Sydney Tokyo Toronto

Mosby
Dedicated to Publishing Excellence

A Times Mirror
Company

Publisher: Geoff Greenwood
Executive Editor: Robert A. Hurley
Editorial Assistant: Jori Matison
Project Manager: Chris Baumle
Production Editor: Eric Van Gordon
Designer: Carolyn O'Brien
Manufacturing Manager: William A. Winneberger, Jr.
Cover Design: Gail Hudson

First Edition

Printed in the United States of America
Composition by Bi-Comp, Inc.
Printing/binding by Maple-Vail Book Manufacturing Group

Mosby, Inc.
11830 Westline Industrial Drive
St. Louis, Missouri 63146

Library of Congress Cataloging in Publication Data

Comprehensive management of spine trauma / [edited by] Daniel A. Capen, Willi Haye. — 1st ed.
p. cm.
Includes bibliographical references and index.
ISBN 0-8151-1463-X
1. Spinal cord—Wounds and injuries—Treatment. 2. Spine—Wounds and injuries—Treatment. I. Capen, Daniel A. II. Haye, Willi.
[DNLM: 1. Spinal Injuries—therapy. 2. Spinal Injuries—diagnosis. 3. Spinal Cord Injuries—therapy. 4. Spinal Cord Injuries—diagnosis. WE 725 C7375 1998]
RD594.3.C65 1998
617.4'82044—dc21
DNLM/DLC
for Library of Congress 97-42383
CIP

98 99 00 01 02/9 8 7 6 5 4 3 2 1

This book reflects the work of my teachers at UCSF, my partners at Southwestern Orthopedic, the spirit of Rancho Los Amigos Medical Center, which has become a victim of the for-profit corporate HMO "Reform" of U.S. healthcare, and my Rancho colleagues and friends, Drs. Garland, Waters, Rothman, and Zigler. A special thanks to all the contributors for their diligent and important work and to my wife Deborah for her patience and support.

This book is dedicated to Nicholas Capen, Matthew Capen, and Camryn Montalvo, three very special young people.

PREFACE

Since Egyptian and Greco-Roman civilizations, writings on spine trauma have existed. Advances from these time periods to modern medicine have permitted diagnosis and treatment of spinal problems in a much more successful manner. This text brings together information on all current technological advances. Injuries that were once hopeless now are treated with great success. The text offers some historical perspective together with the state-of-art thinking on the management of minor injuries to the most major devastating spinal cord injuries.

In this era of health-care reform, there have been several treatment protocols that have been changed, including drastic reduction in hospitalization and a remarkable shift toward outpatient care and treatment. Physician time and energy, as well as reimbursement, have changed drastically. However, in terms of the management of spinal trauma, it is difficult to completely omit intrahospital care because, as you will read, many treatments for spinal trauma involve major surgical intervention.

Unfortunately, the modern era of medicine also has included development of a voracious appetite for malpractice and personal injury litigation in our society. Several of the chapters address these issues, including chapters on whiplash injury, the avoidance of complications, and radiology of spine trauma. In the text, the issue of surgical use of pedicle screws is addressed. One point of this book is to bring the practitioner up to date on the issues surrounding device development and the interfacing of modern American medicine with government bureaucratic agencies, including the FDA.

The media-induced litagation craze surrounding use of pedicle screw fixation is hot, and NASS has attempted to cool it. Fortunately, the vast majority of centers in developed countries rely heavily on pedicle screw fixation for the management of many types of trauma to the thoracolumbar spine, despite ongoing legal maneuvering. Hopefully, the reader will have the opportunity to judge not only the process of development of bone screw fixation for the spine, but actually have sufficient information as to the necessity and the efficacy of its use. Other new device techniques for spine fixation in cervical and thoracic regions also are described.

All the authors hope to provide the modern-day practitioner with a complete source of information concerning identification of spinal column injury, the treatment of these problems, and expected outcomes. Probably the most difficult condition known that a person can survive, spinal cord injury with quadra- or paraplegia, is addressed well from diagnosis to rehabilitation. The practitioner may be faced with specific challenges, and information necessary to provide appropriate treatment to meet these challenges is contained herein.

Although some authors prefer and emphasize specific approaches to problems in the spine trauma arena, the reader has an opportunity to correlate all data presented and judge on an individual basis to select the best treatment. However, all authors emphasize that standard goals of treatment are to appropriately realign the spine when necessary, to adequately protect the spine from further injury either by displacement or inadequate immobilization, and to provide an optimum environment for recovery, both skeletal and neurologic. All authors stress in their individual works the importance of 1) accurate and complete identification of the problem and 2) a well thought out plan of action to treat that problem. Following recommendations in this text will provide the practitioner with a plan to achieve optimum outcomes with a minimum of complications of treatment.

Between identification of the problem and achievement of optimum results, many individual judgments and treatment decisions are required. This text provides the opportunity to use information gathered from generations of practitioners before us, as well as information provided by practitioners among us today. This book also gives a glimpse into the future with respect to recent development of techniques and instrumentation, and treatment regimens for some areas in spinal trauma that represent "the unsolved problem," i.e., spinal cord injury research, research and development in instrumentation, and new approaches to management of spinal trauma.

CONTRIBUTORS

Todd J. Albert, MD
Assistant Professor
Thomas Jefferson University
Department of Orthopaedics
Attending Surgeon
Rothman Institute of Pennsylvania Hospital
Philadelphia, Pennsylvania

Paul A. Anderson, MD
Associate Clinical Professor
Department of Orthopaedic Surgery
University of Washington School of Medicine
Seattle, Washington

Richard A. Balderston, MD
Professor of Orthopaedic Surgery
Allegheny University Hospitals-Graduate
Philadelphia, Pennsylvania

Oheneba Boachie-Adjei, MD
Associate Clinical Professor
Cornell University Medical College
Chief, Scoliosis Service
Associate Attending Surgeon
The Hospital for Special Surgery
New York, New York

Rocco R. Calderone, MD
Staff Physician
Department of Neurotrauma
Rancho Los Amigos
USC Medical Center
Downey, California

Jerome M. Cotler, MD
The Everett J. and Marian Gordon Professor
Department of Orthopaedic Surgery
Jefferson Medical College of Thomas Jefferson University
Thomas Jefferson University Hospital
Philadelphia, Pennsylvania

Christian Hugo Dee, MD
Assistant Professor
Southern Illinois University School of Medicine
Division of Orthopaedics and Rehabilitation
Southern Illinois University School of Medicine
Springfield, Illinois

Rick B. Delamarter, MD
Associate Clinical Professor
UCLA Medical Center
Co-Director, UCLA Comprehensive Spine Center
UCLA Medical Center

Joel A. Finkelstein, MD, FRCS(C)
Assistant Professor
Department of Orthopaedics
University of Toronto
Sunnybrook Health Science Centre
Toronto, Ontario
Canada

Douglas E. Garland, MD
Clinical Professor of Orthopaedics
USC Medical Director
Jacqueline Perry Institute
Rancho Los Amigos Medical Center
Downey, California

Robert Thomas Greenfield, III, MD
Georgia Baptist Medical Center
Atlanta, Georgia
Rockdale Hospital
Conyers, Georgia

Robert E. Henry, MD
Diplomat, American Board of Physical Medicine and Rehabilitation
Director, Physical & Electrodiagnostic Medicine
Downey Orthopaedic Medical Group
Downey, California

Robert D. Harbaugh, MD
Director, Clinical Neurophysiology Laboratory
Cottage Hospital
Adult Neurologist
Neurology Associates of Santa Barbara
Santa Barbara, California

Serena S. Hu, MD
Assistant Professor
University of California, San Francisco
University of California, San Francisco Hospitals & Clinics
San Francisco, California

Mary C. Hume, MD
Assistant Professor of Orthopaedic Surgery
University of Southern California
Director, USC Spine Center
USC University Hospital
Los Angeles, California

Deborah Hyatt
Chicago, Illinois

Samuel S. Jorgenson, MD
Partner
San Ramon Valley Orthopaedic Group
Danville, California

Steven Kirshblum, MD
Assistant Professor
UMDNJINJ Medical School
Director of Spinal Cord Injury Services
Kessler Institute for Rehabilitation
West Orange, New Jersey

David Kramer, MD
Spine Fellow
Rothman Institute of Pennsylvania Hospital
Thomas Jefferson University
Philadelphia, Pennsylvania

John E. Lankenau, MD
Spinal Fellow
Rancho Los Amigos Medical Center
Downey, California

John M. Larsen, MD
Attending Physician
Southwestern Orthopaedic Medical Group
Department of Neurotrauma
Rancho Los Amigos Medical Center
Downey, California

Allan D.O. Levi, MD, Ph.D., FRCS(C)
Assistant Professor of Neurological Surgery
University of Miami
Jackson Memorial Hospital
Miami Veteran's Administration Medical Center
University of Miami Hospitals and Clinics
Miami, Florida

Steven Nagelberg, MD
Clinical Instructor
University of Southern California
Los Angeles, California

William C. Neal, MD
Assistant Clinical Professor of Orthopaedic Surgery
University of California at Los Angeles
Los Angeles, California

Russell W. Nelson, MD
Clinical Instructor
Neurotrauma Service
USC-Rancho Los Amigos Medical Center
Downey, California

Christopher O. Neubuerger, MD
Chief Resident
Department of Orthopaedic Surgery
Harbor-UCLA Medical Center
Torrance, California

Sean E. Nork, MD
Orthopaedic Trauma Fellow
University of Washington School of Medicine
Harborview Medical Center
Seattle, Washington

Kristjan T. Ragnarsson, MD
Dr. Lucy G. Moses Professor of Rehabilitation Medicine
Mount Sinai Medical Center
Chairman, Department of Rehabilitation Medicine
Mount Sinai Medical Center
New York, New York

Scott E. Reeg, MD
Clinical Instructor
East Carolina University School of Medicine
Eastern Orthopaedic Group, Inc.
Greenville, North Carolina

Reynold L. Rimoldi, MD
Clinical Instructor
University Medical Center of Las Vegas
Las Vegas, Nevada

James T. Robertson, MD
Department of Neurosurgery
Memphis, Tennessee
University of Tennessee-Memphis

Stephen L.G. Rothman, MD
Spinal Imaging Service
Rancho Los Amigos
Rothman-Chafetz Medical Group
Torrance, California

Christopher P. Silveri, MD
Clinical Instructor
George Washington University Medical Center
Washington, DC
Fairfax Hospital
Fair Oaks Hospital
Fair Oaks Orthopaedic Associates
Fairfax, Virginia

Volker K.H. Sonntag, MD
Clinical Professor of Surgery, Neurosurgery
University of Arizona, Tucson
Vice Chairman, Division of Neurological Surgery
Director, Residency Program
Chairman, BNI Spine Section
Barrow Neurological Institute
Phoenix, Arizona

Hillel Sperling, MD
Fellow American Academy of Orthopaedic Surgeons
Member North American Spine Society
Private Practice
Sherman Oaks Community Hospital
Encino Tarzana Regional Medical Center
Sherman Oaks, California

Adam B. Stein, MD
Assistant Professor
Mount Sinai School of Medicine
Attending Physician
Mount Sinai Hospital
New York, New York

Alexander R.Vaccaro, MD
Associate Professor
Thomas Jefferson University School of Medicine
Rothman Institute
Philadelphia, Pennsylvania

Jeffrey Wang, MD
Assistant Professor
UCLA Department of Orthopaedic Surgery
Los Angeles, California

Robert L. Waters, MD
Director
Regional Spinal Cord Injury Care System of Southern California
Rancho Los Amigos Medical Center
Downey, California

Gregory M. Yoshida, MD
Director, Orthopaedic Spine Service
Harbor-UCLA Medical Center
Director, Spine Fellowship
Rancho Los Amigos Medical Center
Clinical Instructor
UCLA School of Medicine
Los Angeles, California

Jack E. Zigler, MD
Clinical Professor of Orthopaedic Surgery
USC School of Medicine
Chief, Spinal Injury Service
Division of Neurotrauma
Rancho Los Amigos Medical Center
Downey, California

CONTENTS

1 Epidemiology and Costs of Spine Trauma, 1
Douglas E. Garland/John E. Lankenau

2 Spine Anatomy and Surgical Approaches, 6
Rocco R. Calderone

3 Emergency Management of Spine Trauma, 33
Daniel A. Capen

4 Imaging of Spinal Trauma Pearls and Pitfalls, 39
Stephen L.G. Rothman

5 Soft Tissue Injuries to the Spine from Acceleration-Deceleration Trauma, 96
Daniel A. Capen

6 Spinal Cord Injuries from Minor Trauma, 105
Mary C. Hume/William C. Neal

7 Patient Positioning in Spinal Trauma, 111
Samuel S. Jorgenson/John M. Larsen

8 Role of Spinal Cord Monitoring in Spine Surgery, 119
Robert D. Harbaugh/Robert E. Henry

9 Nonsurgical Management of Cervical Spine Instability, 134
Russell W. Nelson

10 Surgical Management of Cervical Instability, 144
Joel A. Finkelstein/Paul A. Anderson

11 Surgical and Nonsurgical Treatment of Vertebral Fractures to the Upper Thoracic Spine, 185
Reynold L. Rimoldi

12 Nonsurgical and Surgical Management of Fractures at the Thoracolumbar Junction, 199
Alexander R. Vaccaro/Christopher P. Silveri/Richard A. Balderston

13 Lumbar Fractures of the Spine, 214
Jeffrey Wang/Rick B. Delamarter

14 Fractures of the Sacrum and Coccyx, 235
Steven Nagelberg/Hillel Sperling

15 Pediatric Injuries of the Spine: Diagnosis and Management, 241
Christian H. Dee/Sean E. Nork/Serena S. Hu

16 Recognition and Avoidance of Complication in Surgery for Spine Trauma, 276
Daniel A. Capen

17 Osseous Healing in Spinal Injuries, 283
Robert T. Greenfield III

18 Pseudarthrosis as a Complication of Spinal Fracture, 291
John M. Larsen

19 Penetrating Spinal Trauma, 298
Christopher O. Neubuerger/Gregory M. Yoshida

20 Spinal Injuries in the Elderly, 310
Jack E. Zigler/John E. Lankenau

21 Management of Late Deformity after Spine Trauma, 315
Scott E. Reeg/Oheneba Boachie-Adjei

22 Neurosurgical Procedures in Spine Trauma, 331
Allan D.O. Levi/Volker K.H. Sonntag

23 The Spinal Cord and Its Reaction to Traumatic Injury: Implications for the Timing of Surgical Intervention, 345
David L. Kramer/Todd J. Albert

24 Recovery and Functional Outcome in Spinal Trauma, 350
Christopher P. Silveri/Jerome M. Cotler

25 Rehabilitation and Comprehensive Care of The Person with Spinal Cord Injury, 365
Kristjan T. Ragnarsson/Adam B. Stein/Steven Kirshblum

26 Concepts and Issues of Spine Device Development and Regulation, 414
James T. Robertson/Deborah Hyatt

Index, 427

INTRODUCTION

RECOVERY FOLLOWING SPINAL CORD INJURY

Robert L. Waters, MD

Spinal cord injury (SCI) is the most devastating sequelae of severe spinal trauma. Decision making in the treatment of spine trauma requires complete understanding of the diagnosis and prognosis of the SCI to predict outcome and to potentially avoid unnecessary surgery. Since 1974 at Rancho Los Amigos Medical Center, there has been great emphasis placed on treatment according to diagnosis.

Prognostication of outcome following SCI is based on clinical information obtained by neurologic examination. In the past, there was no universally accepted classification system for measuring the severity of SCI. Not only was it difficult to compare outcomes of different published series because different definitions and testing procedures were employed, but it was difficult for physicians to communicate with one another or accurately track a patient's progress.

The Frankel score, or modified Frankel score, was the most commonly used classification system.[1] Patients were divided into five broad categories based on motor and sensory examination. This system, however, was insensitive to changes within each category and depended on broad categories that were not well defined. Treatment based on this score was too often made upon surgeon "intuition."

In 1982, the American Spinal Injury Association (ASIA) initially developed Standards for Neurological Classification of SCI. Revised standards were published in 1992[2] and subsequently endorsed by the International Medical Society of Paraplegia in Barcelona. These standards provide an accurate way of quantifying motor recovery and represent the most valid, precise, and reliable minimum data set to assess SCI.

By using a systematic neurologic examination of key dermatomes and myotomes, the surgeon can define completeness of SCI, which is critical in surgical decision making.[3] Completeness is defined by presence or absence of sacral sparing.[2,3]

Neurological level of injury (NLI) refers to the most caudal segment of the spinal cord with normal function on both sides of the body. Segments with normal function frequently differ by side and in terms of sensory versus motor testing. Therefore, four different components may be identified in the neurologic level: right sensory level, left sensory level, right motor level, and left motor level.

A state of spinal shock, which may result in areflexia for varying periods, develops immediately after SCI. During this initial postinjury period, a patient may have no motor or sensory function below the neurologic level of injury but may still regain excellent recovery. The longer an injury remains complete, however, the potential for motor and sensory recovery progressively diminishes. The requirement for decompression also diminishes.

An incomplete injury is defined as partial preservation of sensory and/or motor functions below the neurologic level and includes the lowest sacral segment. Sacral sensation includes sensation at the anal mucocutaneous junction and deep anal sensation. The test of motor function is the presence of voluntary anal sphincter contraction upon digital examination. A complete injury is one in which there is an absence of sensory and motor function in the lowest sacral segment.

It is often difficult to perform an accurate motor or sensory examination immediately following injury. The patient may be undergoing acute medical stabilization or surgery, may be sedated, intoxicated, confused, or in pain, or have the limbs restricted by intravenous lines or splints. Furthermore, regardless of when the first accurate examination is performed, neurologic recovery or deterioration may have occurred between injury and the time of that initial examination. Brown, et al. demonstrated that examinations conducted between 72 hours and 1 week after injury more accurately predicted short-term functional muscle recovery (up to 3 months) than examinations conducted within the first 24 hours after injury.[4] Understanding this is critical for the surgeon in the decision-making process.

Motor and sensory scores are numerical representations of neurologic deficit. The motor score is calculated by summation of the strength grades for each of the 10 key muscles bilaterally. The total possible motor score is 100 points. The sensory score is derived from the summation of sensory grades for each of the 28 dermatomes tested bilaterally for both pinprick and light touch. The total possible sensory scores are 56 each for light touch and pinprick for a total of 112. Differences in sequential motor and sensory scores are often used to monitor changes in neurologic status.

Rates of recovery can be calculated from changes in the motor and sensory scores between successive examinations. The amount of recovery per day is determined by dividing the change in scores for two successive examinations by the interval (in days) between the examinations. The annual rate of recovery is determined by multiplying the recovery per day by 365 days for the rate of recovery during a particular interval that would have been expected if it was to have continued over the course of a year. Patients with incomplete injuries have higher initial motor recovery rates than those with complete injuries in both the upper and lower extremities. Rates of motor recovery for both complete and incomplete SCI rapidly decline in the first six months after injury, and the amount of recovery after one year is minimal. The decline in the rate of sensory scores parallels motor recovery.

At Rancho we studied 54 cases of incomplete paraplegia,[6] 61 patients with complete tetraplegia,[7] 50 with incomplete tetraplegia,[8] and 142 with complete paraplegia.[5] In the group with complete paraplegia above T9, all remained complete. Below T9, however, 38% of cases showed some motor recovery in hip flexors and knee extensors without surgery. Conventional orthotic and crutch use was achieved in 5%. Four percent of cases with initial complete paraplegia scores became incomplete without surgery.

Table 1. Prediction of Lower and Upper Extremity Motor Recovery

Prediction of Lower Extremity Motor Recovery

Manual Muscle Strength at One Month*	Percent with Functional ≥3/5 Strength at One Year: Complete Paraplegia	Incomplete Paraplegia	Incomplete Tetraplegia
0/5	5%	26%	24%
1/5, 2/5	64%	85%	82%

Prediction of Upper Extremity Motor Recovery

Manual Muscle Strength at One Month*	Percent with Functional ≥3/5 Strength at One Year: Complete Tetraplegia	Incomplete Tetraplegia
0/5	20%	54%
1/5	90%	73%
2/5	100%	100%

* ASIA key muscles.

Complete tetraplegia is clearly more restricted in terms of nonsurgical recovery. On average, there was a 9-point increase on the ASIA motorscore regardless of level of injury. Incomplete tetraplegia also demonstrated some capacity for nonsurgical recovery with 46% of patients regaining ambulatory capacity. As expected, the greatest recovery capability was seen in the incomplete paraplegic group; 75% of these patients regained community ambulation status with no surgical intervention. Table 1 summarizes this data.

Our finding[5–8] at Rancho confirm results found by Crozier in 27 anterior cord patients.[9] It is necessary to consider these findings when weighing the possibility of surgery. Strength gains, which other investigators have found in the upper extremity,[10,11] also emphasize the importance of initial diagnosis and expectations before planning and performing surgery.

Several clinical syndromes have specific findings and prognoses. Central cord, Brown-Sequard,[12] anterior cord, posterior cord, and sacral plexus injuries all provide specific information for the surgeon that must be recognized and considered before surgery is undertaken.

EFFECT OF SURGERY ON NEUROLOGIC RECOVERY

The effects of spine surgery on neurologic recovery in individuals with SCI have caused much study and debate. Several recent studies have suggested that decompressive surgery does not necessarily enhance recovery in individuals with thoracolumbar burst fractures.[13,14] Furthermore, the natural remodelling of retropulsed fragments can result in a canal that is nearly equivalent to a surgically decompressed canal.[15] Surgical decompression of bullets has, however, been demonstrated to enhance motor-score recovery if the bullet is located at or below the T12 vertebral level.[16]

Waters, et al. studied 269 individuals and concluded that when patients were divided according to level and completeness of injury, there were no differences in motor-score recovery between those who received surgical treatment and those who were treated without surgery.[17] Furthermore, among patients with cervical distractive flexion injuries, there were no differences in motor-score recovery between those whose dislocations were reduced and those who did not improve. The investigators speculated that this may be due to the relative delay in reduction for those injuries that improved. The average time to reduction was 14 days, which may be outside the interval during which reduction would be beneficial. Tator and colleagues reported similar results when studying 208 individuals.[18] These investigators found no differences in neurologic recovery between patients treated with surgery and those treated without surgery.

SUMMARY

- Motor and sensory recovery can be monitored through sequential neurologic examinations using the ASIA standards.
- In individuals with complete paraplegia, the amount of motor recovery is dependent on the NLI. Patients with a NLI above T9 demonstrated no recovery of lower extremity function.
- Technologic advances in surgical treatment of slight, moderate, or severe spine trauma must not supplant the understanding of all implications of an accurate diagnosis and prognosis. The text addresses all areas of spine trauma, and the reader will note that diagnosis of the patient is the cornerstone of successful treatment.

REFERENCES

1. Frankel HL, Hancock DO, Hyslop G, et al: The value of postural reduction in the initial management of closed injuries of the spine with paraplegia and tetraplegia, *Paraplegia* 7(3):179–192, 1969.
2. American Spinal Cord Injury Association/International Medical Society of Paraplegia: *International Standards for Neurological and Functional Classification of Spinal Cord Injury,* Chicago, 1966, ASIA.
3. Waters RL, Adkins R, Yakura J: Definition of complete spinal cord injury, *Paraplegia* 29:573–581, 1991.
4. Brown PJ, Marino RJ, Herbison GJ, Ditunno JF: The 72-hour examination as a predictor of recovery in motor complete quadriplegia, *Arch Phys Med Rehabil* 72:546–548, 1991.
5. Waters RL, Adkins RH, Yakura J, Sie I: Motor and sensory recovery following incomplete paraplegia, *Arch Phys Med Rehabil* 75:67–72, 1994.
6. Waters RL, Yakura JS, Adkins RH, Sie I: Recovery following complete paraplegia, *Arch Phys Med Rehabil* 73:784–789, 1992.
7. Waters RL, Adkins RH, Yakura J, Sie I: Motor and sensory recovery following complete tetraplegia, *Arch Phys Med Rehabil* 74:242–247, 1993.
8. Waters RL, Adkins RH, Yakura J, Sie I: Motor and sensory recovery following incomplete tetraplegia, *Arch Phys Med Rehabil* 75:306–311, 1994.
9. Crozier KS, Graziani V, DiTunno JF, Herbison GJ: Spinal cord injury: prognosis for ambulation based on sensory examination in patients who are initially motor complete, *Arch Phys Med Rehabil* 72:119–121, 1991.
10. Ditunno JF, Stover S, Freed M, Ahn Y: Motor recovery of the upper extremities in traumatic quadriplegia: a multicenter study, *Arch Phys Med Rehabil* 72:431–436, 1992.
11. Waters RL, Adkins RH, Yakura JS, Sie I: *Recovery following spinal cord injury. A clinician's handbook,* Downey CA, 1995, Los Amigos Research and Educational Institute.
12. Roth EJ, Park T, Pang T, et al: Traumatic cervical Brown-Sequard and Brown-Sequard-plus syndromes: the spectrum of presentations and outcomes, *Paraplegia* 29:582–589, 1991.
13. Dendrinos GK, Halikias JG, Krallis PN, Asimakopoulos A: Factors influencing neurological recovery in thoracolumbar fractures, *Acta Orthopaedica Belgica* 61(3):226–234, 1995.
14. Limb D, Shaw DL, Dickson RA: Neurological injury in thoracolumbar burst fractures, *J Bone Joint Surg Br* 77-B:774-7, 1995.
15. Kinoshita H, Nagata Y, Ueda H, Kishi K: Conservative treatment of burst fractures of the thoracolumbar and lumbar spine, *Paraplegia* 31:58–67, 1993.
16. Waters RL, Adkins RH: The effects of removal of bullet fragments retained in the spinal canal. A collaborative study by the National Spinal Cord Injury Model Systems. *Spine* 16:934–939, 1991.
17. Waters RL, Adkins RH, Yakura JS, Sie I: Effect of surgery on motor recovery following traumatic spinal cord injury. *Spinal Cord* 34:188–192, 1996.
18. Tator CH, Duncan EG, Edmonds VE, et al: Comparison of surgical and conservative management in 208 patients with acute spinal cord injury, *Can J Neurol Sci* 14:60–69, 1987.

Comprehensive Management of Spine Trauma

1

EPIDEMIOLOGY AND COSTS OF SPINE TRAUMA

Douglas E. Garland
John E. Lankenau

Public concern over health care expenditures in the United States continues to rise. Spinal cord injury (SCI), despite having a much lower incidence than other types of injuries or diseases, carries staggering direct and indirect costs. Increased initial survival and the near normal life expectancies of SCI patients have contributed to a large direct cost. Further, SCI is a "disease" of youth unlike most chronic illnesses which are prevalent in the elderly population; thus, the lost productivity of these individuals results in very high indirect cost, which often exceed the direct cost.

The overall health care environment continues to change in the United States. The public appears reluctant to support tax increases generally and specifically for social programs. Lack of public support for higher taxes coupled with the continued high federal budget deficits will increase scrutiny on social, health, and welfare programs as the government searches for ways to contain spending. For profit health maintenance organizations (HMOs) will also continue to emphasize reduction of health care spending.

Who will and how to pay for these costs become paramount with future budgetary restrictions. Public funding must be spent in as efficient a manner as possible. The National Spinal Cord Injury Model System Database was initiated to provide a better estimate of these costs and to suggest avenues for improving the quality of life for SCI patients while reducing costs. These efforts to control costs must also include prevention activities. By understanding the causes and demographics of spinal trauma, these prevention measures can be focused in the most effective manner. Prevention represents the best measure for controlling costs of spine trauma, whether caused by a compression fracture from a fall at home requiring 2 days hospitalization and follow-up or quadriplegia from a car crash costing in excess of 2 million dollars over a lifetime.

SCOPE OF TRAUMATIC SPINAL CORD INJURY

Trends in traumatic SCI have become better understood over the past 20 years. One element contributing to this improved understanding was the development of the National Spinal Cord Injury Model System Database in the early 1970s. This program has evolved from a single research project into 18 regional model systems. As part of this program, a national standardized database exists. The National SCI Database includes only persons treated at Model System locations and is thus not designed to determine either incidence or prevalence; however, numerous estimates of traumatic SCI prevalence in the United States have been made. These estimates range from 525 cases per million population to 1124 cases per million based on data from the National Health Interview Survey.[1,2] These studies have some drawbacks, which result from the use of mathematical relationships, and are highly dependent on assumed or calculated incidence and mortality rates. More recently a study was based on sampling in the United States.[3] This survey, specifically designed to identify the SCI population, estimated the traumatic SCI prevalence rate to be 721 cases per million in the United States. Based on this prevalence, it is estimated that there were between 183,000 and 230,000 SCI patients in the United States in 1992.

The most frequently cited SCI incidence was 32 cases per million population at risk.[4] An additional 21 cases per million population per year died before reaching the hospital. Two nationalized studies have generated higher estimates of incidence; however, study design flaws have been noted in each case.[5,6] Recently, DeVivo in 1989 calculated the annual incidence rate including hospitalized cases and deaths before hospital admission to be 53.4 cases per million at risk.

While the actual incidence remains unknown, the cited studies provide a good cross section from which to draw inferences. It is likely that the actual rate of hospitalized cases is about 30 to 40 per million population at risk; therefore, there are about 7,000 to 10,000 new cases annually. Population-based studies have shown that SCI generally occurs in teenagers and young adults between 16 and 30 years of age.[7] Spinal cord injury occurs in this group more than all other groups combined. The average (mean) age at injury is 30.7 years, the median age is 26 years, and the most frequently occurring age (mode) is 19 years. The majority of patients (60%) are in the 16 to 30 year age group. Overall about 82% of all patients are males. There is an overrepresentation of minorities with SCIs when compared with the general population.

Causes of traumatic SCI generally fall into three main categories: motor vehicle accidents (MVA), violence, and falls.[7] The distribution for these categories is 44.5% for MVA, 16.6% for violence, and 18.1% for falls. Several trends in the causes of SCI have been noted since the inception of the Model System program in 1973.

Because of various prevention programs the proportion of SCIs caused by MVAs has declined from 47.2% in 1980 to 38.1% in 1990. The proportion of SCI from falls has increased slightly from 15.3% to 20.2% over the same period. The proportion of SCIs from acts of violence has grown considerably over the same period rising from 13.9% to 25.1%. Gunshot wounds (GSWs), mostly from hand guns, account for more than 90% of violence-induced SCI. At an urban institution in Los Angeles, violence as a cause for traumatic SCI has increased from about 15% in the late 1970s to 24% by 1992. The number of GSWs treated at the Spinal Injury Service at Rancho Los Amigos Medical Center has increased steadily since 1987. The number seen in 1991 was double that seen in 1987. The national trend is similar. Gunshot wound causalities have been younger than the overall SCI population with an mean age of 25.

Violence as a cause of SCI appears more commonly in facilities with primarily urban versus rural catchment areas.[7] Estimates of injuries from violence in urban areas range from 21.1% to 50% versus 6.6% to 21.2% in rural areas. Of those patients, nationally 62.1% of SCIs secondary to GSW have been nonwhite leading to overrepresentation of minorities in this area.

The severity of SCI can be evaluated based on the neurologic level of injury and the neurologic category. The neurologic level of injury is defined by the American Spinal Injury Association (ASIA) as the lowest (most caudal) segment of the spinal cord with normal sensory and motor function on both sides. Overall, about 53% of patients in the Database are tetraplegics and 46% are paraplegics. The remaining 1% experienced complete neurologic recovery by the time of discharge. The most common neurologic category is incomplete tetraplegia at 31.2%. Complete paraplegia accounted for 26% of the Model System with 21.9% complete tetraplegia and 20% incomplete paraplegia. There have been trends in declining complete tetraplegia and increasing incomplete paraplegia between 1977 and 1990. Complete tetraplegia has declined from 26.3% to 17.5% while incomplete paraplegia has risen from 17% to 23.1%.

Most persons who sustain SCIs are white males in their late teens or 20s who are high school graduates and have never been married.[7] These injuries occur most frequently on the weekends and during the summer and result from automobile crashes. Violence demographics demonstrate that most of the injured are minorities. For penetrating injury, death rates for Hispanic and black males are 2 and 4 times the rate for non-Hispanic white males. These rates were highest in the core urban counties.

Based on these demographics, it appears that injury because of MVA will continue to decline slowly based on the continued effectiveness of current public health prevention strategies. Injury caused by falls will continue to increase slowly because of the rapid growth in the geriatric population. Most shocking is the rapid growth in violent SCI. The Center for Disease Control and Prevention estimates that by 2003, gunshot wounds will surpass MVAs as the leading cause of injury deaths in the United States. Given these changes in demographics, the overall incidence of SCI will probably remain about the same while some sources of injury will increase while others decrease. To decrease the overall incidence and to control costs, emphasis must be placed on violence prevention strategies and strategies to prevent falls in the elderly.

COSTS OF SPINAL CORD INJURY

Considerable data has been collected addressing individual components of SCI; however, until recently these studies were generally not adequate to determine either total individual costs of SCI or the aggregate costs to society. More current studies by DeVivo et al and Berkowitz and colleagues have helped to better define the economic impact of SCI.[8,9]

The National SCI Database of the Model System was initially designed to collect data to document both initial and long-term direct and indirect costs for persons with SCI. Because of limited resources many costs were deleted from the study in 1983. The study by DeVivo et al was undertaken to fill the gap created by changes in the Model System Data Collection. Using the Model System a random sample of patients from the National SCI Database were selected by

DeVivo. The actual costs incurred by each study participant were then compiled.

Costs are divided into direct and indirect components. Direct costs are defined as the changes incurred as a direct result of the injury. The indirect costs of SCI involve the loss of future wages, fringe benefits, and productivity. The majority of direct costs occur during the first year after injury period. These changes show a wide distribution based primarily on the severity of injury. The mean and median total direct costs for the first year after injury, based on injury level and on using the Frankel Neurologic Classification to grade injury severity, as adapted from DeVivo are shown in Table 1-1. There were four groups: (1) injury between C1 and C4 with Frankel grade A, B, or C; (2) injury between C5 and C8 with Frankel grade A, B, or C; (3) thoracic, lumbar, or sacral injury with Frankel grade A, B, or C; and (4) Frankel grade D regardless of injury level. All charges are adjusted to 1992 dollars. Costs range from a high in group 1 of $417,067.00 for ventilator dependent quadriplegics to a low of $122,914.00 in group 4 for patients with near normal neurologic function. The direct costs collected for each of these groups included charges for emergency medical service, acute care, rehabilitation, rehospitalizations, durable equipment, environmental modifications, and attendant care. The mean and median charges incurred annually after the first postinjury year are shown in Table 1-2. Again these costs are broken down by neurologic groups. The mean costs range from a high of $74,707.00 in group 1 to a low of $8,614.00 in group 4. The charges include rehospitalizations, nursing home care, outpatient services, durable equipment, and attendant care.

At Rancho Los Amigos Medical Center, the number of gunshot wounds treated on the Spine Injury Service has mirrored the national trends.[10] The number has increased steadily since 1987. The total number of GSWs treated at Rancho between 1980 and 1994 was 669. The total cost of care was approximately 90 million dollars. Acute care costs are usually about 20% to 25% of lifetime care costs. Given this, the total cost of GSWs treated at Rancho during this period was about 350 to 450 million dollars. Based on these costs and estimates of GSW incidence rates from the National SCI Model Systems and national incidence estimates the annual costs of acute care and rehabilitation would exceed 200 million dollars with associated lifetime costs of over 1 billion dollars.

Models have been developed to translate the direct costs into average values of lifetime direct costs. These estimates of the present value of average lifetime direct

Table 1-1. First-Year Post-Injury Costs (1992) by Neurologic Category

	Frankel Grade A, B, or C			Frankel Grade D
	Group 1 (C1–C4)	Group 2 (C5–C9)	Group 3 (T1–S5)	Group 4
Mean	$417,067	$269,324	$152,396	$122,914
Median	$404,033	$249,264	$137,756	$116,694

Table 1-2. Annual Costs after First-Year Post-Injury by Neurologic Category

	Frankel Grade A, B, or C			Frankel Grade D
	Group 1 (C1–C4)	Group 2 (C5–C9)	Group 3 (T1–S5)	Group 4
Mean	$74,707	$30,602	$15,507	$8,614
Median	$36,794	$21,967	$7,235	$2,281

Table 1-3. Present Value of Average Lifetime Direct Costs for Persons with SCIs by Age at Injury, Neurologic Category, and Discount Rate of 4%

	Frankel Grade A, B, or C			Frankel Grade D
Age at Injury	Group 1	Group 2	Group 3	Group 4
25	$1,349,029	$748,234	$427,733	$287,001
50	$876,287	$528,021	$326,272	$231,018

Table 1-4. Annual Forgone Earnings by Neurologic Category

	Frankel Grade A, B, or C			Frankel Grade D
	Group 1	Group 2	Group 3	Group 4
Mean	$50,470	$39,753	$35,783	$34,375
Median	$36,003	$32,649	$30,538	$27,867

Table 1-5. Present Value of Average Lifetime Indirect Costs by Age at Injury, Neurologic Category, and Discount Rate of 4%

	Frankel Grade A, B, or C			Frankel Grade D
Age at Injury	Group 1	Group 2	Group 3	Group 4
25	$1,289,005	$1,015,451	$914,312	$878,334
50	$611,872	$481,512	$433,814	$416,249

cost (1992 dollars) is shown in Table 1-3. These costs are calculated for SCI patients based on age at injury, neurologic category, and various discount rates. These estimates demonstrate the direct costs particularly for younger SCI patients in the higher neurologic categories.

The indirect costs of SCI result primarily from losses in wages, fringe benefits, and productivity. These annual costs shown in Table 1-4 are broken down by neurologic category. The differences in normal forgone earnings between the groups are primarily a function of differences in the likelihood of returning to work. In a manner similar to estimating the direct costs, the average lifetime indirect costs can be estimated. Estimates of these costs by discount rate, age at injury, and neurologic category are shown in Table 1-5. The numbers underscore the magnitude of the costs associated with SCI especially for young patients in higher neurologic categories. Interestingly the indirect costs often greatly exceed the direct costs.

IMPLICATIONS FOR THE FUTURE

Theoretically, the easiest way to control costs is through maximum effort for prevention. Through various prevention modalities, deaths caused by MVAs began to decline in 1969. This trend should continue. It is estimated that GSWs will replace traffic accidents as the nation's leading cause of death and SCI within the next 10 years.

As awareness of the problem with violent injury and death caused by firearms increases, strategies have emerged to combat this growing epidemic. The most cost-effective way to control a disease is through prevention. A model system, similar to the prevention modalities used for motor vehicle injuries, may prove to be the most effective strategy. In general, these measures modify the potential for injury or modify the environment in which the injury occurs. These strategies include waiting periods, restrictions on the type of weapons and ammunition, stiffer penalties for violent crimes and school-based education programs. These strategies attempt to (1) alter gun uses or storage; (2) change gun allocation; (3) reduce the lethality of guns; and (4) reduce the number of guns.

The safety issue for minor trauma has been addressed by the American Academy of Orthopedic Surgeons in the "Live-It-Safe" Program. Reduction of home accidents especially for the elderly, would be effective in reducing spine trauma. The Rancho Los Amigos Medical Center experience of a 10-year decrease in swim- and dive-related spine trauma has been directly linked to student education programs concerning the perils of surf and shallow diving spine injuries. Drivers training and education in the past 20 years has made a great impact on the public awareness of the hazards of drinking and driving. These programs should help reduce future incidence of severe spine trauma.

REFERENCES

1. Collins JG: Types of injuries and impairments due to injuries. In *Vital and Health Statistics*. Series 10, No 159. U.S. Department of Health and Human

Services Publication (PHS)I-87-1587, Hyattsville, MD, 1987, National Center for Health Statistics, pp 48–49.
2. Kurtzke JF: Epidemiology of spinal cord injury, *Exp Neurol* 48:163–236, 1975.
3. Harvey C, Rothschild BS, Asmann AJ, et al: New estimates of traumatic SCI prevalence: a survey-based approach, *Paraplegia* 28:537–544, 1990.
4. Kraus JF, Franti CE, Riggins RS, et al: Incidence of traumatic spinal cord lesions, *J Chronic Dis* 28:471–492, 1975.
5. Bracken MS, Freeman LH, Hellenbrand K: Incidence of traumatic hospitalized spinal cord injury in the United States, 1970–1971, *Am J Epidemiol* 113:615–622, 1981.
6. Kalsbeek WD, McLaurin RL, Harris SSH, et al: The National Head and Spinal Cord Injury Survey, major findings, *J Neurosurg* 53(Suppl):519–531, 1980.
7. Stover SL, DeLisa JA, Whiteneck GG: Spinal cord injury: clinical outcomes from the model systems. Maryland, 1995, Aspen Publishers.
8. Berkowitz M, Harvey C, Greene CG, et al: Spinal cord injury: clinical outcomes from the model systems, Maryland, 1995, Aspen Publishers.
9. DeVivo MJ, et al: Trends in spinal cord injury demographics and treatment outcomes between 1973 and 1986, *Arch Phys Med Rehab* 73:424–430, 1992.
10. Garland D, Wharton G: Spinal cord injury care: funding for the future, *Orthopedics* 17:675–678, 1994.

2

SPINE ANATOMY AND SURGICAL APPROACHES

Rocco R. Calderone

EMBRYOLOGY

Development of the spine begins in the third week of gestation.[1] The notochord forms are followed by formation of somites around the notochord. Each somite forms around a segmental artery. They then separate into individual sclerotomes. The majority of formation and segmentation of the spine occurs during the first trimester of gestation. This represents a period of high susceptibility to teratogenic effects. It is a period to which failure of formation and failure of segmentation defects are attributed.

Around the tenth week of gestation ossific nuclei form surrounded by cartilage cells. Each vertebral body is separated by notochord remnants. These remnants and the surrounding fibrocartilage become the intervertebral discs separating each osseocartilagenous sclerotome. This cartilage anlage then separates into the vertebral body and a cephalad and caudad ring apophysis. Basic formation of the spine is complete by 24 weeks of gestation. Each segment is composed of three ossific nuclei. One accounts for the vertebral body and one forms each side of the posterior elements and pedicle. The apophyses remain open and allow for growth of the spine through to skeletal maturity when they fuse to the vertebral body around ages 16 to 20.[2]

CIRCULATION OF THE SPINE

Arterial

The blood supply to the spine follows a single scheme. The arterial circulation to the spine is analogous to that in the cervical, thoracic, and lumbar regions. The aorta feeds three major divisions to the spine: the vertebral, the intercostal, and the lumbar arteries. Paired vertebral arteries in the cervical spine, the intercostal arteries at each segment of the thoracic spine, and the lumbar arteries at each segment of the lumbar spine supply blood to the vertebrae directly with perforators and through branches. The sacrum is vascularized with the middle sacral artery arising from the bifurcation of the aorta into the common iliac arteries and the lateral sacral arteries from the internal iliac arteries (Fig. 2-1). Small arterioles penetrate directly into the vertebral body as the artery crosses over the bone. The second source of arterial blood comes from posterior spinal branches that divide off the main arteries and enter the canal through the intervertebral foramen.[3] Small branches also continue through to the posterior spine where they serve as a supply to the paraspinal musculature and posterior elements (Fig. 2-2).

Within the spinal canal arterioles form an anastomotic network posterior to the vertebral body. This network donates nutrient arteries to each vertebral body through a centrally located nutrient foramen in the posterior wall of the vertebral body (see Fig. 2-2).[4] Also arising from the vertebral, intercostal, and lumbar arteries are the anterior and posterior radicular arteries. These radicular arteries follow the nerve root and subsequently the anterior and posterior ramus beneath the dura to form an anastamosis with the circulation of the spinal cord. Located beneath the dura is the main circulation to the spinal cord consisting of the anterior spinal artery and the paired posterior spinal arteries (Fig. 2-3). The term *artery of Adamkiewicz* refers to a dominant anterior radicular artery generally arising from one of the intercostal arteries in the midthoracic region. Intercostal artery ligation during surgery has been shown to be safe in a large series by Winter et al, although ligation is best performed far from the foramen and only unilaterally if possible.[5]

Venous

The venous system of the spine is unique in that it is a valveless plexiform network from the dural sinuses in the cranium down to the sacrum. The first accurate

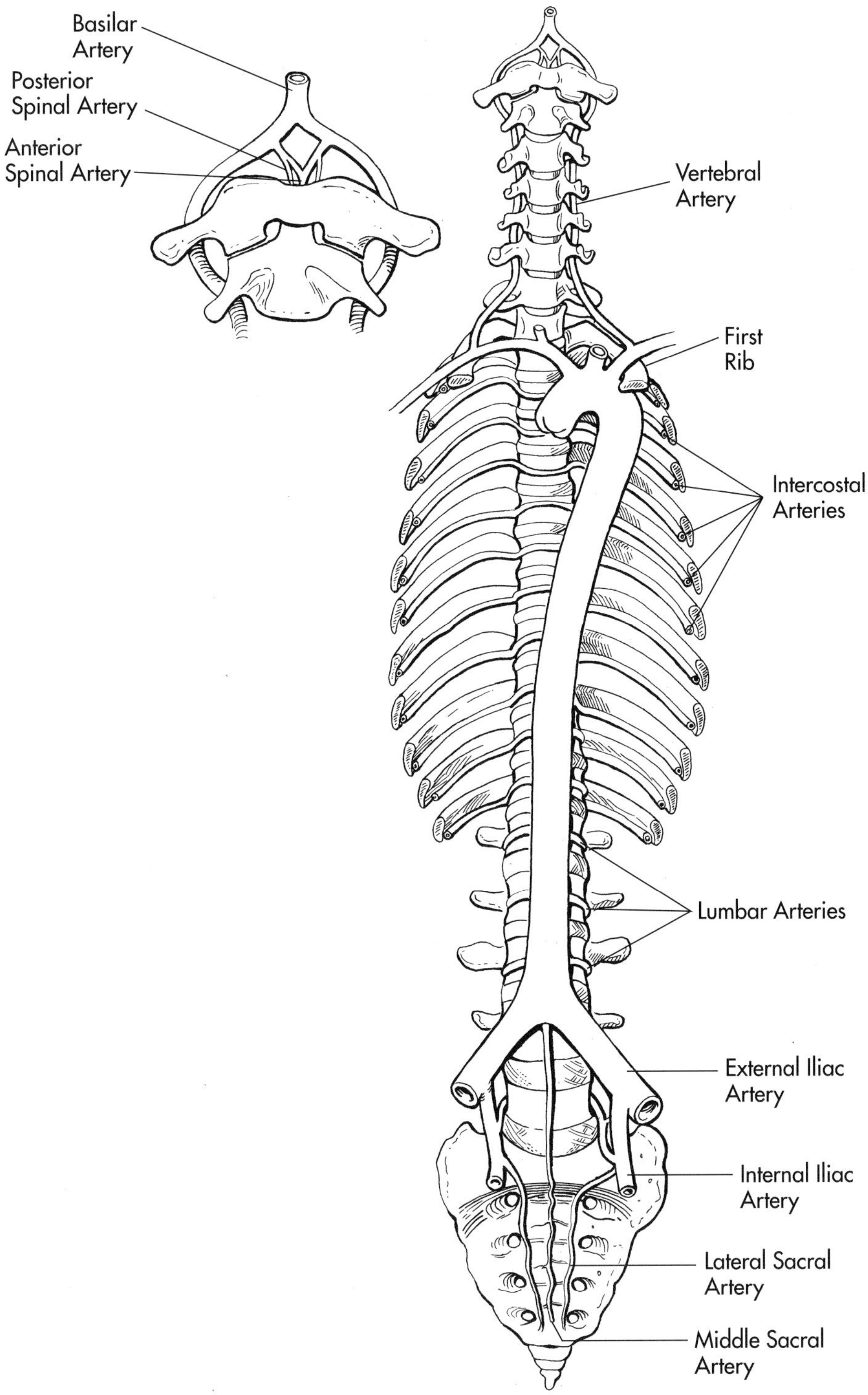

FIGURE 2-1

Arterial supply to the spinal column.

description of this vertebral vein system was by Breschet in 1819.[6,7] Batson in 1957 studied this further and popularized it in his lectures.[8] The original depiction consists of three main divisions: the venous channels within the bone of the vertebral body, the epidural veins surrounding the dura within the canal, and the venous network surrounding the vertebral column within the soft tissues of the paraspinal and paravertebral spaces (Fig. 2-4).[9] Venous capacity of Batson's three divisions greatly exceeds the volume of blood brought in through the arterial system. Of the three divisions, the epidural veins have the largest volume

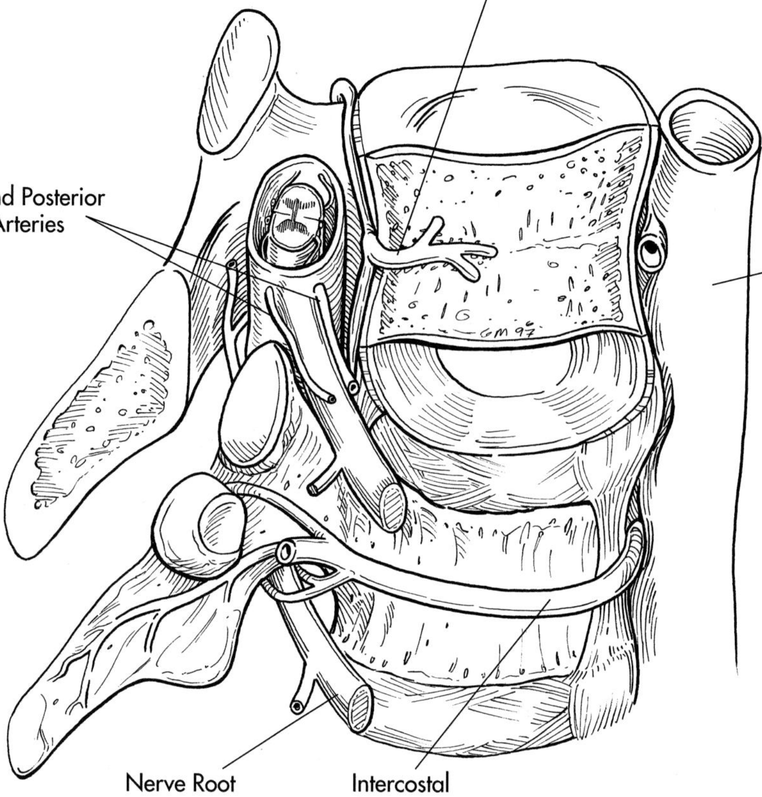

Figure 2-2

Circulatory supply to the spinal column and spinal cord.

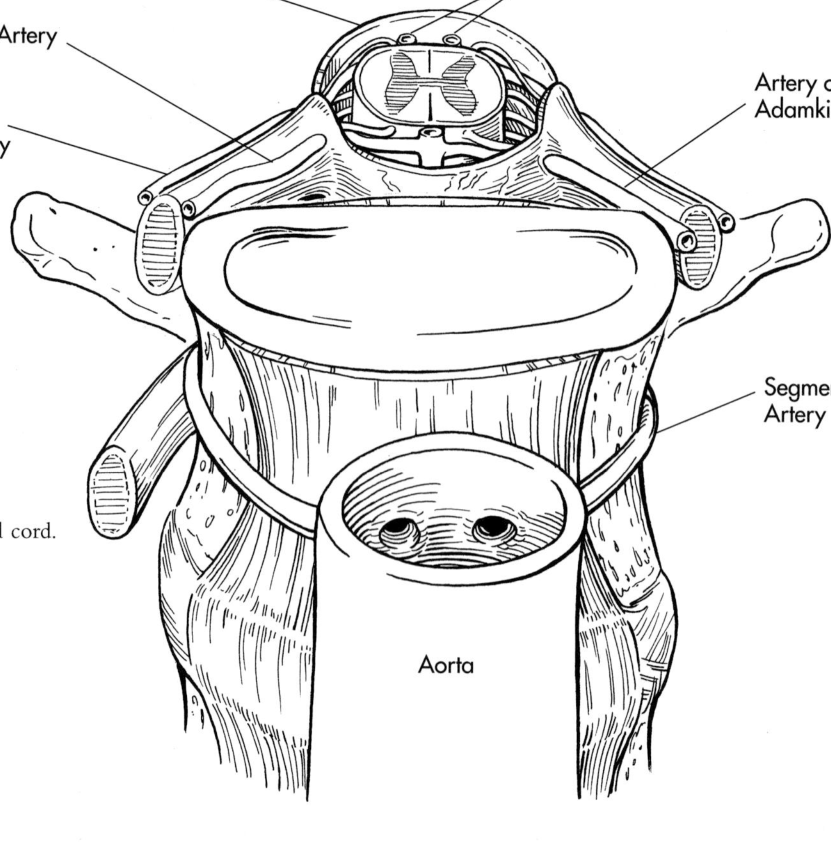

Figure 2-3

Arterial supply to the spinal cord.

capacity. There is an alternate route of circulation established by Batson's plexus which runs parallel to the vena cava system and communicates with the vena cava both cephalad and caudad. Valveless, it can bypass the vena cava with blood returning back to the heart.

BOX 1. ANTERIOR CERVICAL APPROACH TO SUBAXIAL SPINE

Make transverse incision two to four finger breadths above clavicle
Left side avoids recurrent laryngeal nerve beyond operative site
Right side preferred by some right-handed surgeons
Make longitudinal or transverse incision through platysma
Dissect plane lateral to trachea, medial to sternocleidomastoid
Protect carotid sheath laterally
Confirm retroesophageal/retropharyngeal
Identify esophagus medially (may use nasogastric tube)
Confirm level on radiograph with needle marker in disk space
Elevate longus colli muscle bilaterally and place retractor
Incise prevertebral fascia and anterior longitudinal ligament
Perform disc excision, corpectomy, etc.
Use Trendelenburg's position to improve visualization in disc space

CERVICAL SPINE

Accompanying each surgical approach is a summary box.

ANTERIOR SUBAXIAL CERVICAL SPINE

The anterior surgical approach to the lower cervical spine, C3 to C7, was pioneered by Robinson and Smith[10] and Southwick[11] in 1955 and 1960. It involves an anteromedial approach through the interval between the sternocleidomastoid muscle and carotid sheath, laterally and the trachea, larynx, strap muscles, and esophagus medially. This approach allows access to the anterior cervical spine from C3 through C7. The incision for the approach to C5 through C7 should be centered about two to three finger breadths above the clavicle. For levels C5 through C3, the incision should be more cephalad to the clavicle by about three to four finger breadths. The cricoid cartilage marks C5-C6 generally and skin markers can be utilized for radiographic confirmation.

The side of the approach is usually surgeon preference based upon training. Approach on the left side of the patient is more common. Less risk to the recurrent laryngeal nerve has been cited in support of a left-sided approach. On the left side of the body the recurrent laryngeal nerve is carried down and around the arch of the aorta as the great vessel descends during development. The nerve ascends from around the arch of the aorta in close proximity to the trachea and larynx away from the field of surgery. On the right side the course of the recurrent laryngeal nerve is more variable. Those who advocate approach on the right side cite surgeon's

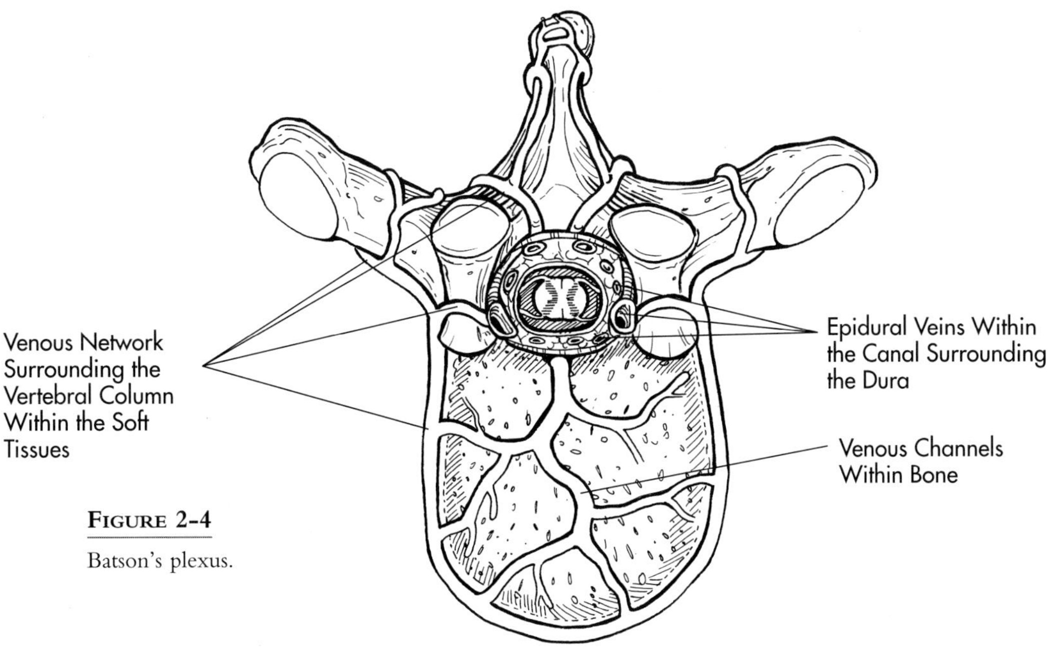

FIGURE 2-4

Batson's plexus.

comfort. Being right-handed and operating from the right side allows easier use of the right hand during delicate maneuvers and is more natural. In addition, recurrent laryngeal nerve injury on the right side has been recognized as rare and infrequent. Revision approaches or making a second approach on the contralateral side may increase laryngeal complications.

A transverse skin incision is more cosmetic. A longitudinal incision is required only to achieve exposure to multiple segments, such as three or more. The incision should be centered over the medial border of the sternocleidomastoid muscle at the appropriate level. Just beyond the subcutaneous tissues lies the platysma muscle. This is incised transversely in line with the skin incision. It can also be divided longitudinally along its muscle fibers according to preference. Small veins are found beneath the platysma requiring attention for proper hemostasis as the approach proceeds. Next, the plane between the sternocleidomastoid muscle and trachea is developed. Carefully and easily the cervical fascia is divided revealing this plane. The trachea, larynx, thyroid, and strap muscles gently and easily move medially as a unit. The sternocleidomastoid muscle and carotid sheath move laterally. The pulse of the carotid artery is easily palpable as a landmark (Fig. 2-5). Identification of the pulse aids in establishing the direction of dissection and avoids inadvertently opening the sheath. Hand-held blunt retractors are most convenient at this point in the dissection. It is important to identify the position of the esophagus. Generally, it moves medially with retraction of the trachea and larynx. Careful blunt dissection is performed along the plane lateral to the esophagus and onto the prevertebral fascia. Confirmation of location is done by palpating the anterior surface of the cervical spine. The endplate ridges of the vertebral segments are easily palpated. The overlying esophagus obscures the vertebra and is mobilized as a thickened muscular layer. Position of the esophagus can be confirmed by palpation of a nasogastric tube placed in the esophagus by the anesthesiologist. Once the path is clear, the pretracheal fascia is incised and bluntly spread to reveal the anterior cervical spine. Identification of anatomic level is now required. A needle is inserted one-half centimeter into an intervertebral disk and a lateral cervical spine radiograph is taken. If desired this needle can be bent 90 degrees one-half centimeter from the tip and then back again 90 degrees one-half centimeter more proximal to create a configuration that would block the needle from inadvertently advancing while the radiograph is taken.

After the appropriate level is identified with certainty, the field is expanded. This is first done with blunt dissection of the prevertebral fascia. Next, subperiosteal reflection of the longus colli muscle is done. The longus colli is reflected laterally to the uncoverte-

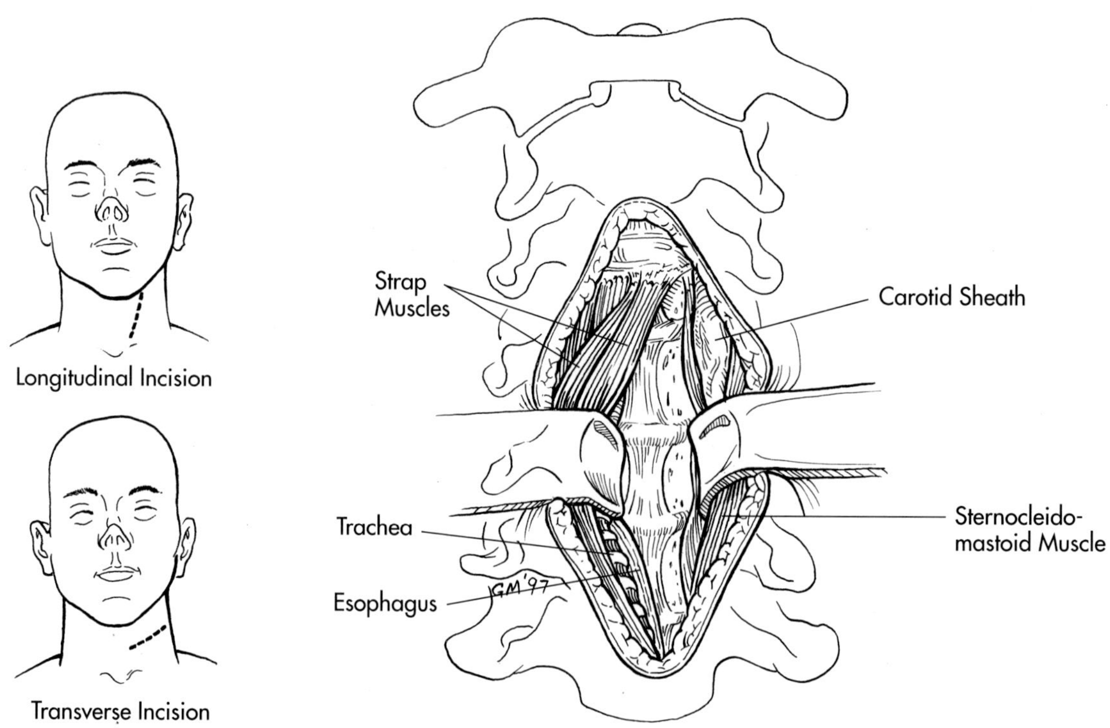

FIGURE 2-5

Transverse skin incision is more cosmetic while a longitudinal incision is required only to achieve exposure to multiple segments. Anterior cervical approach is illustrated here and in Fig. 2-7 E.

bral joint. Dissection beyond this comes into close proximity of the vertebral artery between the vertebral artery foramen. There is anatomic variability to the vertebral artery. Most commonly it enters the vertebral artery foramen at the sixth cervical vertebra and lies anterior to the vertebral artery foramen at the level of the C7 vertebra. A pitfall is failure to identify the midline of the vertebral body resulting in dissection too far laterally on one side.

Once the longus colli have been reflected, self-retaining retractors can be anchored into place underneath the longus colli muscle. The operation can proceed with intervertebral disk excision, corpectomy, decompression, arthrodesis, or fixation. With intervertebral disc excision, visualization back to the level of the posterior longitudinal ligament can be aided by tilting the table into Trendelenberg's position. This allows the path of site to follow the natural slope of the vertebral endplates.

Closure involves allowing the structures to fall naturally back into position with removal of the retractors. A drain is placed to prevent hematoma within this space. A large hematoma can press upon and obstruct the airway. The platysma requires reapproximation followed by routine closure of skin and subcutaneous tissues.

ANTERIOR UPPER CERVICAL SPINE

Anterior approaches to the upper cervical spine have a higher morbidity and are less frequently performed. Three approaches have been described. The two most common are the anterior transoral and the anterior retropharyngeal approaches. The third is an extensile approach through a maxillotomy or partial maxillectomy, dislocation, or osteotomy of the mandible. These techniques are used in tumor surgery and provide greater access anteriorly to the base of the skull and distally to the lower cervical spine. The techniques are beyond the scope of this discussion, and the expertise of an otorhinolaryngologist is required as part of the surgical team.

Transoral Approach. The transoral approach was described by Scoville and Sherman in 1951.[12] Later, Fang and Ong in 1962 reported six cases in which the anterior transoral approach is used.[13] Their infection rate was 67%. Four of the six patients developed pharyngeal wound infections. Wound infection in the transoral approach became recognized as one of the major complications.

More recently Bonney and Williams reported complications of meningitis in two patients and delayed pharyngeal wound healing in three patients of 16 cases reviewed.[14] In a review of 45 cases, however, Marks reported only one infection, a case of meningitis.[15] Similarly, three additional studies have noted low incidences of infection; Louis noted two infections in 76 patients,[16] Hadley et al reported five wound problems in 53 cases,[17] and Merwin et al had no infections or wound problems in 16 cases.[18]

Hadley and Merwin both noted that prevention of the formation of cerebrospinal fluid (CSF) fistula is mandatory. If the dura is opened, a lumbar drain to divert CSF is necessary with wound closure. Inadvertent durotomy requires closure often with a fascial patch. Good surgical technique and perioperative management are very important when using the transoral approach to the upper cervical spine. Wound closure is a critical factor in infection prevention. A watertight closure of the pharyngeal wall is essential. Postoperatively, the wound is bathed in saliva and all its oral flora. Merwin describes a three-layered approach using a horizontal H incision. The three distinct layers, mucosal, pharyngeal constrictor muscle, and anterior longitudinal ligament are each closed separately (see Fig. 2-6 A).[18,19]

The approach begins with the patient supine on a Mayfield head rest. PhisoHex and Betadine are recommended for preparing the oropharynx. The uvula is retracted cephalad out of the operative field with red rubber catheters passed through the nostrils and sutured to the uvula (Fig. 2-6 B). The endotracheal tube and the tongue are retracted caudad with a McGarver retractor. A longitudinal incision is preferred along the back of the oropharynx through the mucosa. The anterior ring of the atlas, the axis, and C3 is easily palpated. The incision is carried down through the thin muscular layer, which is peeled back revealing the anterior longitudinal ligament. After incision through the anterior longitudinal ligament, dissect subperiosteal cortex from the anterior vertebral rings. Working space in the transoral approach is very cramped, and retraction is difficult. An operative microscope is often necessary. Traction sutures are often required instead of conventional retractors.

Closure is performed in layers after copious irrigation. Close the anterior longitudinal ligament and periosteum as one distinct layer, followed by the muscular layer and then the mucosa. A watertight closure is the goal. No drain is placed within the wound. Swelling is accommodated by leaving the endotracheal tube in place until it can be safely removed. Usually this requires 24 hours of intubation to assess the extent of maximal swelling of the oropharynx. If the endotracheal tube is removed too early, a tracheotomy may be required to reestablish the airway. Swelling precludes oral reintubation.

Retropharyngeal Approach. The retropharyngeal approach to the upper cervical spine has been described by McAfee et al.[20] The advantage of this approach is that it is extramucosal. It also permits a larger field of exposure. The disadvantage is that it is more complex

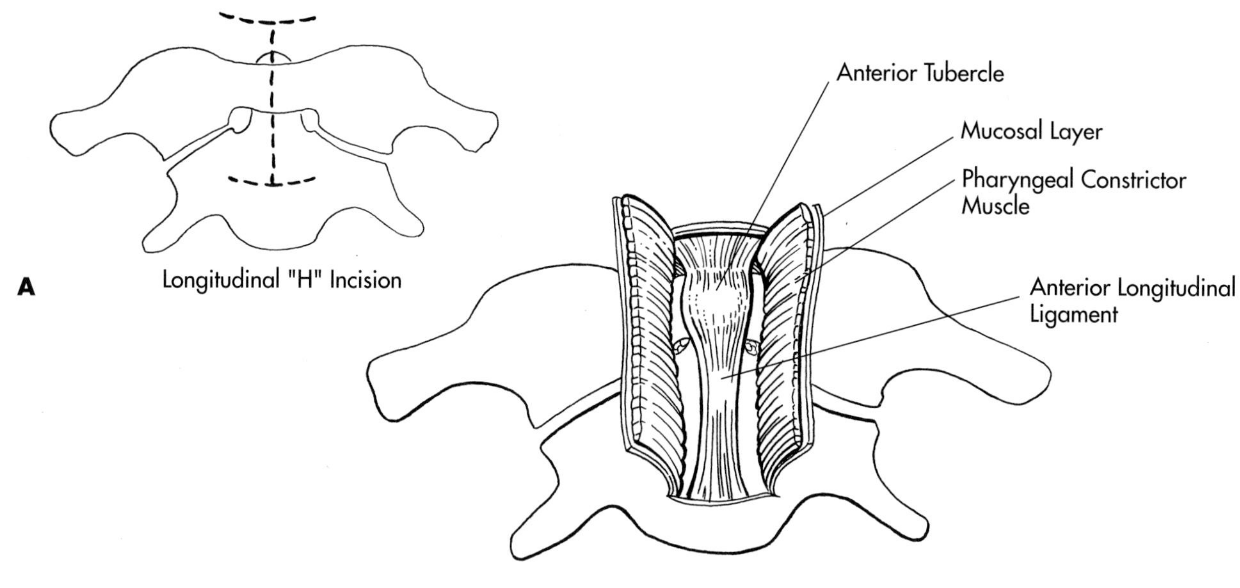

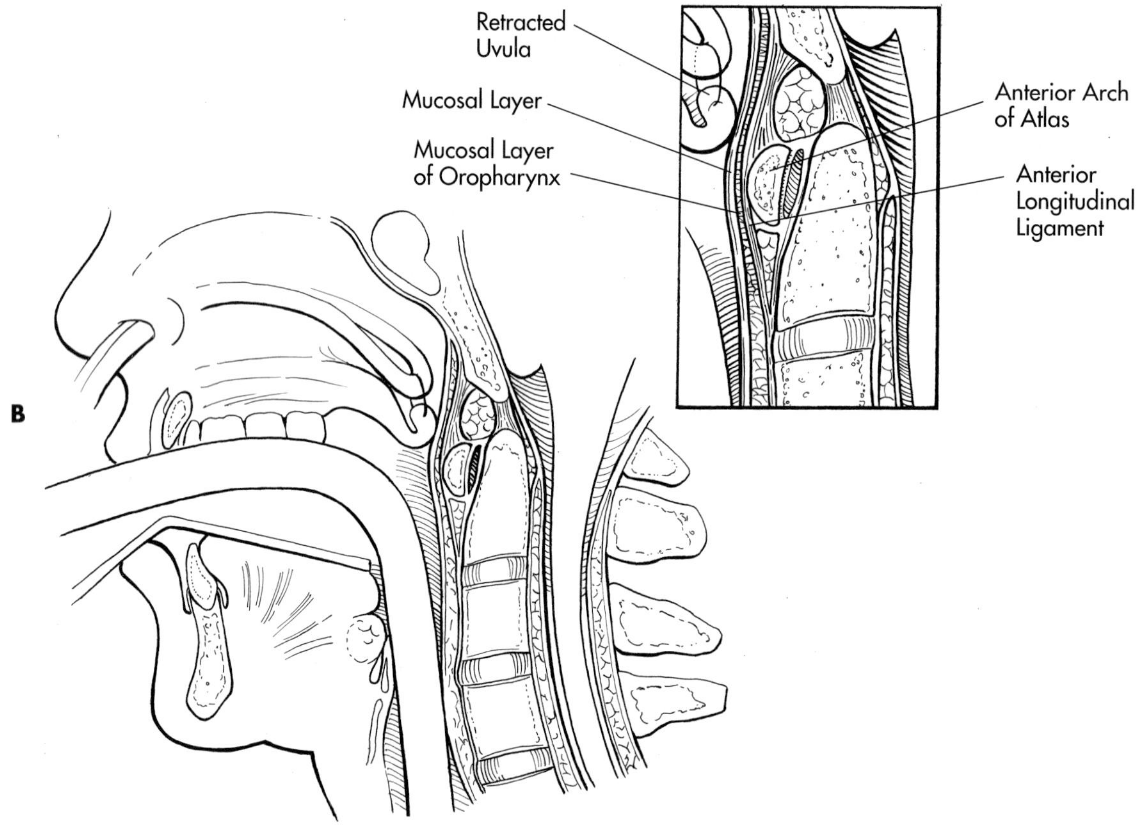

Figure 2-6

A, Transoral approach to the upper cervical spine. Here is the three-layered approach using a horizontal H incision. The three distinct layers, mucosal, pharyngeal constrictor muscle, and anterior longitudinal ligament, are each closed separately. **B**, Transoral approach to the upper cervical spine. The uvula is retracted cephalad out of the operative field with red rubber catheters passed through the nostrils and sutured to the uvula.

involving dissection around additional significant structures. It is reported to have few infections and neurologic injuries.

With the patient positioned supine, a nasotracheal tube allows the jaw to remain closed for increased area of submandibular exposure. If the neck can be safely extended, exposure is facilitated. The incision is based on the right side transversely in the submandibular region (Fig. 2-7 A) and is extended distally in a longitudinal fashion from the middle of the transverse incision.

This increases the exposure. The incision is made through the platysma down to the superficial fascial layer of the neck. The flaps of this T-shaped incision are retracted.

Three nerves within the field of dissection must be carefully avoided. The recurrent laryngeal nerve is located distally and must be avoided if the incision is extended down to the level of the fifth cervical vertebra. Cephalad in the incision, the branches of the fascial nerve and the hypoglossal nerve are within the field of dissection. Identify the marginal mandibular and cervical branches of the fascial nerve, and carefully dissect them away from the field. A nerve stimulator is helpful in identifying them (Fig. 2-7 B). The retromandibular vein may be ligated as it connects to the internal jugular vein. Carefully retract the sternocleidomastoid posteriorly with the carotid sheath. The submandibular gland is resected, and the duct is ligated. Failure to ligate the duct may lead to formation of a salivary fistula.

Proceed to identify the digastric and stylohyoid muscles. The digastric muscle is divided through its tendinous midportion at the hyoid bone (Fig. 2-7 C). Carefully divide the insertion of the stylohyoid from the hyoid bone. Note that the inferior branches of the facial nerve are located in the vicinity of the stylohyoid muscle. Avoid excessive retraction in this area. Once separated from the hyoid bone, the larynx, pharynx, and esophagus can be mobilized medially. The hypoglossal nerve can then be located in the cephalad area of the exposure. Retract it superiorly further away from the field (Fig. 2-7 D).

Continue dissection through the retropharyngeal space. Increase the area of dissection by retracting the sternocleidomastoid and carotid sheath laterally. Small connecting branches including the facial, lingual, and superior thyroid arteries and veins from the carotid artery and vein are ligated as necessary. Medially mobilize and retract the pharynx and trachea (Fig. 2-7 E). Identify and protect the superior laryngeal nerve. With adequate exposure the prevertebral fascia is divided. The longus colli is now identified and subperiosteally dissected from the midline of the first vertebra and down through the exposed area. Avoid dissection too far laterally as the vertebral artery may be injured.

Closure requires a drain to prevent hematoma. The deep tissues are allowed to fall back into place. The stylohyoid and digastric tendons are repaired at the hyoid bone. The platysma layer and skin layer are then closed. As with the transoral approach, intubation is maintained for 24 to 48 hours because of swelling around the airway.[24]

Posterior Cervical Spine

The posterior approach to the cervical spine is among the most common in cervical spine trauma. This approach begins in the midline as a longitudinal incision centered over the spinous processes. The incision is carried down through the fascial plane with electrocautery. The extension of the trapezius is divided from the superficial layer along the midline fascial plane (Fig. 2-8 A). The median raphe weaves its way down to the spinous processes. It does not course straight down but rather deviates to the right or left. Staying within the nuchal ligament assures better hemostasis. Deviating into the trapezius or paracervical muscles creates more bleeding into the wound. Also the greater occipital and third occipital nerve are located laterally in the muscle. Injury to these may cause areas of numbness or neuroma to the posterior scalp and neck.

Box 2. Transoral Approach to the Upper Cervical Spine

Retract uvula cephalad with red rubber catheters
Make longitudinal incision along the oropharynx through the mucosa
Make incision in pharyngeal muscular layer and peel back
Make longitudinal incision through anterior longitudinal ligament
Dissect subperiosteal cortex from the anterior vertebral rings
Place traction sutures

Box 3. Retropharyngeal Approach to the Upper Cervical Spine

Submandibular transverse incision with longitudinal T extension through the platysma and the superficial fascial layer of the neck
Retract marginal mandibular and cervical branch of the facial nerve
Ligate retromandibular vein
Resect the submandibular gland
Ligate the duct to the submandibular gland
Divide the tendons of the digastric and stylohyoid at the hyoid bone
Retract the hypoglossal nerve superiorly
Ligate the facial, lingual, and superior thyroid arteries and veins
Retract the sternocleidomastoid and carotid sheath laterally
Identify and protect the superior laryngeal nerve
Mobilize larynx, pharynx, and esophagus medially
Divide prevertebral fascia longitudinally
Dissect longus colli subperiosteally from the vertebra

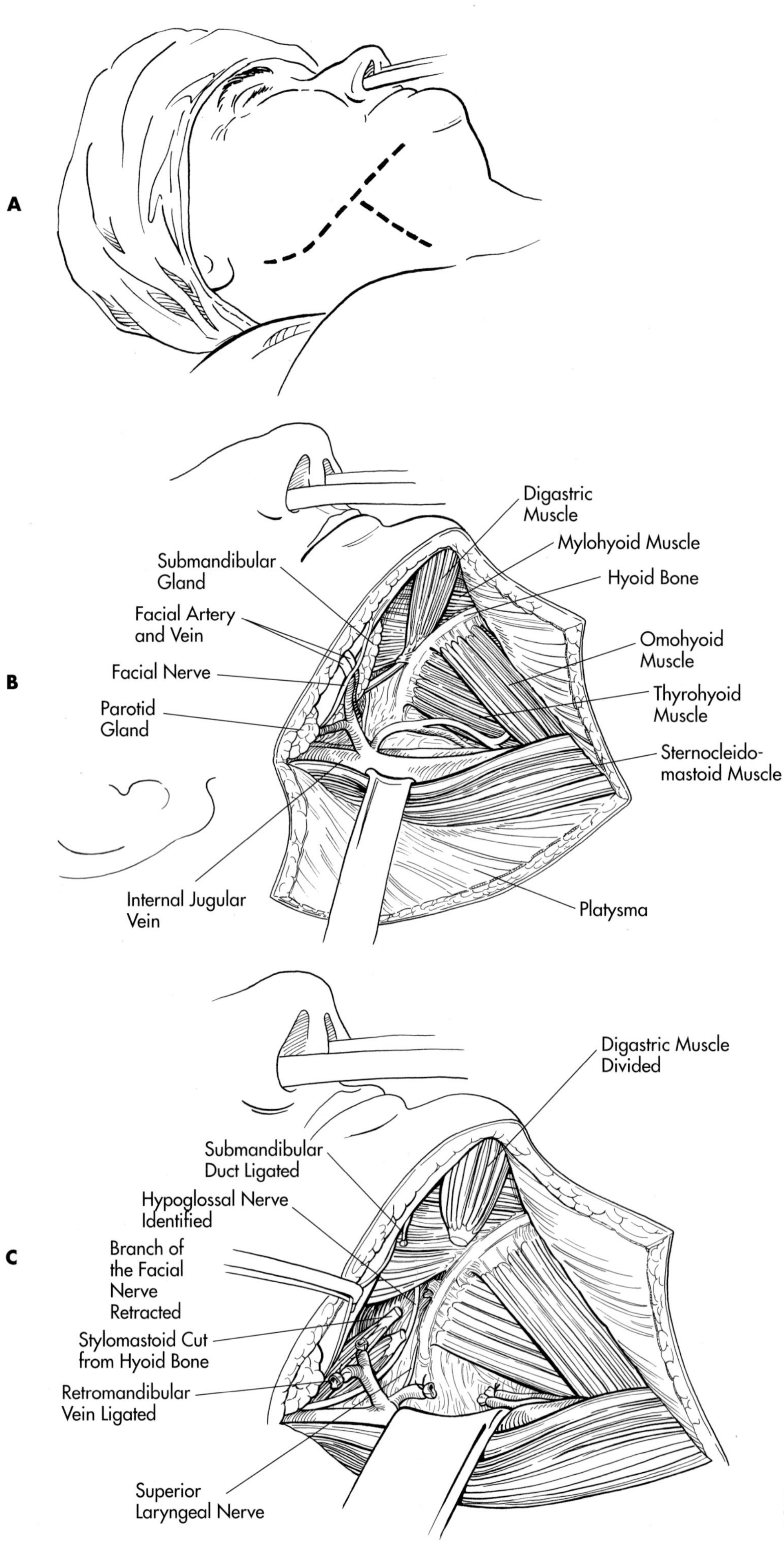

FIGURE 2-7

For legends see opposite page.

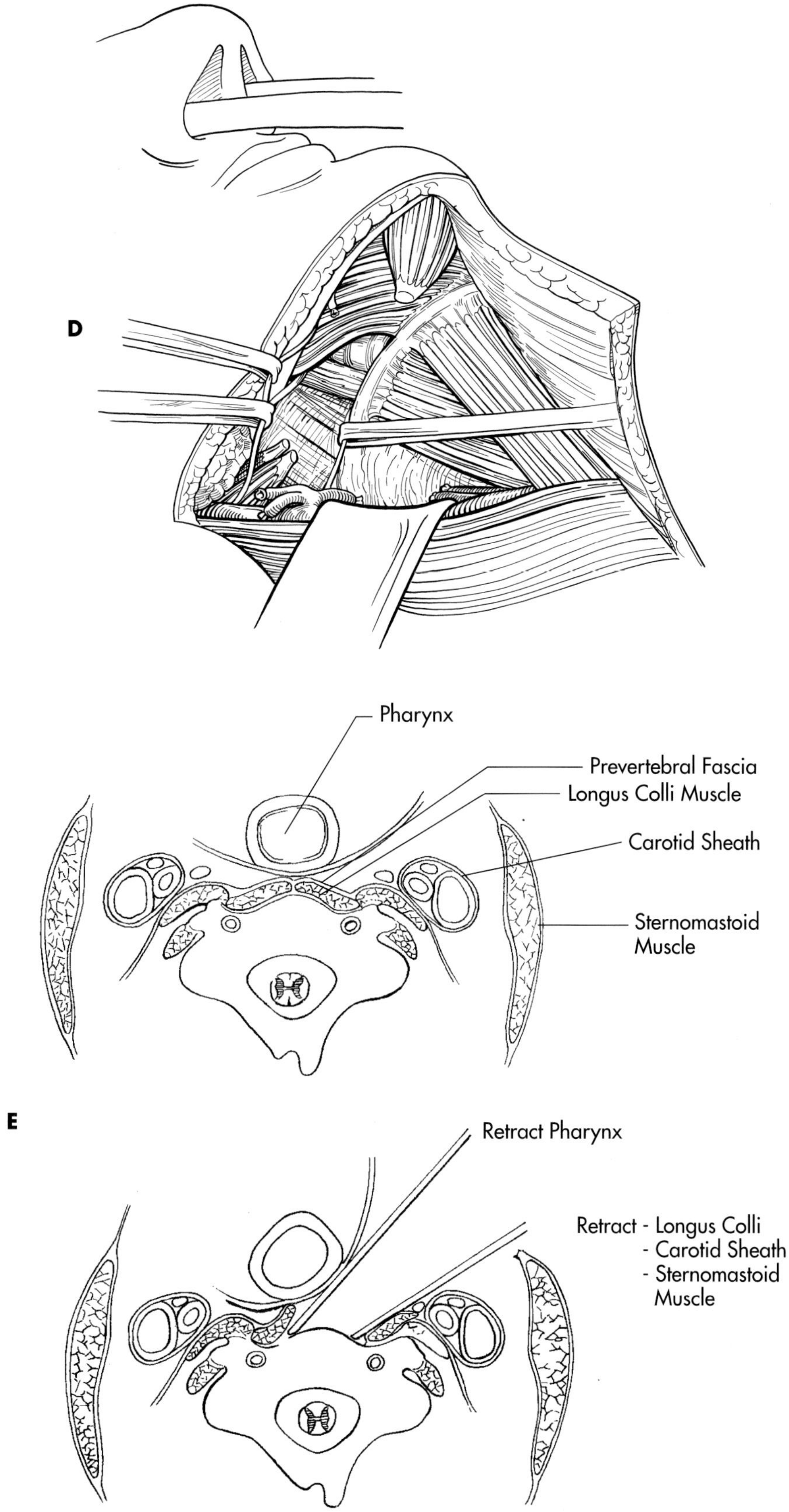

FIGURE 2-7

A, Retropharyngeal approach—incision. **B**, Identify the marginal mandibular branch and cervical branch of the facial nerve and carefully dissect them away from the field. The retromandibular vein may need to be ligated as it connects to the internal jugular vein. **C**, Proceed to identify the digastric and stylohyoid muscles. The digastric muscle is divided through its tendenous midportion at the hyoid bone. **D**, Locate the hypoglossal nerve in the cephalad area of exposure. Retract it superiorly further away from the field. **E**, Medially mobilize and retract the pharynx and trachea. Identify and protect the superior laryngeal nerve.

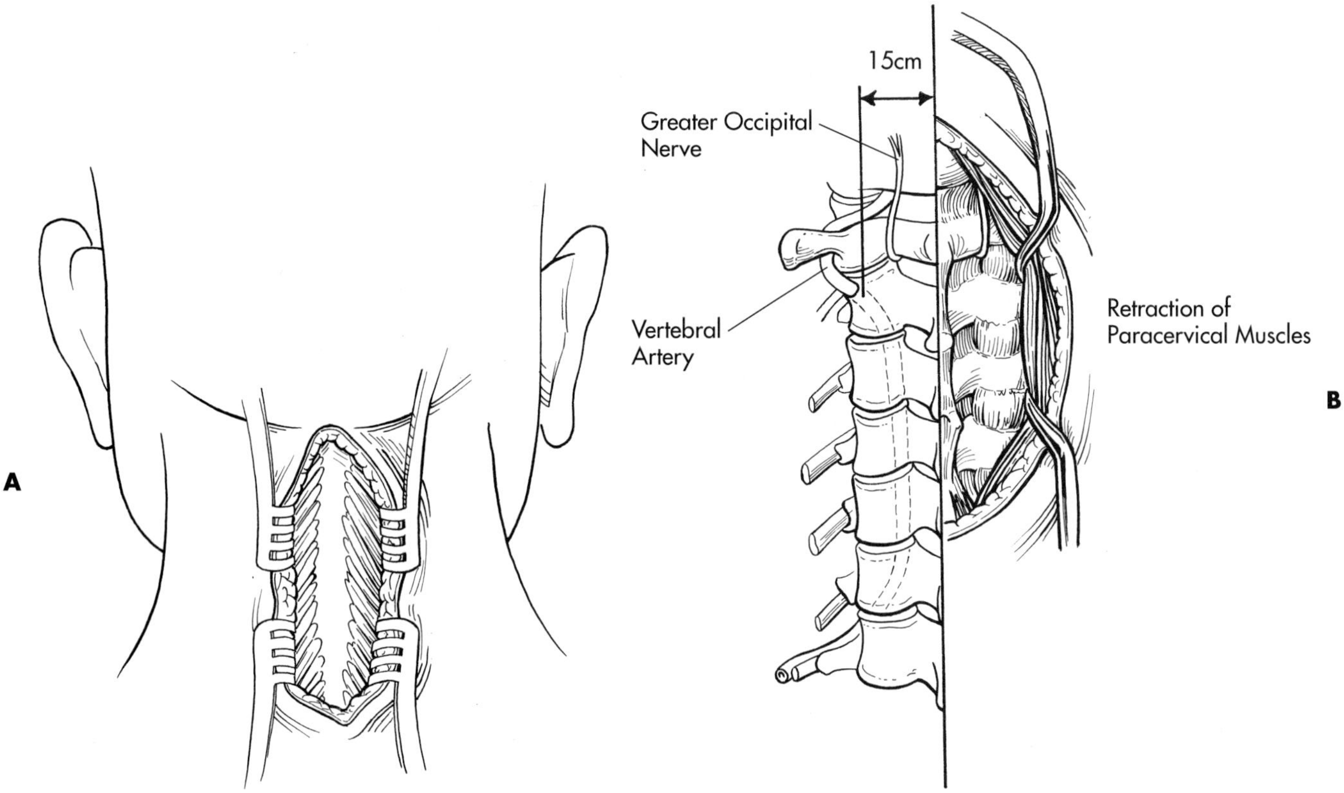

FIGURE 2-8

Posterior approach to the cervical spine.

Upon reaching the spinous processes, the intermediate layer of the paracervical muscles consisting of the semispinalis capitis, splenius capitis, and splenius cervicis are retracted (Fig. 2-8 B). The subperiosteal dissection is carried out laterally. This consists of detaching the deep musculature of the interspinalis cervicis between spinous processes and the rotatores cervicis between spinous processes and transverse processes. By detaching musculature and remaining below the periosteum hemostasis can be maintained. Avoid going beyond the lateral masses as injury to the cervical nerve roots may occur.

This approach can be extended distally the entire length of the cervical spine. In the upper cervical spine the deep layer contains the rectus capitus minor and major from occiput to the spinous processes of C1 and C2, respectively. There is also the superior and inferior obliquus capitus from occiput to transverse process of C1 and from transverse process of C1 to spinous process of C2. Exposing the upper cervical spine and suboccipital area involves identification of the spinous process of the second cervical vertebra and the occiput. The posterior ring of the atlas lies lower than the spinous process of C2. Carefully dissect anteriorly down onto the posterior ring of C1. While advancing palpate and locate the posterior ring to avoid penetrating the atlantooccipital membrane between the occiput and C1. Note that the vertebral artery loops up onto the atlas as it curves into the foramen magnum. Limit the lateral subperiosteal dissection on C1 to about 1.5 centimeters. Going beyond this risks injury to the vertebral artery cervical nerve roots. Note that exposing additional levels may lead to extension of the fusion mass to unintended cervical levels. This phenomenon occurs with an abundant fusion mass, especially in children.

Wound closure involves reapproximating the muscle layer followed by the fascial layer and then the subcutaneous and skin layer. The posterior cervical spine is highly vascularized. There tends to be

BOX 4. POSTERIOR APPROACH TO THE CERVICAL SPINE

- Make longitudinal posterior incision through skin and subcutaneous
- Follow median raphe down to the spinous processes
- Retract the paracervical muscles
- Carry the subperiosteal dissection out laterally
- Limit the lateral subperiosteal dissection on C1 to about 1.5 centimeters
- Limit subperiosteal dissection to levels of fusion

prolonged drainage and much oozing so drain placement is recommended.

UPPER CERVICOTHORACIC SPINE

ANTERIOR CERVICOTHORACIC JUNCTION

Reaching the cervicothoracic junction anteriorly can be a challenge because of the great vessels, the heart, and the depth of the wound with the kyphotic transition of the thoracic spine. There are, however, four common approaches to the cervicothoracic junction. The first two are related: a low anterior cervical approach above the clavicle and an anterior cervical approach involving claviculotomy or partial sternotomy. The third approach is the transsternal approach used in cardiac surgery, and the fourth route is a transthoracic approach through the first, second, or third rib. Assistance of a thoracic surgeon is recommended for all but the low anterior cervical approach.

The low anterior cervical approach is similar to the anterior approach to the cervical spine as described earlier. The difference is that the transverse incision begins one finger breadth above the clavicle. The incision here is carried across the midline as the sternocleidomastoid and carotid sheath approach the midline (Fig. 2-9 A). Care must be taken with the lower cervical spine in the vicinity of the thoracic duct as it links to the internal jugular and subclavian vein. The exposure allows one to reach the first thoracic vertebra. Beyond this region an extended approach involves claviculotomy, separation of the sternoclavicular joint, or partial sternotomy.[22] Chylothorax can result from thoracic duct injury.

Using a longitudinal skin incision with osteotomy of the head of the clavicle,[23] make an incision through the sternoclavicular joint[24] or partial sternotomy of the manubrium. Then cut laterally to the left through the synostosis between the manubrium and the body of the sternum. This allows for an extended anterior cervical approach to the upper thoracic spine (Fig. 2-9 B). These techniques allow access to an area approximating T3.

TRANSSTERNAL APPROACH

The transsternal approach involves an approach similar to that used for cardiac surgery. A longitudinal incision along the sternum is made (Fig. 2-9 C). Cephalad the incision is curved to the left along the sternocleidomastoid muscle as needed for proximal exposure. The parietal pleura is then reflected from the undersurface of the sternum. The sternum is then split from suprasternal notch to xiphoid process using a Gigli saw passed through underneath. Caudally taken care to stay within the thoracic cavity and not enter into the peritoneum. The sternum is spread with retractors. Careful blunt dissection above the arch of the aorta leads back to the spine. The left brachiocephalic vein crosses the field caudally. This vein can be divided if need be for additional exposure. As dissection proceeds further distally, ligation of this vein may avoid rupture from excessive retraction.[13] Ligation of the brachiocephalic vein results in enlargement of the left upper extremity from slowed venous return.

TRANSTHORACIC APPROACH

A transthoracic approach permits a more direct approach to the kyphotic anterior thoracic spine. The approach begins with a periscapular incision through the latissimus and trapezius muscles (Fig. 2-9 D). Part of the rhomboideus major muscles may also require release from the medial border of the scapula. The scapula is elevated. Removal of the first, second, or third rib depending on the exposure desired allows transthoracic access of approximately C6 to T4. Incise over the rib. Subperiosteally elevate over the cephalic edge, behind, and then under. Protect the intercostal neurovascular bundle traveling below the rib. Remove the rib. Incise through the parietal pleura. Pack off the lung or deflate if possible with bifurcated endotracheal tube. Expose and identify the desired segment of spine.

THORACIC SPINE

ANTERIOR THORACIC SPINE

This approach is also called the transthoracic approach. The level of the approach can be varied with the limits of the exposure cephalad to T2 and caudad to T12. The spine is accessed through the chest. The patient is in the lateral decubitus position with the left side up. Put a sand bag or padded bump under the right side and flex the table to allow the ribs on the left side to open up (Fig. 2-10). Patient positioning produces a scoliotic curvature to the right. This must be taken into account and undone during fixation if the surgery is to correct deformity.

The left-sided approach is favored by most for several anatomic reasons. On the left side the aorta is easier to maneuver around than the much more fragile vena cava. The heart is also easier to retract anteriorly on the left side. On the right side the liver may obstruct the exposure. In the upper thoracic spine the right side gives the surgeon the advantage of avoiding the carotid and subclavian artery. On the right side these vessels emanate from the brachiocephalic or innominate artery, which is more cephalad above the upper thoracic spine.

Selection of the appropriate rib level for the incision depends on the exposure desired. For isolated exposure

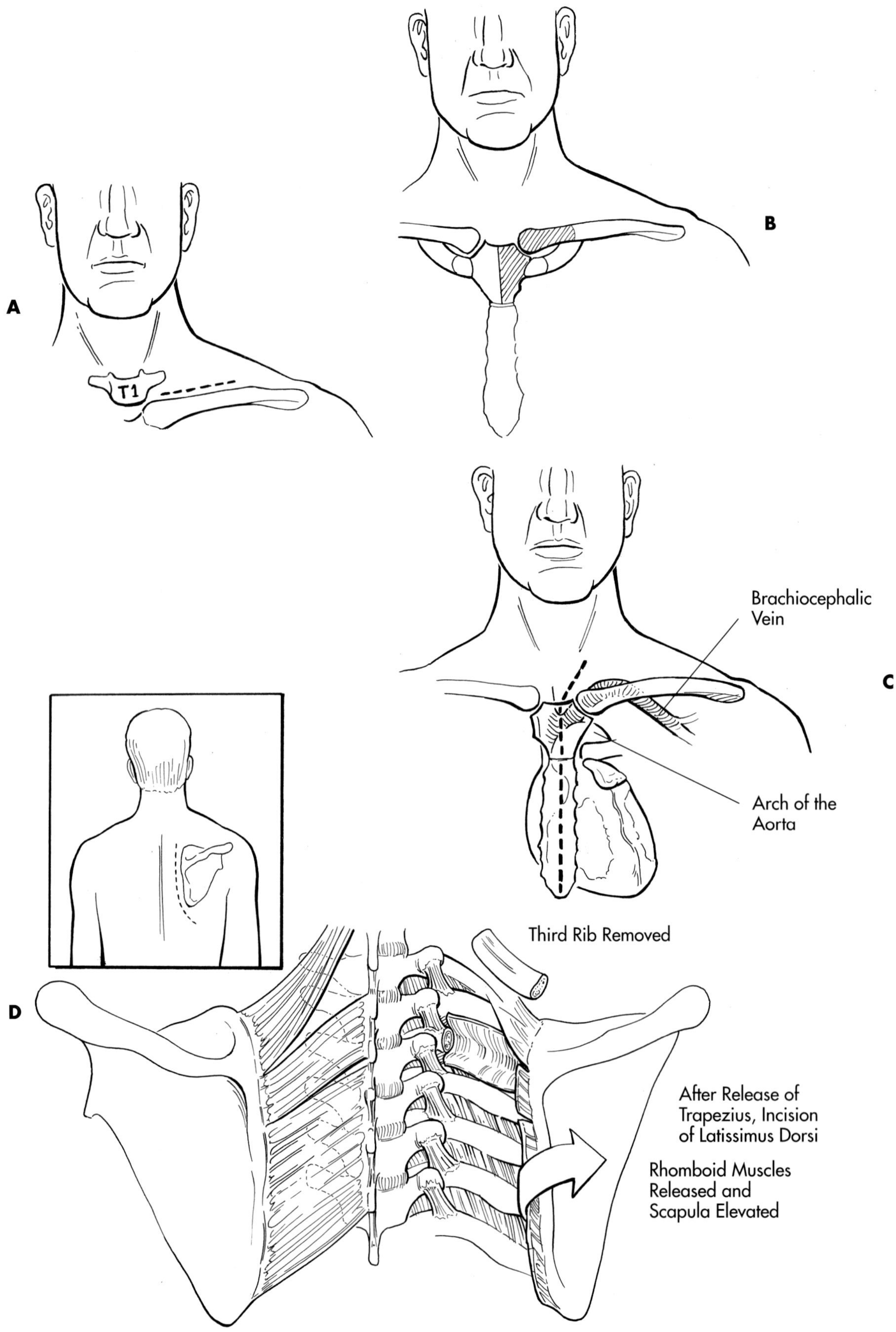

Figure 2-9

A, Low anterior cervical approach. **B**, Anterior cervical approach with claviculotomy and partial sternotomy. **C**, Transsternal approach to the cervicothoracic junction and upper thoracic spine. **D**, Transthoracic approach to cervicothoracic junction.

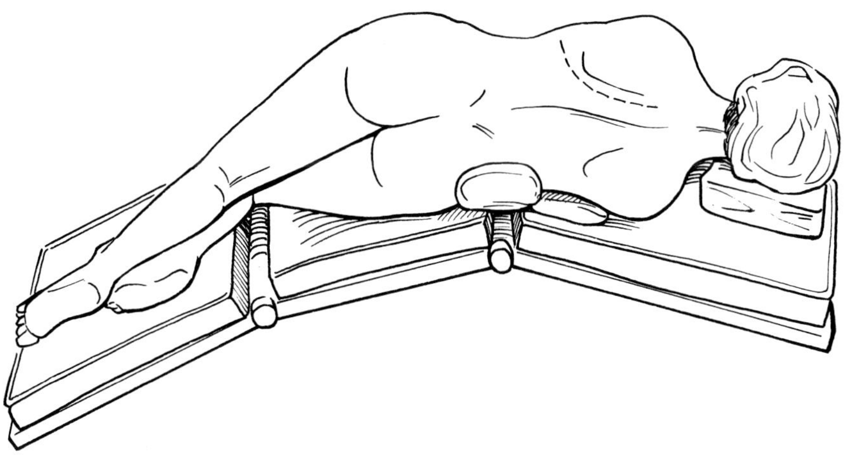

FIGURE 2-10

Patient position for left transthoracic approach.

BOX 5. ANTERIOR APPROACH TO THE CERVICOTHORACIC SPINE

For high transthoracic approach, use left periscapular incision
Incise through latissimus and trapezius
Elevate scapula and scapular musculature
Locate upper ribs and level of access desired
Incise and strip first, second, or third rib
Remove rib at desired level
Pediatric patients may require removal of two adjacent ribs
Reflect or deflate lung and proceed with exposure of vertebrae

of one segment, such as in a biopsy, the incision can be centered over the rib at that level. Generally, a larger exposure is needed. For this, it is easier to begin at the rib one or two levels above the desired vertebral level and work cephalad to caudad. Because the ribs slope distally as they curve laterally and anteriorly around the chest wall, it is better to begin at a rib level above the main vertebral level. Also, for the upper thoracic levels a periscapular incision is first used as described previously. The scapula and periscapular muscles overlie the ribs of the upper thoracic spine. By incising around the scapula, through from posterior medially around to anterior laterally the trapezius, latissimus, and serratus anterior muscles, the scapula can be retracted and upper ribs identified for the next level of the approach.

The incision should follow the selected rib level around from posterior to anterior. Carry the incision through the skin and subcutaneous tissue. Using cautery for hemostasis, carry the approach down through the periosteum of the rib. With subperiosteal dissection detach the intercostal muscles from over the top of the rib. The intercostal nerve, artery, and vein run underneath the rib so that the approach should proceed first over the superior edge of the rib. The intercostal muscles are composed of three adjacent layers; the external intercostal, the internal intercostal, and the innermost intercostal muscles. The intercostal nerve, artery, and vein run between the innermost intercostal muscle and the internal intercostal muscle layers. Rib spreading retractors are inserted and limited exposure may be obtained. More commonly, a larger area of exposure is required. This necessitates removal of a rib (Fig. 2-11).

Subperiosteal dissection then proceeds over the top of the rib and around to the inner and under surface. Gaining access to the under surface requires dissecting above the neurovascular bundle and staying against the bone. Once the intercostal muscles and neurovascular bundle have been taken away from the undersurface of the rib, a rib stripper may be inserted and used to carry the subperiosteal plane around to the remainder of the rib. The section of rib is then cut proximally and distally and that portion removed. Depending on the exposure, additional rib can be removed all the way back to the vertebra by detaching its articulation with the transverse process and demifacets of the vertebral body. The rib articulates with the anterior lateral aspect of the tip of the transverse process in an area termed the transverse costal facet. It is also anchored to the posterior lateral aspect of the vertebral body above and below through superior and inferior costal facets. It is important to protect the intercostal neurovascular bundle. The intercostal nerve also serves as an important localizer. It can be followed back into the neuroforamen. (Excised ribs can be used as a source of bone graft although it is not as strong and abundant as tricortical iliac crest bone graft.)

A Finochietto rib retractor facilitates exposure. A

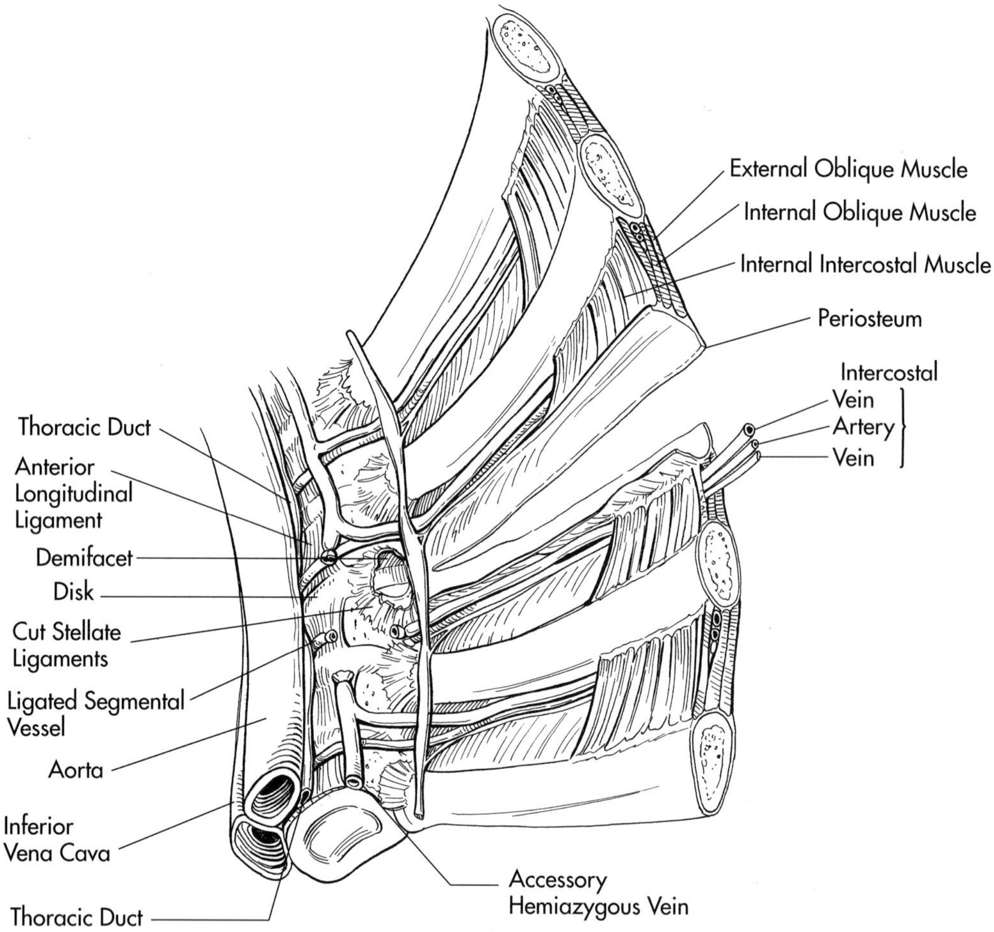

Figure 2-11

Left-sided transthoracic approach.

lung may be retracted by sponge packing or deflating. This is done with a bifurcated endotracheal tube through which the anesthesiologist may selectively deflate the left side. Next identify the area by inserting a needle into the disk space and taking a radiograph to confirm the position. Incise through the parietal pleura and reflect it away. Locate the segmental artery and veins. These are found crossing the mid portion of the vertebral body. These are ligated with sutures or clips and dissected off the spine. Cauterization can also be used although it usually is inadequate. Impeding the blood supply to the spinal cord with resultant paralysis is a very rare occurrence. Winter et al have documented 1,197 cases involving anterior vessel ligation without resultant paralysis.[5] There is an abundance of collateral circulation from the right side and from vessels proximal and distal to the area of dissection. Subperiosteal dissection can then expose the vertebral body, disks, and pedicle. The aorta is visualized overlying the anterior lateral aspect of the vertebral body on the left. The anterior longitudinal ligament is under the aorta. The intervertebral disks are removed using a scalpel or cautery with Cobb elevators and ring curettes. The pedicle identifies the limit of the posterior vertebral body. Corpectomy can now be accomplished. Straighten the table and reposition the patient if necessary when spinal fixation is performed.

Wound closure requires insertion of a chest tube to drain oozing and prevent pleural effusion and to eliminate pneumothorax as the wound heals. The chest tube is sutured into the skin. A purse string suture is added if desired for later site closure when the tubes are pulled. Establishing stability of a bone graft or fixation is all that is necessary deep within the wound. There is generally no periosteal, pleural, or deep layer to close over the spine. Sponges and packing are removed and the lung is reinflated. Lung inflation is enforced intermittently by the anesthesiologist to eliminate areas of atelectesis. The rib above and below the area of dissection are reapproximated. The table and patient are taken out of a side-flexed position to bring

BOX 6. ANTERIOR APPROACH TO THE THORACIC SPINE

Incise skin along the path of chosen rib level
Divide latissimus and serratus anterior muscles
Elevate scapula as needed, incise down onto rib
Begin subperiosteal dissection over top and around rib
Elevate under rib avoiding intercostal nerve and vessels
Strip rib proximally and distally detaching intercostal muscles
Excise rib by cutting distally and cutting or detaching from vertebra proximally
Deflate lung, pack off, and insert rib spreading retractors
Reflect pleura from vertebra and ligate segmental vessels
Subperiosteally dissect and expose vertebral body, disks, and left pedicle

the ribs together. Maintenance of chest wall closure can be aided by passing a few sutures below the lower rib taking care to avoid the neurovascular bundle above the upper rib. The intercostal muscles above and below are then brought together in a watertight fashion with a running suture. Serratus anterior, latissimus, and trapezius muscle layers are brought together. Subcutaneous and skin layers are closed in routine fashion.

Postoperative management includes frequent and regular use of incentive spirometry, coughing, and deep breathing techniques. The chest tube is managed in routine fashion and pulled when drainage sufficiently decreases and risk of pneumothorax no longer present.

COSTOTRANSVERSECTOMY APPROACH

Costotransversectomy is a less common approach. Its usefulness lies in accessing the anterior spine from the posterior route. The incision begins 2 to 3 inches lateral to the midline in a longitudinal direction. The incision is centered between the spinous process and the rib apex (Fig. 2-12 A). The dissection is carried down through the trapezius muscle cephalad and latissimus muscle caudally. Cautery is needed for hemostasis in the muscle layers. The erector spinae muscles are divided longitudinally. The muscular insertions of the deep layer of paraspinal muscles are detached from the transverse processes and ribs. Subperiosteally elevate from the transverse process and posterior rib. Carefully resect 2 to 3 inches of posterior rib along with the transverse process. Elevate from the rib and protect the intercostal artery and nerve. Bluntly dissect the parietal pleura away from injury. Proceed subperiosteally along the pedicle following the plane around to the lateral aspect of the vertebral body. Elevate the sympathetic trunk and ganglia away from the bone along with the parietal pleura. The nerve roots emanating from the neuroforamina above and below should be well visualized. The anterior spine is thus exposed for the procedure (Fig. 2-12 B).

Closure of the wound demands attention to the pleura as a high risk of pneumothorax is present with this approach. One early way to tell the presence of a defect to the parietal pleura is to fill the wound with water and ventilate the lungs. The presence of bubbles indicates air escaping from the lung. Air leaks require chest tube drainage postoperatively. Allow the pleura, sympathetic trunk, and periosteum to fall back into place. Reapproximate the muscular layers with a drain in place to prevent a postoperative hematoma from forming. Close the subcutaneous layer and skin. A final check for a pneumothorax with a postoperative radiograph of the chest is required.

ANTERIOR THORACOLUMBAR JUNCTION

The challenge of approaching this section of spinal anatomy is that it straddles two major body compartments; the thoracic cavity and the retroperitoneal space. The presence of the diaphragm interrupts the continuity of exposure from thoracic to lumbar spine. The heart and pericardium rests upon its central tendonous portion. The right and left phrenic nerves descend on either side of the heart, through the pericardium, and onto the diaphragm. Then each divide into three major branches and extend peripherally toward the muscular outer portion of the diaphragm (Fig. 2-13). To the right and left sides the lungs rest on the diaphragmatic pleura extending out to the muscular periphery of the diaphragm. On the right side and just posterior to the heart the vena cava ascends through the vena caval foramen in the tendonous portion of the diaphragm. Posteriorly the esophagus and the aorta pass through the diaphragm; the esophagus through the esophageal hiatus and the aorta between the right and left crura. The esophageal hiatus is formed by the right crus, which encircles it on either side before coming together as it descends on to its insertion on the spine. The right and left crura of the diaphragm descend posteriorly, inserting onto the prevertebral fascia of the anterior aspect of L1, 2, and 3. The area between the right and left crus forms the median arcuate ligament through which the aorta passes. Anteriorly the dome of the diaphragm inserts onto the xiphoid process. Its insertion includes the lower six ribs as it extends across the cartilaginous costal junction and onto the eleventh and twelfth ribs. The diaphragm

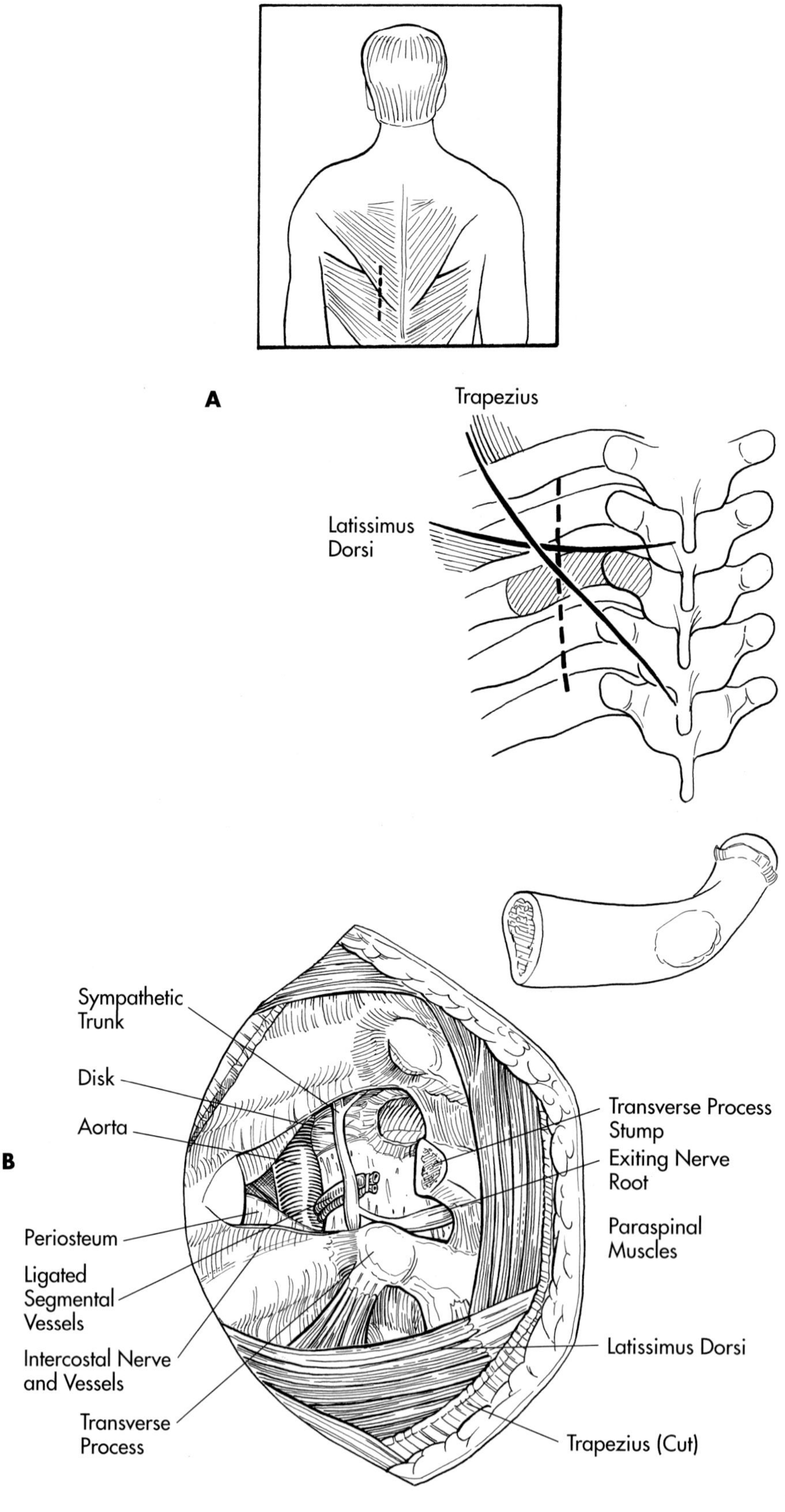

Figure 2-12

A, Costotransversectomy approach. **B**, Costotransversectomy exposure.

then inserts from the twelfth rib onto the transverse processes of L1 forming the lateral arcuate ligament. The tendinous triangular area formed between the ligament and the muscular portion of diaphragm at its periphery is termed the vertebralcostal or lumbocostal trigone. The lateral arcuate ligament is also known as the lateral lumbocostal arch under which passes the quadratus lumborum muscle. From the transverse process of L1 the diaphragm inserts onto the anterior vertebral body of L1. This junction forms the medial arcuate ligament or medial lumbocostal arch. Through this arch passes the psoas muscle and sympathetic trunk. The posterior insertions of the diaphragm, therefore, form three archways: the median arcuate ligament with the aorta, the medial arcuate ligament with the psoas muscle, and the lateral arcuate ligament with the quadratus lumborum. Incisions in the diaphragm should always be in the periphery close to its insertion to avoid injury to any of the branches to the phrenic nerve. Thoracic duct feeders may originate under the crus of the diaphragm.

A limited approach to the lumbosacral spine may be undertaken through only one body compartment. If the exposure requires reaching caudad only to T12 without need to go beyond this vertebra, a very limited exposure of this area may be achieved by a low transthoracic approach as described earlier. Similarly, if the approach requires only limited exposure of L1 without need for a wider exposure, then a retroperitoneal approach as described in the following paragraphs may suffice. Most commonly the thoracolumbar junction requires a wider exposure to safely operate. Decompression, grafting, and fixation all involve visualizing and working above and below the affected vertebra. For this the combined approach is needed.

The thoracolumbar junction is approached from the left side. On the right side the liver may impede

Box 7. Costotransversectomy Approach to the Thoracic Spine

- Make a paraspinal incision through skin, subcutaneous tissue
- Longitudinally divide paraspinal muscles
- Proceed with subperiosteal elevation
- Expose the posterior rib and transverse process
- Excise rib and transverse process
- Protect intercostal artery and nerve
- Dissect pleura and sympathetic trunk away from bone
- Follow pedicle down and around to vertebral body

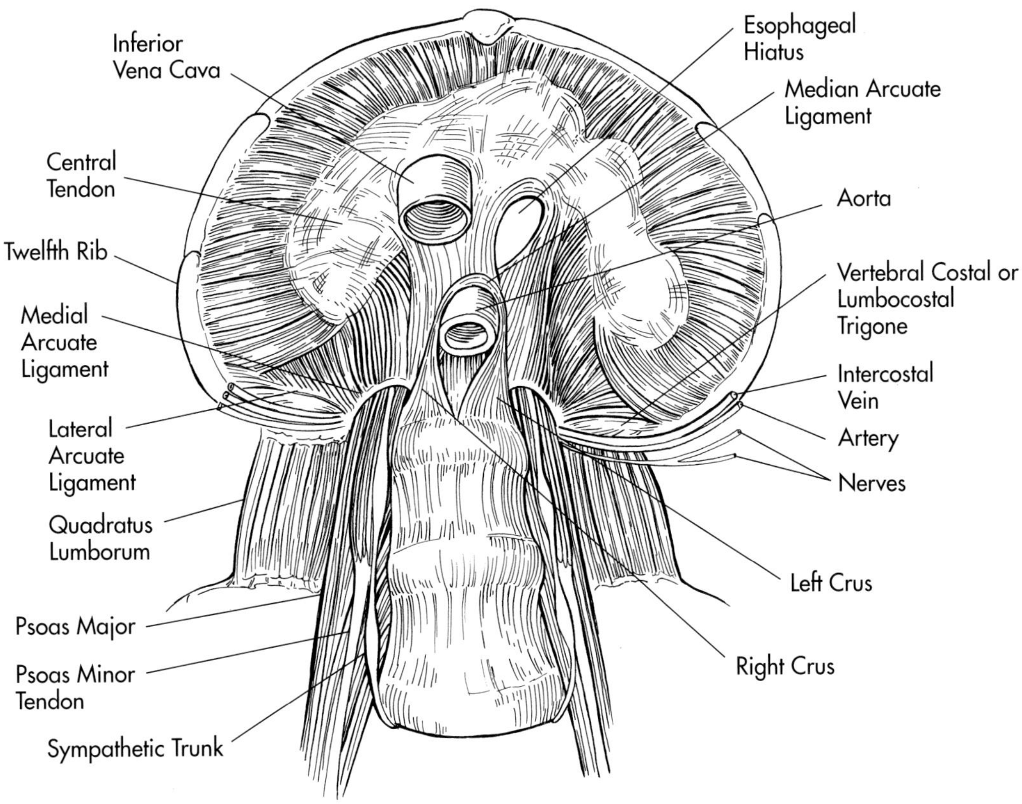

Figure 2-13

Anterior thoracolumbar junction with diaphragm.

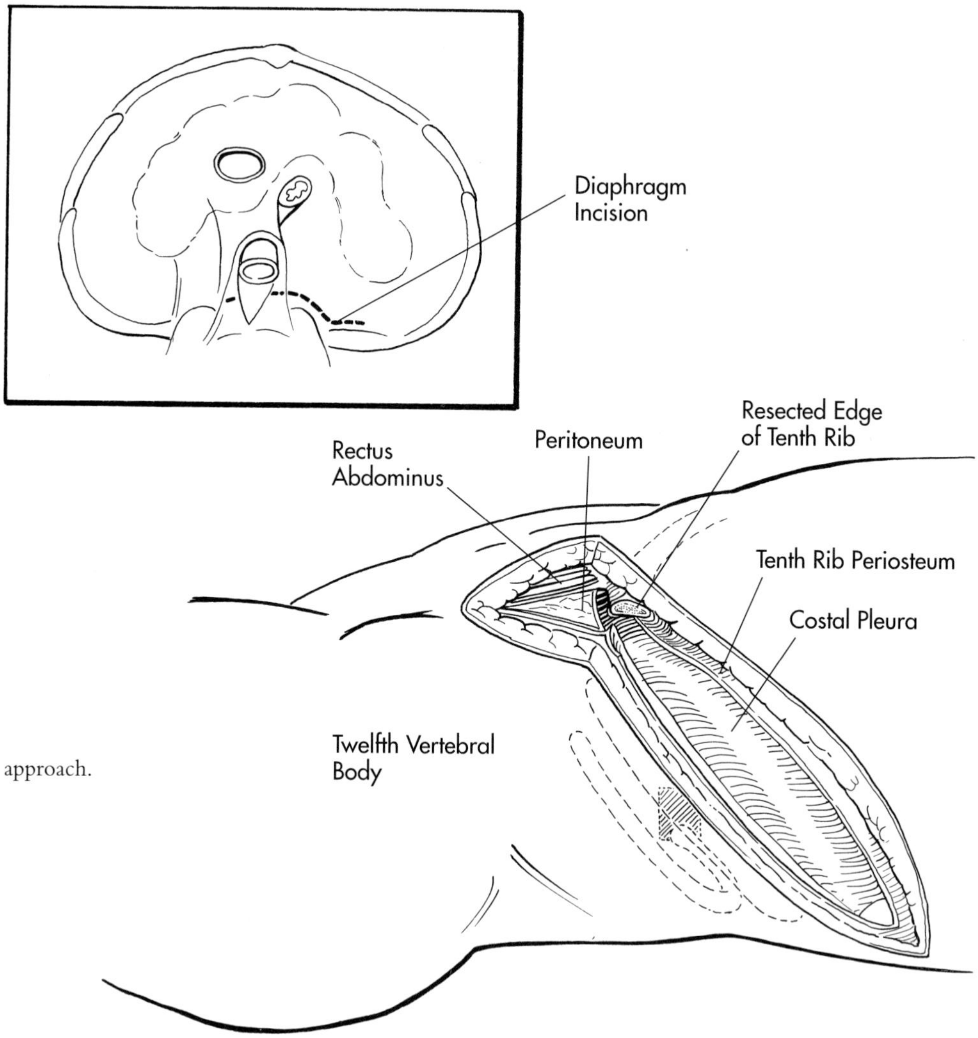

FIGURE 2-14

Anterior thoracolumbar approach.

exposure, and the vena cava is difficult to retract as it is much more fragile with bleeding more difficult to control than in the aorta. A right lateral decubitus position is used. The curvilinear left-sided incision extends from the tenth rib across the midaxillary line and down along the lateral border of the rectus muscle (Fig. 2-14). It is best to begin the exposure as a transthoracic approach. The tenth rib is exposed in routine fashion as described under the transthoracic exposure above. The tenth rib is then resected. Entering the chest at this level requires extra attention as the diaphragm arches inferiorly close to the chest wall. The diaphragm or the lung may lie in close proximity as the incision is continued down to the parietal pleura. Once access to the chest has been achieved the lung may be deflated and packed away from the field. The top of the diaphragm is then visualized. The incision is carried distally. The lateral border of the rectus abdominis is then visualized. The abdominal wall is composed of external abdominal oblique, internal abdominal oblique, and transversus abdominis muscles. Anteriorly the abdominal wall contains the rectus abdominus muscle. The junction between the former

BOX 8. ANTERIOR APPROACH TO THE THORACOLUMBAR SPINE

Incise skin along left side in curvilinear fashion
Begin at the tenth rib cross the midaxillary line
Continue incision down along the lateral border of the rectus muscle
Expose and excise the tenth rib
Proceed through parietal pleura; protect and pack off lung
Carry incision distally along between lateral border of rectus and external oblique
Incise through aponeurosis of the external, internal obliques, and transversus abdominus
Carefully incise through the transversalis fascia
Bluntly dissect peritoneum away proceeding posteriorly into retroperitoneal space
Incise diaphragm 1 to 2 cm from periphery
Reflect diaphragm from lower ribs and anterior spine
Incise prevertebral fascia and ligate segmental vessels
Subperiosteally dissect and expose vertebral body and disks

three and the latter rectus muscle is composed of the aponeurosis of the external oblique, the internal oblique, and the transversus abdominus. It is through this avascular junction of aponeuroses that the abdominal part of the incision passes. Below this, the transversalis fascia is encountered. The retroperitoneal space is entered between the transversalis fascia and the underlying peritoneum. Carefully incise through the transversalis fascia, and bluntly dissect the peritoneum back away from the fascia. Violation of the peritoneum requires repair of this layer. The dissection is carried around to the spine, packing off the peritoneum and opening up the retroperitoneal space. The two cavities are connected by taking down the diaphragm at its periphery. Incise the diaphragm from the inferior ribs around to the anterior spine. Incise one to two centimeters away from its insertion to allow enough for repair. Proceeding through the periphery will avoid denervating a large portion of diaphragm as the larger branches of the phrenic nerve are more central. The anterior thoracolumbar spine is now exposed for incision of prevertebral fascia, ligation of segmental vessels, and subperiosteal exposure and definitive treatment. Repair of any peritoneal entry should be done at the time of diagnosis as the rent can widen during spine surgery with readjustment of retractors.

Wound closure in this approach requires first an accurate repair of the diaphragm. Chest tube drainage must be inserted through the transthoracic portion of the exposure. A drain in the retroperitoneal space may also be used but is not often required. The peritoneum is allowed to fall back into place. The transversalis fascia and aponeurosis of the transversus abdominus, internal oblique, and external oblique are tightly repaired to prevent hernia formation. The intercostal interval between the ninth and eleventh rib is reapproximated. The subcutaneous layer and skin are closed in routine fashion.

Posterior Thoracic Spine

Standard approach to the posterior thoracic spine is straightforward. Skin incision is made longitudinally through the subcutaneous tissues in the midline. A solution of 1:500,000 epinephrine to saline may be used to inject the skin and subcutaneous tissue prior to incision if so desired to aid in hemostasis. Dissection with electrocautery is also used for hemostasis as the incision is carried down through the fascial layer. The longitudinal incision follows the intermuscular plane down to the supraspinous ligament and on to the tips of the spinous processes.

The superficial layer proceeds through the interfascial layer of the trapezius muscle, which extends from occiput to the spinous process of T12. The superficial layer also includes the fascial extension through which the rhomboids attach to the midline. This attachment extends from approximately C7 through T5. Caudally the latissimus extends to the midline through the thoracolumbar fascia from approximately T7 on down to the sacrum.

The intermediate muscular layer of dissection contains the serratus posterior superior from C7 to T3, the serratus posterior inferior from T11 to L2, and the erector spinae muscles. The erector spinae muscles from medial to lateral consist of spinalis, longissimus, and the iliocostalis muscles. Dissection must stay within the midline fascial plane to avoid entering or dissecting through the highly vascular musculature. Cutting directly down onto the spinous processes allows easy access into this next stage of the approach the subperiosteal dissection. The aforementioned musculature is retracted through subperiosteal elevation from the spinous processes (Fig. 2-15 A).

The next layer involves detaching the deep musculature of the back from the posterior elements of the spine. The semispinalis thoracis and rotatores thoracis muscles attach from the transverse processes to the spinous processes several levels above and one level above, respectively. They are detached and elevated in routine fashion to expose the posterior thoracic spine (Fig. 2-15 B).

Closure proceeds with reapproximation of the intermediate and deep muscle layers together as one with figure-eight sutures. Often a drain is used in this deep layer to prevent a hematoma from the oozing musculature. The superficial muscle layer is reapproximated through the fascial extensions. This layer is recognized as "the fascial layer." It is a confluent of the trapezial and thoracolumbar fascia. Next the fat and subcutaneous tissues are reapproximated and the skin closed in routine fashion.

Box 9. Posterior Approach to the Thoracic Spine

- Make a midline incision through skin and subcutaneous tissue
- Identify fascial layer with midline plane
- Incise down to the supraspinous ligament and then onto the tips of the spinous processes
- Retract paraspinal erector spinae muscle
- Proceed with subperiosteal elevation
- Detach the semispinalis and rotatores
- Expose posterior elements of the spine

LUMBAR SPINE

Anterior Lumbar Spine

The two approaches to this area are the retroperitoneal approach and the less common transperitoneal

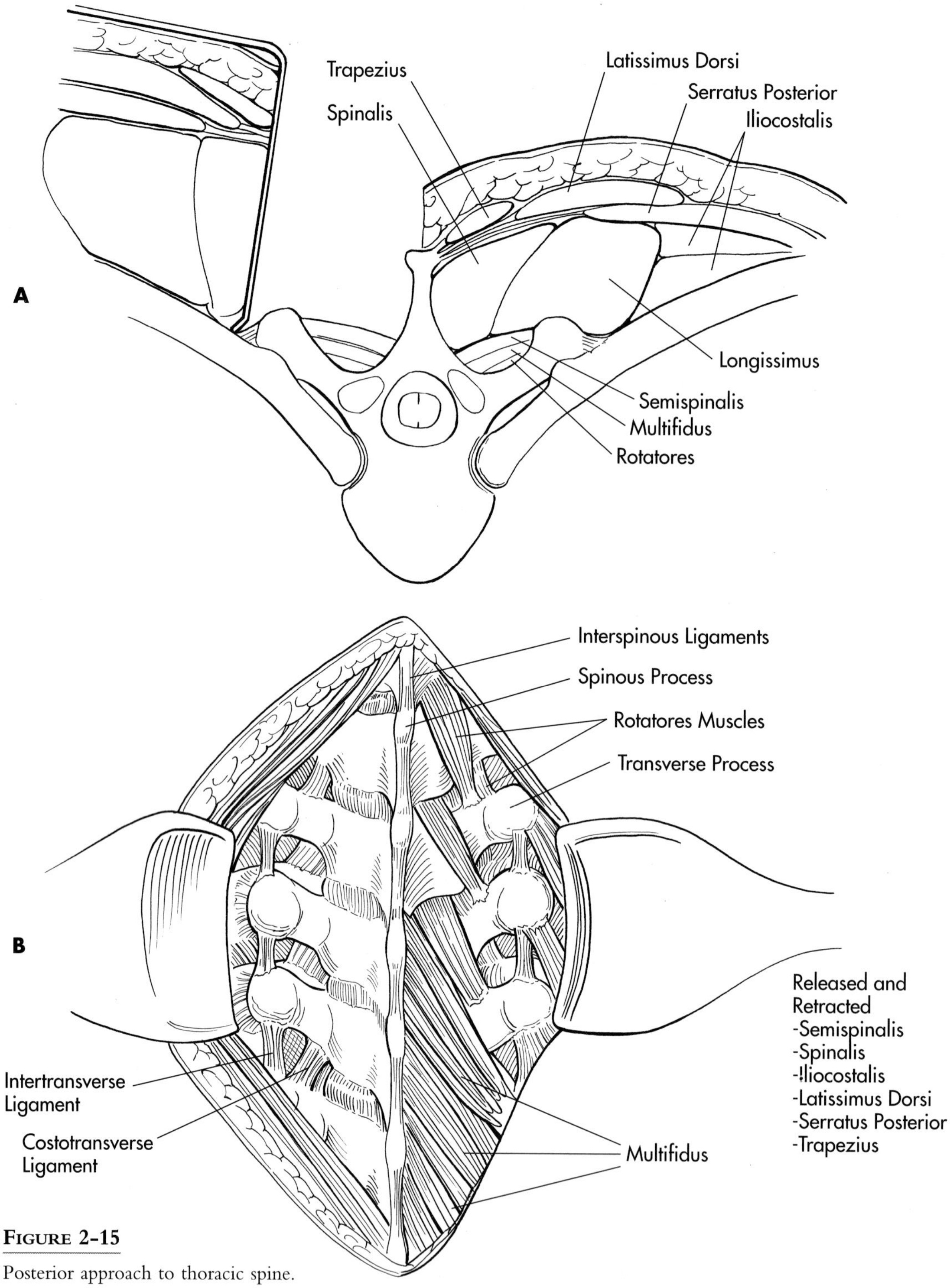

FIGURE 2-15

Posterior approach to thoracic spine.

approach. The anterior retroperitoneal approach allows access to approximately L1 through S1. Again as with anterior approaches described earlier, a left-sided approach is recommended to avoid the liver, which may block exposure, and to avoid the inferior vena cava, which may be injured and difficult to repair. The patient is positioned in a lateral decubitus or a semilateral position lying on the right side leaning 45 degrees posteriorly. Flexing the table allows the body to flex, opening the space between the ribcage and pelvis. Remember this when instrumenting or correcting spinal deformity. The hips should be flexed to relax the psoas muscle. The incision begins midway between the twelfth rib and the iliac crest and proceeds transversely or obliquely to the anterior abdomen. The placement and the obliquity of the incision depends

BOX 10. ANTERIOR RETROPERITONEAL APPROACH TO THE LUMBAR SPINE

Incise skin along left side in transverse fashion
Begin over twelfth rib or below depending on level requiring exposure
Incise around anteriorly to just above umbilicus for upper lumbar
Curve distally below the level of umbilicus for lower lumbar levels
Incise through the muscle of latissimus, external and internal obliques, and transversus abdominus
Begin at border of erector spinae and quadratus lumborum posteriorly
Extend to border of rectus abdominus anteriorly
Incise through the transversalis fascia
Continue incision down along the lateral border of the rectus muscle
Carefully incise through the transversalis fascia protecting the peritoneal layer
Bluntly dissect peritoneum away anteriorly, proceeding posteriorly into retroperitoneal space
Gently bring the ureter and surrounding retroperitoneal fat anteriorly off the psoas muscle
Elevate the psoas muscle from the vertebral body
Retract the psoas muscle laterally toward the transverse process
Ligate lumbar segmental vessels
Subperiosteally dissect and expose vertebral body and disks

on the level of the spine requiring exposure. For the upper lumbar spine, begin over the twelfth rib and proceed transversely around to the anterior abdomen above the level of the umbilicus. For lower levels begin one or two finger breadths below the costal margin and proceed obliquely and distally around to the anterior abdomen below the level of the umbilicus (Fig. 2-16).

Proceed through the skin and subcutaneous tissue. Cautery maintains hemostasis when proceeding through the muscular layer. Posteriorly the incision is carried through the lateral aspect of the latissimus muscle and around anteriorly through the external oblique, internal oblique, and transversus abdominis muscles. Anteriorly the incision stops at the lateral border of the rectus abdominis muscle. Posteriorly the incision stops at the lateral border of the erector spinae and quadratus lumborum muscles. The transversalis fascia is then divided while carefully protecting the peritoneum. Any violations of the peritoneum must be repaired. Bluntly dissect the peritoneum and its contents away anteriorly. Pack it off and insert a self-retaining Finochietto rib retractor and hand-held Deaver retractors as needed.

With dissection through the retroperitoneal space, the ureter and surrounding retroperitoneal fat is gently brought anteriorly off the psoas muscle. Important structures in the area include the aorta lying anteriorly on the vertebral body, the sympathetic chain found between the psoas and the vertebral body, and the genitofemoral nerve lying on top of the psoas muscle. These structures must be protected while working in the area. The psoas muscle is retracted laterally to the transverse process after elevating it from the vertebral body. The lumbar vessels in the area of dissection are ligated. They cross the field transversely at the midaspect of the vertebral body branching from the aorta. Subperiosteal dissection and exposure of vertebral body, pedicle, and neuroforamen proceed in routine fashion (Fig. 2-16 C).

ANTERIOR LUMBOSACRAL SPINE

Exposing the L5-S1 area can also be performed through a standard retroperitoneal approach as described previously. Dissecting further caudally one encounters the common iliac arteries and veins. Retract the peritoneum and expose between the bifurcation of the iliac vessels. The L5-S1 intervertebral disk lies within this bifurcation. The middle sacral artery and vein descends from the bifurcation and require coagulation. The left common iliac vein crosses over the L5-S1 disk and must be carefully retracted and protected. Subperiosteal dissection and disk excision can proceed in routine fashion (Fig. 2-17).

Closure is accomplished by allowing the peritoneum to fall back into place and repairing the transversalis fascia. A drain is inserted into the retroperitoneum. The muscle layer is repaired with a running suture followed by the subcutaneous layer and skin in routine fashion.

Alternately, a pararectus retroperitoneal approach may be used for the L5-S1 region. This involves a midline incision in the skin beginning just proximal to the umbilicus curving around the umbilicus to the left and extending approximately 4 centimeters below the umbilicus. The incision is carried through the anterior rectus sheath. Retract the rectus abdominus muscle medially. Identify and protect the inferior epigastric artery and vein. Incise through the posterior rectus sheath. The posterior rectus sheath ends at the arcuate line. Carefully incise through the transversalis fascia protecting the peritoneal layer. Bluntly dissect the peritoneum to the right working around to the retroperitoneal space on the left. Once arriving at the bifurcation of the common iliac vessels proceed as described previously.

Drainage is not often required as peritoneal contents obliterate the space. The posterior rectus sheath and then the anterior rectus sheaths are closed followed by the subcutaneous and skin closure.

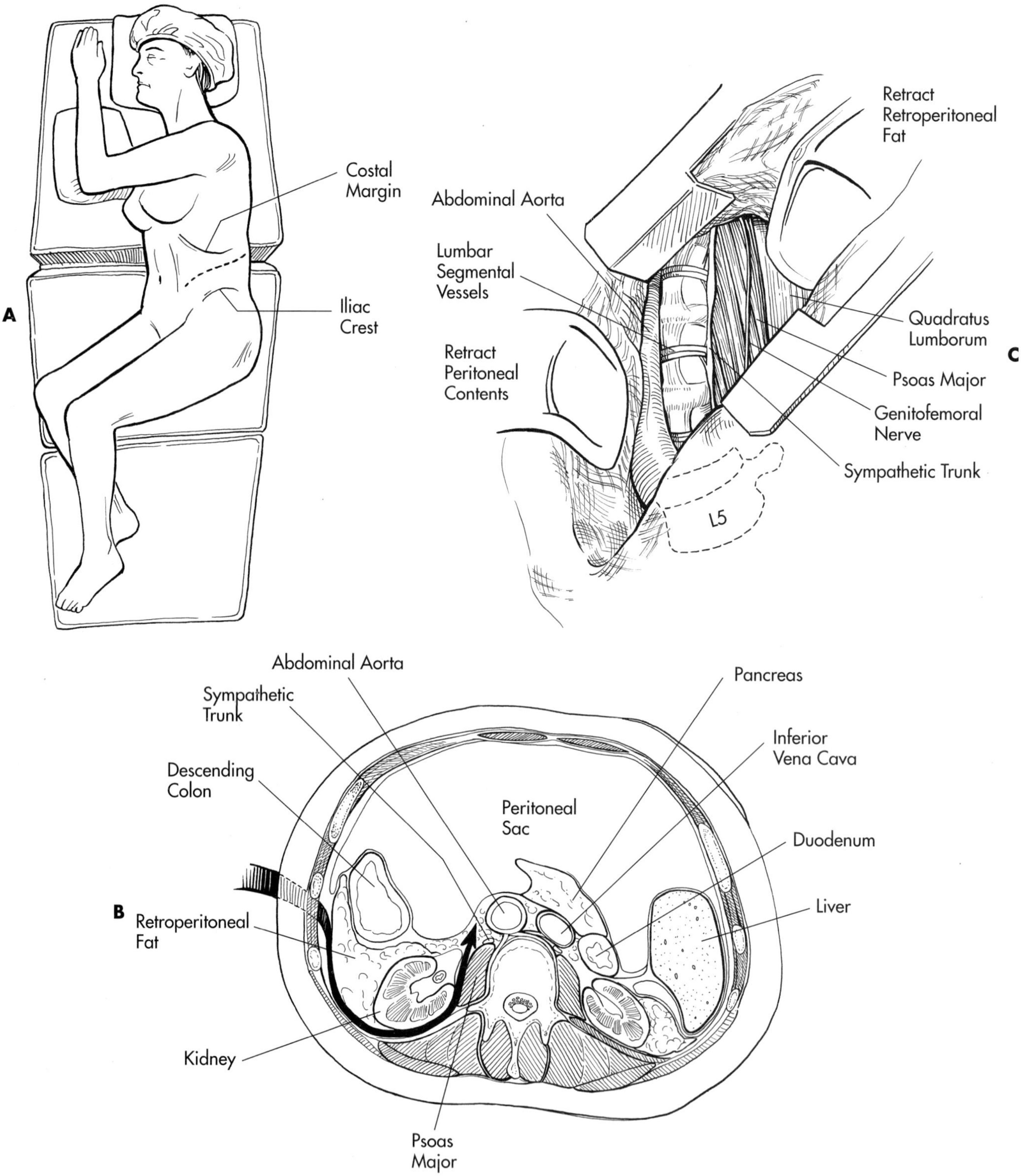

FIGURE 2-16

A, Patient positioning–retroperitoneal approach to the anterior lumbar spine. **B**, Anterior retroperitoneal approach to the upper lumbar spine—coronal view. **C**, Retroperitonal approach—exposure.

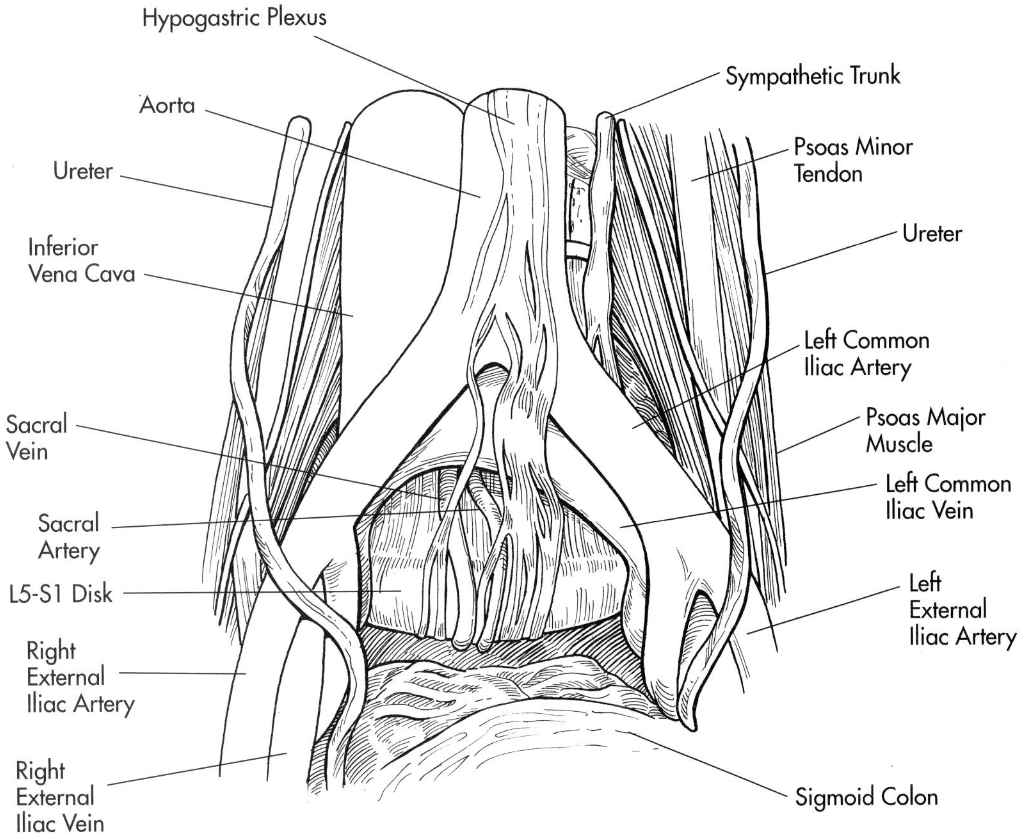

FIGURE 2-17

Anterior lumbosacral spine.

An alternate approach to the L5-S1 area of the spine is through the transperitoneal approach. For this approach a longitudinal incision over the anterior abdominal wall is used. Less commonly a transverse incision may be used for cosmesis. Incise through the anterior and posterior rectus sheath through the midline linea alba. Proceed through the transversalis fascia. Next carefully incise the peritoneum protecting the bowels from injury. The intestines must be packed off above the field of exposure. Identify the posterior peritoneum overlying the aortic bifurcation. Incise through the posterior peritoneum without endangering any of the structures posterior to it. The superior hypogastric nerve plexus overlies the great vessels and the lumbosacral junction in the retroperitoneal space. This supplies sympathetic function to the urogenital system. Blunt dissection through this area is necessary. The ureters cross over the common iliac vessels at about the area of their bifurcation into internal and external branches. Spread bluntly through this prevertebral tissue. Injury to the hypogastric plexus may result in retrograde ejaculation in males although this is not common.[25] Use bipolar cautery to coagulate the middle sacral artery if necessary. This avoids thermal injury to the plexus. The left common iliac vein often crosses directly over the L5-S1 intervertebral disk within the bifurcation of the aorta. Gently retract the vein and proceed with exposure of the disk and vertebrae.

Wound closure requires closure of the posterior and anterior peritoneal layers. Repair the transversalis fascia followed by the rectus sheath, subcutaneous layer, and skin.

POSTERIOR LUMBAR AND LUMBOSACRAL SPINE

The posterior approach to the lumbar spine is similar to the posterior approach of the thoracic spine. A midline longitudinal incision is used. Dissection proceeds through the subcutaneous adipose layer encountering next the thoracolumbar fascial layer. The midline fascia of the trapezius extends caudally to approximately the spinous process of T12. The thoracolumbar fascia, which is confluent with the latissimus dorsi musculature extends cephalad underneath the trapezial fascia to about T7. Caudally the thoracolumbar fascia extends to the sacrum and coccyx. This represents the superficial muscular layer. The intermediate layer of the lumbar spine include the erector spinae muscles. The erector spinae extend from upper thoracic spine to the sacrum and are composed of the spinalis medially and the iliocostalis laterally with the longissimus between those two. These three muscles are collectively referred to as the erector spinae muscles. They are also referred to in general terms as the paraspinal musculature. The fascial insertion of the serratus posterior inferior muscle cross over just superficial to the erector spinae on their way from the inferior four ribs to the spinous processes of T11 through L2. Staying within the midline avoids encountering the vascular musculature. The incision is carried down through the supraspinous ligament and on top of the spinous processes. Subperiosteal dissection then carries the approach through the deep muscular layer. This layer consists again of the multifidus muscle, the rotatores

BOX 11. ANTERIOR PARARECTUS RETROPERITONEAL APPROACH TO THE LUMBOSACRAL SPINE

Make a leftsided periumbilical longitudinal incision in anterior abdomen
Incise through the anterior rectus sheath
Retract the rectus abdominus muscle medially
Incise through the posterior rectus sheath and transversalis fascia
Carefully protect the peritoneal layer, bluntly dissect peritoneum away medially
Proceed around laterally and posteriorly into retroperitoneal space
Ligate the middle sacral artery, retract the left common iliac vein
Subperiosteally dissect and expose vertebral bodies and disk

BOX 12. ANTERIOR TRANSPERITONEAL APPROACH TO THE LUMBOSACRAL SPINE

Incise skin longitudinally along the anterior abdominal wall
Continue through the anterior and posterior rectus sheath in the midline
Incise through the transversalis fascia
Carefully incise through the peritoneum protecting the bowels beyond
Pack off the intestines above field of exposure
Carefully incise through the posterior peritoneum
Bluntly spread through the prevertebral tissue
Retract the left common iliac vein
Expose the L5-S1 intervertebral disk and vertebrae

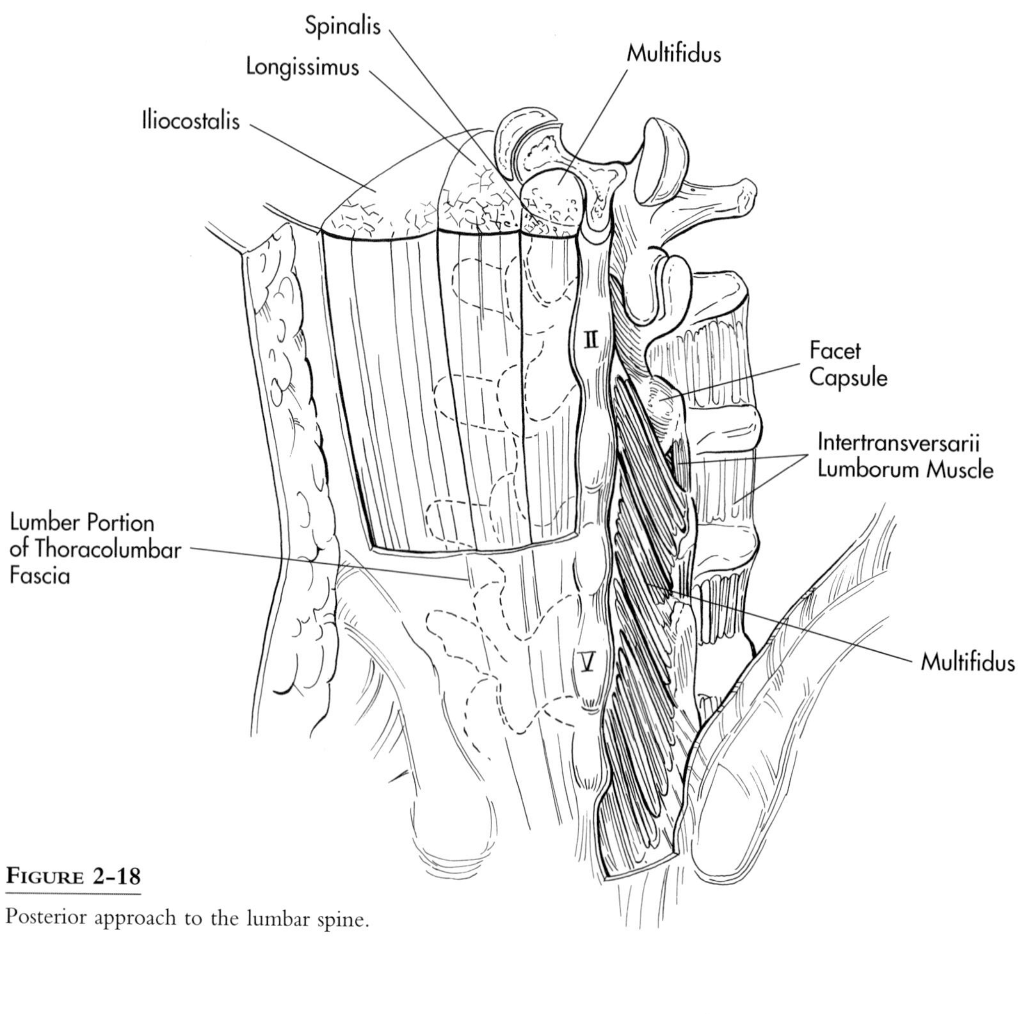

FIGURE 2-18

Posterior approach to the lumbar spine.

longus and brevis muscles, and the lateral intertransversi muscles. These are detached from the spinous and transverse processes while developing the subperiosteal plane. Exposure of the posterior elements is thus achieved (Fig. 2-18).

Closure of the wound requires reapproximation of the musculature. A deep drain at this level reduces hematoma formation. The thoracolumbar fascial layer is then closed tightly. Subcutaneous adipose layer and skin are then closed in routine fashion. Postsurgical cooling therapy can be utilized to assist in pain control and to reduce hematoma formation.

PARASPINAL LUMBAR APPROACH

The posterior paraspinal approach to the lumbar is a variation of the posterior midline approach. It is often called the Wiltse approach after his description and pioneering of this technique.[26,27] It begins as a midline incision longitudinally over the lumbar spine as described above. After arriving at the fascial layer the adipose layer is elevated away from the midline on either side to allow longitudinal paraspinal incisions through the fascia. These incisions should lie approximately two finger breadths from the midline on either

BOX 13. POSTERIOR APPROACH TO THE LUMBAR SPINE

Make a midline incision through skin and subcutaneous tissue
Identify fascial layer proceed in the midline plane
Incise down to the supraspinous ligament then onto the tips of the spinous processes
Retract paraspinal erector spinae muscles
Proceed with subperiosteal elevation
Detach the multifidus and rotatores
Expose posterior elements of the spine

BOX 14. POSTERIOR PARASPINAL APPROACH TO THE LUMBAR SPINE

Make a midline incision through skin and subcutaneous tissue
Identify fascial layer elevate laterally
Incise fascia longitudinally 2 finger breadths from the midline
Bluntly develop plane between multifidus and longissimus
Proceed with subperiosteal exposure
Expose facet joints and transverse processes

A

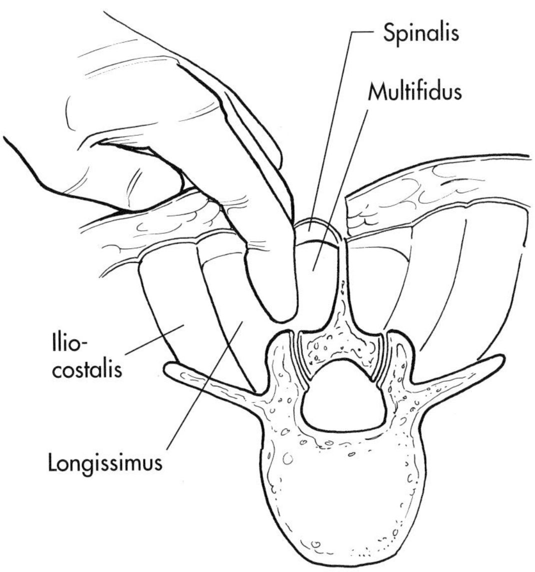

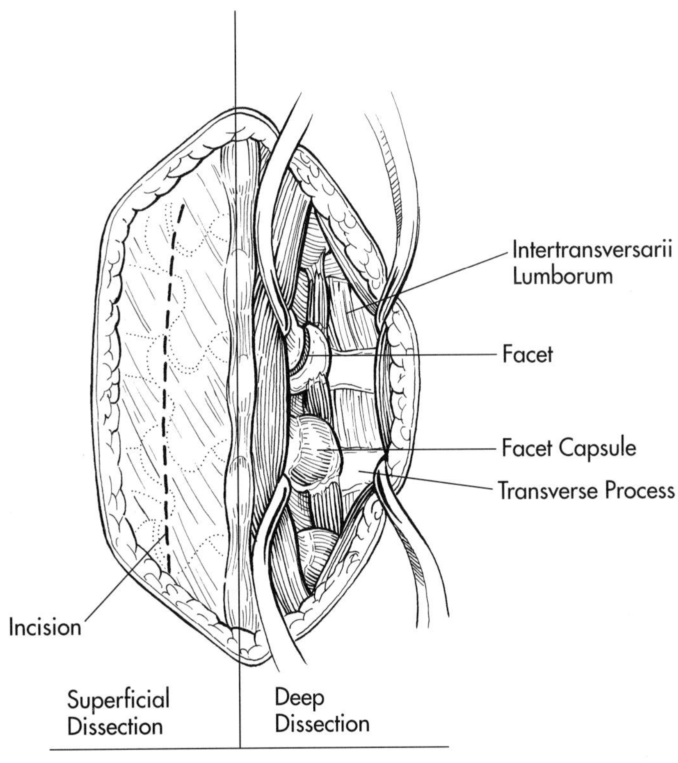

B

FIGURE 2-19

Posterior paraspinal approach to the lumbar spine. **A**, Blunt finger dissection can be used to locate the cleavage plane and palpate down onto the facet joints to assure proper location.

side. After incising the fascia, an intermuscular plane is developed between the medial lying spinalis and multifidus muscles and the lateral lying longissimus muscles. Blunt finger dissection can be used to locate the cleavage plane and palpate down onto the facet joints to assure proper location (Fig. 2-19 A). Cautery is needed for adequate hemostasis. Approach to both right and left sides of the spine requires alternate retraction. A self-retaining retractor is inserted into the developed muscle plane as subperiosteal exposure is performed. This muscle splitting approach arrives at the facet joints and transverse process on either side. This approach is useful for posterior lateral lumbar fusion and pedicle screw fixation. It is not useful for posterior spinal decompression for which a midline approach is necessary. Periodic relaxation of retraction is suggested to reduce muscle ischemia (Fig. 2-19 B).

When closing the wound the muscle is allowed to fall back into place. The fascial incisions are then tightly closed. A drain is often used just above the fascial layer where it is common for a seroma to form postoperatively in the adipose layer. The space created by elevating the skin flaps and adipose from the thoracolumbar fascia is contained by suturing the subcutaneous layer to the fascial layer. The skin is then closed in routine fashion.

REFERENCES

1. Rothman RH, Simeone FA: *The spine*, vol 1, ed 2, Philadelphia, 1982, WB Saunders.
2. Weinstein SL, Buckwalter JA, editors: *Turek's Orthopedics*, ed 5, Philadelphia, 1994, JB Lippincott. p 42–67.
3. Waldvogel FA, Medoff G, Swartz MN: Osteomyelitis: a review of clinical features, therapeutic considerations and unusual aspects (second of three parts), *N Engl J Med* 282(5):260–266, 1970.
4. Hollinshead WH: *Anatomy for surgeons,* ed 3, vol 3, Philadelphia, 1982, Harper & Row.
5. Winter RB, Lonstein JE, Denis F, et al: Paraplegia resulting from vessel ligation, *Spine* 21:1232, 1996.
6. Breschet G *Essai sur les veines du rachis,* Paris, 1819, Mequignon-Marvis.
7. Breschet G *Recherches anatomiques, physiologiques et pathologiques sur le systeme veineux et specialement sur les cavaux veineux des os,* Paris, 1828–1832, Villaret et Cie.
8. Batson OV: The vertebral vein system. *Amer J. Roentgenol Rad Ther Nucl Med,* 78(2):195–212, 1957.
9. Hollinshead WH: *Anatomy for surgeons,* ed 3, vol 3, Philadelphia, 1982, Harper & Row.
10. Robinson RA, Smith GW: Anterolateral cervical disc removal and interbody fusion for cervical disc syndrome, *Bull Johns Hopkins Hosp* 96:223, 1955.
11. Robinson RA, Southwick WO: Surgical approaches to the cervical spine, In American Academy of Orthpedic Surgeons Instructional Course Lectures, vol XVII, 1960, pp 299–330.
12. Scoville WB, Sherman IJ: Platybasia, *Ann Surg* 133:496, 1951.
13. Fang HSY, Ong GB: Direct anterior approach to the upper cervical spine, *J Bone Joint Surg* {Br} 44A:1588, 1962.
14. Bonney G, Williams JAR: Transoral approach to the upper cervical spine, *J Bone Joint Surg* {Br} 67:691, 1985.
15. Marks RJ, Forrester PC, Calder I, et al: Anesthesia for transoral craniocervical surgery. *Anesthesia* 41:1049, 1986.
16. Louis R: Anterior surgery of the upper cervical spine, *Chirurgia Deli Organi di Movimento* 77:75, 1992.
17. Hadley MN, Spetzler RF, Sonntag VK: The transoral approach to the superior cervical spine, *J Neurosurg* 71:16, 1989.
18. Merwin GE, Post JC, Sypert GW: Transoral approach to the upper cervical spine, *Laryngoscope* 101:780, 1991.
19. Wheeler MK, Merwin GE: Transoral surgical approach to anterior vertebrae C1-C3, *Surg Forum* 31:523, 1980.
20. McAfee PC, Bohlman HH, Riley LH Jr, et al: The anterior retropharyngeal approach to the upper part of the cervical spine, *J Bone Joint Surg* 69-A:1371, 1987.
21. Fang HSY, Ong GB: Direct anterior approach to the upper cervical spine, *J Bone Joint Surg* 44-A:1588, 1962.
22. Darling GE, McBroom R, Perrin R: Modified anterior approach to the cervicothoracic junction, *Spine* 20(13):1519–1521, 1995.
23. Standefer M, Hardy RW, Marks K, Cosgrove DM: Chondromyxoid fibroma of the cervical spine—a case report with a review of the literature and a description of an operative approach to the lower anterior cervical spine, *Neurosurgery* 11:288–292, 1982.
24. Sundaresan N, Shah J, Feghali JG: A transsternal approach to the upper thoracic vertebrae, *Am J Surg* 148:473–477, 1984.
25. Faciszewski T, Winter RB, Lonstein JE, et al: The surgical and medical perioperative complications of anterior spinal fusion surgery in the thoracic and lumbar spine in adults, *Spine* 20:1592, 1995.
26. Wiltse LL: The paraspinal sacrospinalis-splitting approach to the lumbar spine, *Clin Orthop* 91:48, 1973.
27. Wiltse LL, Spencer CW: New uses and refinements of the paraspinal approach of the lumbar spine, *Spine* 13:696, 1988.

3

EMERGENCY MANAGEMENT OF SPINE TRAUMA

Daniel A. Capen

Eventual outcome for the spine trauma patient frequently depends upon actions taken by the emergency team in the first 6 to 12 hours after injury. Developed nations have continued to improve care and treatment for traumatic conditions. While it is difficult to argue that in some spine trauma the severity of the damage is determined by the forces applied to the spine at the time of injury, there are many cases in which initial injury occurs and what health care professionals do immediately after injury has a direct effect on the outcome, good or bad. In most cases of spine trauma, the spinal surgeon is one of a team of personnel responding to the patient's needs.

Advances in emergency care have arisen out of necessity. The Emergency Medical Services Act of 1973 established guidelines in America concerning care and delivery systems to the hospital. Since that time there has been a steady improvement in emergency services in the United States. Other developed countries have similar plans. Toscano cited initial severe complication rates associated with transfer.[1] We have improved from the 26% neurological complication rates generated from field care and transport to the hospital.

The process, many times, begins with transportation from the site of injury to the hospital. Field emergency personnel are well trained in initiating treatment by (1) protecting the vital functions of the patient by maintaining airway, (2) supporting and assisting in the respiratory effort, and (3) establishing intravenous (IV) lines to support the circulatory system. Most emergency technicians, especially in developed countries, are well-trained in the critical phases of protecting the spine from further damage. Collars and cervical supports are applied so that neck motion is greatly reduced. The trauma patient is almost always transported on a rigid bedboard. In regions of this country where ambulance transport to a nearby hospital is not possible, there exists a network of airplane and helicopter transportation so that a minimum amount of time elapses until the patient is at a medical facility equipped to deal with severe trauma.

Another area in which the practitioner may be called upon to assist in the field assessment of spine trauma is in the athletic arena. Many states require the presence of a physician to supervise the athletic competitions involving contact. In this instance, while there may be no clear blueprint for treatment, the author suggests prudence and abundance of caution in determining the nature and extent of injury. The patient's well being, not athletic outcome, should be first and foremost on the mind of any team or treating physician. Contact injuries involving central nervous system or spinal cord symptomatology, regardless of the severity, should require immediate cessation of playing until complete and accurate evaluation can take place. Reentry into competition is not only to be discouraged but should be recognized as being fraught with danger. Concussion or radicular type symptomatology of a transitory nature should convey to the physician a "red flag" that requires immediate attention. Not every athletic event is a professional event in which a team of medical personnel is available before, during, and after the game. Many times the physician must communicate with parents to insure adequate follow-up and radiographic evaluation take place. Textbooks are available on evaluation and management of many athletic related injuries, and suggestions with respect to accurate perimeters for determination of the extent of injury are available in these texts.[2]

Significant spine trauma in this nation most frequently results from high-energy injury, which in almost every case requires multispecialty treatment. Vehicular trauma and gunshot wounds almost always involve multisystem injury. The emergency doctor can triage, evaluate, and begin treatment. Once again, the critical phases in many cases involve advanced life-support techniques. Treatment of the spine trauma may be delayed for care and treatment of multisystem injury. One of the first goals of the spine surgeon is to interact with the treatment team. Any unconscious or intoxicated trauma victim should be presumed to have spinal trauma with cord injury until proved otherwise. Protection of spinal elements during life-saving intervention must be the first goal of the spinal specialist.

Triage in the emergency department focuses on

basic life support. Airway establishment, circulatory support, and monitoring are foremost. Obvious spinal cord injury requires attention to the cervical, thoracic, and lumbar spine, in a manner that permits the maintenance of the airway and the circulatory system without placing any further mobilization stress on the cervical spine. Assembly of the treatment team is next. The beginning of basic trauma treatment is accomplished as information is gathered. A checklist is shown on Table 3-1.

It is obvious that life threatening injuries take precedence; however, in the very early phases of emergency management, there are several critical factors to consider. The first is to apply appropriate support to the spinal elements. If it appears that diagnostic work-up and life support in the emergency room requires an extensive period of time, the spine surgeon and the trauma team must get the patient off the rigid bedboard. Any kyphotic deformity or any inability on the patient's part to communicate a sensation of pressure may result in development of late sequelae, including pressure sores that result in skin necrosis and increased incidence of infection. If skin necrosis occurs directly on the spine midline, it could preclude or delay surgery for a significant period of time. Pressure sores from prolonged bedboard time have occurred on the coccyx, trochanters scapulae, and elbows. Sores are always multiorganism infection and pose an expensive long-term treatment especially if muscle necrosis is present. The expense level for these sores can reach a staggering level, and they are often preventable by the early institution of log rolling and removal from the bedboard.[3]

Table 3-1. Basic Trauma Treatment

1. Contact and consult with field team
2. Prepare emergency area for victim
3. Establish airway and begin respiratory support if needed
4. Establish fluid replacement to restore circulation; treat shock
5. Evaluate and reevaluate physical status
   - Neurologic
   - Chest
   - Abdomen
   - Extremities
6. Foley catheter for drainage and monitoring
7. Chest tube, prn
   - Abdominal tap, prn
   - Nasogastric tube
8. Evaluate
   - CNS
   - Spine
   - Long bones
9. Spinal protection
   - Skeletal traction
   - Neck bracing
10. Methylprednisolone for spinal cord injury
11. In coma, everything is injured or fractured until proved otherwise
12. Plan appropriate treatment for spine injury

Evaluating the ability of temporary immobilization to adequately support the spine is critical. If it is at all possible, an accurate assessment of the spine and spine function must be performed. Obviously, the practitioner cannot make an adequate or a complete neurologic assessment if the patient has any brain injury or is intoxicated. In suspected cervical injury, tongs or a halo may be necessary before surgery. Accurate placement of tongs or halo may prevent later complications of the devices. This is well described by Garfin et al.[4]

The *New England Journal of Medicine* study of the effects of methylprednisolone on the spinal cord recovery generated some important information. Bracken and coworkers clearly established the benefit of methylprednisolone in cord trauma in this double-blind, randomized research sponsored by the National Acute Spinal Cord Injury Study Group.[5] Except for gunshot trauma to the spine, corticosteroid protocol for any spinal cord injury must be implemented immediately. This is effective only if it is instituted within 12 hours of the injury. This protocol is standard treatment in all U.S. trauma centers. The dosage profile, described in the primary study, involves a loading IV dose of 30 mg/kg for 15 to 30 minutes, followed by 5.5 mg/kg/hr for 23 hours. This procedure arguably creates the environment for stress ulceration and other systemic complications, but with documented or suspected neurologic injury it has a clear and beneficial effect on recovery and must be administered. This treatment must not be used in children under the age of 13, during pregnancy, and in patients with diabetes or infection, and it must be used with caution in patients with compound fracture.

Life-threatening injuries may require consultation and interaction by the general surgical team. Other patients may have emergency triage and may have clearance for very early management and supervision by the spine surgeon alone. In any case of blunt abdominal trauma in which surgery is not necessary, fluid management is critical for establishing circulatory support. Prevention and treatment of shock is absolutely imperative because this directly influences the outcome in spinal cord injury. All zones of potential recovery can be adversely affected by hypoperfusion from shock.

If no spinal cord injury is present, and if the patient is cleared for early supervision by the spinal surgeon, it then becomes extremely important to evaluate the entire spine because multilevel spine fractures frequently occur.[6,7] The treating spinal doctor must understand that in multiple trauma, fractures and injuries can be missed. The literature is replete with information on the diagnosis of peripheral fractures in the extremities at very late periods.[6,7] Many authors have described multiple injuries that have been recognized after initial emergency care and treatment. There is variability of frequency, up to 15%, of noncontiguous spinal fractures. A complete musculoskeletal examination should be carried out in the emergency theater. Repeated examinations over the next 24 to 48 hours should be performed especially in the initially unconscious patient who regains consciousness. Swelling, edema, and ecchymosis may be a clue to long-bone fractures. Sudden changes in neurologic conditions can be a hint of noncontiguous fractures.[6,7]

If there is head trauma, if the patient awakes from intoxication, or if emergency surgery is performed, repeat physical examinations are very important. In an emergency setting, especially if a patient has spine trauma and a single long-bone fracture, the sensory inputs from this type of trauma are going to outweigh by far a minimally displaced fracture to the wrist or other extremity injuries. The "fine-toothed comb" theory of examination is the only theory to follow to avoid delay in diagnosis and treatment of all injuries.

In the assessment of the spine, noncontiguous spinal fractures must be ruled out. In many cases in the peripheral referral center, multilevel, noncontiguous fractures have been uncovered. In the past 5 years at Rancho Los Amigos Medical Center, there have been four cases in which a higher spinal cord injury became neurologically symptomatic after initial emergency evaluation.

EVALUATING STABILITY

In the work-up of spinal instability, there may be many instances in which full detection of instability cannot be accomplished with plain radiographs. However, understanding mechanistic classifications of instability for the cervical, thoracic, and lumbar spine is important. There are well-described classifications of fractures and dislocations that enable the practitioner to detect the nature and extent of instability from plain radiographs.[8] There are, however, many exceptions to this rule. Suspicion of spinal trauma and instability must be maintained in high energy trauma. Even in patients in whom there is no immediate apparent spine injury, the practitioner must obtain radiographs of the entire spine with adequate visualization of all spine segments. Other chapters in this text contain many different methods for classification of spine fractures and instability and information on appropriate radiographic studies.

The practitioner must thoroughly evaluate areas difficult to radiograph completely, such as the thoracic region and the cervical, cervicothoracic, and upper cervical spine. The occiput and first and second cervical vertebra can have injuries that are difficult to detect, and they may not initially present any neural deficit. Any suspicious rotation of the occiput on the upper cervical spine on plain radiographs must lead to imaging studies. Maintaining immobilization until instability is ruled out is the only "rule of thumb" in multiple trauma, coma, or intoxication. Later neurologic disaster can result from early failure to recognize the spine injury.

When skeletal radiographs do not detect instability, and there appears to be neurologic compromise, a more detailed study may be required. Computed tomography (CT) scanning can detect spinal column injury not detectable by plain radiographs. Magnetic resonance imaging (MRI) scans can be extremely helpful, especially when ligamentous injury is present. Emery and coworkers, have eloquently described the black stripe sign detecting torn posterior ligaments.[9] This may be required to diagnose instability.

ANESTHESIA

In spinal trauma, emergency anesthesia may be required for life threatening cardiovascular, abdominal, or intracranial injury. The spinal surgeon may not be a direct member of the surgical team, but he or she must ensure safe transport and transfer to the operating room along with the effective maintenance of spinal alignment during the procedure.

Most trauma centers are experienced in dealing with spinal trauma and cord injury. In centers where the problem is less frequently seen, however, the spinal surgeon must be aware of potential problems for the patient. If spinal cord injury is present or suspected, preservation of blood flow and oxygenation of the cord is critical. The anesthesiologist may be required in the emergency ward for maxillofacial injury and head trauma. Drummond's information on hyperglycemia and cord trauma may not be known, so the spinal surgeon may have to ensure that during resuscitation overdosing the patient on glucose is avoided.[10]

EMERGENCY PROCEDURE FOR REALIGNMENT OF THE CERVICAL SPINE

In many cases the patient has a fracture, fracture dislocation, or a pure dislocation of the cervical spine. These can be present without neurologic injury, especially in the upper cervical spine. Fractures of the odontoid, unilateral facet dislocations, or bilateral perched facets with a wide spinal canal can be present requiring the application of skeletal traction and reduction procedures. It is imperative that the physician do this with a minimum amount of sedation and analgesia so that the patient can provide instant, continuous, and accurate neurologic feedback.

One of the pitfalls of this emergency procedure is the failure to maintain complete, ongoing contact with the patient. A serious complication can occur if there is no contact with the patient after traction. Adding weights, leaving, and coming back an hour later to take a radiograph is fraught with the risk of overdistraction or worsening of the neurologic status because of edema or hypoperfusion. The recommended procedure is to have either a lateral radiograph available or a C-arm present and to gently, steadily add weights. Protection against overdistraction or worsening of the alignment is instantaneous. The patient can be given a muscle relaxant and gentle, reversible IV analgesia during the procedure. If C-arm is present, gentle traction manipulation or changing the angle of pull through the halo or tongs to allow flexion or extension in a safe, effective manner can assist in reducing the spine. General anesthesia to allow for manipulation increases risk of neurologic injury in the manipulation procedure.

If it is not possible to relocate the spine, posterior surgical intervention can be considered for some injuries. This can be done in a safe, effective manner under local anesthesia, especially if the patient has absolutely no neurologic deficit whatsoever.[11] If the patient has a complete cord injury, the surgeon must avoid unnecessary injury to functioning nerve roots and to preserve the well-documented potential for root escape at a level at or below the injury. It is the one scenario, however, in which urgent action is required because reduction becomes more difficult with the passage of time, since settling and ligament contracture can prevent relocation of even the seemingly simplest of spinal displacements.

With closed reduction, as with other spinal procedures, the surgeon must keep in mind that there is a certain window of safe surgical intervention followed by a period in which surgical intervention is fraught with increased risk of neurologic complication because of cord edema and changes in the blood flow to the neural elements. Intervention can occur in the first 48 to 72 hours; however, a "closed-window" then exists for approximately 7 days during which the cord is extremely refractory to any manipulation because of edema and circulatory changes. Marshall and coworkers suggest surgery on an elective basis is not recommended during this period.[12] The window remains open after this period.

EMERGENCY SURGERY IN SPINE TRAUMA

Authors in this text present various approaches with some individual preferences concerning the parameters for emergency spinal surgery. To avoid complications and to insure successful outcome, the practice at Rancho Los Amigos Medical Center has been to use emergency surgery only for those cases where clear neurologic deterioration is documented. Surgery for a patient in spinal shock neither permits accurate neurologic diagnosis nor does it allow the practitioner to determine if neurologic improvement is going to occur independent of surgery. Some authors cite the animal study of Delamarter and coworkers as showing early surgery being extremely beneficial in facilitating neurologic recovery.[13] This must be considered in light of the time parameters. In that experimental study, surgery done within an hour of constriction was statistically beneficial. It is indeed rare for the patient to have surgery within an hour of spinal cord injury.[13]

The debate as to what exactly constitutes a spinal surgical emergency continues. Some centers advocate immediate spinal cord decompression. Most evidence, however, points to the fact that an emergency spinal cord decompression does not have scientific support for a positive effect on overall outcomes. There are, however, some undeniable scenarios in which emergency spinal cord decompressive surgery is required, such as clear neurologic worsening.

There is no rationale for emergency spinal stabilization unless (1) the patient is systemically stable and can tolerate the additional surgery, and (2) if all other multiinjured systems do not contraindicate surgery. In some cases in which operative intervention is obligatory, such as for abdominal trauma or long bone stabilization, it clearly may be safe and advisable to stabilize the spine. In those cases, it should be kept in mind that the appropriate support staff and team should be available. Other authors in this text express their feelings on emergency stabilization and emergency decompression.

The one clear emergency condition in which decompression would be required is the presence of an ascending intraspinal epidural hematoma. This can be diagnosed by a combination CT scanning, myelography, and the appropriate documentation of deterioration of neurologic function. This can be life threatening in the cervical spinal cord injured patient and can require surgery even if it is clear that the patient has a complete neurologic injury. Untreated ascension of compression can lead to respiratory failure and death; therefore, decompression is essential.

The second clear scenario in which emergency decompression would be required is in the presence of an incomplete neurologic injury where there is clear sequential documentation over a short period of time of worsening of the neurologic condition. If neurologic loss is present, urgent operative intervention offers the best opportunity for recovery and protection of the zone in the spinal neural elements that is ischemic but not necrotic. It is imperative for all patients to have appropriate imaging to locate the area of compression early and in the event that neurologic worsening does occur. Time could be lost in an attempt to obtain appropriate imaging if it is not already available.

The third scenario in which urgent surgical intervention is required is in the lumbar spine where the development of a cauda equina syndrome is documented. Sudden loss of bowel and bladder control, perineal sensation, or the development of a neurologic injury early in the course of trauma indicates emergency action.

SPINE TRAUMA CORD INJURY AND EMERGENCY PROBLEMS

With 10,000 new spinal cord injury cases per year, in triage the spinal surgeon may be the only treating physician.[14,15] It is imperative for the surgeon to maintain awareness of potential abdominal, urologic, and circulatory disaster. Although the primary age group for such injuries is 19 to 34, there is a mortality rate of 10% to 15% in the first year, which suggests impact injury and multisystem involvement.[16]

Diagnosis and treatment of the delayed development of an acute condition in the abdomen may be very difficult. In flaccid paresis above the T6–T8 area, minimal to no signs or symptoms are present. Penetrating and nonpenetrating injuries to the liver, small and large bowel, pancreas, and stomach may be difficult to detect. Obvious peritoneal signs will not be present, and fever, hypotension, and abnormal lab values may be the only tip off for the spinal surgeon that disaster looms and urgent consultation is required.[17]

Deep venous thrombosis and subsequent pulmonary embolism are a very real threats.[18,19] The practitioner must be aware and use thromboembolic disease support (TED) hose, early extremity ranging, and, if not contraindicated, anticoagulation. Loss of mobility and muscle function in spinal cord injury predisposes the patient to stasis. In addition, in the early stages of shock and recovery from hyperperfusion, extremity blood flow vacillates. Watson described an astronomical 81% incidence of deep vein thrombosis in complete cord injury patients in the first month postinjury.[18]

Hypercoagulability may contribute to the problem early after trauma. Awareness is critical, so any extremity swelling should be swiftly recognized. I prefer Lovenox and mobilization, but mechanical compression and full anticoagulation are options. No treatment is proved superior.[19] Awareness is often the best prevention.

SUMMARY

Early supervision of spine care in the multiple trauma patient must focus on prevention of neurologic injury. Treatment of all life-threatening injuries preceeds spinal intervention, but spinal alignment should not be ignored.

Rapid diagnosis of all spinal trauma prior to surgical intervention may prevent a missed injury. Methylprednisolone protocol implementation is necessary in the first 8 hours. Outcome is dependent upon emergency measures for most spine trauma victims.

REFERENCES

1. Toscano J: Prevention of neurologic deterioration before admission to a spinal cord injury unit, *Paraplegia* 26(3) 143–150, 1988.
2. Watkins RG, editor: *The spine in sports*, Philadelphia, 1996, Mosby–Year Book.
3. Richardson RR, Meyer PR: Prevalence and incidence of pressure sores in acute spinal cord injuries, *Paraplegia* 19:235, 1981.
4. Garfin SR, Bott MJ, Waters RL, Nickel VL: Complications in the use of the halo fixation device, *J Bone Joint Surg (Am)* 68:320–325, 1986.
5. Bracken MB, Shephard MJ, Collins WF: A randomized controlled trial of ethylprednisolone or naloxone in treatment of acute spinal cord injury, *N Engl J Med* 322:1405, 1990.
6. Calenoff L, Chessara JW, Rogers LF, et al: Multiple level spinal injuries; the importance of early recognition, *Am J Roentgenol* 130:665–669, 1978.
7. Keenen TL, Antony J, Benson, BR: Non-contiguous spinal fractures, *J Trauma* 30(4):489–491, 1990.
8. Allen BL, Ferguson RL, Lehman TR, O'Brien RP: A mechanistic classification of closed-indirect fractures and dislocations of the lower cervical spine; *Spine* 7:1–27, 1982.
9. Emery SE, Pathria MN, Wilbur RG, et al: Magnetic resonance imaging of post–traumatic spinal ligament injury, *J Spin Disord* 2(4):229–233, 1989.
10. Drummond JC, Moore SS: The influence of dextrose administration on neurologic outcome after temporary spinal cord ischemia in the rabbit, *Anesthesiology* 70:64, 1989.
11. Capen DA, Zigler JE, Rockowitz N, et al: Posterior cervical fusion with local anesthesia, the awake patient as the ultimate spinal cord monitor, *Spine* 12:206–208, 1987.
12. Marshall LF, Knowlton RS, Garfin SR, et al: Deterioration following spinal cord injury: a multi center study, *J Neurosurg* 66:400–404, 1987.
13. Delamarter RB, Sherman J, Carr JB: Pathophysiology

of spinal cord injury, *J Bone Joint Surg (Am)* 77A:1042–1049, 1995.

14. Fine PR, Kuhlemeier KV, De Vivo MJ, Stover SL: Spinal cord injury: an epidemiologic perspective, *Paraplegia* 17:237–250, 1979.
15. Eisenberg MG, Tierney DO: Changing demographic profile of the spinal cord injury population: implications for health care support systems, *Paraplegia* 12:335, 1985.
16. Stover SL, DeLisa JA, Whiteneck GG: Spinal cord injury: clinical outcomes from the model systems, Gaithensberg, 1995, Aspen Publishers.
17. Davis JH: Initial operative management of multiple abdominal organ injury. In Najarian JS, Delaney JP, editors: *Emergency medicine—Trauma-Shock-Sepsis-Burns*. Chicago, 1986, Mosby–Year Book.
18. Watson N: Venous thrombosis and pulmonary embolism in spinal cord injury, *Paraplegia* 16:113–121, 1978–1979.
19. Wessler S: Prevention of venous thromboembolism: rationale, practice and problem prevention of venous thrombosis and pulmonary embolism. NIH Consensus Development Conference, Bethesda MD, March 24–26, 1986, pp 15–18.

4

IMAGING OF SPINAL TRAUMA PEARLS AND PITFALLS

Stephen L.G. Rothman

The diagnosis and treatment of spinal injuries may require utilization of a wide range of imaging examinations. Imaging is so integrated into the topic of spinal trauma that almost every chapter in this and every other book must contain spinal radiograph, magnetic resonance imaging (MRI) and computed tomography (CT) scans. This chapter, therefore, attempts an overview of spinal imaging from the perspective of the spinal radiologist as consultant to the spinal surgeon. An attempt is made to summarize the most important imaging manifestations of most of the common and some uncommon traumatic lesions of the spine. The standard mechanistic approach is used broadly dividing each anatomical zone into compression, flexion, and hyperextension injuries. Interspersed with the pictorial demonstration of the typical manifestations of the various lesions is a series of comments labeled as *Pearls* or *Pitfalls*. These small segments are meant as useful vignettes alerting the reader to common problems of omission or commission, which can easily be avoided by the radiologically sophisticated clinician. Whenever possible, common anatomic variations that may masquerade as fractures are included in the appropriate sections.

We live in the MRI-CT era. These two modalities have become of paramount importance in the diagnosis of spinal injuries. One must not neglect, however, the basic radiologic skills, which have been paramount for generations. Little is written in the current scientific literature on radiographic diagnosis. Many wonderful, radiologic texts are becoming hard to find. Interested readers are referred to the classic text books listed in the references as a complete dissertation on the radiology of spinal trauma is beyond the scope of this chapter. Although it is often tempting to perform both MRI and CT on spinal injured patients, one or both are often unnecessary. In this chapter, I attempt to define which single imaging study is most useful in the evaluation of each entity.

Dividing patients into two categories is useful; those with gross anatomic injuries that can be diagnosed by imaging studies, and those with real symptoms but no diagnosable anatomic lesion. Severe spinal trauma is defined as an episode that causes some type of anatomic derangement, which is obvious in an objective imaging study. When such a patient presents to an acute care facility, most often it is clear that the patient is severely injured. If the patient is conscious and not under the influence of drugs or alcohol, pain, muscle spasm, or neurologic deficit is obvious. When the patient is incoherent, unconscious, or has many other severe injuries spinal injury may not be as obvious. Appropriate spinal imaging is critical in either instance.

PLAIN FILM RADIOGRAPHY

The vertebral column performs several functions: it supports the weight of the head and upper body; it allows controlled flexibility with rotation, tilting, and bending; and it provides a protective bony ring for the spinal cord and exiting nerve roots. The diagnostic evaluation of the spine must assess all three of these functions. Integrity of the vertebral body and vertebral joints are primarily associated with weight bearing. Ligamentous integrity and the zygapophyseal joints affect flexibility, and an intact bony ring is the primary factor in protecting the neural elements.

After life-saving procedures, the spine should be immobilized and high-quality emergency radiographs should be taken without moving the patient. In patients suspected of having cervical injuries, take frontal, cross table lateral, and open mouth views of the dens.[1,2] When a lumbar or thoracic fracture is suspected, frontal and cross table lateral radiographs should be obtained on the immobilized patient. A more complete examination can be delayed if these radiographs are normal. These should always be evaluated in a timely fashion by a qualified radiologist. If there is a hint of structural injury in the physical examination, a complete set of spine radiographs should be obtained. Bony integrity and vertebral alignment must be evaluated and a preliminary diagnosis made. If the patient is a surgical candidate or if additional anatomic information is necessary, a high-quality, thin section CT scan should be performed with complete sagittal and coronal reformations. It is much easier to deal with a sick or severely injured patient in a CT scanner rather than in an MRI machine, and CT is ideal for the evaluation of spinal integrity.

Stability of the spine is best evaluated with conventional flexion and extension films. In unusual cases of suspected cervical spine instability, dynamic MRI can be performed using a sequence of midline, gradient echo-type images with the head in flexion and extension. This can be performed easily with a variety of scanners. Vertebral ring and joint integrity is best evaluated on axial CT images. It is rarely necessary to perform CT myelography. If it is crucial to see the spinal cord, MRI is the procedure of choice. If myelography is necessary, it should be done through a lateral C1-C2 puncture with the patient in the supine position.

TECHNIQUE OF SPINAL CT

Virtually all currently operating CT scanners are capable of producing adequate images of the traumatized spine. Scan slices should always be as thin as possible. The ideal thickness in cervical spine scanning is $1\frac{1}{2}$ mm.[3,4,5] If that is impossible technically, the narrowest setting should be used. It is rarely necessary to scan with 1 mm slices, although the images produced in this manner are remarkably sharp. It is not necessary to overlap the slices to get high-quality reformations as long as slice thickness remains below 3 mm. In our practice, we never use slices thicker than 2 mm in the cervical spine.

Lumbar and thoracic CT can be done with contiguous 3 mm slices or with 5 mm slices with 2 mm overlap. This latter technique produces images of high signal-to-noise ratio and smooth reformations. Newer scanners can perform as many as 30 slices per minute. This allows the entire examination to be completed in minutes.[6] No spinal CT examination is complete without a full series of sagittal and coronal reformations. Ideally, the coronal reformations should be curved to follow the contour of the spine. All studies should be photographed for soft tissue and bony detail. Good quality CT images can diagnose cord hemorrhage, mass effect, and acute disk herniation.

TECHNIQUE OF SPINAL MRI

The MRI scanner is capable of a producing many different types of images. It is not necessary to list the possible benefits and drawbacks of all commonly used sequences. Each examination should include at least one T1-weighted sagittal sequence, a sagittal sequence with water displayed bright (T2 spin echo, fast spin echo, or gradient refocused image), and a series of axial images. T1-weighted views show anatomy a bit crisper than comparable T2 images and far better than most gradient echo-type images. Often a sequence producing 1-mm thick sections can be used to reformat oblique and coronal images of good quality, especially in the cervical spine.[7]

THE CRANIOVERTEBRAL JUNCTION

The craniocervical junction includes the spine from the superior endplate of C3 through the foramen magnum. This area is frequently traumatized, often with devastating neurological consequences.

Dislocation of the craniovertebral joint is a rare and nearly universally fatal injury most often caused by autos hitting pedestrians, typically children.[8] Survival has been reported when victims received very early cardiopulmonary resuscitation.[9] The diagnosis is obvious on routine radiographs because the skull and the cervical spine do not align properly. Retropharyngeal soft tissue swelling is very dramatic (Fig. 4-1).

Fracture or fracture subluxation of one or both of the atlantooccipital joints is also uncommon. Because it is reasonably likely that patients with such injuries will survive once they arrive at an emergency facility, proper diagnosis is critical.

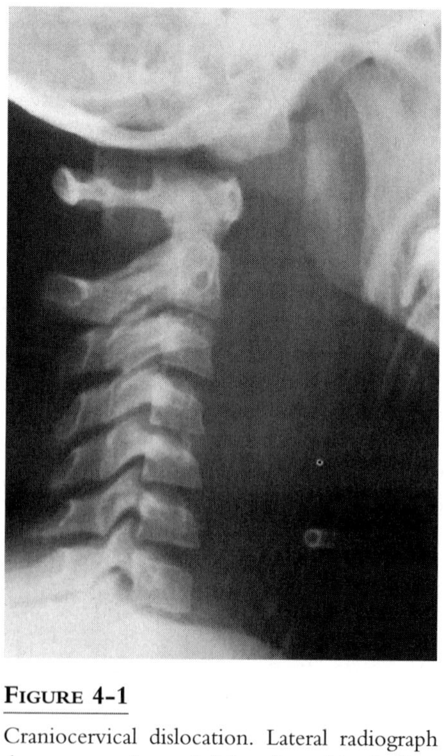

FIGURE 4-1

Craniocervical dislocation. Lateral radiograph demonstrates forward dislocation of the skull on the cervical spine. Note profound prevertebral swelling.

> **PEARL**
>
> There is never any normal rotation between C1 and the skull. Consequently the maxilla must always align with the C1 ring. The demonstration on axial CT of even minor rotation between C1 and the maxilla indicates anatomic abnormality (Fig. 4-2 A).

The anatomy of the craniooccipital facets is best seen on thin-section sagittal CT reformations. Note the subtle compression fracture of the occipital condyle in Figure 4-28 C.

There are three types of occipital condyle fracture.[10,11,12] Type I, an impact fracture, is produced by axial load with lateral bending. Type II is a basilar skull fracture, which extends through the condyle, and type III fracture is an avulsion of the medial portion of

A

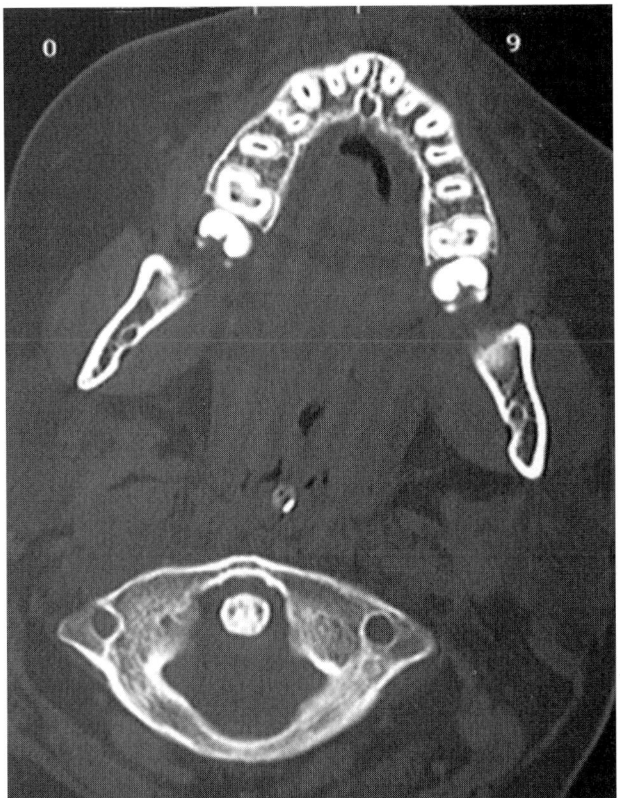

B C

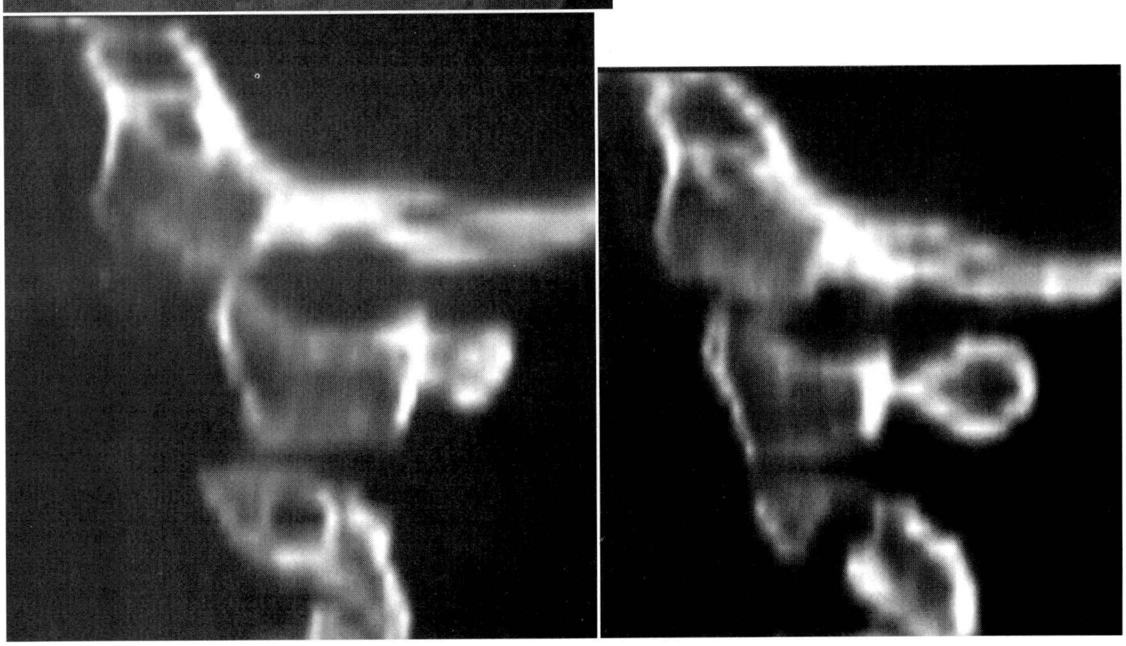

FIGURE 4-2

Craniocervical subluxation. Axial CT scan **A** reveals rotation of the jaw with respect to the atlas. **B**, Sagittal CT reformation through the dislocated right occipital condyle. **C**, Sagittal CT reformation through the subluxed left condyle.

the condyle (Fig. 4-3). Depending on the amount of subluxation, regular radiographs may show little bony displacement. Soft tissue swelling in the prevertebral space is prominent. Abnormal rotation between C1 and the occipital bone is common because the joint injury is usually asymmetric.

Severe compression of an occipital condyle or medial subluxation of the foramen magnum edge may injure the eleventh cranial nerve within the hypoglossal canal. Deviation of the tongue is an important physical sign, which necessitates CT scanning. It is much less likely for an occipital condyle to fracture than for the C1 ring to burst.

Direct axial compression to the craniovertebral junction produces downward and outward force vectors on the superior articular processes of C1. This is caused by transmission of forces by the occipital condyles, which are shaped like a pair of opposing facing chisels. The C1 ring usually bursts in two places, just anterior to and just posterior to one of the articular pillars. These are classic indications of a "Jefferson fracture." Diagnosis is generally made on the open mouth radiograph in which the lateral masses of C1 appear separated from the dens with bilateral lateral offset of the articular processes (Fig. 4-4). There may be asymmetry of the spaces between the dens and the lateral masses.[13,14]

A

B

C

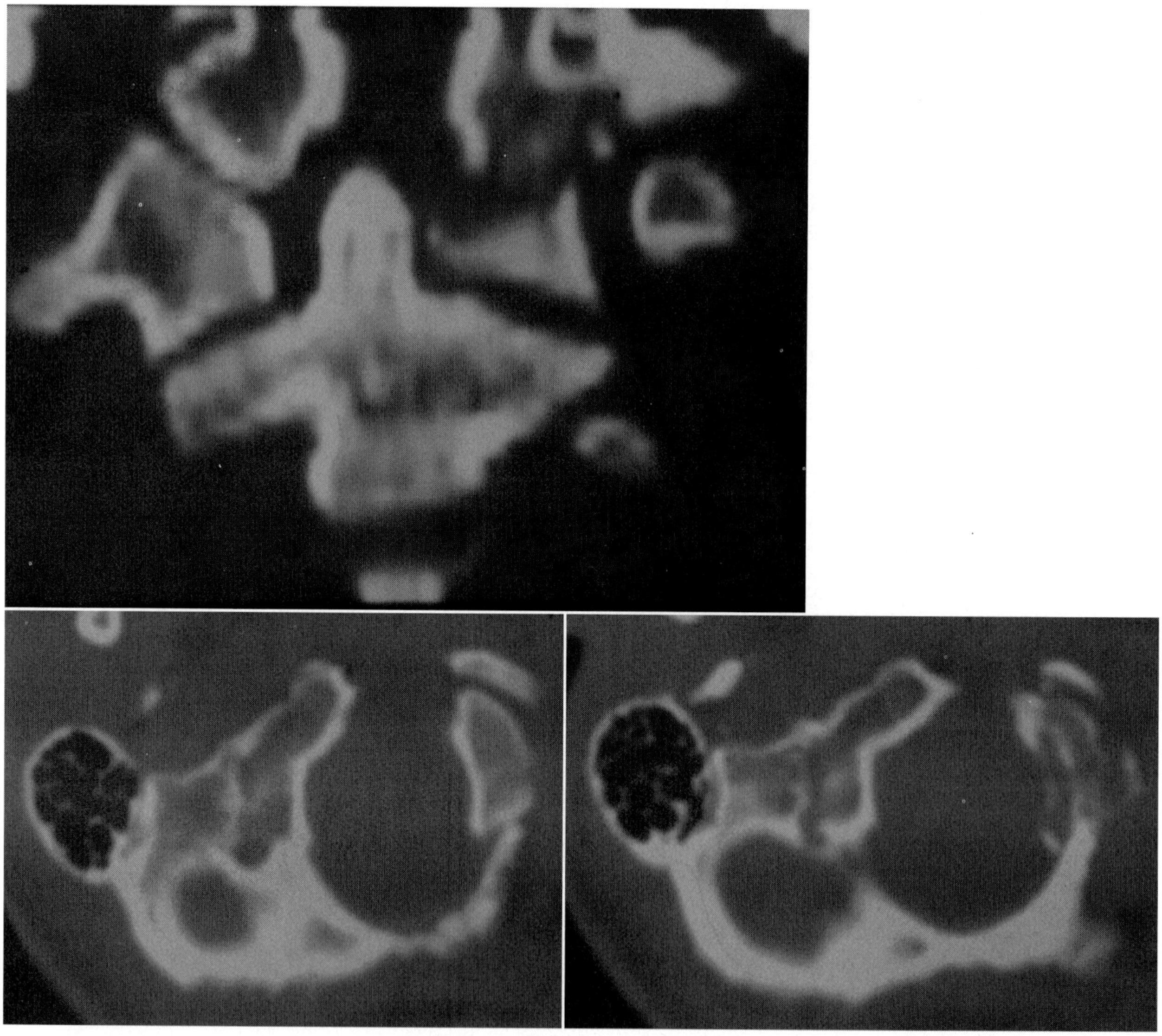

FIGURE 4-3

Fracture of the craniooccipital facets: **A**, Type I fracture. Coronal CT reformation demonstrating compression of the left occipital condyle and superior facet of the atlas. **B&C**, Consecutive axial CT scans of a patient with Type III occipital condyle fracture with medial displacement of the rim of the foramen magnum.

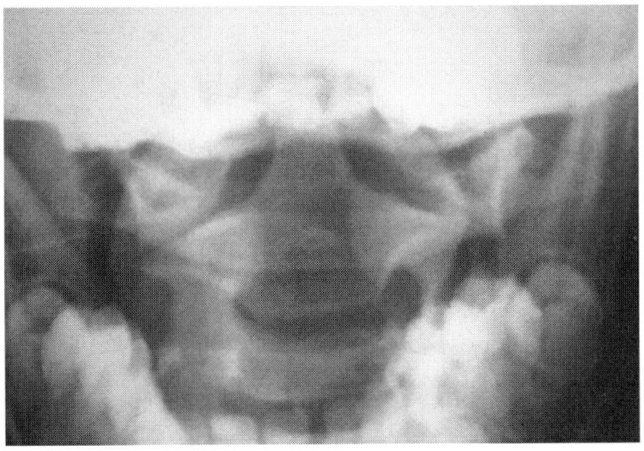

FIGURE 4-4

Jefferson fracture. Frontal radiograph reveals bilateral offset of the lateral masses of C1 with the C2 spinous process in the midline.

> **PITFALL**
>
> Not all patients with bilateral lateral offset of the C1 condyles have Jefferson fracture. Patients with torticollis, with lateral bending of the neck and contralateral rotation of the head, appear to have bilateral offset caused by a complex set of rotations. These two conditions can be differentiated radiographically by the position of the spinous process of C2. To make the diagnosis of Jefferson fracture the spinous process must be in the midline. In patients with torticollis and rotation, the spinous process of C2 is deviated away from the offset articular process. A conventional anteroposterior (AP) tomogram, therefore, is not a good tool to investigate the injury, because spinous processes are out of the plane of the pertinent cuts.

Occasionally, fracture of the lateral portion of the C1 ring is obvious in regular lateral radiographs (Fig. 4-5 A). More commonly, however, the lateral radiograph may appear completely normal. In uninjured people, the tip of the dens should crest at the same height as the superior margin of the anterior ring of C1.

> **PEARL**
>
> If the tip of the dens projects superior to the arch of C1, a Jefferson fracture is likely even in the absence of any other finding. This is because of upward herniation of the dens into the widened C1 ring. A CT scan should always be performed if this subtle abnormality is noted (Fig. 4-5 B).

The CT scan is the imaging procedure of choice for the evaluation of C1 fractures. The CT scan defines the ring fractures and often demonstrates avulsion of the insertion of the transverse ligament (Fig. 4-6 A). The bony attachments of the transverse ligament are avulsed more frequently than ruptured. Instability of the anterior atlantoaxial joint, because of avulsion of the attachment of the transverse ligament, is the cause of the upward migration of the dens. An MRI scan is generally unnecessary in the evaluation of C1 fractures, because they are self-decompressing injuries. The spinal cord is easily visualized at the craniovertebral junction on good quality CT scans even without the injection of intrathecal contrast.

Lateral compression fractures of C1 are seen less frequently than Jefferson fractures. Occasionally both types are present in the same vertebra. Lateral compression forces produce comminution of the lateral mass on the concave side of the torticollis. Occasionally, relatively minor trauma to the craniovertebral junction can cause subtle fracture of one or both of the articular surfaces. These fractures are not usually visible on conventional radiographs. Routine CT with thick axial scans are often inadequate to identify minor articular irregularities. These fractures may produce degenerative arthritis and chronic neck pain. This condition may be difficult to diagnose (Fig. 4-7). Fractures of the occipital condyles, C1, and C2 may coexist further complicating the deformity. A CT scan with coronal reformation is the diagnostic procedure of choice to evaluate the articular pillars and facets.

Abnormal flexion or extension forces to the craniovertebral junction can cause fracture of the dens or stretching or rupture of the transverse ligament. Subluxation of the C1-C2 joint caused by tearing of the transverse ligament is very rare. Usually the ligament avulses its attachment to C1 (Fig. 4-8). Lateral radiography demonstrates widening of the AP distance between the arch of C1 and the dens. This distance should be less than 3 mm in adults and 4 to 5 mm in young children in whom the ligaments are more lax and the bone is not as well developed.[16,17] This finding, however, does not always indicate acute traumatic subluxation. It is important to note the clinical signs and symptoms of the patient. Although unusual, some patients have a wide anterior joint space without acute injury. Immobilizing a patient on the basis of abnormal radiographs may be tempting, but it is often inappropriate. A person with recent trauma with widening of the anterior C1-C2 joint caused by acute ligamentous rupture must have significant localized clinical signs and symptoms.

The diagnosis of subtle C1-C2 subluxation is usually made on the lateral view of the cervical spine. Identifying the posterior cortical plate of the dens is often difficult, and fracture subluxation of the dens with C1

A

B

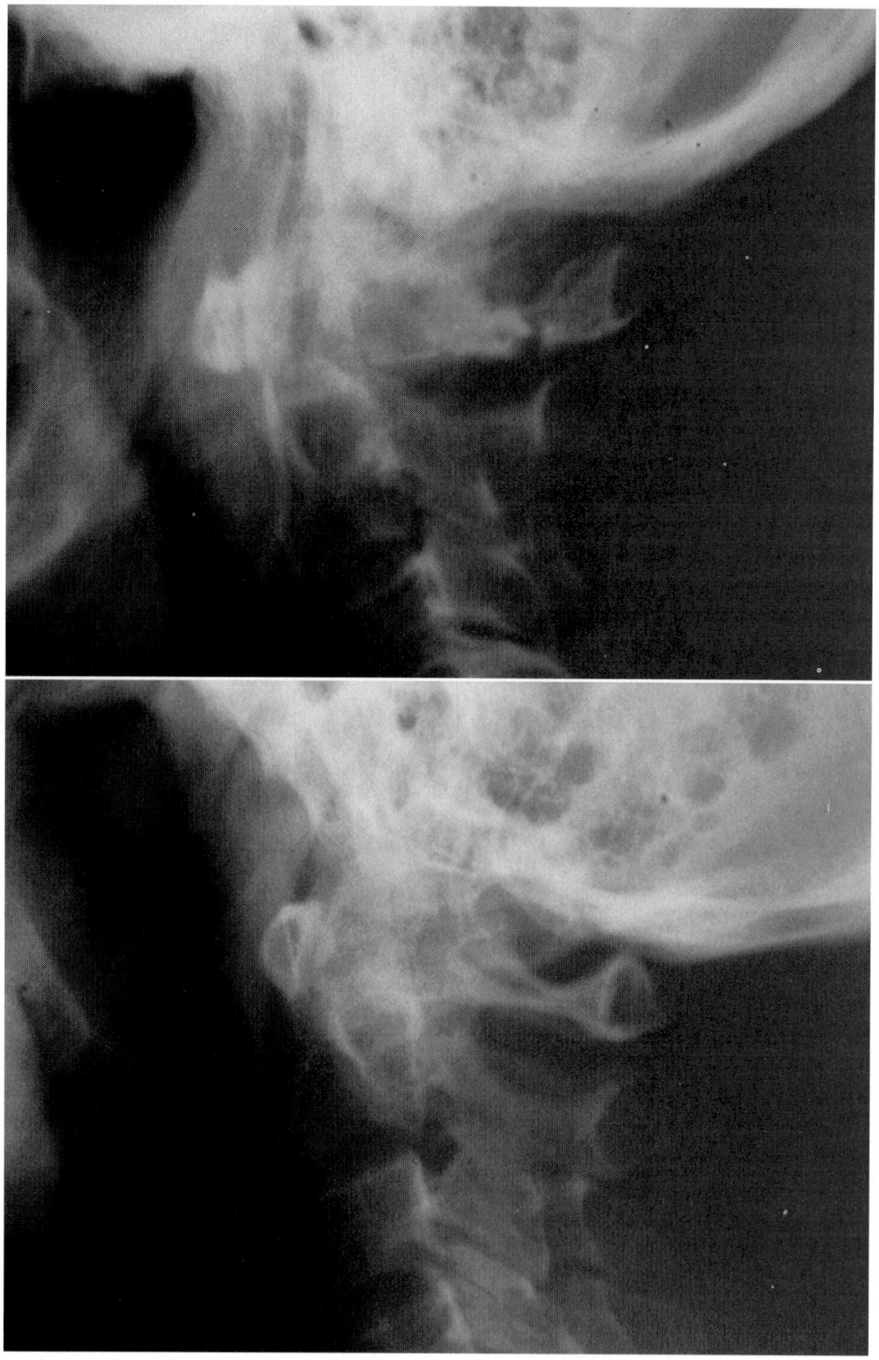

FIGURE 4-5

Jefferson fracture. **A**, Lateral radiograph demonstrating fracture line through the lateral arch of the atlas. **B**, Lateral radiograph demonstrating upward herniation of the dens into the atlas ring. The tip of the dens projects well above the superior edge of the anterior arch of the atlas.

subluxation may be missed. There is another way to make this diagnosis.

PEARL

The internal cortex of the posterior ring of C2 appears as a crescentic dense bony line on the lateralradiograph. The posterior ring of the foramen magnum is identifiable as the point of intersection of the dense bones of the internal and external tables of the skull. This appears as a horizontal V on the lateral radiograph. In uninjured individuals the internal cortical margin of the posterior C1 ring should fall along the line projecting superiorly in the inner margin of the C2 ring of the posterior lip of the foramen magnum (Fig. 4-9 A,B). Deviation either anterior or posterior to this line often indicates fracture or dislocation.

PITFALL

Not all cases in which the posterior ring fails to fall along its usual course are caused by fracture or subluxation. In rare instances the C1 ring is unusuallyshort in AP diameter. This causes the posterior ring to project much further forward of the previously mentioned line. More commonly the posterior arch of C1 is incomplete with no identifiable cortical bone. This anomaly appears on the lateral radiograph because the end of the unfused ring has a smooth cortical margin (Fig. 4-10). Anomalies of fusion of the C1 ring are very common, and they must not be confused with acute fractures. Small bony remnants of the occipital vertebra often occur either just inferior to or just superior to the anterior margin of C1. These also must not be confused with fracture (Fig. 4-16 C,D).

There are two related entities caused by abnormal rotation of the atlas on the axis. Rotary subluxation, the more severe of the two is diagnosed on routine radiographs by misalignment of the two vertebrae. On a lateral radiograph of the skull, C1 is properly aligned but C2 is abnormally rotated with respect to C1 and appears obliquely oriented (Fig. 4-11 A). The diagnosis is not always easy to make on regular films because the presence of torticollis makes it very difficult to produce good quality radiographs. When the distance between the anterior arch of C1 and the dens is increased in any of the views the diagnosis can be made with certainty. When the facets are completely subluxed, the head may become rotated 90 degrees to the long axis of the body. This is easily seen on axial CT scans (Fig. 4-11 B). Rotary fixation is a rare entity, but is usually seen in children. There is an abnormal relationship between the atlas and the axis, which does not change upon rotation of the head.

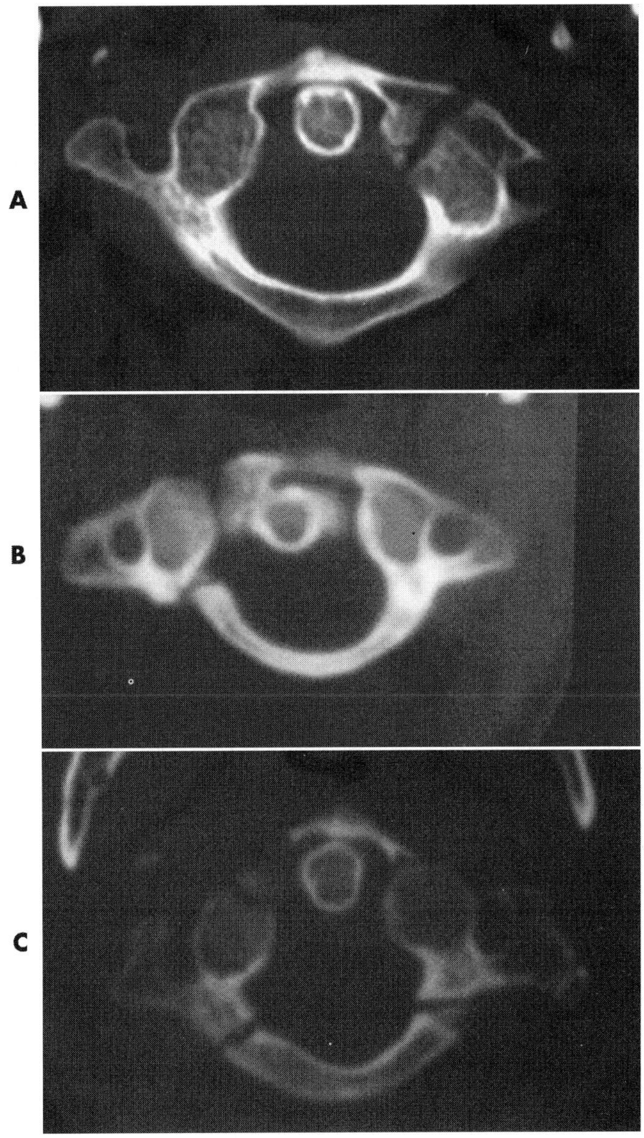

FIGURE 4-6

Jefferson fracture, four different patients. **A**, Axial CT scan: A single fracture is present through the lateral mass of the atlas on the right. There are no contralateral fractures. This is very unusual. **B**, Axial CT scan revealing two fractures of the right side of the atlas ring, one anterior to, and one posterior to, the articular process. **C**, Axial CT scan: four fractures are seen two on each side of the ring; two just anterior to, and two posterior to, the lateral masses.

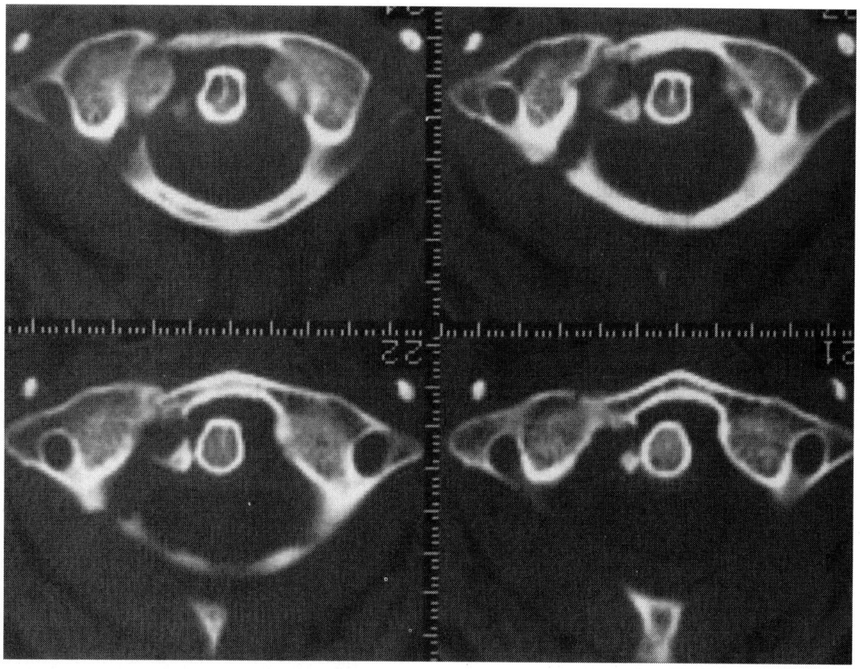

Figure 4-6 *Continued*

D, Axial CT scan on a patient with Jefferson fracture with avulsion of the tubercle onto which attaches the transverse ligament.

> **Pearl**
>
> The diagnosis is made by comparing open mouth radiographs of C1-C2 taken with the head slightly rotated to each side. In uninjured patients rotation of the neck narrows the space between the dens and the lateral mass of C1 on the side to which the spinous process rotates.[15] Consequently, when the head is rotated to the right, the spinous process rotates to the left, and the left lateral mass of C1 glides forward on the parallel facet of C2. The space between the lateral mass on the left and the dens narrows. Rotation of the head to the left produces the opposite effect. In patients with rotary fixation, C1 can not rotate on C2. Consequently the relative position of the lateral masses of C1 and the dens does not change when the head is rotated slightly to each side. Radiographs produced in the frontal plane through the open mouth show narrowing of the lateral mass–dens space on the same side regardless of which side the spinous process of C2 projects (Fig. 4-12).

DENS FRACTURES

Dens fractures are usually visible on well-positioned lateral radiographs.[16–21] Producing adequate lateral radiographs in a severely injured, unconscious, or intoxicated patient is a problem.

> **Pearl**
>
> To obtain optimal lateral radiographs of C1-C2, center the X-ray beam on the skull and not the neck. A true lateral radiograph of the skull produces an image with the C1 ring parallel to the skull base and, therefore, is an ideal visualization of C1-C2 (Fig. 4-13).

All three types of dens fractures are best evaluated on CT scans with sagittal and curved coronal reformations.

Type I fractures of the dens are quite rare. The fracture line is through the dens above the junction with the C2 body. These injuries should be conceptualized as avulsions of the tip of the dens with intact alar ligaments (Fig. 4-14).

Type II fractures extend through the attachment of the dens to the body of C2. They may be caused by hyperflexion forces whereby the transverse ligament forces the dens forward faster than the bone can accommodate or by hyperextension forces whereby the anterior arch of the dens propels the dens posteriorly (Fig. 4-15).

In type III dens fractures, the fracture line extends into the C2 body (Fig. 4-16). Differentiation of the three types is important because type III fractures usually heal while pseudarthrosis is more common in true

Text continued on p. 53

E

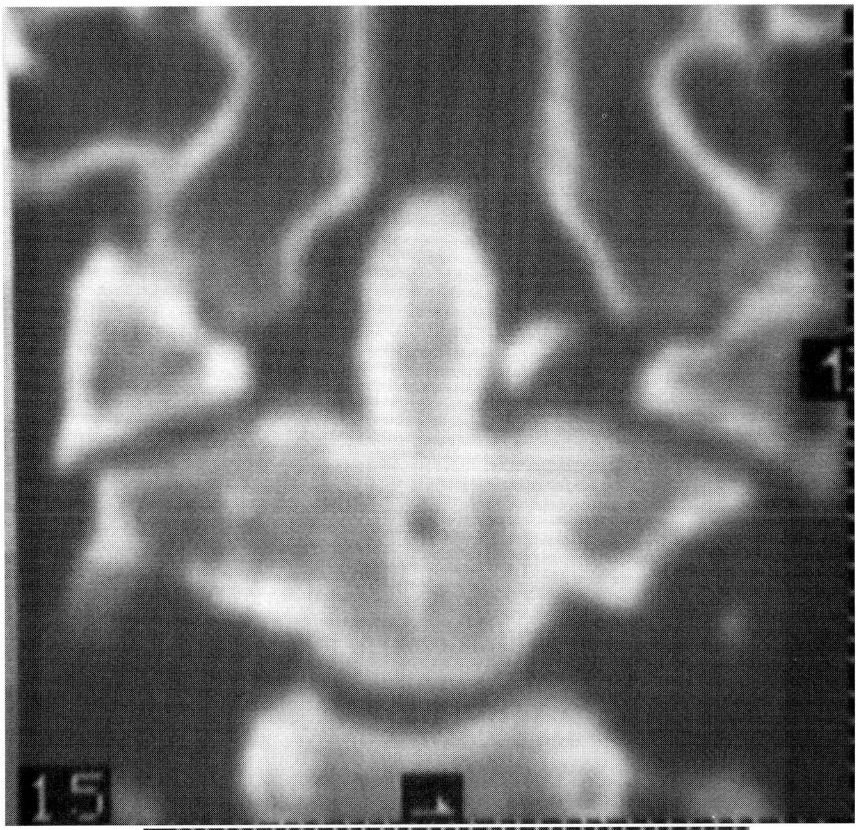

F

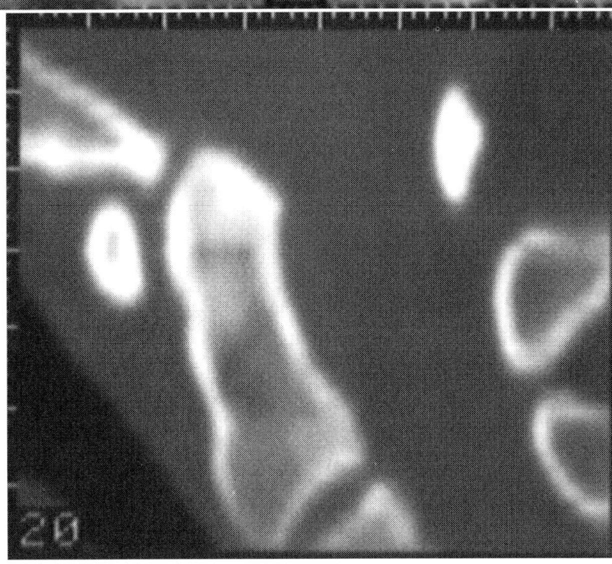

FIGURE 4-6 *Continued*

E, Coronal reformation. **F**, Sagittal reformation: note upward migration of the dens.

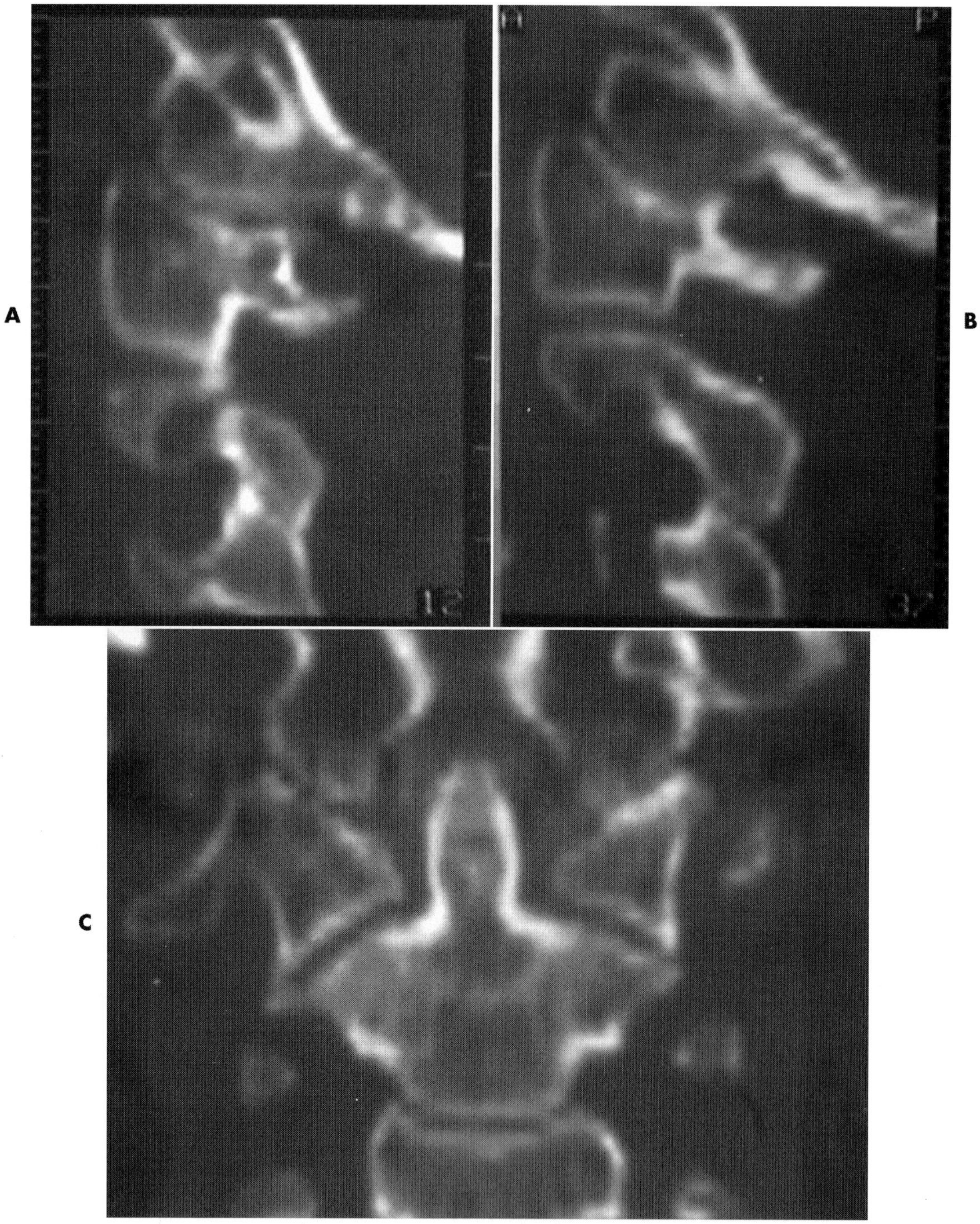

FIGURE 4-7

Posttraumatic arthritis craniooccipital joint. **A**, Sagittal CT reformation through the normal occipital condyle. **B**, Sagittal CT reformation through the narrow, sclerotic joint. **C**, Coronal CT reformation; note the asymmetry of the joint spaces.

A

B

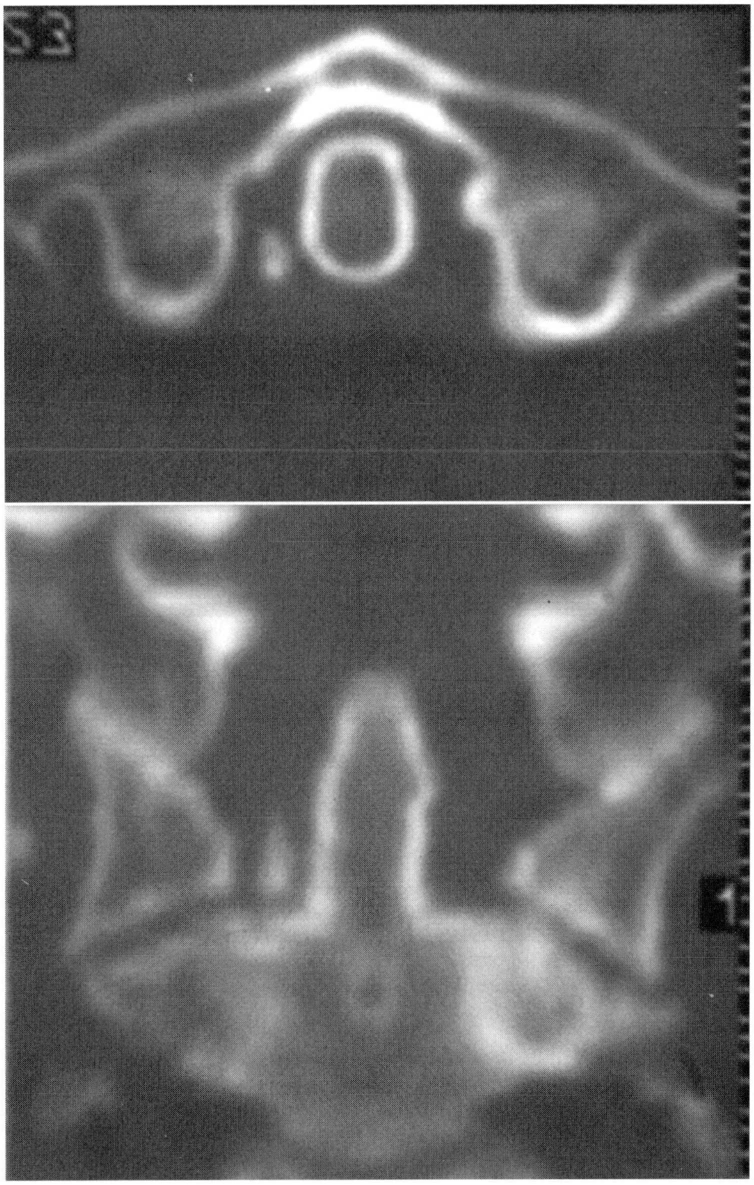

FIGURE 4-8

Traumatic subluxation of atlantoaxial joint. **A**, Axial CT scan shows avulsion of the right tubercle. **B**, Coronal CT reformation same patient.

A

B

C

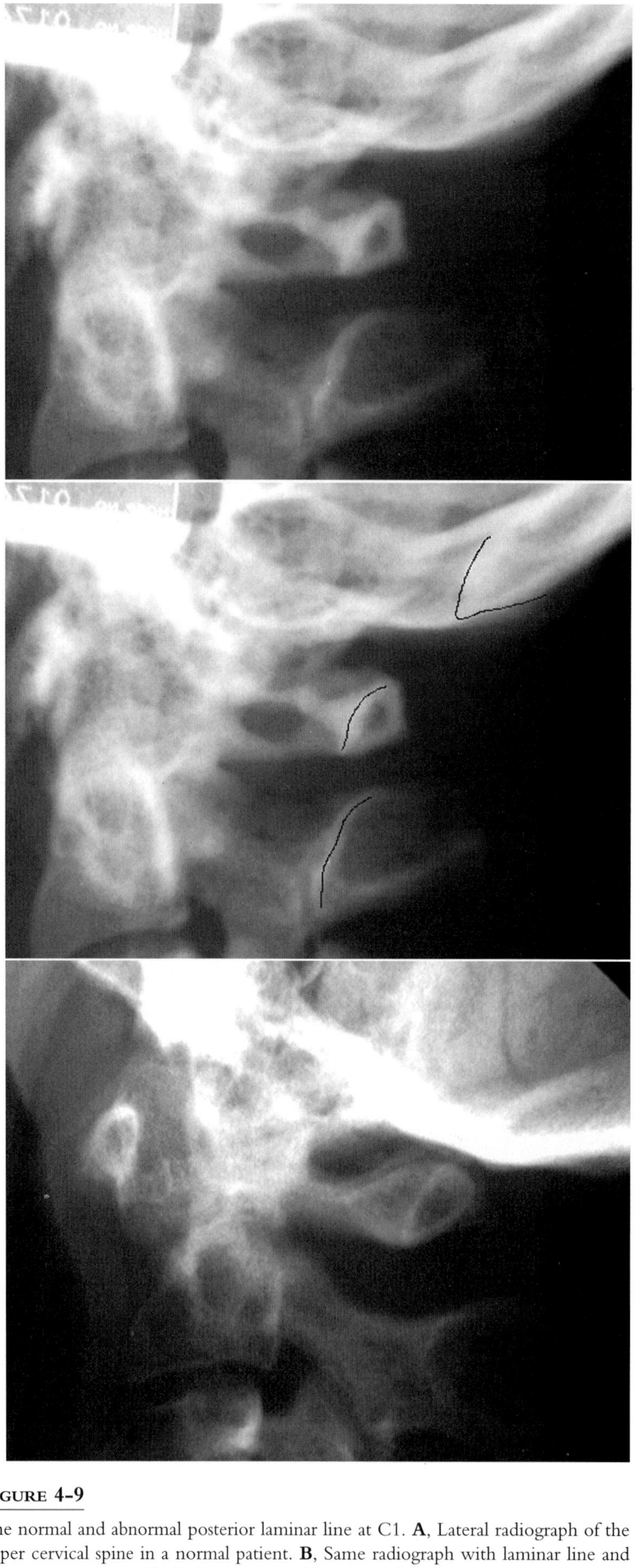

Figure 4-9

The normal and abnormal posterior laminar line at C1. **A**, Lateral radiograph of the upper cervical spine in a normal patient. **B**, Same radiograph with laminar line and foramen magnum marked. **C**, Forward subluxation of the atlas.

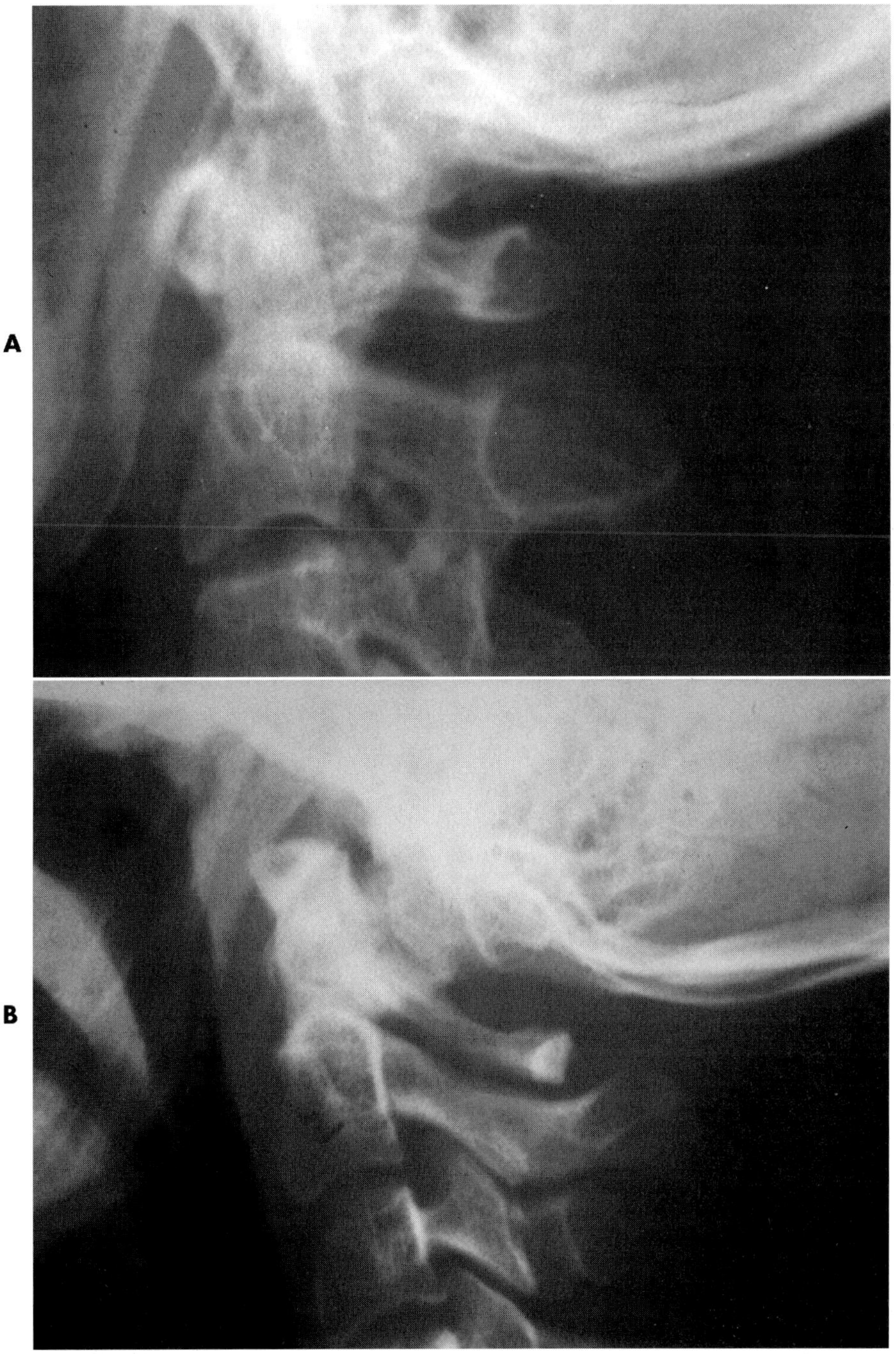

FIGURE 4-10

Anomalies of the atlas ring. **A**, Congenitally short atlas ring. **B**, Unusually high position of the anterior facet of the dens with a sloping atlas ring.

C

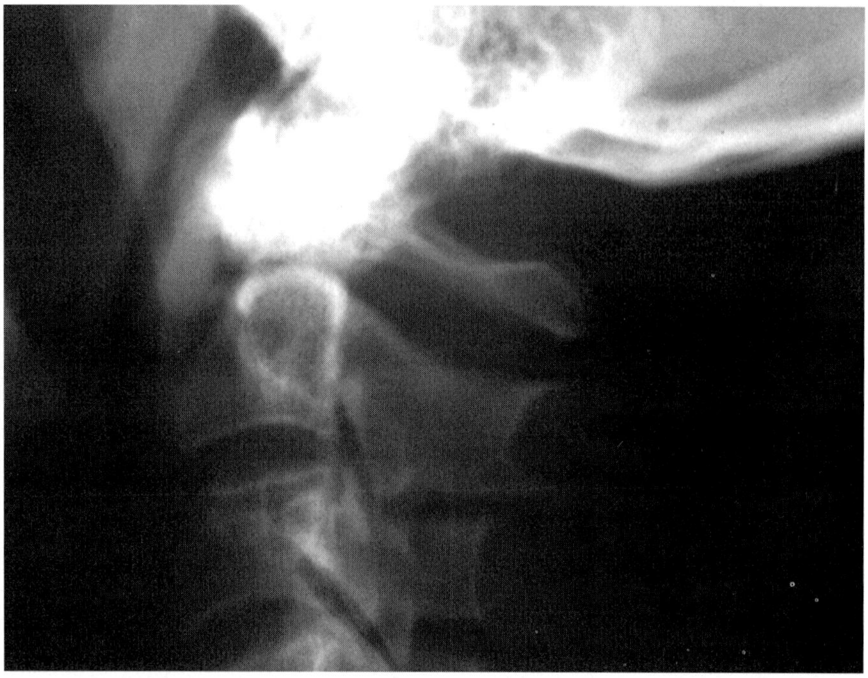

Figure 4-10 *continued*

C, Incomplete ossification of the posterior atlas ring. The distal portions of both halves of the unfused arch look like a chicken drumstick on its side. There is no posterior laminar line because there is no posterior lamina.

A

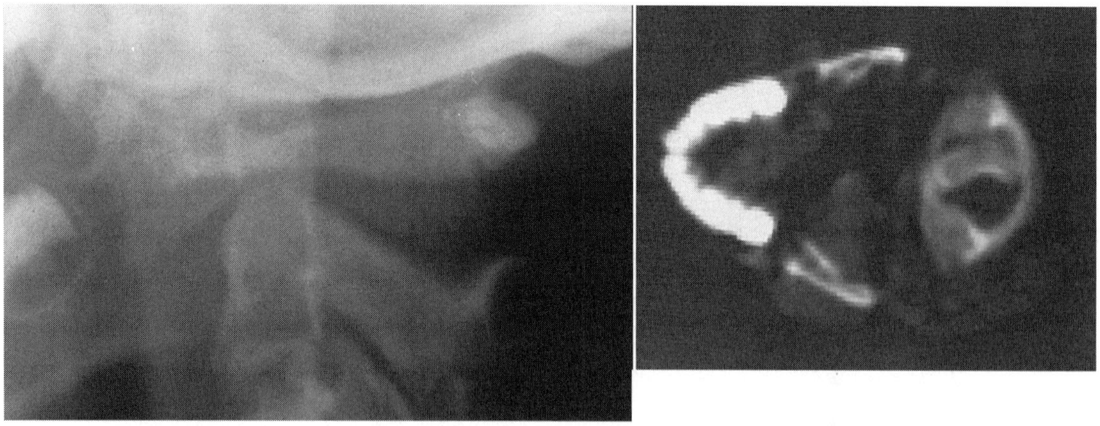

B

Figure 4-11

Rotary subluxation. Lateral radiograph of the craniocervical junction **A** reveals the ring of C1 to be properly oriented with respect to the base of the skull but there is abnormal rotation between C1 and C2. Axial CT scan **B** on another patient who crashed into a tree on a snow sled shows that the head is oriented 90 degrees to the cervical spine because of facet subluxation.

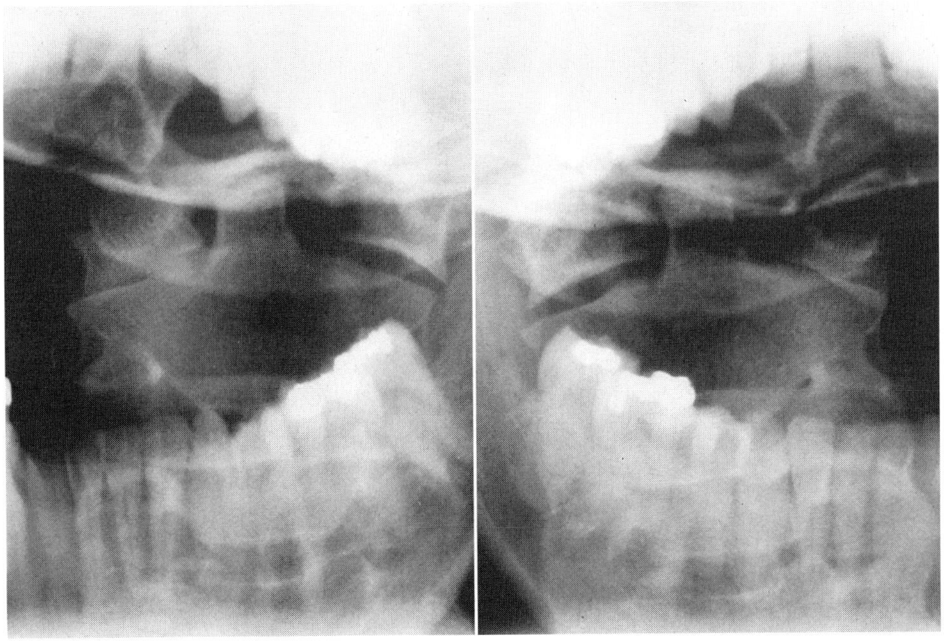

FIGURE 4-12

Rotary fixation. Frontal radiographs of the craniovertebral junction through the opened mouth with the patients head turned to the right **A** and to the left **B** reveal constant malposition of the dens with respect to the lateral masses of C1. The distance between the dens and the lateral mass is narrow on the same side regardless of the direction of rotation of the head.

type II lesions even with an adequate course of treatment in a halo. It is much easier to diagnose a nondisplaced pseudarthrosis of C2 on a thin section reformatted CT than on MRI. When residual subluxation is present, however, either study is diagnostic, although the MRI is much more difficult to evaluate (Fig. 4-15 B).

Type II dens fractures must be differentiated from the subluxing congenital os odontoideum.[23–26] It is generally accepted that the os odontoideum anomaly is a congenital maldevelopment of the three different somites that form the C2 vertebra. The body of C2 forms from the C2 somite; the main portion of the dens is derived from paired C1 ossification centers. The single terminal ossicle that fuses to the tip of the dens is formed from the cartilage of the fourth occipital somite. In the adult C2 vertebra the fusion zone between the C1 and C2 somites is the remnant of the vestigial disk, which appears as a sclerotic line within the vertebral body. Occasionally cartilage is noted within the disk space remnant. A vertical line down the center of the dens marks the plane of fusion of the paired C1 ossification centers. On frontal images the fusion plane between the terminal ossicle and the C1 portion is identified as a V-shaped cortical bony line (Fig. 4-17). Older literature regards os odontoideum anomaly as a pseudarthrosis of a childhood dens fracture.[22] Indeed, relatively silent dens fractures can occur. If the diagnosis of dens fracture is missed, acute pseudarthrosis is common. There may be no symptoms of dens pseudarthrosis, and, consequently, many years may elapse before a radiograph of the spine is taken and an abnormality identified. This may appear very similar to the congenital os odontoideum. Reformatted CT and MRI allow the differentiation of these two abnormalities in most cases.

PEARL

In patients with pseudarthrosis, the separated dens is properly formed from its usual three ossification centers; therefore, the internal architecture of the mobile fragment resembles a normal dens.

The mobile dens fragment is made up of the two fused C1 segments and the attached fourth occipital terminal ossicle. The sclerotic bone of the fusion plane between the C1 halves and the terminal ossicle are, therefore, distinctly identifiable (Fig. 4-17 A). A congenital os odontoideum, being formed from a single ossification center, shows little internal structure. Occasionally, some internal dense bone is visible but the fusion planes are not present. The os odontoideum also tends to be more spherical than a fractured dens.

Text continued on p. 56

A

B

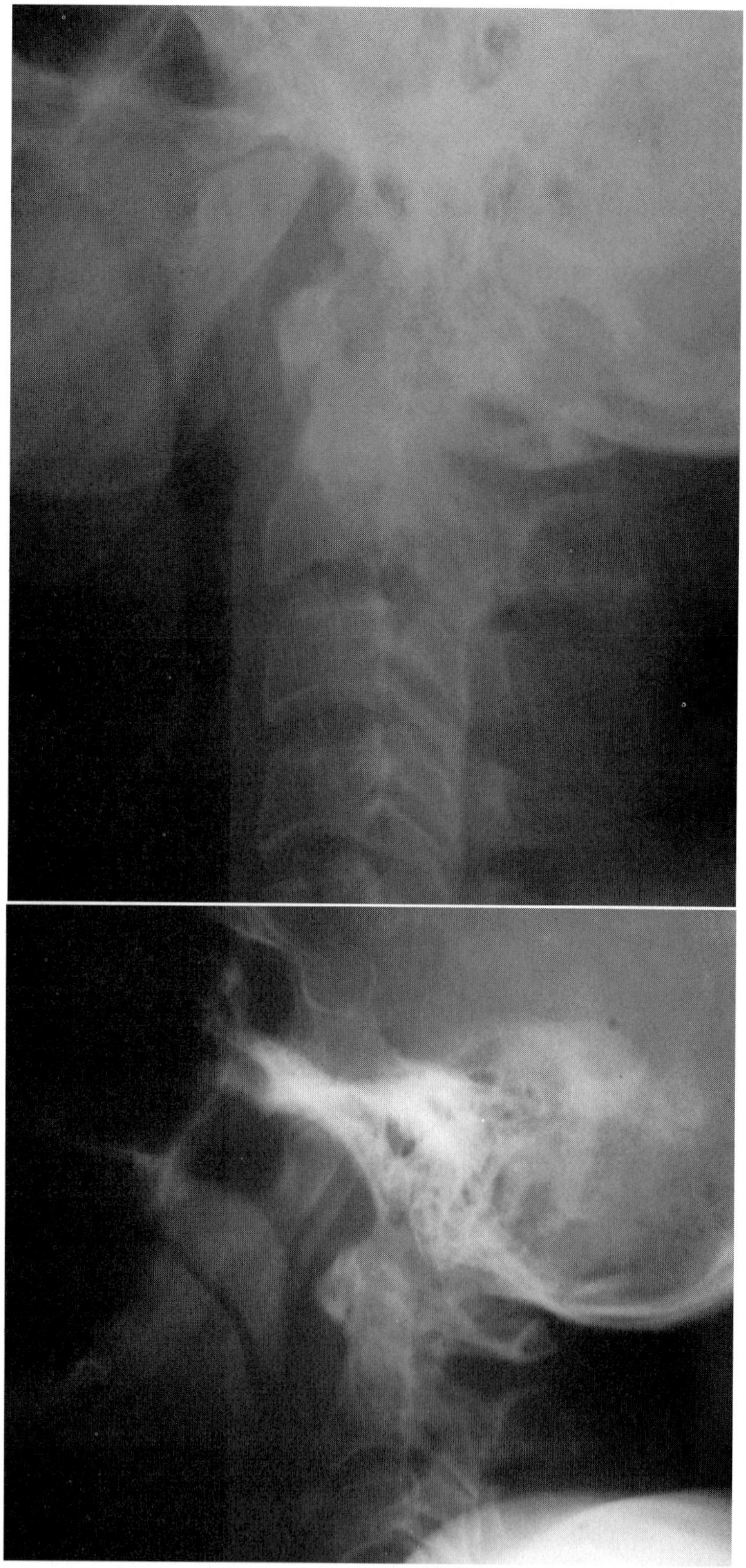

FIGURE 4-13

A, Lateral view of a the cervical spine on a patient with torticolis. The atlas ring is tilted and the anatomy of C1-C2 is difficult to evaluate. **B**, Lateral view of the skull causes the atlas ring to be perpendicular to the plane of the film and consequently the atlantoaxial relationship is obvious.

A

B

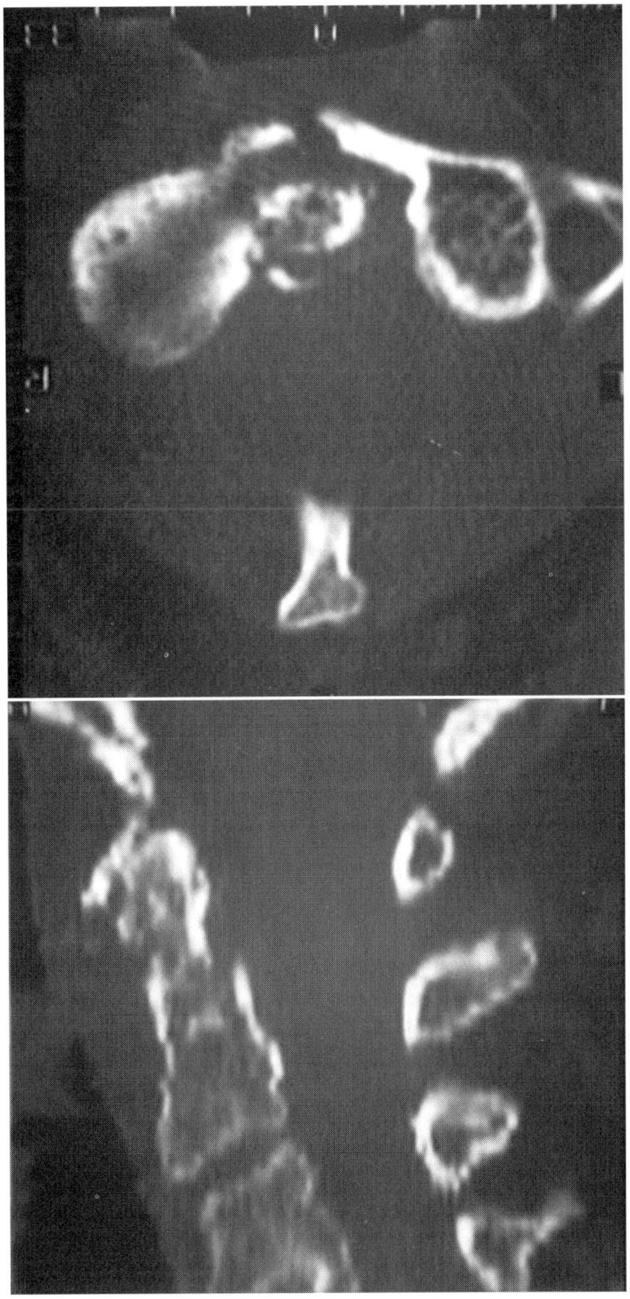

FIGURE 4-14

Type I dens fracture. **A** Axial CT and **B** sagittal reformation. Note the distal fragmentation of the dens. The C1 ring is fractured anteriorly.

A

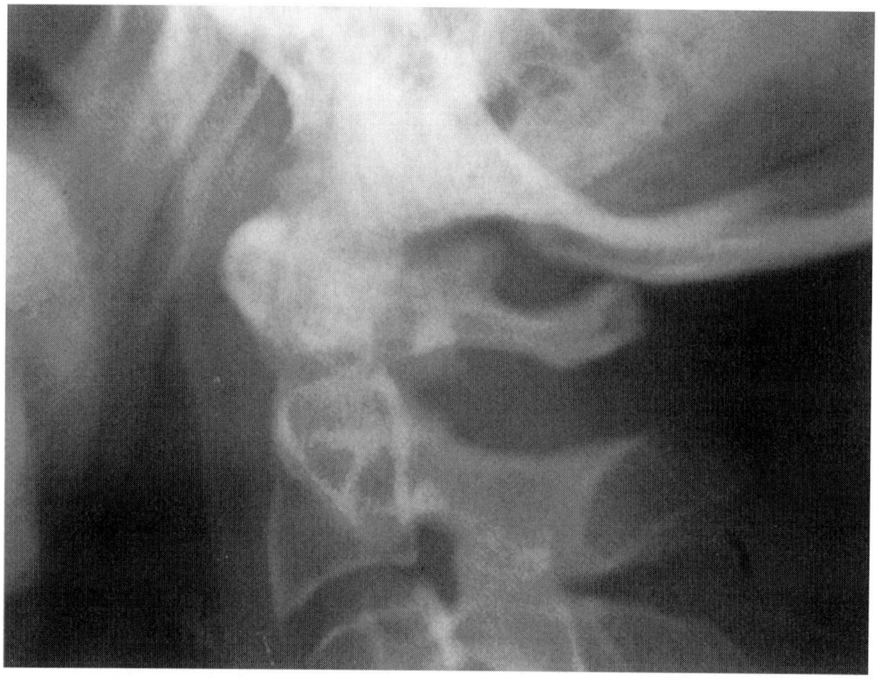

FIGURE 4-15

Type II dens fracture. **A**, Plain film shows a very subtle fracture of the base of the dens.

The anterior arch of C1 is often wider in cross-sectional diameter and more bulky in patients with os odontoideum. This is clearly visible on routine lateral radiographs and on sagittal CT reformations (Fig. 4-17 B–D). The differentiation between these two abnormalities may be clinically irrelevant if there are clinical signs of craniovertebral instability, because a fusion may be indicated in either instance. There is, however, extraordinary medical and legal significance. Often os subluxation is found by happenstance in routine cervical radiographs taken after minor whiplash trauma. These may be misdiagnosed as fractures and inappropriately be the basis for very large damage claims.

An understanding of the embryology of the craniovertebral junction allows the diagnosis of some strange and unusual abnormalities. Perhaps one of the most bizarre is demonstrated in Figure 4-18. The patient was seen in the emergency room following cervical trauma, and on routine radiographs the dens projected anterior to the arch of C1. Subluxation of the dens was diagnosed and a posterior fusion performed. Conventional tomograms and a three-dimensional (3D) CT scan proved the diagnosis to be different. On conventional tomograms (Fig. 4-18 B) the tip of the dens is smooth and regular and is V-shaped rather than jagged as one might expect if there were an acute fracture. The CT scan (Fig. 4-18 C,D) demonstrates a small ossicle located behind the anterior arch of C1 within the confines of the transverse ligament. The most telling image is the 3D CT scan (Fig. 4-18 E), which demonstrates a V-shaped deformity at the tip of the dens. This complex series of observations allows the diagnosis of an extraordinarily rare lesion. The patient has subluxation of a persistent terminal ossicle of Bergmann. In rare instances the terminal ossicle of the dens fails to form a bony connection to the C1 portions of the dens. A fibrous connection is present instead. Frontal images show the V shape of the C2 portion of the dens with the terminal ossicle separated from the dens. This ossicle is not enlarged as in the os odontoideum anomaly, and there is no dysplasia of the C1 portion of the dens. In this particular patient, hyperextension forces caused separation of the fibrous connection between the terminal ossicle, which remained in situ, and the rest of the dens, which subluxed under the anterior arch of C1. Unfortunately, the complex anatomy was not recognized preoperatively, and the spinal cord injury occurred in the postoperative period, perhaps because of cord compression during the operative procedure.

HANGMAN FRACTURES

Although judicial hanging is a thing of the past in most parts of the world, hangman's fracture remains a common traumatic lesion.[27] The originally described fracture was caused by rapid hyperextension of the neck by the upward jerking of a submentally placed knot below the jaw of the victim. This produced bilateral fracture of the neural arch of C2 usually near the

Text continued on p. 61

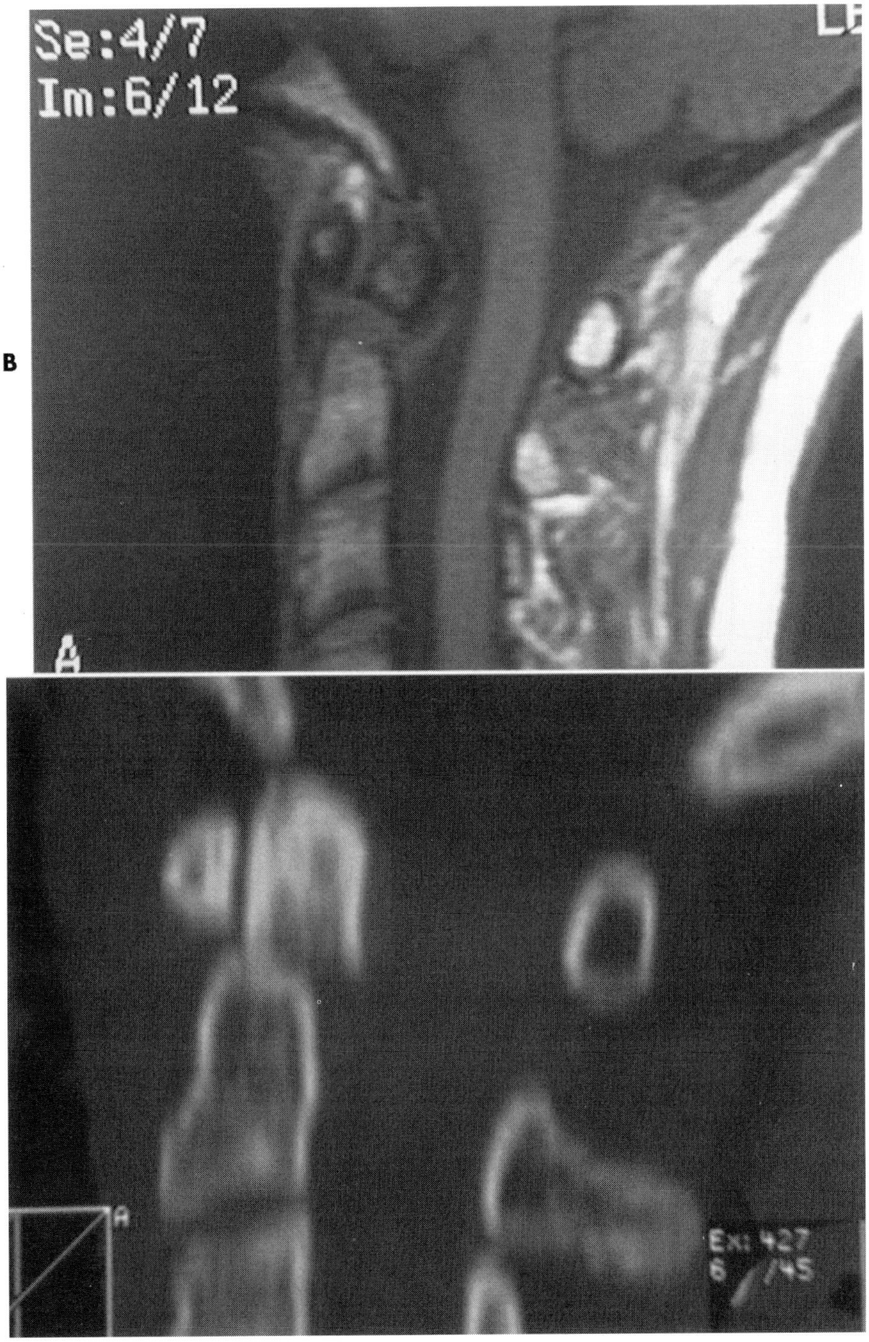

FIGURE 4-15 *continued*

B, Pseudarthrosis of a dens fracture. T1-weighted MRI scan performed 7 months following an acute fracture of the dens reveals fibrosis within the space between the dens and the body of the axis. **C**, Reformatted CT showing similar pseudarthrosis.

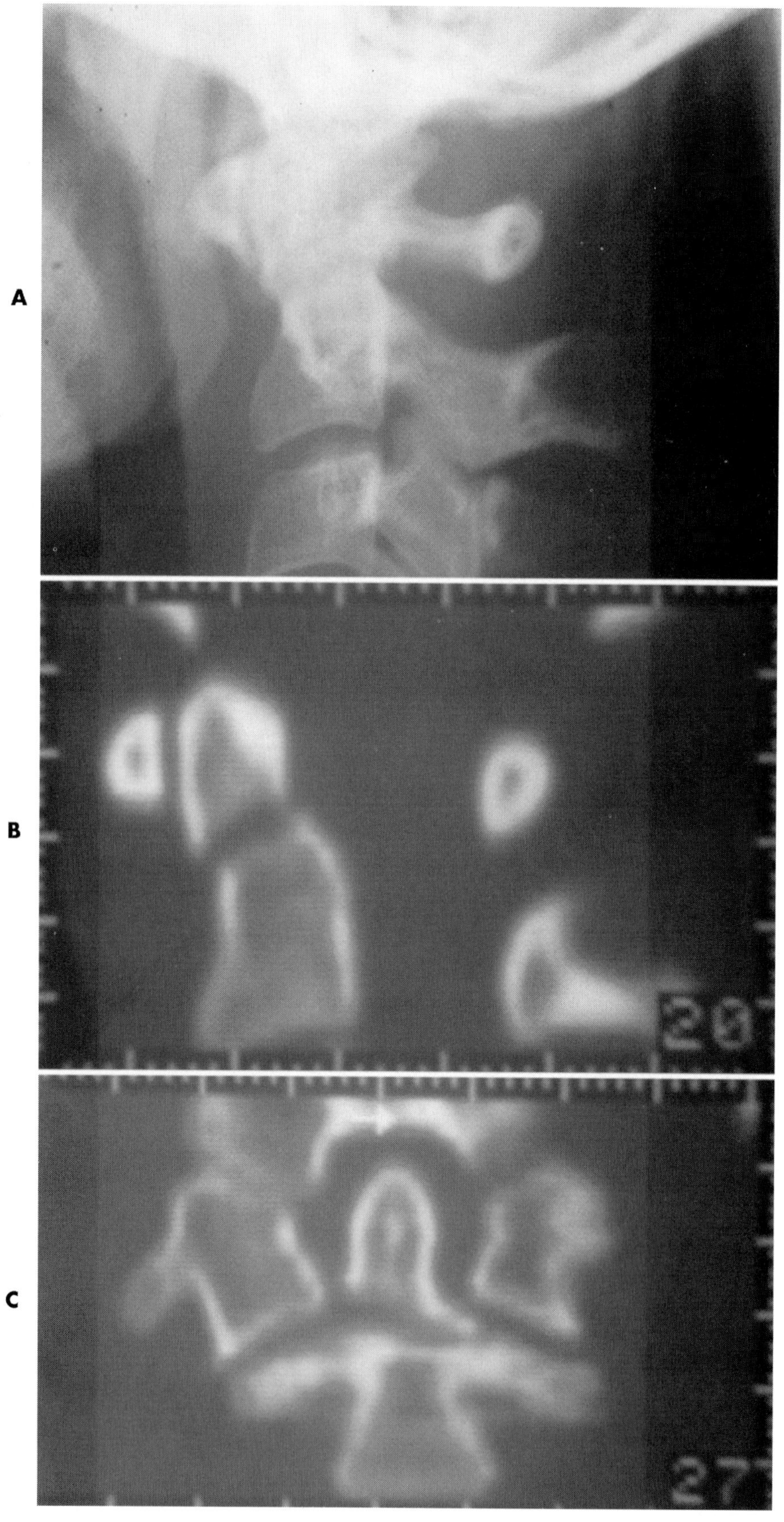

Figure 4-16

Type III dens fracture. **A**, Plain radiograph reveals forward deviation of the dens and the atlas. **B**, Sagittal CT reformation shows an acute fracture line at the base of the dens. **C**, Coronal CT reformation reveals the fracture to extend into the body of the axis on the right.

A

B

C

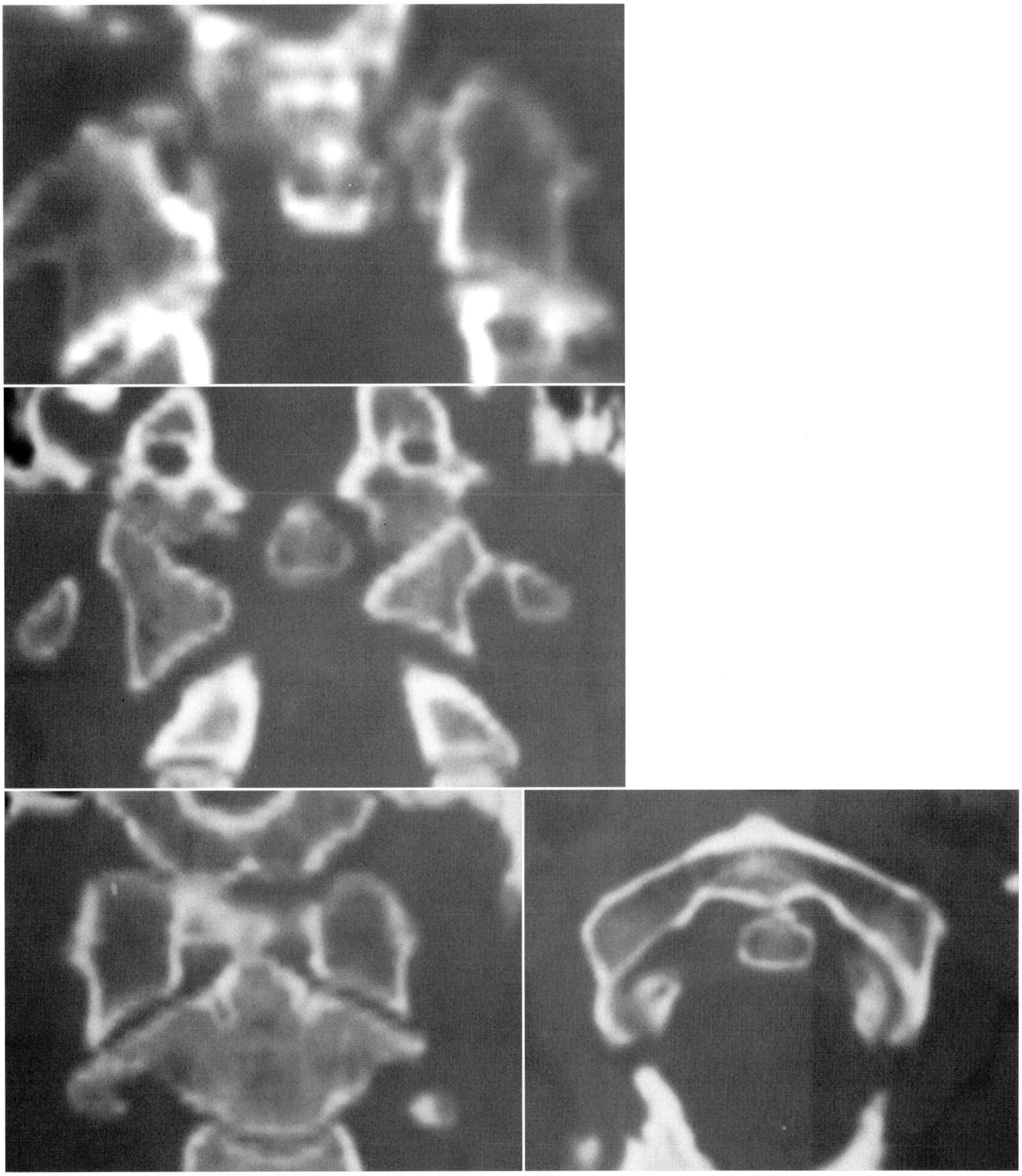

D

FIGURE 4-17

Differentiation between pseudarthrosis and congenital os odontoideum. **A**, Coronal CT reformation through a previously fractured dens demonstrating the normal internal anatomy of the dens. Note the central sclerotic line of the fusion zone between the two ossification centers of C1. **B&C**, Sequential coronal CT reformations on a patient with os odontoideum. The internal architecture of the distal ossicle is not that of a normal dens. There is no central sclerotic line. The fragment is larger in diameter than a normal dens. **D**, Axial CT scan shows the anterior arch of the atlas to be larger than normal.

A B C D

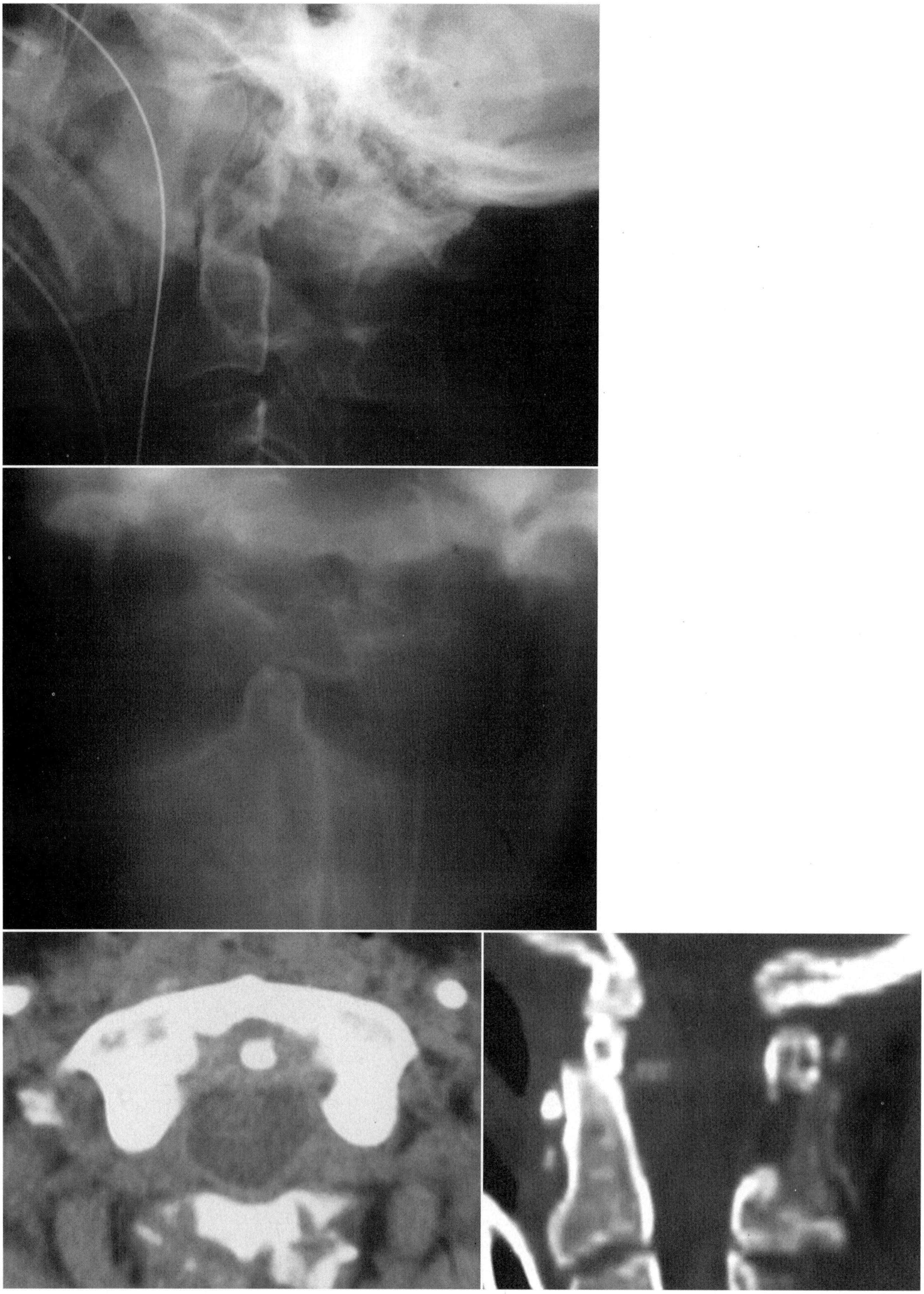

Figure 4-18

For legends see opposite page.

E

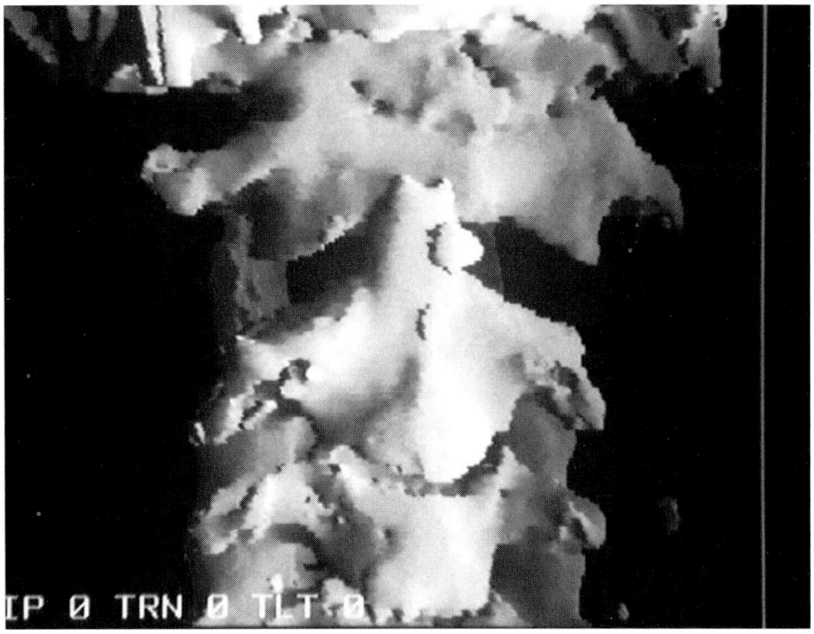

FIGURE 4-18

Subluxation of a terminal ossicle of Bergmann. **A**, Routine radiograph of the cervical spine reveals displacement of the dens anterior to the arch of the atlas. Conventional tomogram performed immediately following trauma. **B**, shows the tip of the dens to be smooth and sclerotic not jagged as one would expect in an acute fracture. **C**, Axial CT scan and **D**, sagittal CT reformation prove the dens to be anteriorly displaced, but also shows two unusual, small ossicles, one tucked behind the transverse ligament and the second anterior and inferior to the dens apex. Both of these ossicles are derived from the fourth fetal occipital ossification center. The anterior one is a normal variant, the posterior one is the terminal ossicle of Bergmann, which has separated from its normal location atop the dens. **E**, 3D CT reformation showing the V-shaped apex of the dens typical of the junction of the C1 portion of the dens and the terminal ossicle of Bergmann.

insertion of the arch into the vertebral body. Today, hangman's fracture is most often caused by vehicular accidents. Typically the chest hits the steering wheel, and the forehead hits the windshield producing hyperextension. Lateral radiographs demonstrate backward displacement of the dens and fracture of the neural arch. The CT scan is the imaging examination of choice.

Bilateral neural arch fractures of C2 can also be caused by hyperflexion. These are self-decompressing injuries as the patient performs the equivalent of bilateral laminar osteotomies in the trauma (Fig. 4-19).

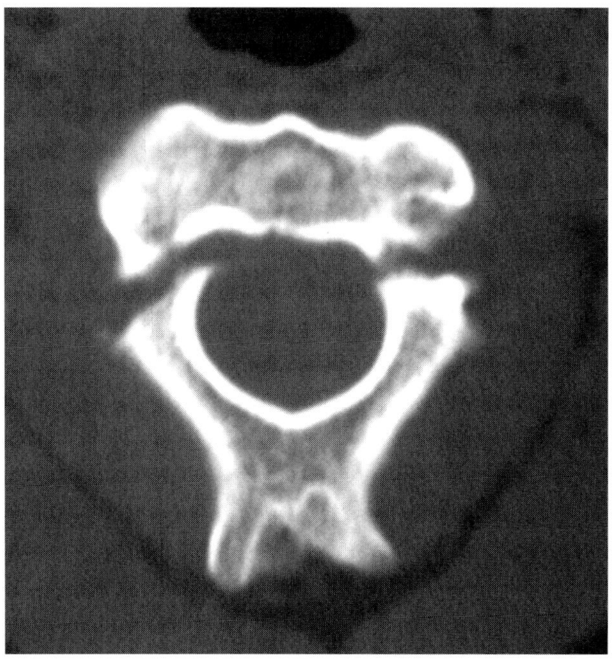

FIGURE 4-19

Hangman's fracture. Axial CT scan shows traumatic spondylolysis of the two sides of the neural arch just posterior to the body of the axis.

MISCELLANEOUS FRACTURES OF THE CRANIOCERVICAL REGION

Thus far the fractures included in this chapter conform to well-described entities. Often, however, lesions do not fall cleanly into the standard categories. Occasionally, fractures may be associated with unusual congenital variations, which explain their unusual appearance and sometimes complicate their treatment. Two examples suffice to illustrate these phenomena.

Trauma to the articular processes at C1-C2 usually occurs in association with other more obvious fractures. In rare instances, isolated fracture of a facet may

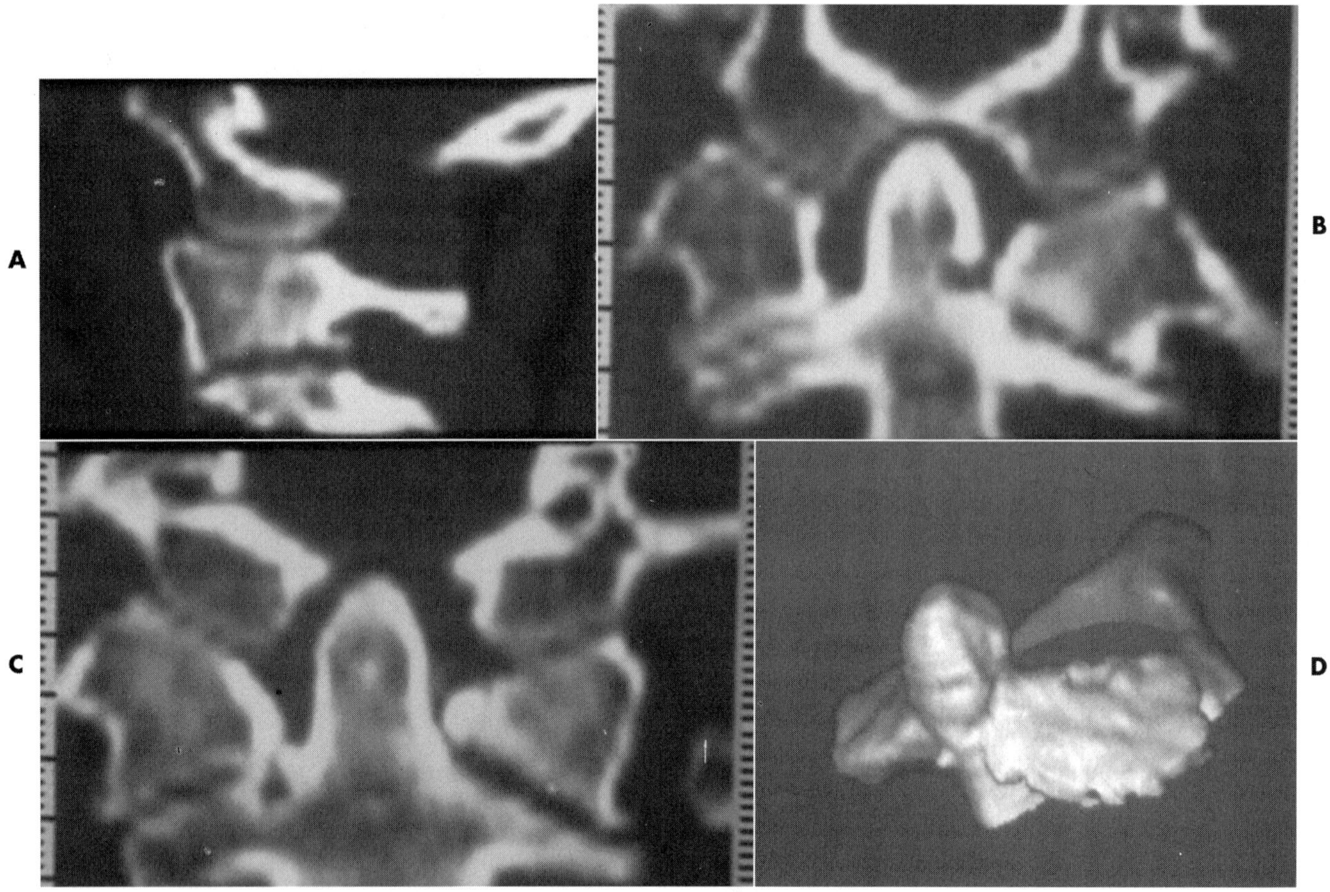

FIGURE 4-20

Posttraumatic arthritis at the lateral atlantoaxial joint. **A**, Sagittal CT reformation through the lateral atlantooccipital joint shows erosion, sclerosis, and bony overgrowth of the left facet. **B&C**, Sequential coronal CT reformations reveal atlantoaxial rotary subluxation with two areas of bone erosion and degenerative cyst formation. **D**, 3D CT reformation of the axis with the atlas removed. The irregularity and bony overgrowth of the superior facet is obvious.

occur. The patient depicted in Figure 4-20 developed severe neck pain following cervical manipulation. Reformatted CT demonstrates very subtle fragmentation of the right facet joint at C1-C2. Small degenerative osteophytes developed about the joint. Rotary subluxation caused the lateral surface of the dens to become eroded by the displaced lateral mass of the atlas. Posttraumatic arthritis is one of the most important complications of occult articular fractures.

The patient in Figure 4-21 was injured in an automobile accident. An astute radiologist noted forward displacement of the laminar line of the posterior arch of the atlas. The fracture that produced this subluxation is extremely difficult to identify on the routine radiographs. The CT scan reveals an oblique fracture extending through the body of the axis on the left side and the junction of the body of C2 and the neural arch on the right. The left side looks like a type III dens fracture and the right like a hangman's fracture. The probable cause for this unusual fracture is hidden on the routine lateral radiograph and elucidated on the more rostral CT scans. This patient has a large paracondylar process hanging down from the base of the skull, which articulates with a tubercle projecting down from the lateral mass of the atlas. This may stabilize the upper segment and probably directed the force vector inferiorly through the contralateral neural arch.

THE LOWER CERVICAL SPINE

The cervical spine is rarely injured by direct trauma to the neck. Most injuries occur because of acceleration or deceleration forces, which cause the head to be placed in motion.[28] The cervical spine, a chain of movable, linked bones, is not optimally suited to bear the forces generated by the rapid motion of such a massive structure as the head. As velocity of acceleration or deceleration increases or decreases, respectively, the forces on the cervical motion segment increase according to standard physical laws. Depending on the precise vectors, the neck fails at its weakest point.

A

B

C

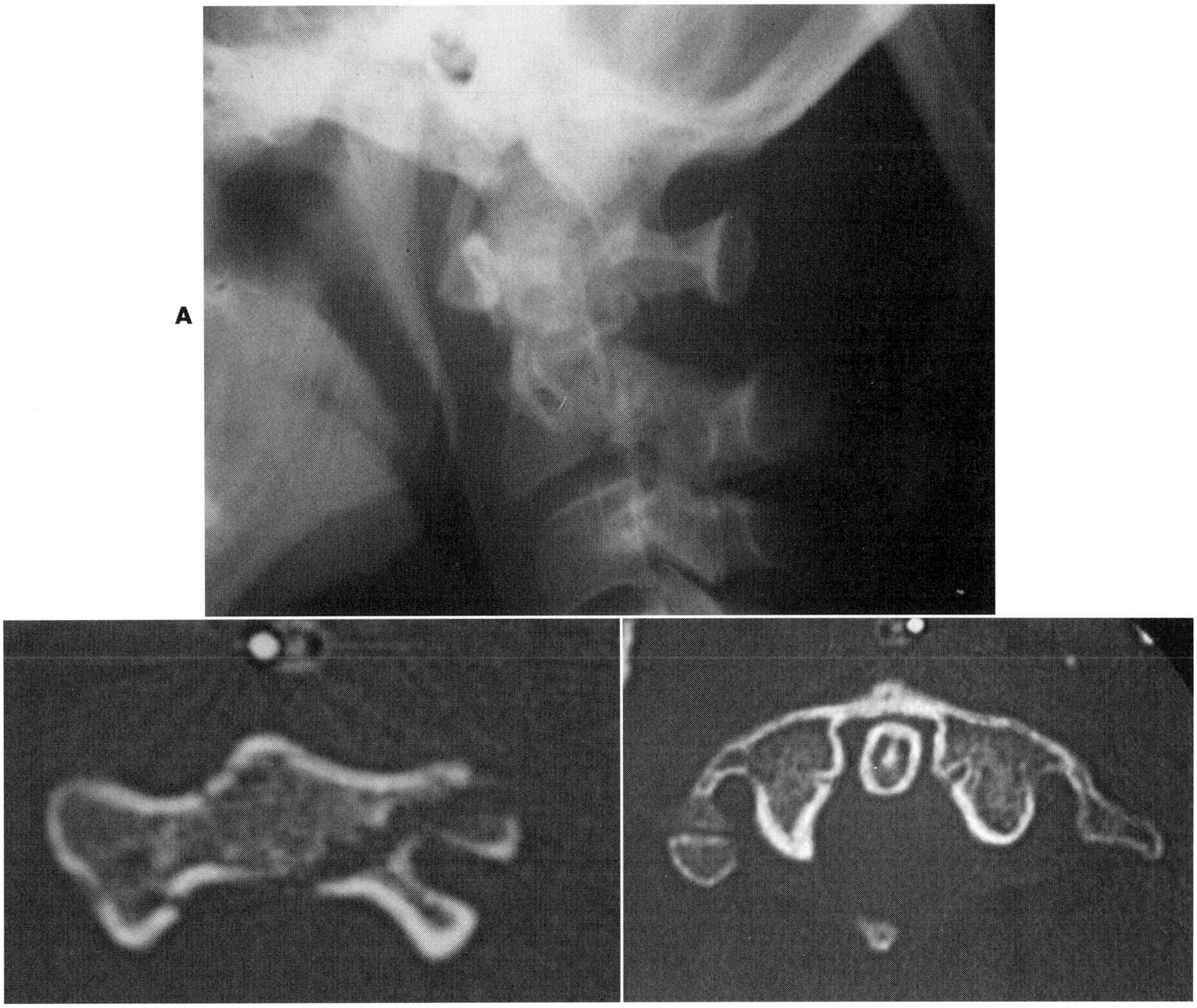

FIGURE 4-21

Unusual fracture of the axis. **A**, Lateral radiograph of the upper cervical spine revealing a very subtle fracture line at the base of the dens. A large stalagmite of bone projects down from the base of the skull and articulates with a tubercle on the inferior surface of the atlas. **B**, Axial CT scan shows a fracture line extending through the body of the axis on the right and the junction of the neural arch on the left. **C**, Axial CT scan through the anomalous articulation between the epitransverse process and the transverse process of the atlas.

Forces are often complex combinations of flexion, rotation, bending, axial loading, or distraction. The mechanism of bony or soft tissue injury can often be deduced from the pattern of anatomic disruption.

FLEXION INJURIES

Flexion injuries can occur with distraction or compressive forces. Compression-flexion injuries tend to fragment the vertebral bodies with little subluxation of the zygapophyseal joints. Distraction-flexion injuries cause less vertebral body fragmentation but more facet distraction with subluxation or dislocation. The diagnosis is obvious in most compressive injuries as the fractured vertebral bodies are usually evident on routine radiographs and CT scans (Fig. 4-22).

> **PITFALL**
>
> It is critical that proper emergency room radiographs include the C7-T1 level. This is the most difficult portion of the spine to see, especially in patients with thick, short necks. No examination of the cervical spine is complete unless the integrity of the C7-T1 disk and facets can be established. In difficult cases, thin-section reformatted CT should be performed to exclude a destabilizing injury prior to moving the patient.

Distraction injuries are much more difficult to diagnose than compression injuries. Significant soft-tissue

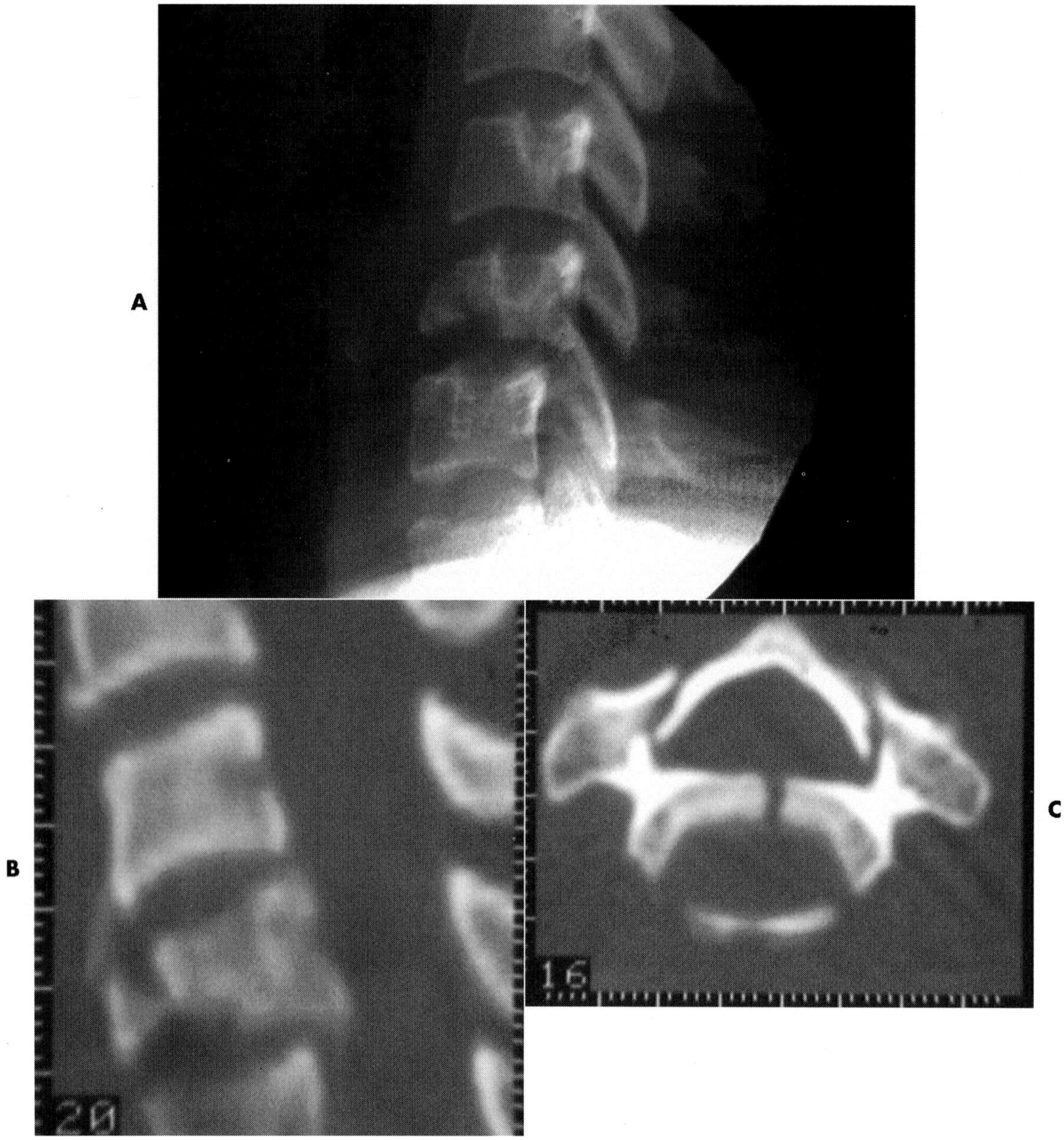

Figure 4-22

Flexion compression injury. **A**, Lateral radiograph with the patient in traction. Fragmentation of the vertebral body is obvious. There is retropulsion of a portion-of the inferior endplate of C5 and widening of the facet joint space indicating some instability. **B**, Sagittal CT reformation on a different patient with a similar fracture. **C**, Axial CT scan demonstrates a central cleavage plane within the vertebral body and bilateral laminar fractures.

joint injury can occur with little or no bony fracture. In the acute phase muscle spasm may maintain the alignment of the spine even with torn joint capsules. As the acute spasm diminishes and the patient moves about, a devastating dislocation may occur. If severe ligamentous injury is suspected in the absence of fracture, MRI may be useful in defining objective ligamentous rupture.[29] Acute ligamentous rupture is associated with hemorrhage in the interspinous ligament. This will appear bright on T1-weighted images and bright on T2-weighted images after several days. Acute injury of the interspinous ligament appears bright on T2-weighted images (Fig. 4-23).

When facet dislocation or subluxation is present, injury to the intervertebral disk *must* have occurred. Laceration of the disk can be identified on MRI scans. There is abnormal bright signal within the disk on T2-weighted images (Fig. 4-24). The lacerated annulus may be visible as well. Acute nuclear herniation may be present.

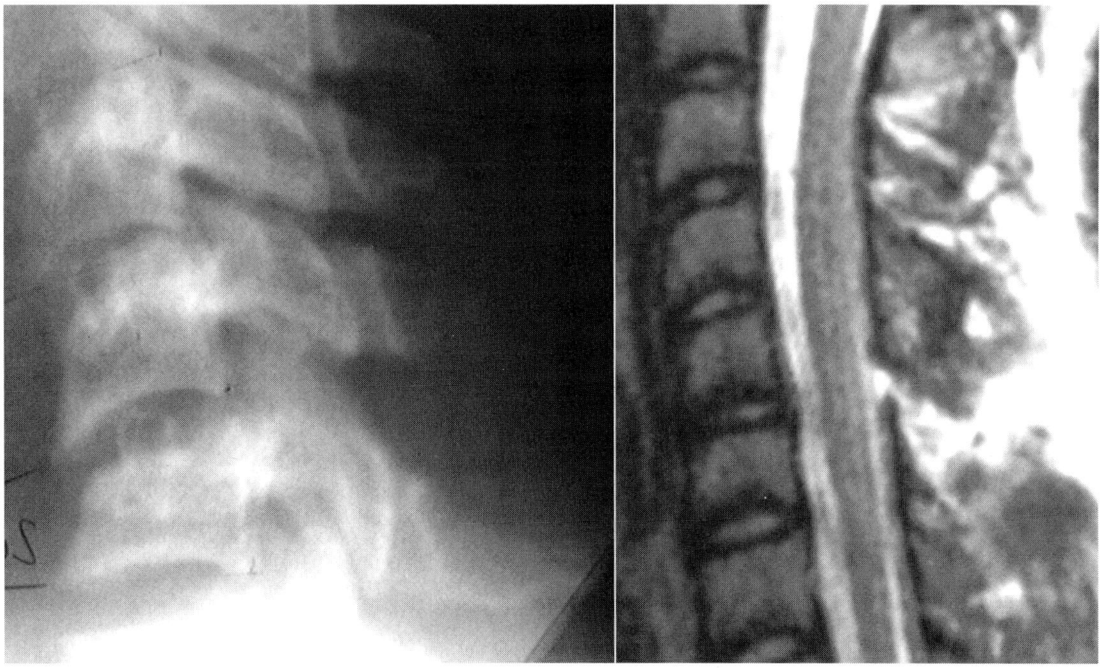

FIGURE 4-23

Flexion distraction injury. **A**, Lateral radiograph shows widening of the posterior portion of the C5-6 disk space and separation of the spinous process indicating tearing of the intraspinous ligament at C5-6. **B**, T2-weighted sagittal MRI scan on another patient with a similar injury. Note the disruption of the posterior ligaments.

PITFALL

It is important to recognize that the disk is injured in patients with flexion injuries. Manipulation of the spine may further expel nuclear material from the disk and compromise the spinal cord or nerveroots.[30] It is, therefore, critical to do any manipulation or reduction of the articular lesions in an alert, cooperative patient with adequate neurologic monitoring. Nonsurgical reduction can often be accomplished by traction.

PEARL

An elegant way of monitoring the progress of increasing head traction on reducing a subluxation is to subtly modify the traction protocol outlined by White and Panjabi.[31] The traction protocol is followed except for the substitution of portable image intensified fluoroscopy for routine radiographs. This allows instantaneous visualization of the spine with lower radiation dose than standard radiographs. The patient is placed in a supine position within the portable image intensifier and the fluoroscope is aligned laterally. Periodic fluoroscopic exposures of no more than 1 to 2 seconds, with or without permanent digital images, are taken as traction weights are adjusted allowing the treating physician to note when reduction occurs and will aid in preventing over distraction of the injured disk. Any angulation of the spine can be monitored as well.

The decision whether to perform surgery on a patient with flexion-distraction injury is determined by extent of deformity of the spine, amount and type of instability, and the patient neurological status. This decision rests in the mind and hands of the spinal surgeon and must be predicated on a complete diagnosis and understanding of the injury. Information from complete and accurate imaging is essential to achieve optimal outcome. Visualization of the entire injury area is important as with greater comminution bone fragments compressing the next rostral nerve root are likely.

Reformatted CT is ideal in defining the presence of facet fragmentation, which occurs upon the downward recoil from the primary distractive force. It is occasionally possible to diagnose a compressed nerve root by this method and allow recapture of partial function of one extra neural segment by appropriate late decompression.[32] Partial recapture of even a single nerve root

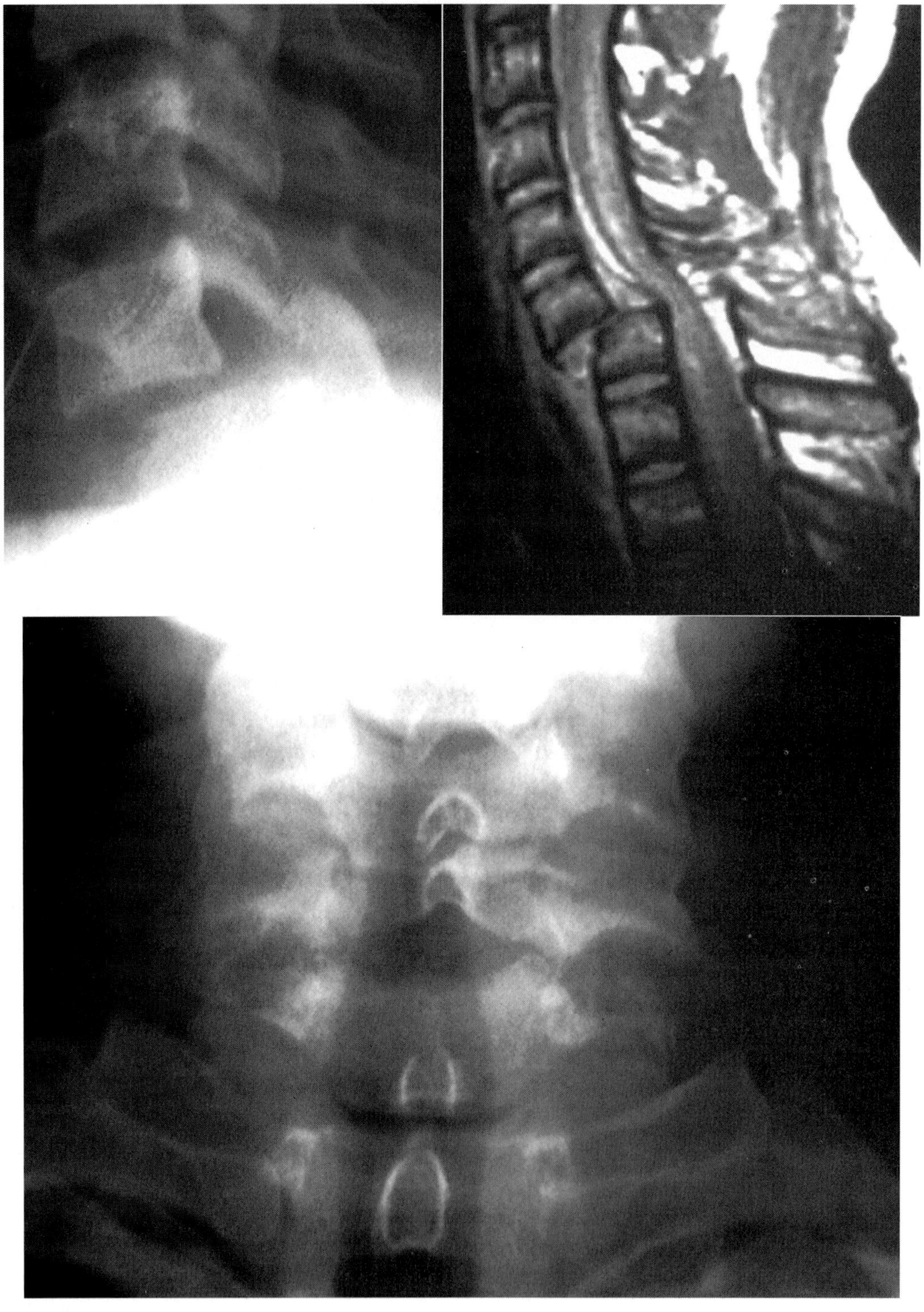

A

C

B

FIGURE 4-24

Flexion distraction injury with facet dislocation. **A**, Routine radiograph. The disk space is narrow and the facets are locked. **B**, Frontal radiograph. It is much more difficult to make the diagnosis of this severe lesion on the frontal film. Only the abnormal relationship between the spinous processes of C5, C6, and C7 indicates subluxation. **C**, T2-weighted MRI scan demonstrates total disruption of the disk with herniation anteriorly and posteriorly. Bright signal within the compressed spinal cord attests to the cord injury.

A

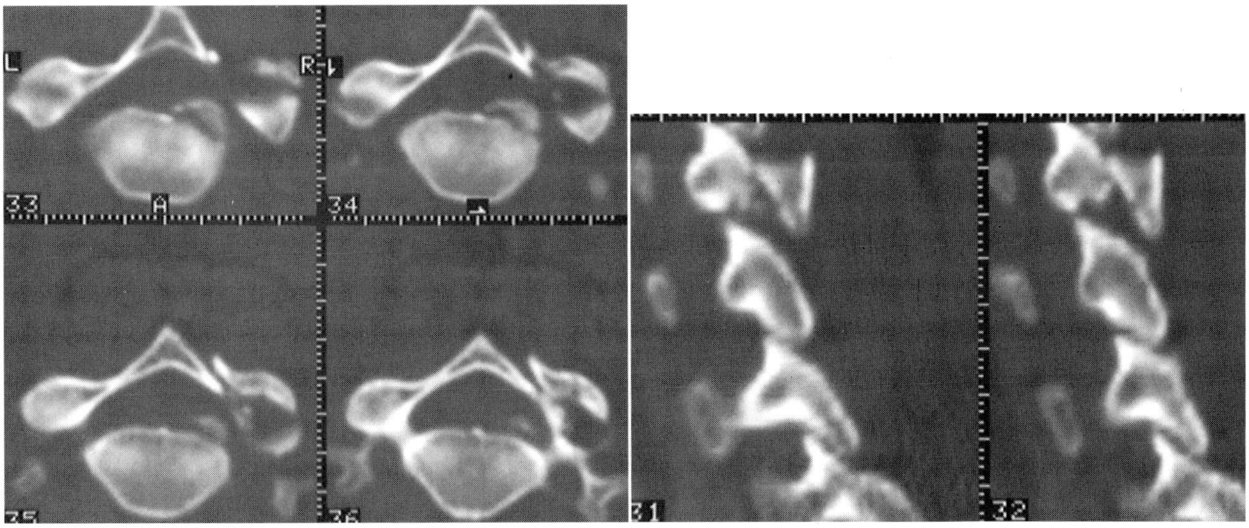

B

FIGURE 4-25

Flexion distraction injury with unilateral facet dislocation. **A**, Axial and **B**, sagittal reformation on a patient with lamina and facet fractures. Decompression of the lateral recess and foramen can allow recovery of the C6 root.

may demonstrably alter the quality of life in a quadriplegic patient (Fig. 4-25).

Disk herniation, when present, is usually at the level of the complete cord lesion. Anterior diskectomy when there is flexion-distraction injury in a complete spinal injury is contraindicated as it causes further instability by weakening the anterior column of the injured segment.

COMPRESSION INJURIES

Axial load classically causes vertebral bursting. Fragmentation of the vertebral body is accompanied by disruption of the neural arch. While fragmented vertebral bodies are generally easy to diagnosis, neural arch fractures are much more difficult to see. This is especially true on MRI scans. Burst fractures tend to be inherently unstable fractures because of complex injuries to the articular processes.

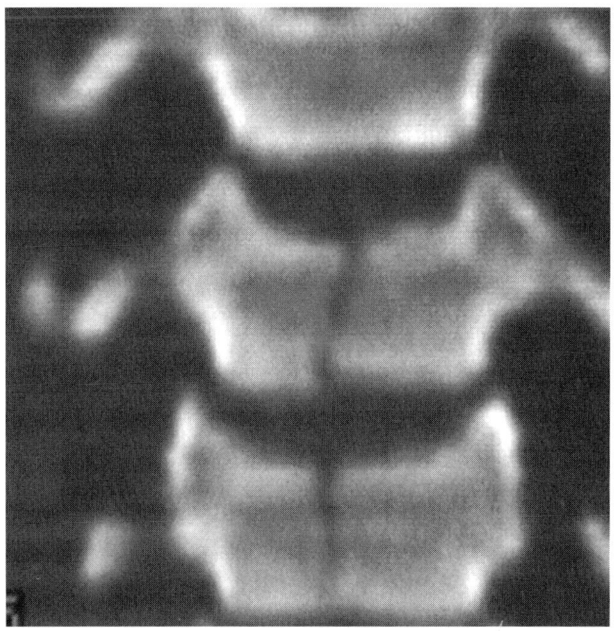

FIGURE 4-26

Cleavage of two contiguous vertebral bodies. Coronal CT reformation shows continuous fracture line through the two adjacent bodies.

PITFALL

Obvious compression of one of the vertebra is often accompanied by midline cleavage fracture of an adjacent vertebra. It is important to diagnose this cleavage fracture because it is usually accompanied by fracture of the neural arch. This fracture may be very subtle. If posterior fusion surgery with interspinous wiring is contemplated, it is critical to prove that the laminae at the proposed surgical sites are intact. Axial CT scans and curved coronal reformations are the images most likely to give the critical information (Fig. 4-26).

PITFALL

In rare instances, congenital failure of development of the various ossification centers of the vertebrae look like compression flexion fractures with wedging of the vertebral bodies with central lucencies. Midline reformatted CT is, therefore, very confusing. The diagnosis can be made with certainty by correlating the images in all three CT planes (Fig. 4-27).

Mild flexion injuries may cause little vertebral fragmentation. Subtle flexion, tear-drop fractures may be produced by either upward displacement of the anterior portion of the inferior endplate at the upper vertebra or downward displacement of the anterior edge of the superior endplate.

PITFALL

The apophyseal plates form from separate ossification centers. These fuse to the vertebral bodies during the second decade of life (Fig. 4-28 A,B). Failure of complete ossification of the anterior margin of the superior apophyseal ring is common. It causes a subtle downward sloping of the superior vertebral edge (Fig. 4-28 C,D). This can be easily misconstrued as a compression fracture. The differ-

A B C

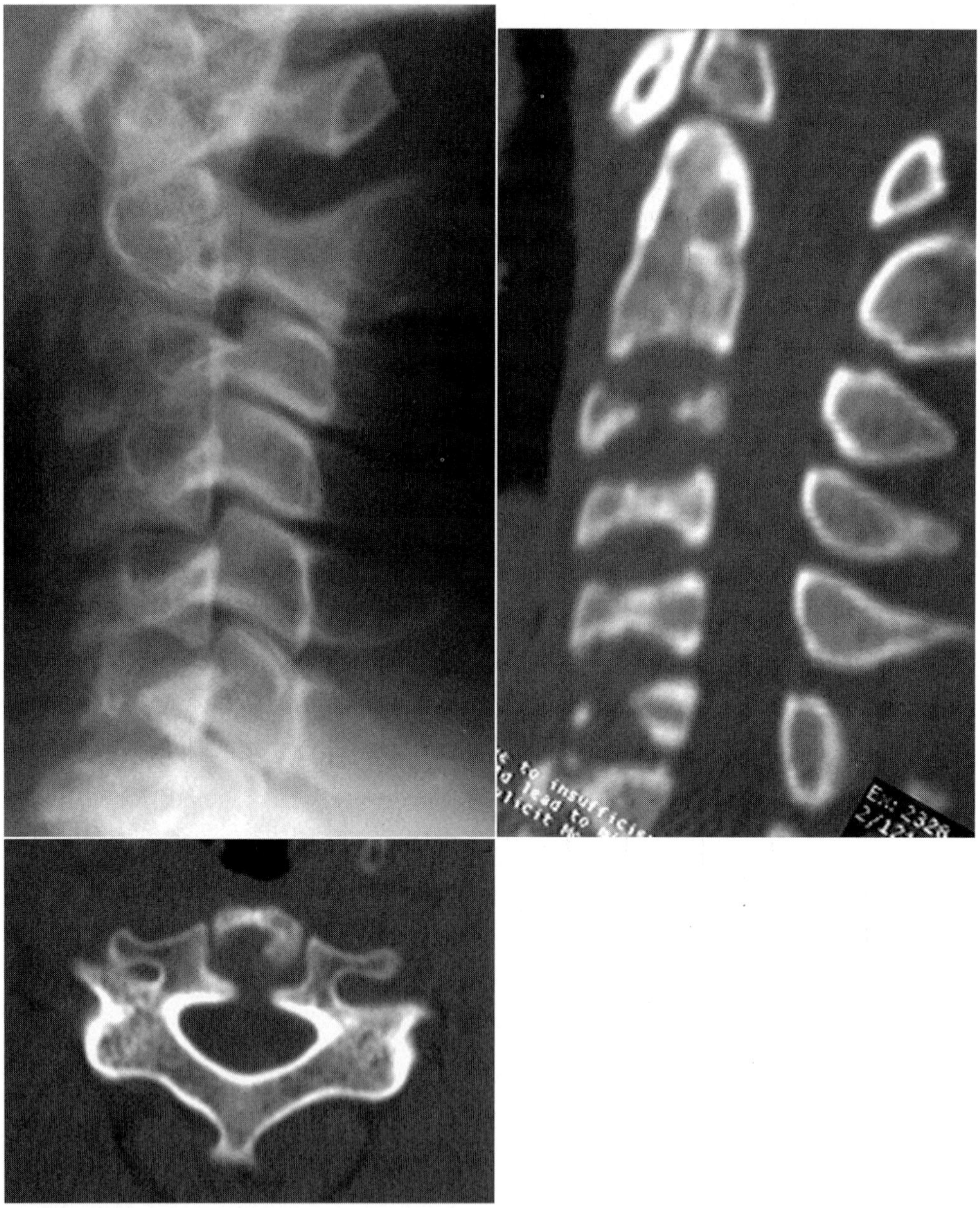

FIGURE 4-27

Congenital failure of ossification of the vertebra. **A**, Lateral radiograph appears to show compression fractures of several vertebrae. **B**, Midsagittal CT reformation shows that the centers of the vertebrae are not ossified. **C**, Axial scan proves that the anterior segment of the vertebral body has not formed.

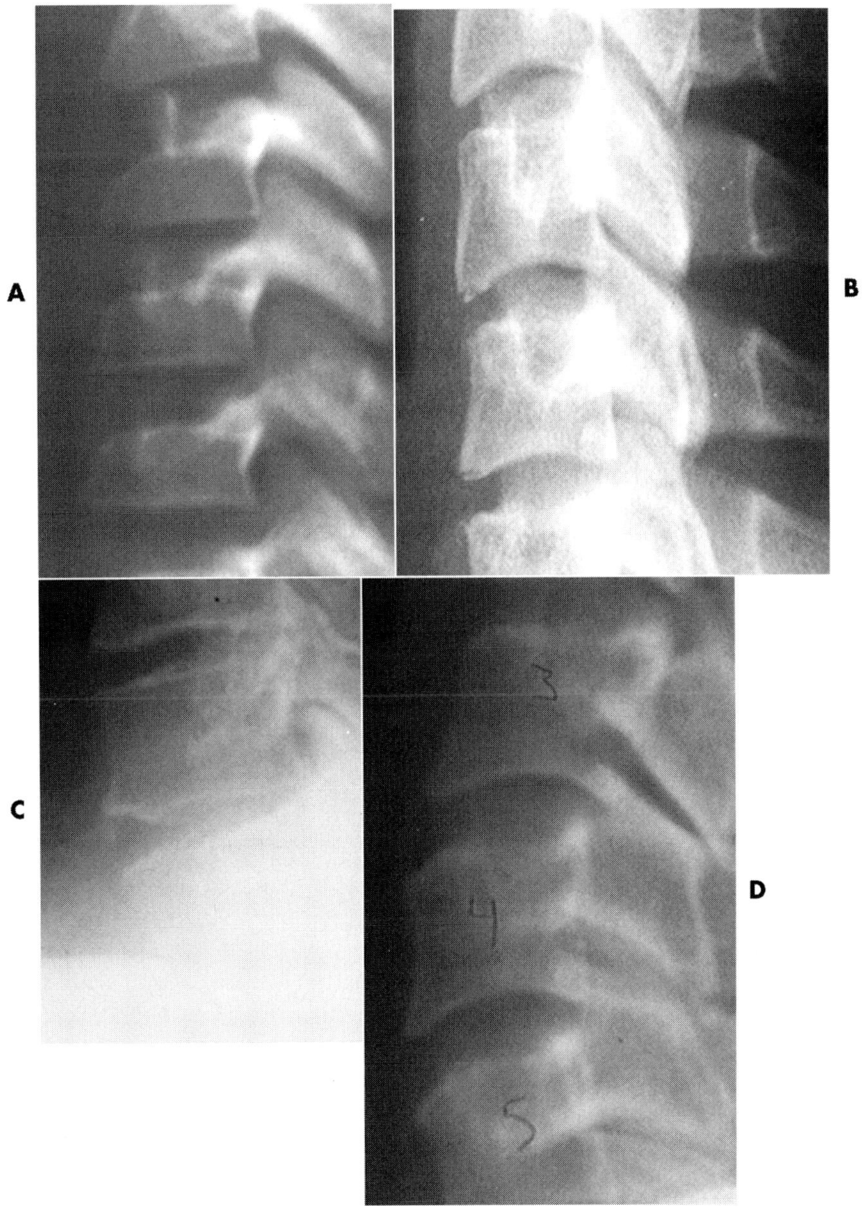

FIGURE 4-28

Variations of the cervical apophyseal endplates. **A**, Lateral radiograph of cervical spine of a child. The ring apophysis have not yet ossified and the anterior, superior border appears to slope downward. **B**, Lateral radiograph of an 18 year old. The apophyseal rings have nearly totally fused the vertebral bodies. A very small cleft is still visible at several levels. **C**, Lateral radiograph demonstrates ossification of the apophyseal ring. The ring has failed to fuse to the vertebral endplate. **D**, Lateral radiograph of a patient with failure of ossification of the superior apophysis.

entiation can be made on high-quality routine radiographs because this type of endplate deformity does not cause displacement of the prevertebral fat stripe. The disk space tends to be slightly wider anteriorly because of the increased height of the cartilage.

Displacement of the prevertebral fat line is a subtle marker of bleeding into the anterior prevertebral space. A conscious effort must always be made to identify it on each lateral cervical spine radiograph in a traumatized patient.

Flexion-compression injuries in the elderly patient with well-established spondylitic spurs can cause fracture and separation of the osteophytes from the verte-

E

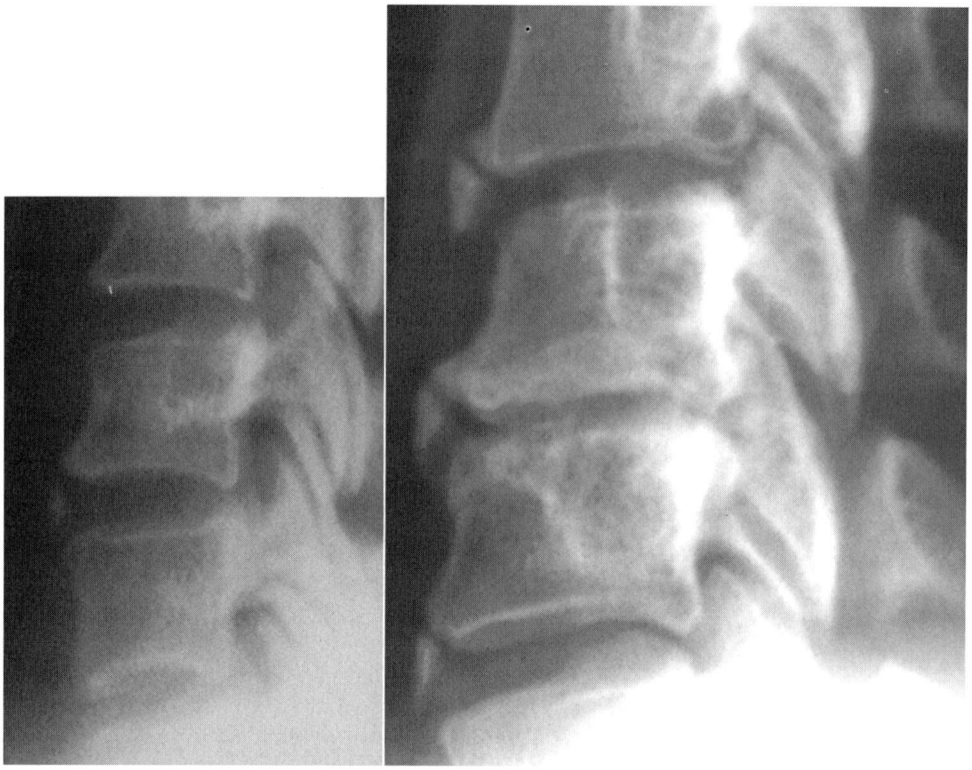

F

FIGURE 4-28 *continued*

E, Lateral radiograph of a patient with a degenerative calcification in the anterior annulus. **F**, Lateral radiograph showing anterior osteophytes.

bra. These need to be differentiated from crescentic ossification within the anterior longitudinal ligament or annulus.

> **PEARL**
>
> Fractured osteophytes have jagged edges at their vertebral attachments. Annular or ligamentous ossification has smooth, well-corticated borders (Fig. 4-28 E,F). Associated prevertebral soft tissue swelling is acutely present.

Retropulsion of bony fragments and disk material in the spinal canal is much more commonly seen in flexion injuries with compression. Surgical decompression in a patient with spinal cord injury can be logically planned when the extent of bony fragmentation is clarified. Multiplanar CT imaging is the procedure of choice.

When rotatory or bending forces are superimposed upon compression-flexion trauma, complex lesions occur. Articular compression with fragmentation occurs from the primary insult with significant fracture of the neural ring. Fixed rotatory deformity is common. Imaging these injuries is challenging because it is difficult or even impossible to obtain cross-sectional scans in the usual physiological planes.

> **PITFALL**
>
> When the neck is tilted, the plane of axial section may traverse more than one vertebra. This causes superimposition of portions of adjacent vertebrae. It is very common for portions of two different lamina to appear on a single axial scan. This may easily be mistaken for a neural arch fracture (Fig. 4-29). Patients with compression injuries absolutely require a high-quality reformatted CT to elucidate the multiple injuries.

HYPEREXTENSION INJURIES

Hyperextension injuries are much more difficult to diagnose by imaging studies than flexion injuries. Fracture of the vertebral bodies are rare except for avulsion

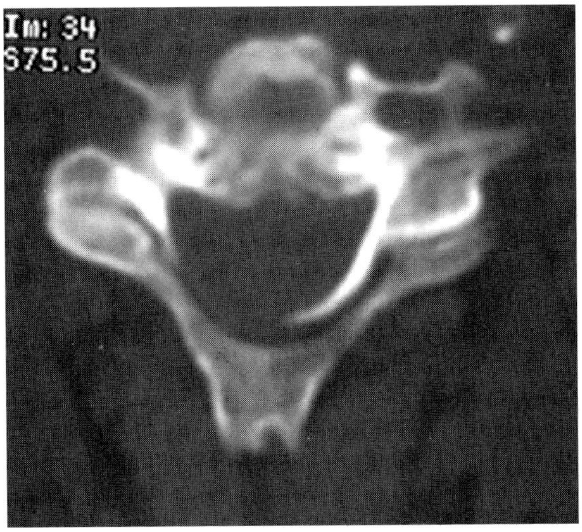

FIGURE 4-29

Axial CT scan traversing portions of two different lamina. This can be misdiagnosed as a fracture.

of a portion of the insertion of the anterior longitudinal ligament. When the head is accelerated posteriorly with sufficient force to cause failure of a motion segment, the anterior longitudinal ligament generally avulses one of its attachments. The disk consequently is lacerated, either partially or completely.

PEARL

This diagnosis is occasionally made on plain radiographs. The anterior fat line is lost or displaced (Fig. 4-30 A). A thin, short line of gas can occasionally be seen adjacent to the vertebral endplate representing gas within a small tear in the fibers of the annulus.[33–36] This is thought to be indicative of hyperextension sprain. It is important to differentiate this thin, anterior "vacuum effect" from the more common "vaccum" found in many patients with degenerative disk disease. A tiny, tear-drop fracture may or may not be present.

The disk space may actually be widened anteriorly because of the distraction forces. An MRI scan demonstrates an abnormal signal within the disk indicative of bleeding and or swelling. High-resolution sagittal views often show the torn annulus and anterior longitudinal ligament (Fig. 4-30 B). When no tear-drop fracture is present, axial CT scans may appear normal.

The lateral masses can be compressed in hyperextension injuires. These fracture are very difficult to diagnoses on standard radiographs.

PEARL

Patients in whom significant hyperextension injury is suspected should have frontal radiographs taken with the central ray of the beam angled caudally parallel to the slope of the articular pillars.[37] These views allow comparison of the heights of the articular pillars, and, consequently, compression fractures can be appreciated. If the patient is able, caudally angled frontal radiographs should also be obtained with the head turned to both sides.

Turning the head removes the shadow of the mandible from over the upper joints. Reformatted, curved coronal CT reformations are the images of choice for delineating the detail of complex lateral mass fractures (Fig. 4-32).

PITFALL

A well-corticated notch or groove often appears along the superior surface of one of the lower articular processes. This is a normal variant and should not be confused with compression fracture.[38] Complex congenital neural arch anomalies may also produce strange-shaped articular processes, which may mimic a fracture (Fig. 4-31).

In severe hyperextension compression injuries the posterior elements may be fractured by being sandwiched on each other. These forces tend to cause bursting decompression of the neural ring rather than bony canal compromise. If there is a significant rotatory component to the hyperextension, the neural arch fractures may be unilateral.

Moderate to severe hyperextension trauma may produce devastating spinal cord injury even though radiographs are normal or nearly normal. This is especially true in elderly patients with chronic disk disease and cervical spondylosis.[39] Typically the spinal cord becomes compressed between the posterior projecting osteophytes at the disk space and the lamina of the next lowest vertebrae. Cord contusion with intramedullary hemorrhage or swelling is the consequence, often resulting in central cord syndrome. These changes are obvious on good quality MRI scans.

Avulsion fracture of the spinous process of C7 is called clay-shovelers' fracture. It is caused by violent traction of the supraspinous ligament upon the spinous process. The bony margins of the fragment and the

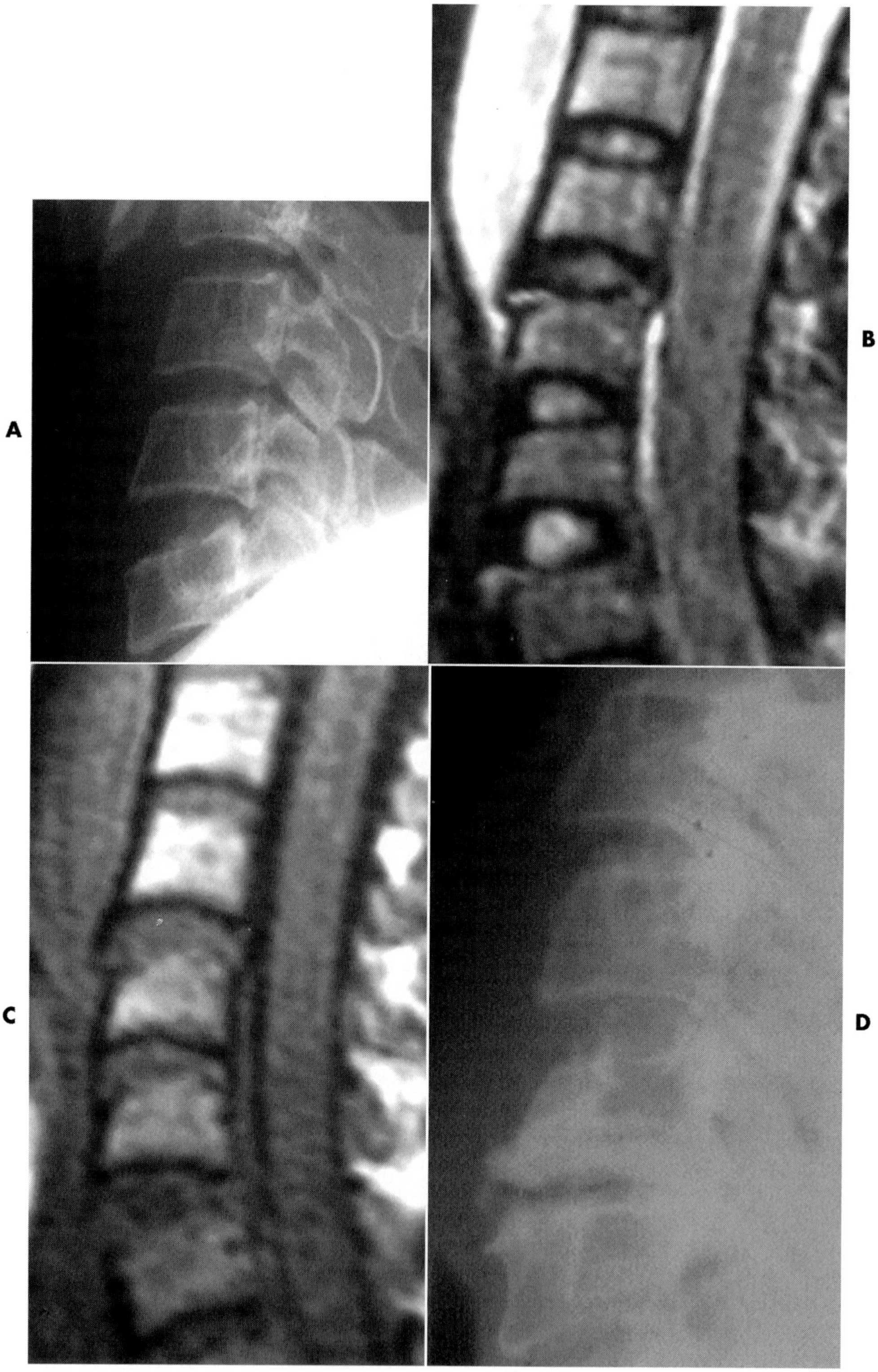

FIGURE 4-30

A, Lateral radiograph showing acute hyperextension sprain with gas within the disc. The anterior annulus is torn, the disc space is widened, and there is swelling of the prevertebral soft tissues. **B**, Sagittal T2-weighted and **C**, T1-weighted scans show abnormal signal anterior to the vertebral bodies representing prevertebral swelling. The C4-C5 and C6-C7 disks are torn. The disc at the C6-C7 level is widened. Abnormal signal is noted adjacent to the endplates. **D**, Lateral radiograph of a patient with to degenerated disks with "vacuum" effect.

A

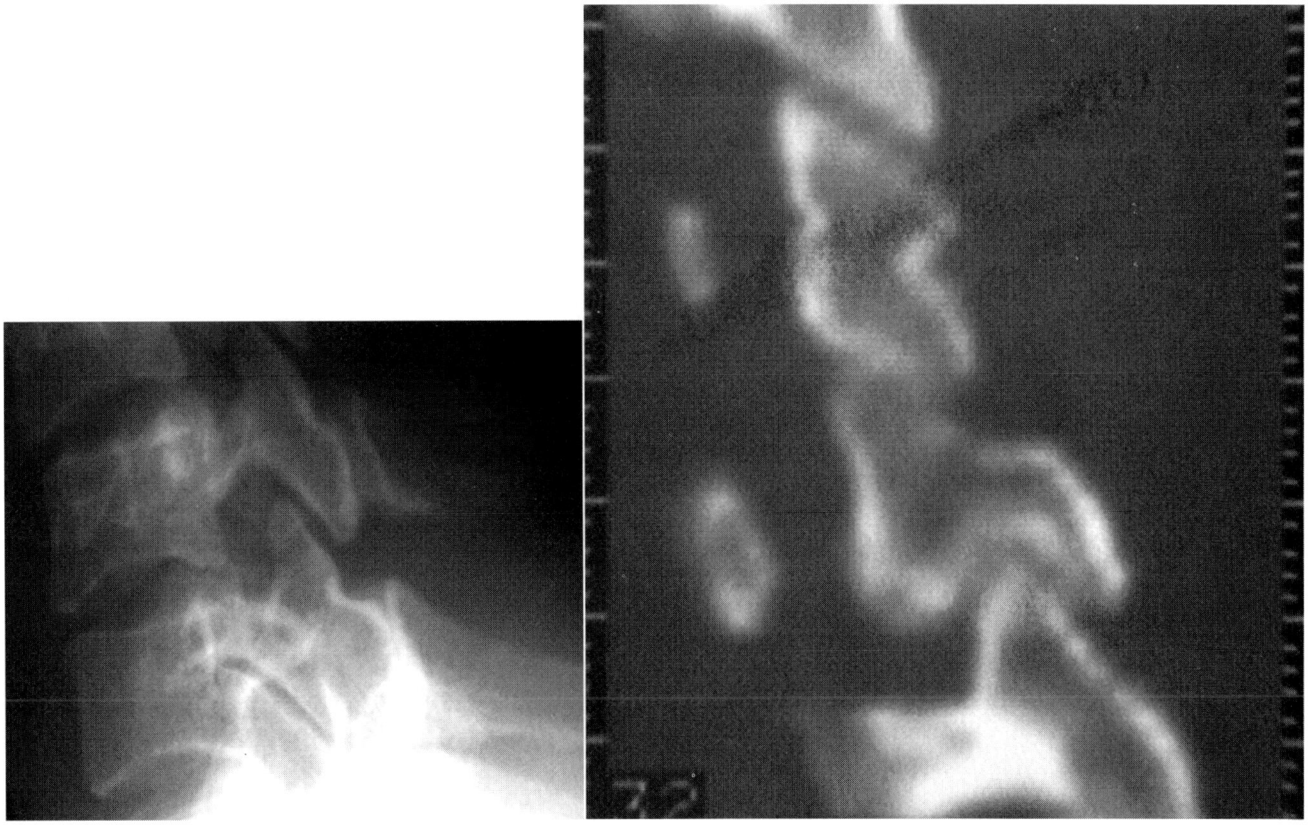

B

Figure 4-31

Notched facets **A**, Lateral radiograph showing typical small superior facet notch. **B**, CT scan on another patient with an anomalous facet with a very prominent inferior notch.

spinous process from which it is torn are rough and jagged.

> **Pitfall**
>
> There is occasionally a separate ossification center for the distal tip of the spinous process, which is often confused with acute fracture. This normal anatomic variant can be differentiated from an acute fracture because its edges are smooth and regular (Fig. 4-32).

Thoracolumbar Injuries

There are numerous systems for classifying thoracolumbar injuries. The most frequently used systems have been based on the morphology of the fracture, vector of injuring force, and spinal stability.[40,41]

Trauma to the thoracic spine tends to produce either devastating, total spinal cord disruption or no neurologic signs at all. The rib cage adds stability to the thoracic spine in all but the most severe anatomic injuries. The mechanism of injury determines the pattern of bony disruption. Flexion-compression trauma is the most common, producing wedge deformity of the vertebrae and retropulsion of vertebral fragments. Because the size of the spinal canal is small compared to the cord within it, bony fragmentation tends to injure the spinal cord. Acute traumatic thoracic disk herniation without fracture dislocation is a great rarity. Flexion-rotation injuries tend to cause the most instability in thoracic and thoracolumbar trauma. Spinal translation in the AP or lateral plane is an important finding on plane radiographs, suggesting a highly unstable injury. Routine radiographs usually define the nature of the bony injury, but on occasion the lateral radiographs may be indeterminate.

> **Pearl**
>
> Subtle fractures that produce paravertebral bleeding widen the paravertebral stripe on frontal views. This should raise the index of suspicion even if the fracture is not obvious (Fig. 4-33).

A

B

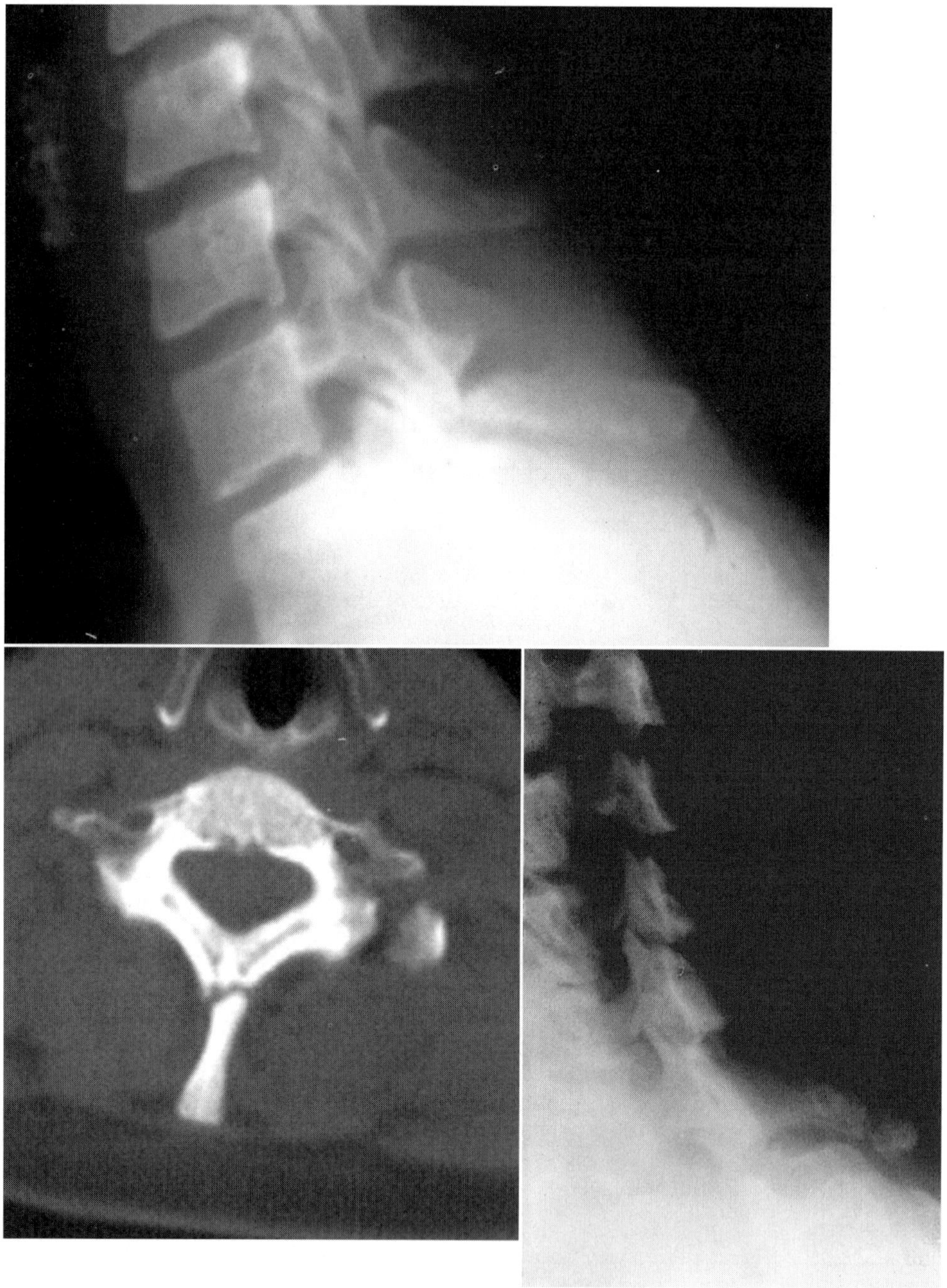

C

Figure 4-32

Clay-shovelers' fracture. Lateral radiograph **A** and axial CT scan **B** demonstrate fracture of the spinous process of C7. Note the irregular edges characteristic of acute fracture. The differential diagnosis of this fracture includes an anomalous, unfused ossification center of the spinous process **C**, which has smooth, regular margines.

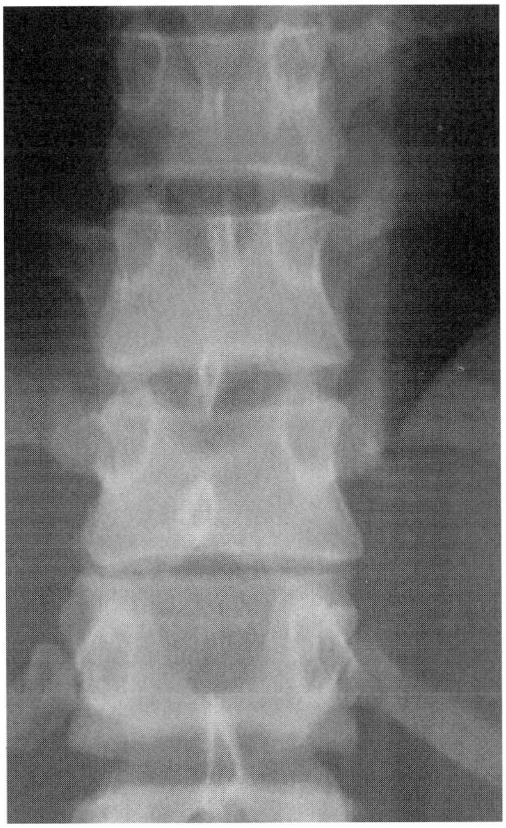

FIGURE 4-33

Paravertebral swelling. Frontal radiograph shows deviation of the paravertebral stripe.

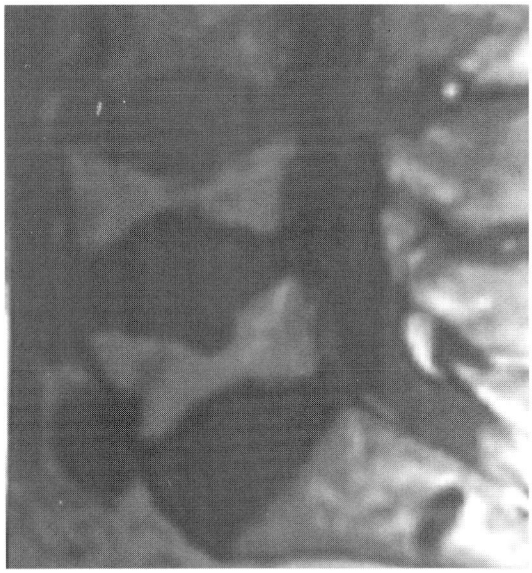

FIGURE 4-34

Old compression fracture. Sagittal T1-weighted MRI scan with a compressed L4 vertebra with normal marrow signal.

On routine radiographs it may be difficult to differentiate subtle compression fractures from similar wedge deformity caused by spondylosis or chronic vertebral end plate disease called adolescent kyphosis (Scheuermann's disease).[42] Scheuermann's disease is of unknown cause and occurs during the phase of vertebral growth, usually between the ages of 12 and 16. It is characterized by multiple anterior Schmorl's nodes usually with sclerotic margins. A majority of the endplate is pitted and compressed producing the wedge deformity generally at more than one segment.

Wedge deformity of the vertebrae is frequent in older people due to osteoporosis. These develop from chronic fractures. In questionable cases nuclear bone scanning or MRI confirms the diagnosis. A technetium 99m nuclear bone scan becomes positive within 24 hours of a fracture and remains positive for months.[43] The MRI scans demonstrate low signal within the bone on T1-weighted images and increased signal on T2 or gradient echo sequences. These signal changes represent replacement of the normal fatty marrow with blood or edema. The MRI scans may also remain positive for many months. The bone marrow signal remains normal in patients with chronic end-plate disease. Any visible signal abnormalities generally relate to chronic irregularities of the end plates because of multiple Schmorl's node type lesions.

PEARL

Wedge compression fractures with normal marrow signal on MRI are not due to acute injury (Fig. 4-34).

Flexion fractures produce anterior wedge deformity of the vertebra, but typically the neural arch remains intact. Stability of the spine depends on the amount and severity of facet joint disruption. Axial CT scans demonstrate "naked" facets when the joints are dislocated. The dislocated superior facets project superior to the inferior facets and are, therefore, visible on different axial cross sections.[44]

If a component of rotation is present in a thoracic injury, producing translation at the unstable level, axial CT images may be very confusing. Coronal reformations usually identify the various components of the lesion (Fig. 4-35).[45,46]

THE LUMBAR SPINE

FLEXION INJURIES—WEDGE COMPRESSION FRACTURE

When the body undergoes abnormal forward flexion, disruption may occur at any portion of the motion

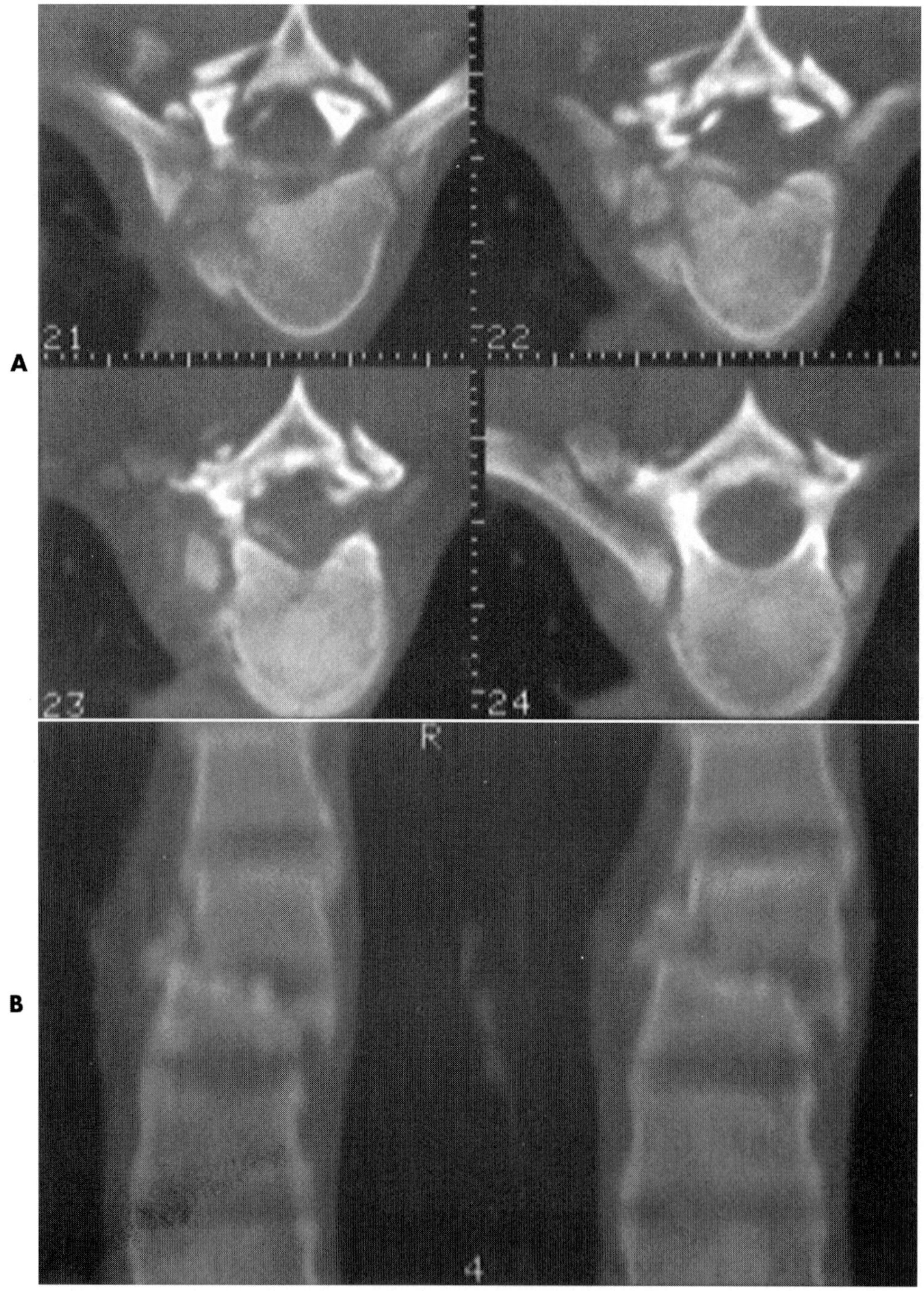

FIGURE 4-35

Comminuted, unstable, thoracic fracture. **A**, Axial CT scan and **B**, coronal CT reformation demonstrate a compression fracture with translation.

segment. Vertebral body compression is common. The neural arch generally remains intact. By definition only the anterior column is fractured. Simple vertebral body wedging can be noted on regular radiographs. In acute fractures, cortical disruption is usually obvious. There is increased bone density along the fracture line because of bony impaction (Fig. 4-36 A). The CT scans show web-like, sharply marginated cracks within the bone. As healing proceeds the fracture lines smooth out and the edges become indistinct. The MRI scans show decreased signal on T1 and increased signal on T2-weighted images indicative of acute bony trauma.

PITFALL

Not all wedged-shaped vertebrae are caused by fractures. Multiple endplate irregularities similar to those seen in the thoracic spine in Scheuermann's disease are often found in upper lumbar endplates. Failure of complete ossification of the anterior ring apophysis is an inconsequential developmental abnormality, which is often confused with compression fracture (Fig. 4-36 B).

In teenagers, the ossifying apophyseal rings appear as thin, short lines of bone at the anterior edges of the vertebral bodies.[47] Occasionally, the anterior apophyseal center fails to completely ossify, producing a normal, wedged vertebrae. These last two entities can be differentiated from acute fracture because the internal architecture of the bone is normal on all imaging studies (Fig. 4-36 C,D).

PITFALL

Congenital butterfly vertebra may be mistaken for a compression fracture. On lateral radiographs the vertebra is often wedge-shaped leading the uninitiated to presume that a fracture is present. Even sagittal reformatted CT scans can be confusing. The axial scans allow definitive diagnosis because the margins of the central vertebral lucency are smooth as they represent a zone of intraosseous cartilage (Fig. 4-36 E).

Compression of a vertebra with fragmentation has been termed a burst fracture. Both the anterior and middle column are disrupted. Burst fractures may be stable or unstable depending on the status of the posterior elements. A specific type of burst fracture with fragmentation of the vertebral end plate and midline splitting of the vertebral body and neural arch is called a crush-cleavage fracture.[48] It is very important to differentiate pure flexion fractures from crush-cleavage injuries or other forms of unstable burst fractures.

PEARL

Anteroposterior plane radiographs may reveal subtle widening of the interpedicular distance. When present, this indicates fracture of the neural arch with bursting of the neural ring with instability (Fig. 4-37 A).

Neural compromise is generally caused by fragmentation of the body with retropulsion into the spinal canal. The position of the bone fragments is best evaluated by reformatted CT. It is well known that patients with thoracolumbar and lumbar compression fractures may have terrible looking CT scans but be intact or nearly intact neurologically (Fig. 4-37 B).

PEARL

One must remember that we treat patients and not imaging studies. It is impossible to make a patient with no neurological deficit better, only worse. There is no indication for early decompression of the intact patient. There is also little benefit to decompress the spine of a patient with complete spinal cord injury who is out of spinal shock as there is no chance of neural recovery, only root escape.

Recent studies have documented that the spinal canal will remodel if left alone. If instability becomes a problem, it can be addressed with an appropriate fusion at a suitable interval.[49,50] If a patient develops intractable back pain or radiculopathy, appropriate therapy can begin at a later date.

Patients with incomplete neurological deficits are those who stand to benefit most from early surgical intervention, provided all compressing elements are identified and decompressed. Posterior distraction and fixation, if performed in the first several days, may produce very dramatic reduction of dislocated fragments by ligamentotaxis (Fig. 4-37 C).

Flexion distraction injuries are caused by forces applied to the spine with a fulcrum anterior to the vertebral body. This injury is typified by the seat belt fracture

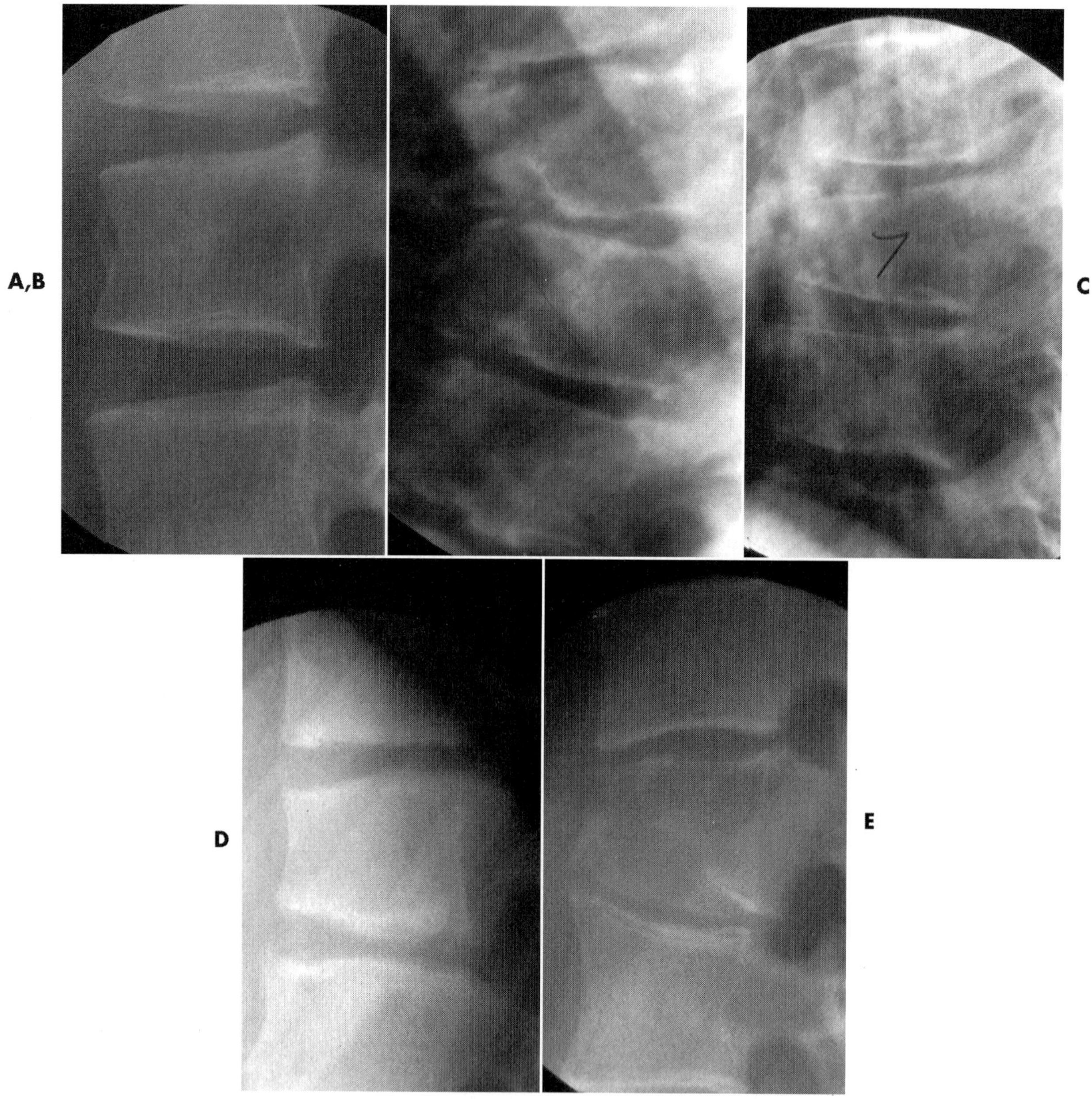

FIGURE 4-36

The Gamut of "wedged-shape" vertebrae. **A**, Acute compression fracture–lateral radiograph of the lumbar spine. There is subtle break in the anterior cortex with sclerosis along the fracture line due to impaction. **B**, Scheuermann's syndrome—there is irregularity of the vertebral endplates at multiple levels with wedge deformity. **C**, Incompletely ossified apophyseal rings with normal wedged appearance of the vertebra. **D**, Failure of ossification of the apophyseal rings in adults leads to a wedged-shaped vertebra. **E**, Congenital butterfly vertebra with abnormal vertebral segmentation. Note compensatory enlargement of the anterior third of the adjacent vertebral bodies.

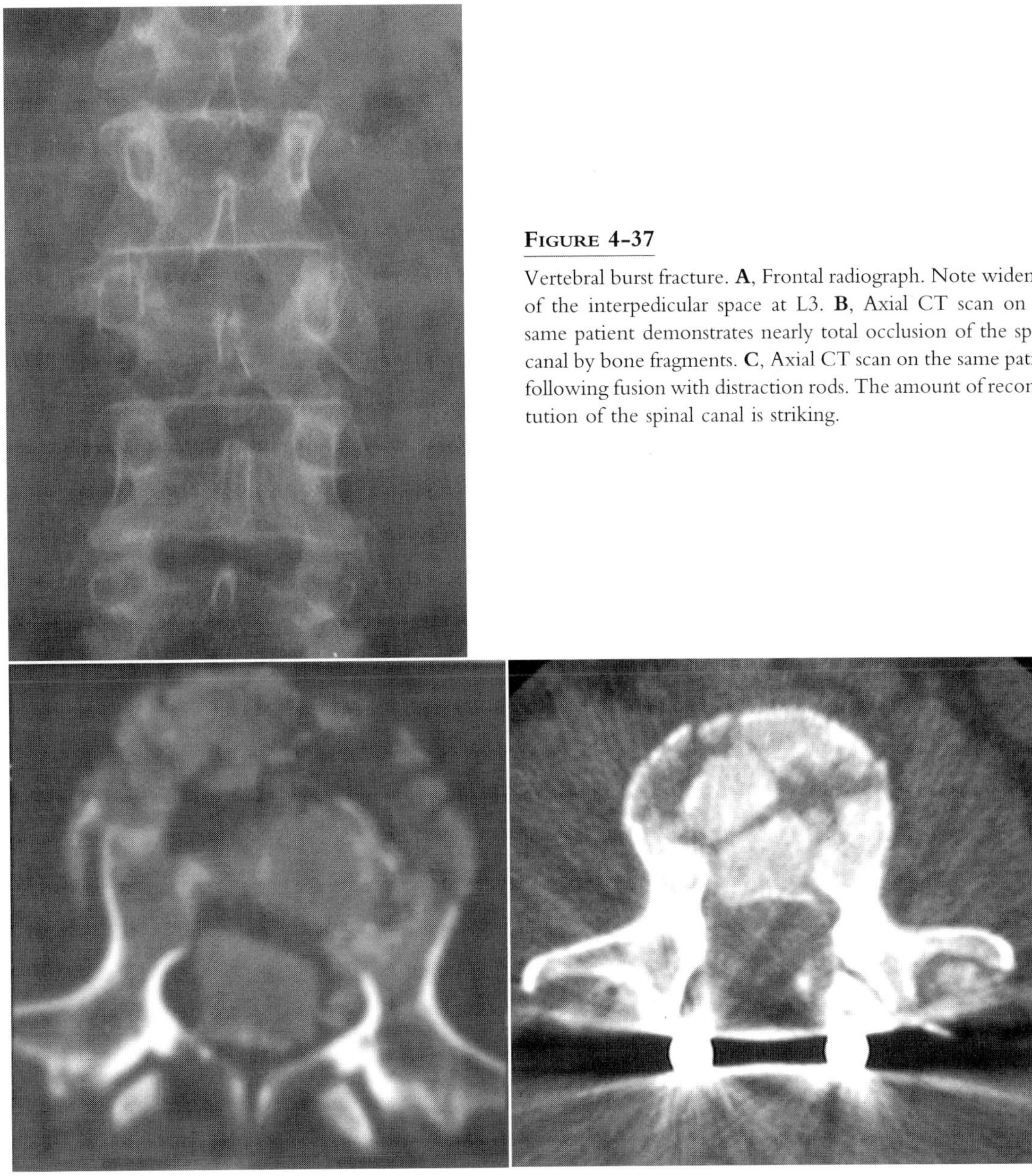

FIGURE 4-37

Vertebral burst fracture. **A**, Frontal radiograph. Note widening of the interpedicular space at L3. **B**, Axial CT scan on the same patient demonstrates nearly total occlusion of the spinal canal by bone fragments. **C**, Axial CT scan on the same patient following fusion with distraction rods. The amount of reconstitution of the spinal canal is striking.

described by Chance.[51] There are several variants of this type of fracture, but all are characterized by a horizontal cleavage of the motion segment. The usual Chance fracture is through all three columns segments. Routine radiographs reveal a horizontal split through the bone from spinous process to the body sparing the anterior longitudinal ligament. Rarely, a soft tissue Chance fracture occurs in which the horizontal cleavage extends through the intraspinous ligament, the facet joints, and the disk. This latter type produces a very unstable spine, because ligamentous structures do not heal as predictably as bone (Fig. 4-38).

The most unstable spines are produced by multidirectional forces adding a component of translation to flexion or extension. The patient in Figure 4-39 sustained a complex distraction flexion injury causing dislocation of the lumbosacral facets with forward slippage of L5 on the sacrum. Note that the pars interarticularis is intact bilaterally and the facets are "naked". The lamina has been fractured by the downward recoil from the initial distraction force.

HYPEREXTENSION FRACTURES

Hyperextension injuries are less common than flexion or compression injuries. They are caused by distraction forces, which may produce shearing and translation. They tend to be quite unstable. Reformatted

A

B

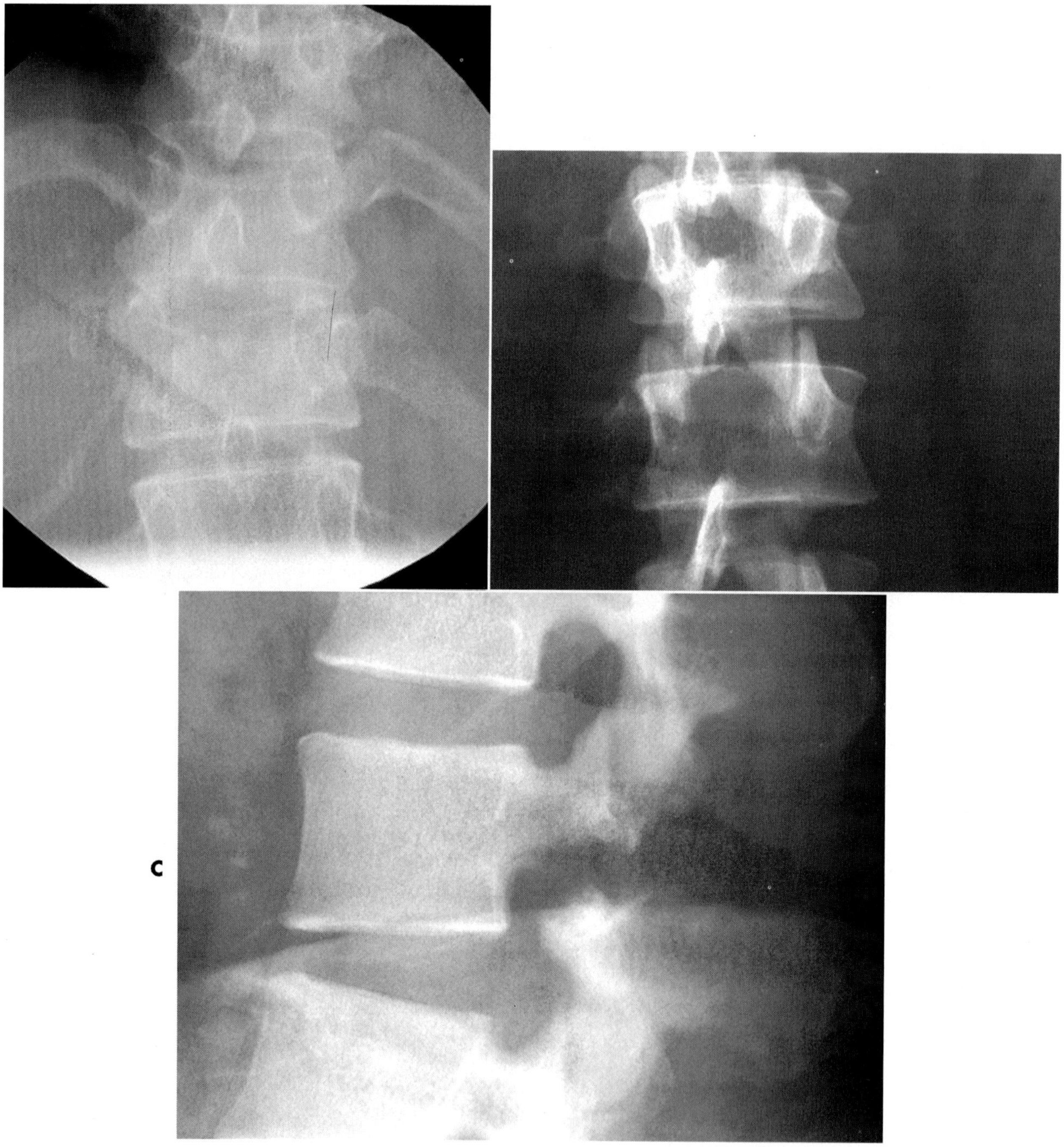

C

Figure 4-38

Chance fractures. **A**, Unilateral Chance fracture; frontal radiograph reveals horizontal fracture through the right pedicle and rib. **B**, Combination soft tissue and bony Chance fracture. Close up frontal radiograph on another patient reveals horizontal fracture through both pedicles. Lateral radiograph **C**, reveals widening of the intervertebral disk because of disk laceration and bilateral pars fractures with separation of the neural arch.

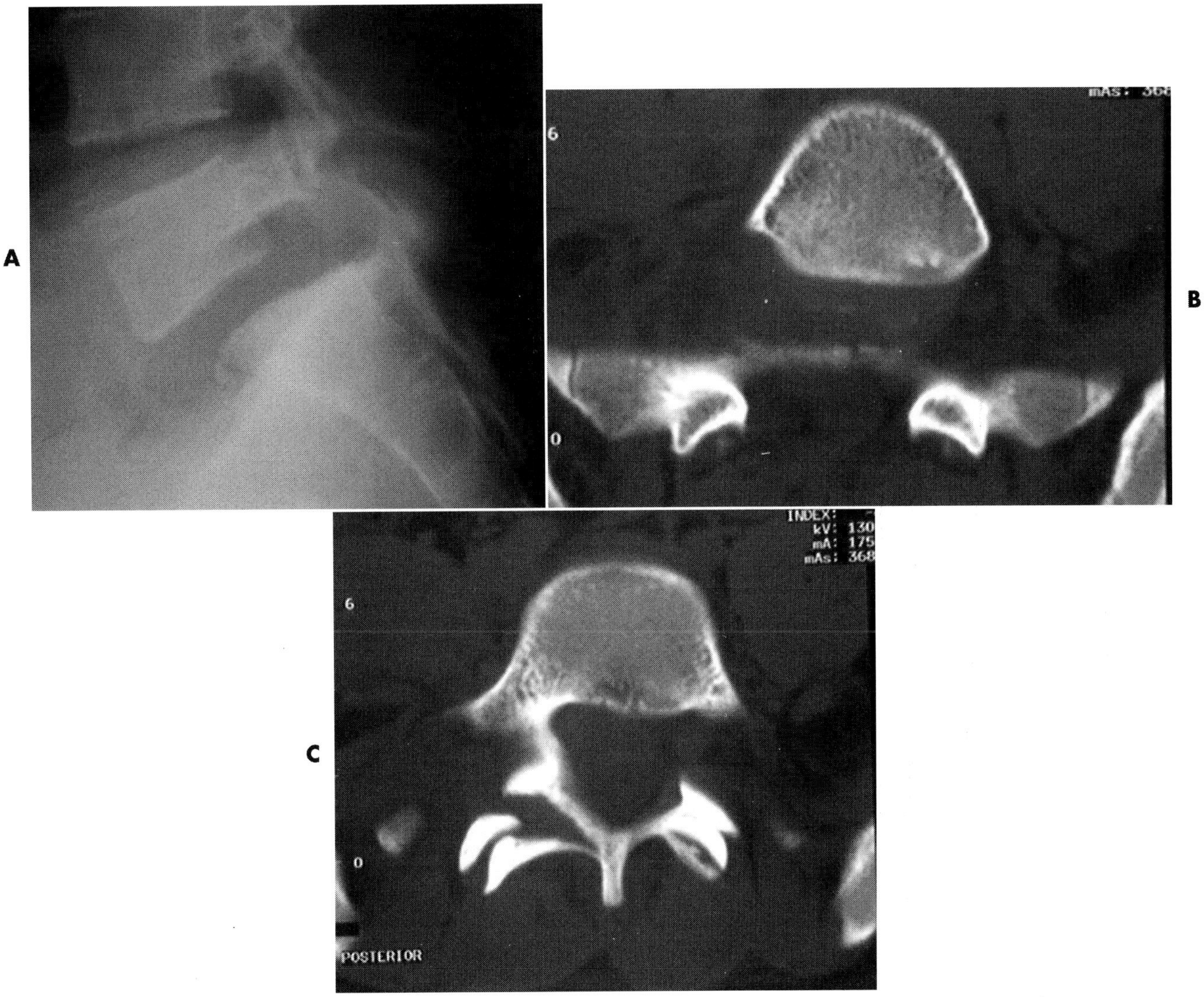

FIGURE 4-39

Fracture dislocation of the lumbosacral junction. **A**, Lateral radiograph reveals the abnormal position of L5 on the sacrum. **B**, Axial CT shows "naked facets". **C**, Adjacent axial CT scan demonstrates an impaction fracture of the lamina as it recoiled down on to the superior articular process of the sacrum.

CT is the diagnostic procedure of choice to evaluate the complex abnormalities typical of this type of injury.

SPONDYLOLYSIS AND OTHER STRESS FRACTURES OF THE LUMBAR SPINE

There is a common misconception that spondylolytic spondylolisthesis is caused by adult trauma. This is not the case. The literature is clear that spondylolysis is a disease of childhood.[52,53] It is a stress fracture probably created by multiple subclinical forces placed on the pars, which breaks. Reformatted CT scans performed shortly after the onset of back pain in such injured children demonstrate typical fracture of the pars. Often the fracture line can be seen traversing only a portion of the pars. It is possible to distinguish acute stress fracture from the more common chronic pars pseudarthrosis.[54,55]

> **PEARL**
>
> Spondylolysis caused by a single acute traumatic episode after the age of 20 is an extraordinary rarity. Nearly all cases diagnosed as "traumatic" spondylolisthesis are actually juvenile spondylolistheses diagnosed by imaging studies.

In patients with acute traumatic subluxation, the pars is intact and the joints sublux or fracture. On occasion the pars interarticularis may break acutely, but such fractures almost invariably are associated with other neural arch fractures.

Subtle stress fractures may occur in any portion of the neural arch. Fracture of the pars interarticularis is, of course, the most prevalent. They are most often bilateral, but unilateral fractures occur often enough to warrant special comment. There is some controversy regarding unilateral spondylolysis. Typically the neural arch on the contralateral side is thickened and sclerotic. The usual explanation is that the thickening is because of increase in the bony stress line on the side opposite form the fracture. While this may occasionally occur, this deformity represents healing of a second pars fracture on the opposite side.[55] On occasion the residual fracture line may actually be visible on high-quality CT images (Fig. 4-40).

There are several neural arch defects that are associated with isthmic spondylolysis. The most common are called the retrosomatic cleft, which is a cleavage plane between the pedicle and the vertebral body, and the retroisthmic cleft, which is a cleavage behind the pars. These two abnormalities have been assumed to be congenital lesions because a theoretic cleavage plane can exist near those sites. Both of these clefts are almost certainly neural arch fractures on the side opposite typical isthmic spondylolysis. The bony edges of these lesions are almost always jagged and irregular with no cortical margins. This finding is typical of a pseudarthrosis and not a congenital cleft. In a series of more than 2,000 patients with spondylolysis or spondylolisthesis, several patients had such lesions that healed. Similar stress fractures have also been identified in the pedicles (Fig. 4-41).

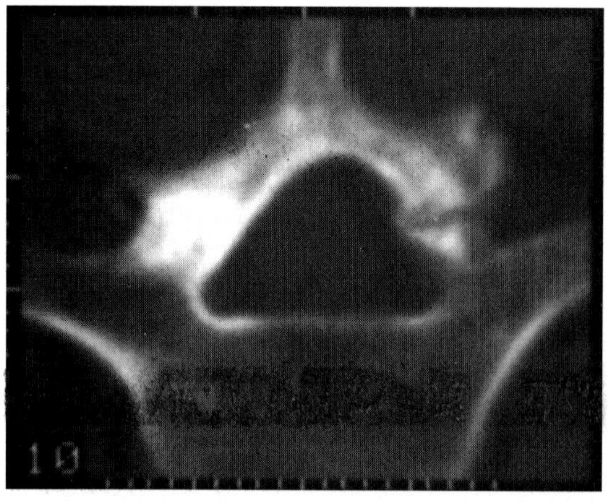

FIGURE 4-40

Unilateral spondylolysis-Axial CT demonstrates a defect on one side and sclerosis of the contralateral pars.

Technically, the posterior apophyseal ring of the vertebral body makes up the anterior border of the neural arch, and fractures of the ring do occur. The most frequent traumatic lesion of the posterior apophyseal ring is called the posterior limbus vertebra. This injury, occuring in teenagers, is a separation of a portion of the vertebral endplate caused by intrabody disk herniation through the cartilage just anterior to the unfused apophyseal ring, (Fig. 4-42).[56,57] When a large segment of the ring is fractured off, the lesion is likely caused by a single traumatic episode. If a very small segment is involved, it is more likely a typical Schmorl's node in an atypical location.

There is considerable controversy as to the role of facet injury as a cause of back pain following minor trauma.[58,59] Facet injection is often done to relieve back pain without objective diagnosis of traumatic lesion. Subtle facet fractures can rarely be identified on CT scans early in the course of injury. They appear like any other fracture. They have sharp borders with no sclerotic edges (Fig. 4-43). More often CT scans are done well after minor trauma, and the acute fracture can not be diagnosed. Often, smooth "ossicles" are identified in association with the articular processes. These have previously been attributed to congenital accessory ossification centers of articular processes. It some instances it is likely that that is correct. In many instances it is more likely that these ossicles are actually *ununited* stress fractures of the articular processes.

INJURY TO THE SPINAL CORD AND NEURAL STRUCTURES.

The advent of the MRI scanner has revolutionized the diagnosis of lesions of the spinal cord and central nerve roots. The spinal cord should be clearly visualized on all MRI scans. Fast spin echo or gradient echo axial images (where cerebral spinal fluid {CSF} is made white) allow direct visualization of the intrathecal nerve roots and their extension peripherally through the neural foramina. It is rarely necessary to perform myelography on spinal injured patients. The procedure should be confined to that small subset of patients with pacemakers and some metallic implants or those with extraordinary claustrophobia. The combination of noncontrast CT and MRI nearly always precludes the need for contrast studies. Perhaps the only absolute indication for myelography is the localization of CSF leak where surgical correction is contemplated.

The MRI appearance of the injured spinal cord is well known.[60–68] It is possible to differentiate acute intramedullary hemorrhage from cord swelling. The contused spinal cord without well-defined central cord hematoma is usually normal on T1-weighted images

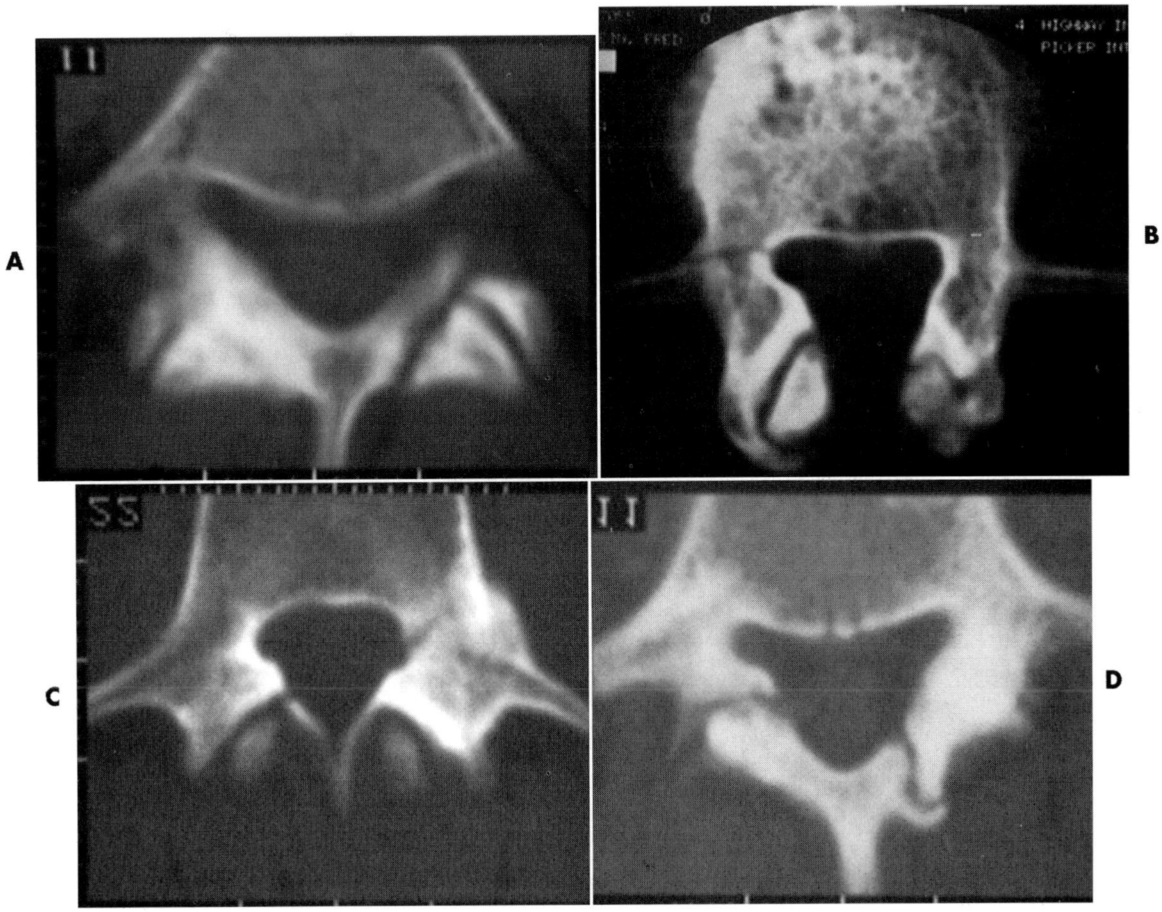

FIGURE 4-41

Stress fractures of the neural arch other than through the pars interarticularis axial CT scans. **A**, Unilateral spiral stress fracture of the lamina. **B**, Unilateral stress fracture through the pedicle. **C**, Healed retrosomatic stress fracture. **D**, Pars defect on the right and retroisthmic defect on the left. This is clearly a pseudarthrosis with callous and not a congenital anomaly.

and bright on T2-weighted scan. Central cord hemorrhage is difficult to identify acutely on T1-weighted images. In the immediate posttrauma period, hyperacute blood appears isointense to cord and is difficult to identify. Within several days, however, recent hemorrhage becomes more obvious. Fresh blood becomes bright on both T1- and T2-weighted sequences (Fig. 4-44). There is also be a zone of swelling surrounding the hemorrhage, which is bright on T2-weighted images. Within several weeks hemosiderin deposition occurs. This may occasionally be identifiable on T2-weighted images as a zone of low signal around the clot. With the passage of time, localized clots liquefy and are ultimately seen as a pool of water in the spinal cord. These posttraumatic cysts appear low in signal on T1-weighted images and bright on T2-weighted scans (Fig. 4-45 A and B). One of the common, treatable causes of delayed, increasing neurological deficit is expansion of an intramedullary cyst or syrinx.[69] Drainage of the cyst with or without shunting is a frequently performed procedure (Fig. 4-45 C). The shunts can be identified within the cord and should not be misdiagnosed as areas of old hemorrhage.

PITFALL

The presence of a cyst within the spinal cord on a scan following minor trauma in neurologically intact patients does not mean that there was a spinal cord hematoma. Not all localized fluid pools within the spinal cord are caused by trauma. Furthermore, it is extraordinarily unlikely for there to be an intramedullary lesion without immediate, obvious neurologic dysfunction.

The severely injured spinal cord may undergo progressive deterioration with increase in neurological

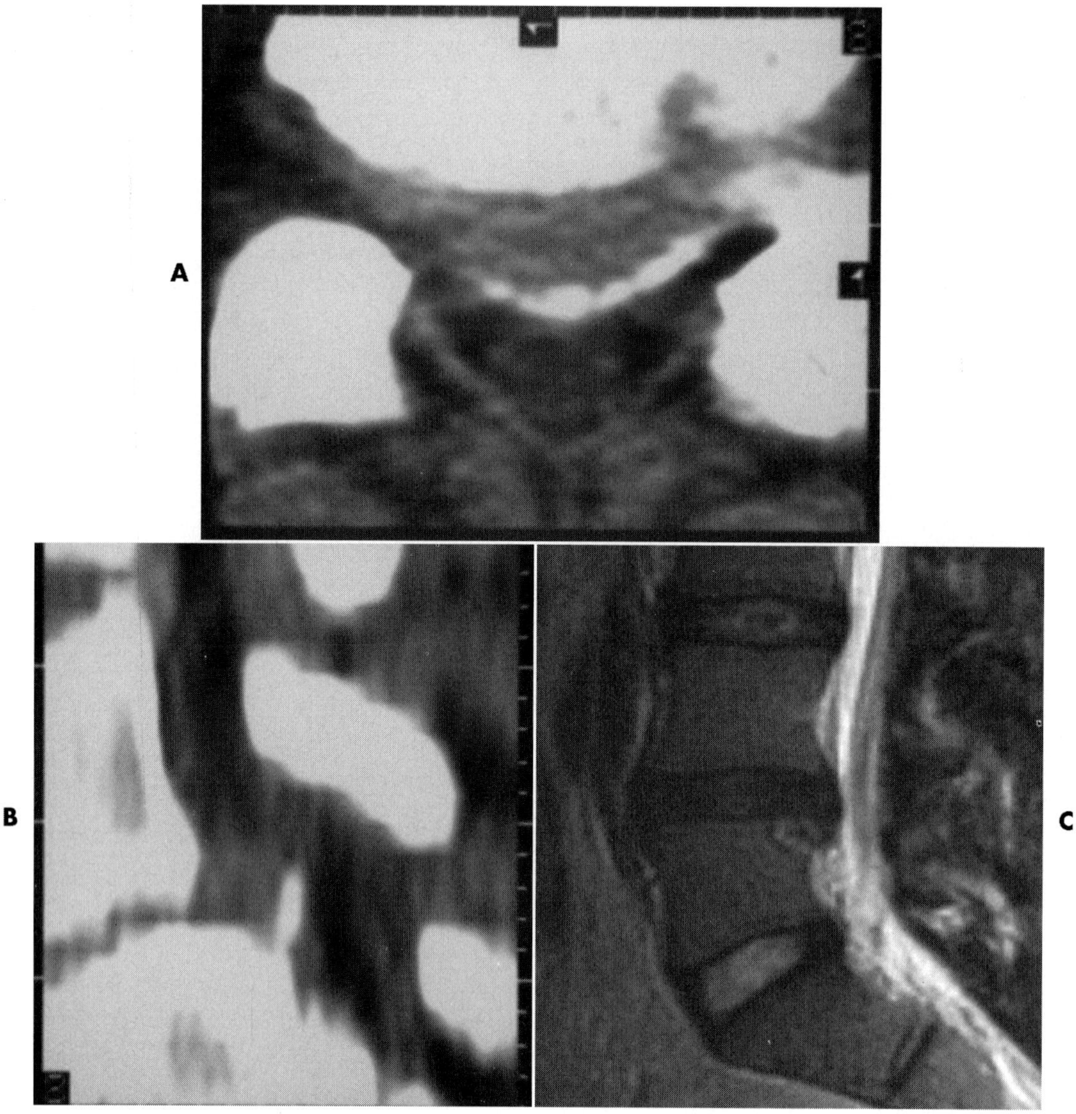

FIGURE 4-42

Posterior limbus vertebra. **A**, Soft tissue axial CT scan and **B**, Sagittal CT reformation, demonstrating disc herniation with separation of the posterior apophyseal ring. **C**, T2-weighted sagittal MRI scan on another similar patient. Note the bright signal anterior to the separated apophyseal ring fragment.

deficit without cyst formation. The continuum of deterioration has been termed progressive posttraumatic myelomalacic myelopathy.[70,71,72] The pathology varies from intrinsic gliosis to a condition in which innumerable very small unshuntable cysts form at the site of injury. These are seen as areas of abnormal MRI signal on T1- and T2-weighted scans in a spinal cord with indistinct edges.

The severely injured spinal cord may ultimately atrophy. The diminutive cord is easily identified on MRI or high-quality CT scans (Fig. 4-46 A). Cord transection can be diagnosed as well. Generally, there is significant intradural bleeding adding to the complexity of the images (Fig. 4-46 B).

While it is intellectually pleasing to differentiate the various types of intramedullary trauma, there is little clinical relevance as it is impossible at this time to intervene surgically if a localized intramedullary clot is present. It is, however, important to differentiate intramedullary from extramedullary clot, which can be surgically removed.

Subdural and epidural hematomas may be seen in cases of blunt trauma as well as penetrating wounds but can also occur spontaneously in patients with coagulopathies. Bleeding into the epidural space occurs more frequently than subdural hematoma. On CT scans, epidural hematomas are well-demarcated, high-density lesions with biconvex edges, which border the

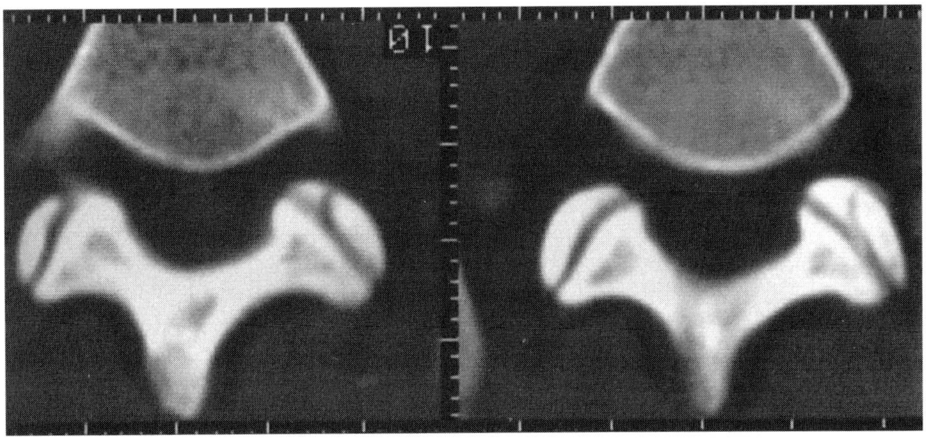

FIGURE 4-43

Axial CT scan performed several days following the acute onset of severe back pain following a gymnastic routine. Acute fracture of the articular process is seen. (From Rothman SLG and Glenn WV *Multiplanar CT of the spine*, Baltimore, 1985, University Park Press)

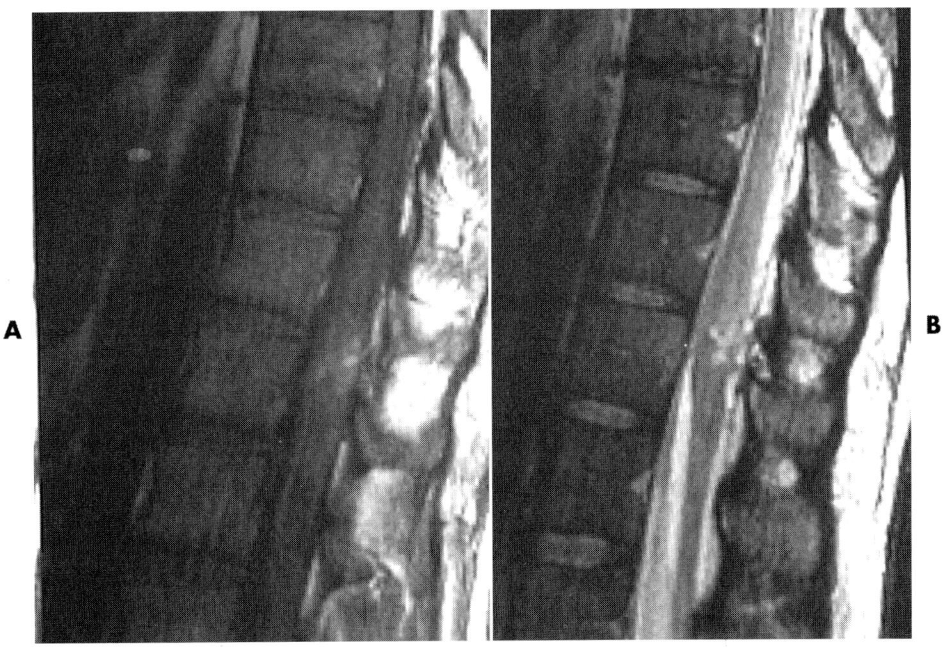

FIGURE 4-44

Acute cord hemorrhage caused by bullet wound. **A**, Sagittal T1-weighted and **B**, Sagittal T2-weighted MRI scans demonstrate high signal blood within the swollen conus medularis.

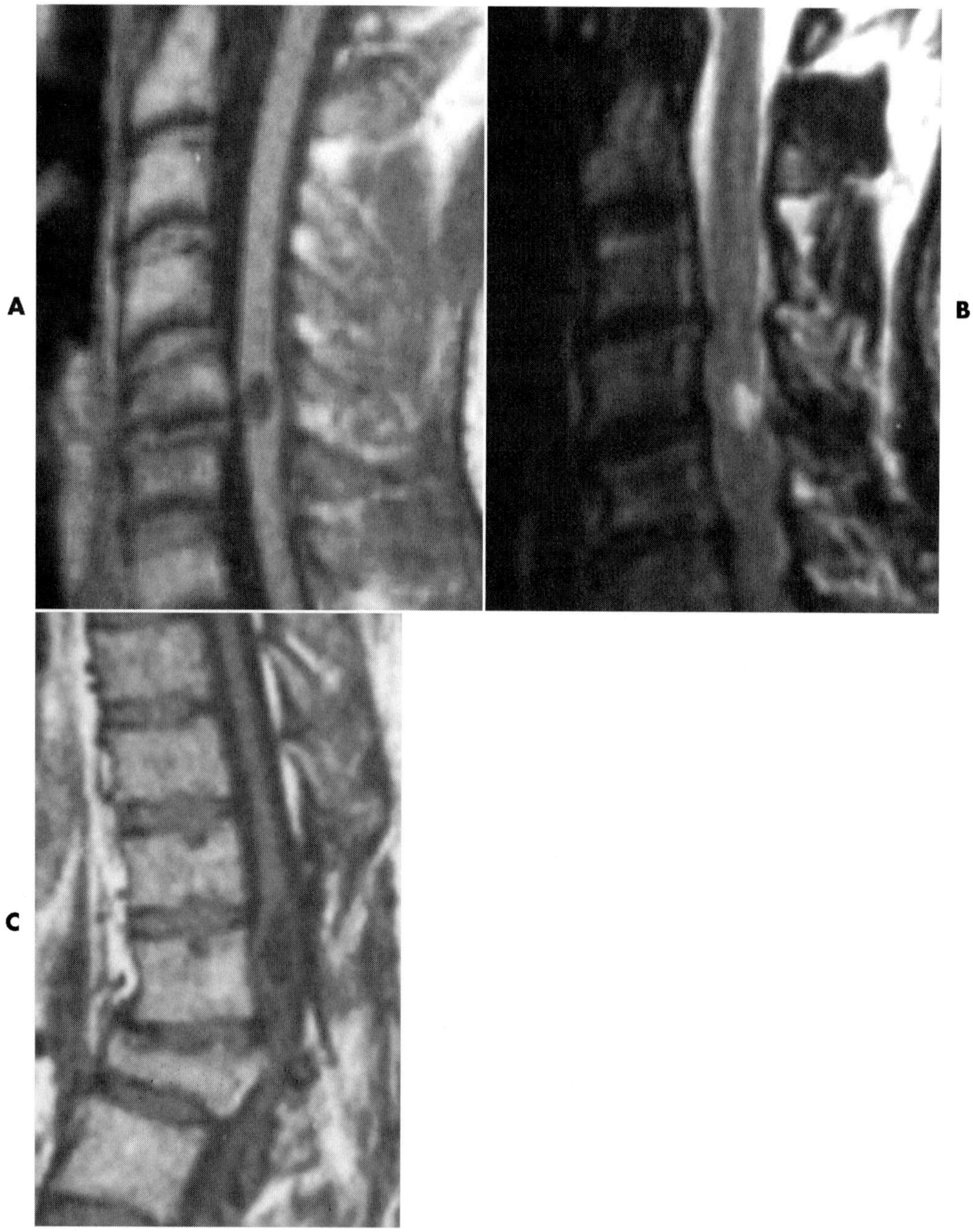

FIGURE 4-45

Posttraumatic intramedullary cyst. **A**, Sagittal T1-weighted and **B**, T2-weighted MRI scans revealing an intramedullary cyst, which has decreased signal on the T1 and increased signal on the T2-weighted scans. **C**, Intramedullary expanding cyst in a patient with increasing neurologic deficit 6 months following spinal injury.

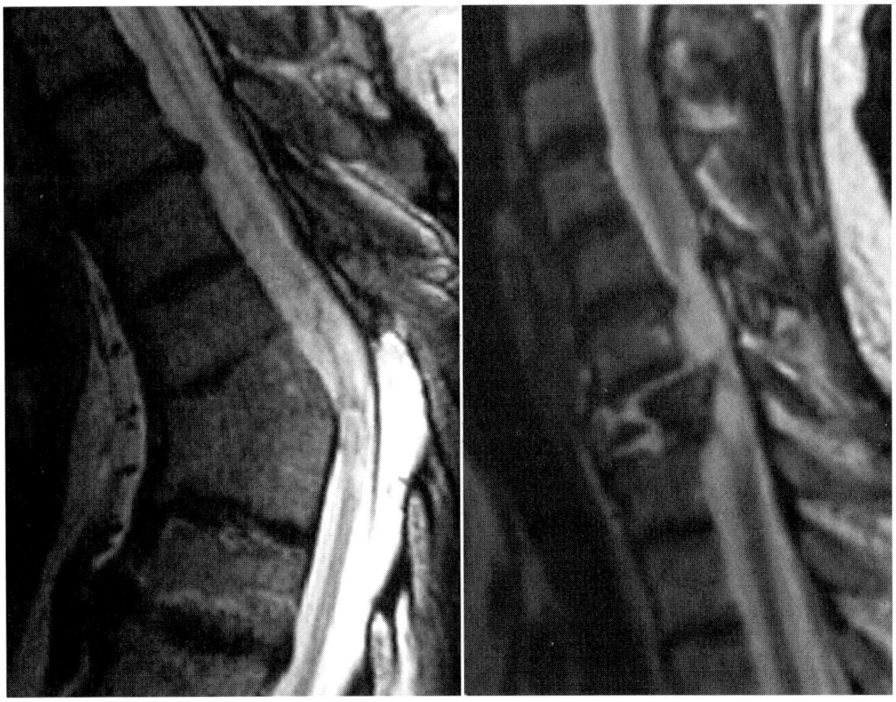

FIGURE 4-46

Posttraumatic atrophy. **A**, T2-weighted MRI scan reveals marked atrophy of the thoracic cord at the level of the healed fracture. **B**, Spinal cord transection. Sagittal T2-weighted MRI scan reveals fracture dislocation at C7 with complete cord transection.

bony spinal canal.[73,74,75] Cerebrospinal fluid and the spinal cord appear lower in density than the more peripheral clot. An MRI scan defines a linear fluid collection with tapering upper and lower margins (Fig. 4-47). The signal characteristics of intraspinal clots develop over time similarly to those seen in intracranial hemorrhage. Subdural hematomas are located within the thecal sac and are separated from the epidural fat and bony neural arch.[76] Very low signal within the clot on T2-weighted sequences is caused by the presence of deoxyhemoglobin and makes the diagnosis of extramedullary clot obvious. On occasion prominent subarachnoid hemorrhage can be seen in the spine. Subarachnoid hemorrhage can produce CT images that look like postmyelographic scans because the bloody CSF acts as a contrast agent. The spinal cord may appear lower in density than the surrounding CSF (Fig. 4-48).

Traction injuries to the upper extremities may cause avulsion of one or more roots of the brachial plexus. This causes a flaccid upper extremity. The diagnosis can be made on axial MR images. The thecal sac appears wider on the side of the avulsion, and the lateral gutter of the sac is empty. The nerve roots that are generally easy to identify are missing. Often there is extension of a dural pouch out beyond the neural foramen (Fig. 4-49). Avulsion of the lumbar roots is rare.

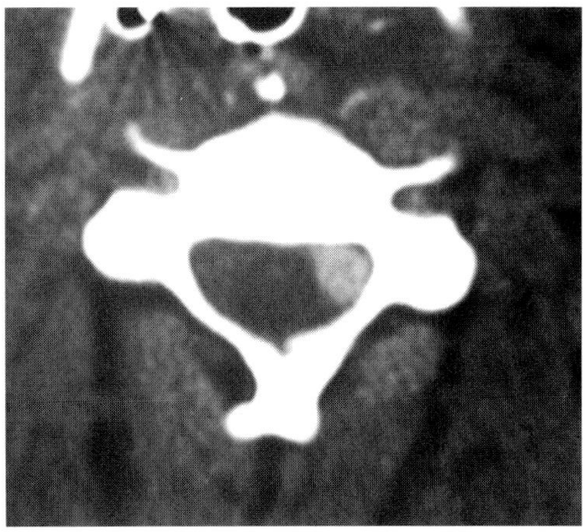

FIGURE 4-47

A patient with epidural hematoma; CT scan demonstrates the high density blood adjacent to the bone.

PENETRATING WOUNDS OF THE SPINE

Penetrating trauma of the spine may cause any of the severe spinal cord lesions described in the previous section. Generally, MRI scanning is the procedure of choice for the evaluation of these lesions. Lead bullet fragments produce disturbing artifacts on CT scans but rarely detract from the image quality of an MRI scan.

Such MRI scans may be disturbingly normal for patients with nonferromagnetic materials in the body. Figure 4-50 demonstrates a very striking example of this phenomenon. Note that the MRI scan is normal while the routine radiograph reveals the presence of more than 50 metalic pieces of shot within the neck.

It is unusual for blunt trauma to cause vascular injury although vertebral or carotid artery disection has been reported with twisting and shearing injuries. It is common, however, for the major vessels to be lacerated by bullets and knives (Fig. 4-51).[77] The evaluation of penetrating wounds of the neck may require emergency carotid and vertebral arteriography. The most important abnormalities demonstrated by angiography are acute active hemorrhage; vascular occlusion, pseudoaneurysm, and arteriovenous fistula formation.

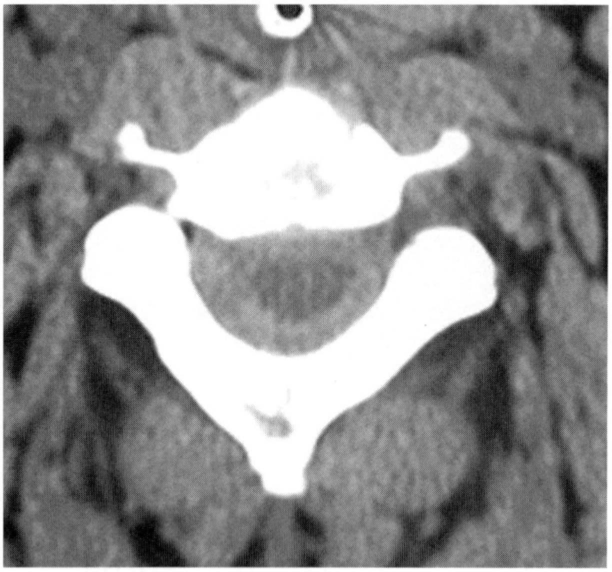

FIGURE 4-48

Subarachnoid hemorrhage. High-density blood totally surrounds the spinal cord within the thecal sac.

THE MEDICAL-LEGAL CLAIM OF SPINAL INJURY

Claims of spinal injury following minor accidents fill the courts of the land. Aggressive attorneys have created an industry with their claims of spinal injury based on poor science and pseudoscience. While it is true that many people involved in falls, automobile accidents and other mishaps do develop back pain following trauma, the contention that these clinical syndromes are caused by lesions of the intervertebral disk is often false. The literature is very clear that disk disease is extremely common in the normal population.[78–85] It is also clear that disk protrusion may be a degenerative disorder of the spine and can be seen in a large portion of asymptomatic individuals. Why has this fact escaped so many plaintiff "experts"? A superficial perusal of any text book of radiology, orthopedics, or neurosurgery reveals that the discussion of disk herniation resides in the chapter on degenerative disk disease and not trauma. Ferooznia and coworkers specifically stated in

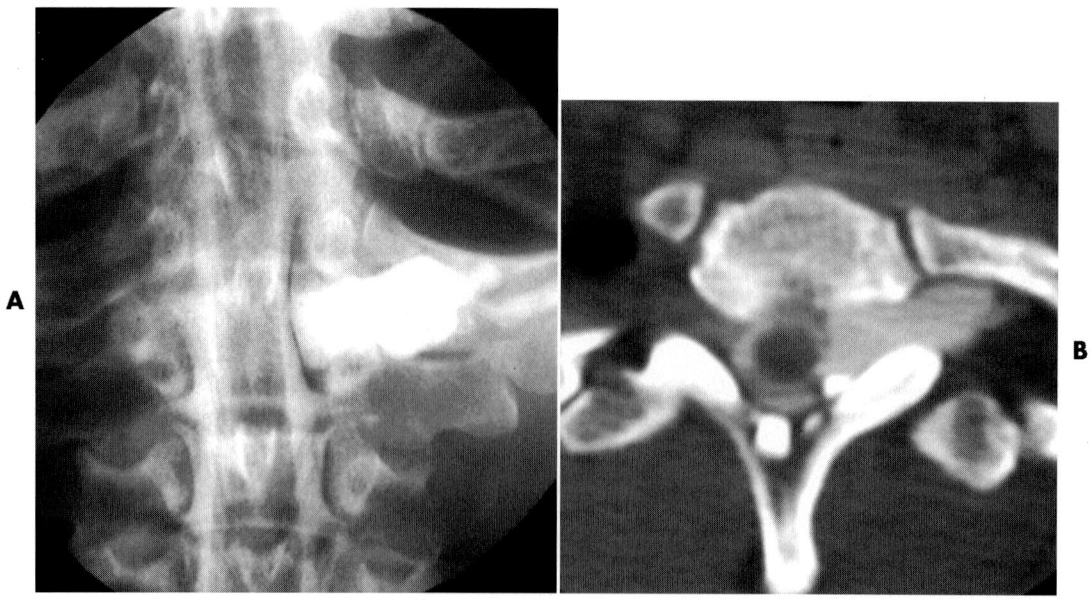

FIGURE 4-49

Traumatic meningocele and avulsion of one of the roots of the brachial plexus. **A**, Frontal myelogram shows an abnormal dural pouch at the site of the tear. Post myelographic CT scan **B** shows the pouch to be void of nerve roots.

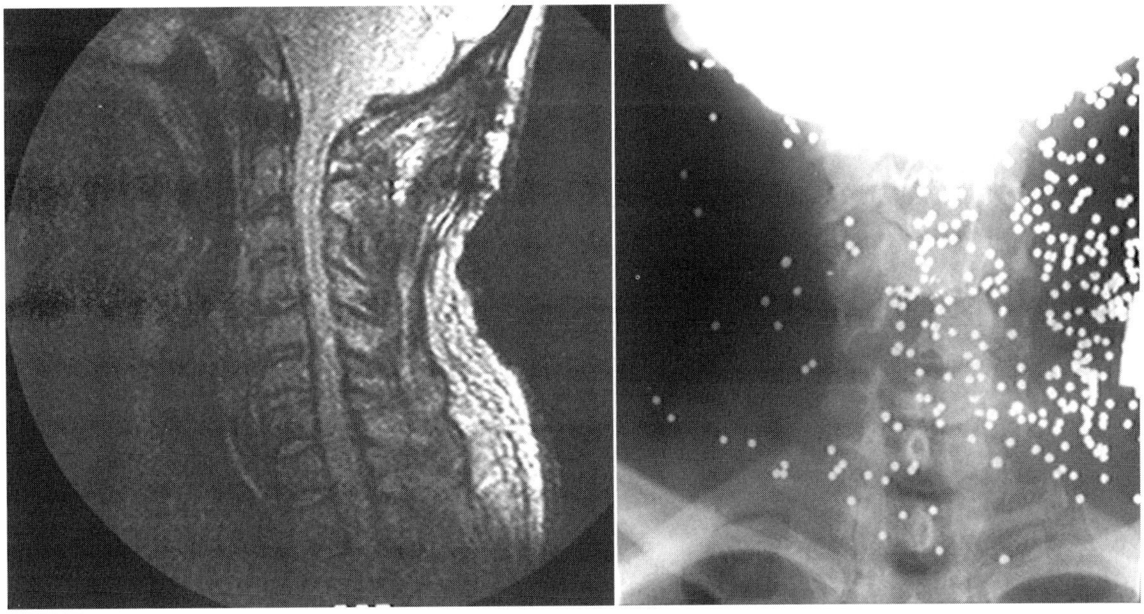

FIGURE 4-50

Shotgun wound of the neck. MRI scan **A** is normal. Routine radiograph of the neck **B** demonstrates innumerable radioopaque foreign bodies.

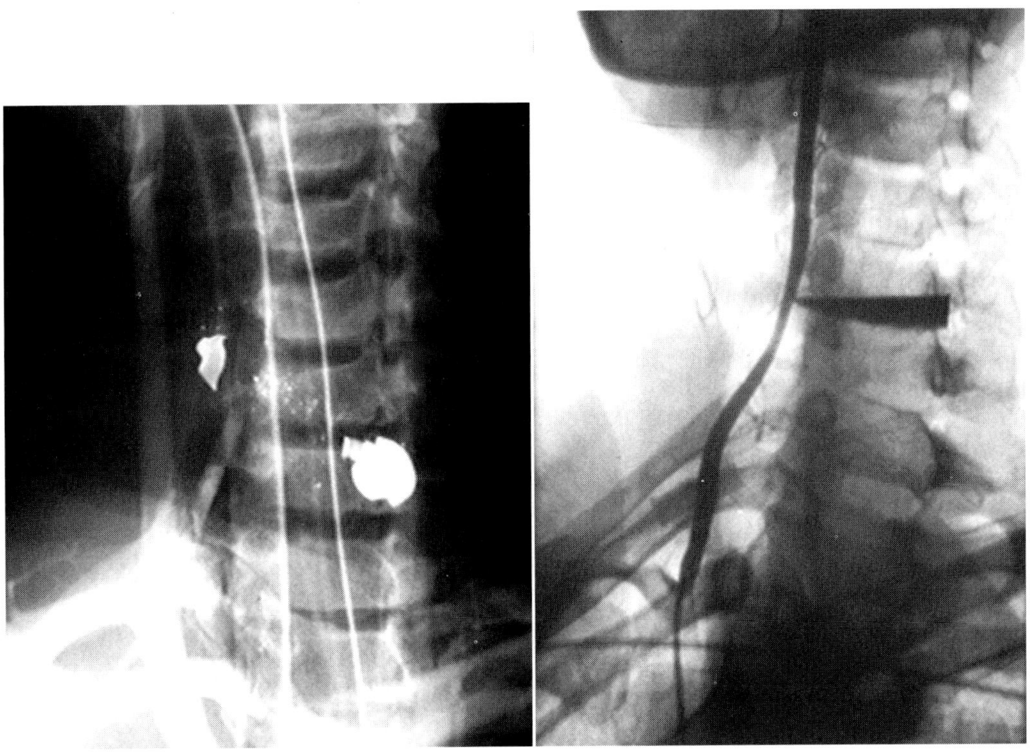

FIGURE 4-51

Penetrating trauma. **A**, Bullet wound to the neck with vertebral artery occlusion noted on an aortogram. **B**, Knife wound to the spine. Arteriography shows that the point of the blade is indenting the vertebral artery and causing some spasm, but the vessel is not occluded.

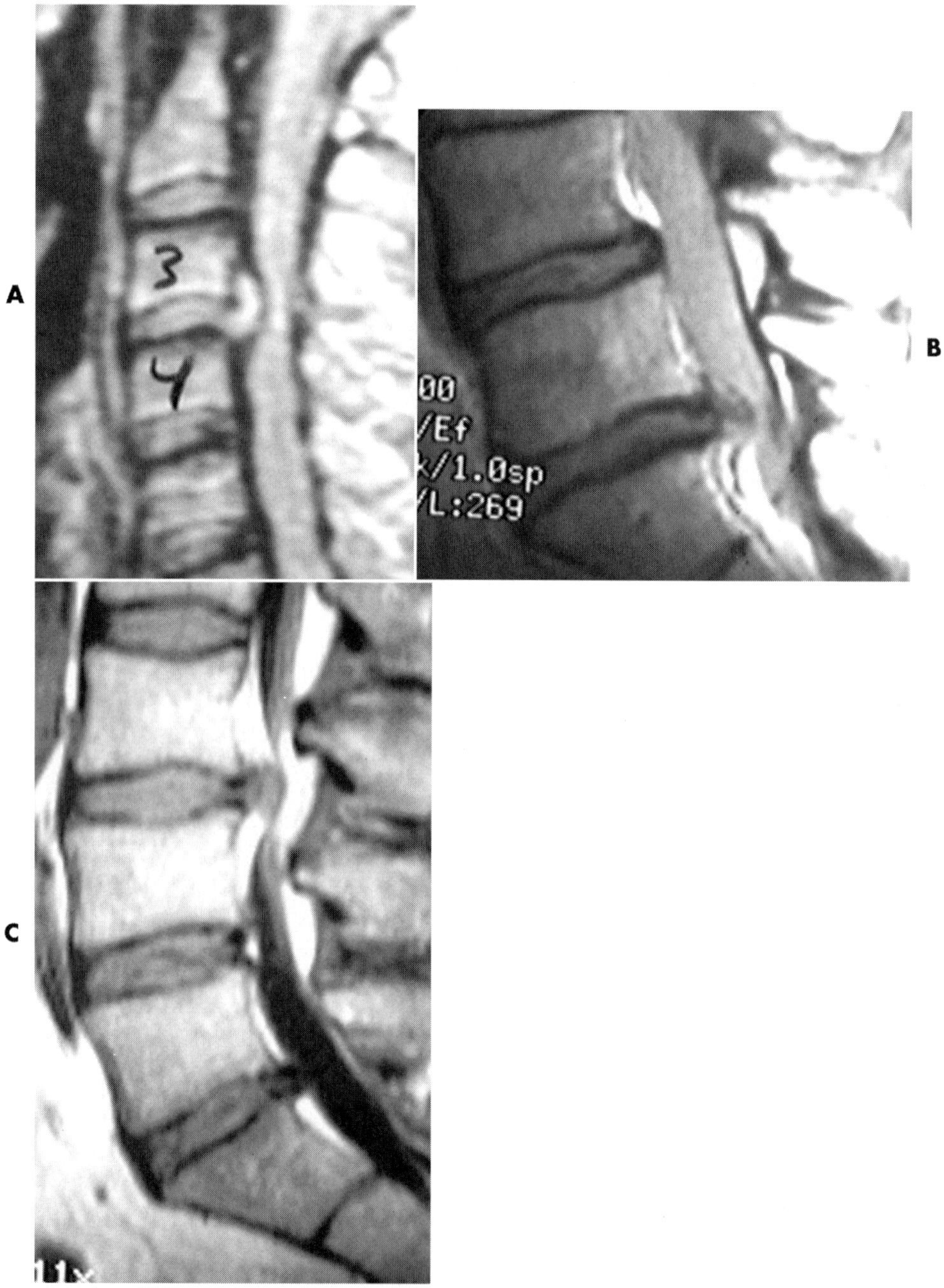

Figure 4-52

Acute and chronic disc herniation. **A**, Sagittal MRI scan of the cervical spine reveals an acute C3-C4 soft tissue disc herniation. Note that the signal within the extruded fragment is much brighter than the disc from which it came. Sagittal MRI scan of the lumbar spine **B** reveals a bright signal acute disc herniation. Contrast enhanced T1-weighted sagittal MRI **C** scan on another patient with an acute disc herniation at L3-L4 and chronic herniation or protrusion at L5-S1. Note the enhancement in the epidural space around the bright signal soft tissue herniation. The signal in the chronic protrusion is low.

their series that of 256 surgically proved disk herniations none were caused by trauma.[86] Previously uninjured individuals, however, can suffer an injury, undergo a scan, and have a diagnosis of disk herniation.

It is very difficult to cause an acute disk herniation in the laboratory without fracturing the adjacent bone. Many experiments have demonstrated that compression trauma fractures the vertebra before it ruptures the disk. Flexion compression force does not cause acute herniation without bony injury.[87–92] Farfan has demonstrated the importance of torsion in the development of disk degeneration, but acute disc herniation was not caused by pure rotational forces.[93,94] Hyperextension ruptures the anterior longitudinal ligament or fracture the articular processes rather than herniate the nucleus into the spinal canal. Only recently Gordon and coworkers showed that producing an acute disk herniation required the simultaneous action of flexion, compression, and torque.[87] It is difficult to produce these forces in the spine of a completely restrained person in a car crash. As of this writing, the author could find no papers in the English language literature in the Medline computer that document acute lumbar disk herniations in restrained persons in automobile accidents. There remains an obligation for clinicians who are caring for patients with back pain following an accident to perform imaging studies, usually MRI scans. This must be done to rule out other potentially serious conditions and to identify possible causes of pain.

It is clear in the literature that the incidence of abnormal disks, disk protrusions, and chronic disk herniation is very high in the general population. In normal teenagers, the incidence of MRI diagnosable disk degeneration has been reported as being as high as 26%.[95] Disk herniation runs in families.[96] The relative risk of developing a lumbar disk change before the age of 21 is estimated to be approximately 5 times greater in patients with a family history of disk herniation than their matched controls.

The abnormal disks seen on imaging studies may have been caused by an accident because the patients were asymptomatic prior to the incident and became symptomatic following the incident. That position is better supported if the imaging studies show changes of acute spinal injury such as ligamentous tear, disk disruption, and acute nuclear herniation. If imaging studies show low intradiskal signal, chronic disk protrusion, bony ridging, and other signs of chronic disk disease, it is more difficult to support the diagnosis of acute traumatic disk injury.

If the incidence of abnormal disks in 40-year-old asymptomatic people is 50%, it becomes difficult to conclude that a patient's back pain is related to visibly abnormal disks unless it is an isolated, single abnormality. While it is certainly possible for a patient to have back pain following an accident, and it is possible that the pain is coming from the intervertebral disk, it is not justifiable to state that MRI or CT alone confirms that diagnosis. Some believe that a localized area of bright signal within the disk on T2-weighted scans correlates with painful disks on diskography; yet, even in their series, 14% of patients had intradiskal bright signal with no back pain.[97,98] Furthermore, even in patients who complain of true radicular signs following trauma, the possibility remains that any visualized lateral disk herniation or bony ridge was present prior to the accident. If the patient's symptoms appear related to the injury, they would likely be caused by traction irritation of the nerve root adjacent to the injured disk or bone.

Acute disk herniations appear brighter on MR images than uninjured disk (Fig. 4-52).[99–102] This is likely caused by the accumulation of inflammatory cells at the periphery of the nuclear fragment.[103,104] The farther away a nuclear fragment migrates from the disk the more likely it brightens on MRI, and even brighten more so following gadolinium infusion.[105] Acute disk herniations with high signal tend to disappear over time.

Chronic disk protrusions generally have the same signal as the intact disk. One should never presume that a disk protrusion with low signal similar to the parent disc is an acute lesion. A disk herniation or protrusion that is isointense or of lower intensity than the uninjured disk is almost certainly a chronic disc herniation regardless of symptoms before the injury. The fact that the disc herniation is chronic in no way suggests that the patient should not be appropriately compensated for pain. The amount of compensation may be lower, however, than if the injury produced a true, acute disabling herniation. The factors producing symnptoms after vehicular trauma are described in the appropriate Chapters. There are many anatomic explanations for pain, and the practitioner must consider all factors, not only the results of imaging studies, before reaching conclusions on causation.

CONCLUSION

Radiological diagnosis of traumatic lesions of the spine is a precise and logical science. Abnormalities that are demonstrated on various imaging studies depend on the forces generated by the trauma. They fall into well-recognized patterns. The most important pitfalls result from carelessness of technique and sloppy thinking. The treating physician must never settle for poor or inadequate plane scan images. Computed tomographic scans must be made with thin sections and resulting data reformatted into a complete set of sagittal and coronal views. Any MRI scans should be obtained from the best possible machines with the smallest fields of view and with T1- and T2-weighted sequences.

One must know what normal is! Imaging studies on most uninjured people do show some abnormalities. Radiographic, CT, and MRI studies are only part of the diagnostic picture.

ACKNOWLEDGEMENT

I would like to acknowledge the contributions of the past and present surgical staff of the spinal injury service of Rancho Los Amigos Hospital. Over the past 11 years they have taught me to think like a surgeon. Special thanks goes to my soulmate and friend Dr. Jack Zigler, one of the smartest and most dedicated spine surgeons I have ever met.

REFERENCES

1. Gehweiler JAJ, Osborne RL, Becker RF: *The radiology of vertebral trauma*, Philadelphia, 1980, WB Saunders.
2. Harris JH Jr, Edeiken-Monroe, B: *The radiology of acute cervical spine trauma*, ed 2, Baltimore, 1987, Williams & Wilkins.
3. Glenn WV Jr, Rothman SLG, Rhodes ML: Computed tomography/multiplanar reformatted (CT/MPR) examination of the spine. In Genant HK, Chafetz NI, Helms CA, editors: *Computed tomography of the lumbar spine*, San Francisco, 1982, University of California.
4. Rothman SLG, Glenn WV Jr: *Multiplanar CT of the spine*, Baltimore, 1985, University Park Press.
5. Olsen WL, Chakeres DW, Berry I, Richaud J: Spine and spinal cord trauma. In Manelfe C editor: *Imaging of the spine and spinal cord*, New York, 1992, Raven Press. p. 407–444.
6. Kalender W, Polacin A, Marchal G, Baert AL: Current status and new perspectives in spiral CT. In Felix R, Langer M, editors: *Advances in CT II*, Berlin, 1992, Spiringer-Verlag.
7. Berry I, Sigal R, Lebas J, Mark AS, Le Bihan D: Magnetic resonance imaging: principles, techniques, and imaging protocols. In Manelfe C, editor: *Imaging of the spine and spinal cord*, New York, 1992, Raven Press.
8. Gerlock AJ, Mirfakhraee M, Benzel EC: Computed tomography of traumatic atlantooccipital dislocation, *Neurosurgery*, 13:316–319, 1983.
9. Zigler J, Waters R, Perry J: Occipito-cervical dislocation with survival treatment with occipito-cervico-thoracic spine fusion, *Spine*, 11:645–646, 1986.
10. Noble ER, Smoker WRK: The forgotten condyle: the appearance, morphology, and classification of occipital condyle fractures, *Am J Neuroradiology*, 17:507–523, 1996.
11. Clayman DA, Sykes, CH Vines FS. Occipital condyle fractures: clinical presentation and radiologic detection, *Am J Neuroradiology* 15:1309–1315, 1994.
12. Levine AM editor: Occipital cranial injuries. In *Orthopaedic knowledge update trauma*, Chicago, 1995, American Academy of Orthopaedic Surgeons, p 311–322.
13. Levine AM, Edwards CC: Fractures of the atlas, *J Bone Joint Surg*, 73A:680–691, 1991.
14. Levine AM, Edwards CC: Traumatic lesions of the occipitoatlantoaxial complex, *Clin Orthop* 239–253, 1989.
15. Shapiro R, Youngberg AS, Rothman SLG: The differential diagnosis of traumatic lesions of the occipito-atlanto-axial segment, *Radiol Clin North Am*, 3:505, 1973.
16. Hinck VC, Hopkins CE: Measurement of the atlanto-dental interval in the adult, *Amer J Radiol*, 84:945–951, 1960.
17. Locke GR, Gardner JL, VanEpps EP: Atlas dens interval in children. A survey based on 200 normal cervical spines, *Amer J Radiol*, 97:135–40, 1966.
18. Anderson LD, D'Alonzo RT: Fractures of the odontoid process of the atlas. *J Bone Joint Surg*, 56A:1663–1674, 1974.
19. Levine AM editor: Fractures of the axis. In *Orthopaedic knowledge update trauma*. Chicago, 1995, American Academy of Orthopaedic Surgeons, p 323–328.
20. Clark CR, White AA: Fractures of the dens: a multicenter study, *J Bone Joint Surg*, 67A:1340–1348, 1985.
21. Ehara S, el-Khoury GY, Clark CR: Radiologic evaluation of dens fractures: role of plain radiography and tomography; *Spine*, 17:475–479, 1992.
22. Wackenheim A: *Roentgen diagnosis of the craniovertebral region*. Berlin, 1974, Springer-Verlag.
23. Von Torklus D, Gehle W: *The upper cervical spine*, New York, 1972, Grune & Stratton.
24. McRae DL: *Craniovertebral junction*. In Newton TH, Potts, DG, editors: Radiology of the skull and brain, vol 1, book 1, St. Louis, 1971, Mosby–Year Book.
25. Gehweiler JA J, Osborne RL, Becker RF: *The radiology of vertebral trauma*, Philadelphia, 1980, WB Saunders.
26. Rothman SLG, Chafetz NI: *The radiological distinction between congenital os odontoideum and post-traumatic pseudoarthrosis of the dens*. Presented at American Society of Neuroradiology meeting, Nashville TN, May (3-7), 1994.
27. Levine AM, Edwards CC: The management of traumatic spondylolisthesis of the axis, *J Bone Joint Surg*, 67A:217–226, 1985.
28. Alan BL Jr, Ferguson RL: Lehmann TR, O'Brien RP: A mechanistic classification of closed, indirect fractures and dislocations of the lower cervical spine, *Spine*, 7:1–27, 1982.

29. Davis SJ, Teresi LM, Bradley WG Jr, et al: Cervical spine hyperextension injuries: MR findings, *Radiology,* 180:245–251, 1991.
30. Robertson PA, Ryan MD: Neurological deteriorization after reduction of cervical subluxation: Mechanical compression by disc tissue, *J Bone Joint Surg,* 74B:224–227, 1992.
31. White AA III, Panjabi MM, editors: *Clinical biomechanics of the spine,* ed 2, Philadelphia, 1990, JB Lippincott.
32. Yablon IG, Palumbo M, Spatz E, et al: Nerve root recovery in complete injuries of the cervical spine, *Spine,* 10 (suppl):S518–S521, 1991.
33. Reymond RD, Wheeler PS, Perovic M, Block B: The lucent cleft, a new radiologic sign of cervical disc injury, *Clin Radiol,* 23:188–192, 1972.
34. Resnick D, Niwayama G, Guerra J, et al: Spinal vacuum phenomena: anatomical study and review, *Radiology,* 139:341–348, 1981.
35. Jonsson H Jr, Bring G, Rauschning W, Sahlstedt B: Hidden cervical spine injuries in traffic accident victims with skull fracture, *J Spinal Disorders,* 4:251–263, 1991.
36. Taylor JR, Twomey LT: Acute injuries to the cervical joints: an autopsy study of neck sprain, *Spine,* 18:1115–1122, 1993.
37. Vines FS: The significance of "occult" fractures of the cervical spine, *Amer J Radiol,* 107:493, 1969.
38. Kattan KR, Pais MJ: Some borderlands of the cervical spine. Part 2: The subtle and hidden abnormal, *Skeletal Radiol,* 8:7–12, 1982.
39. Zigler JE, Capen DA, Rothman SLG: Spinal disease in the aged. *Clin Orthop,* 316:70–79, 1995.
40. McAfee PC, Yuan HA, Fredrickson BE, Lubicky JP: The value of computed tomography in thoracolumbar fractures: An analysis of one hundred consecutive cases and a new classification, *J Bone Joint Surg,* 65A:461–473, 1983.
41. Denis F: The three column spine and its significance in the classification of acute thoracolumbar spinal injuries, *Spine,* 8:817–831, 1983.
42. Schmidt H, Freyschmidt J: *Borderlands of normal and early pathologic findings in skeletal radiography,* Stuttgart, 1993, Georg Theime Verlag.
43. Datz FL, Patch GG, Arias JM, Morton KA: Nuclear medicine a teaching file. St. Louis, 1992, Mosby–Year Book.
44. O'Callaghan JP, Ullrich CG, Yuan HA, Kieffer SA: CT of facet distraction in flexion injuries of the thoracolumbar spine: the "naked" facet; *Am J Neuroradiology,* 1:97–102, 1980.
45. Manaster BJ, Osborn AG: CT patterns of facet fracture dislocation in the thoracolumbar region, *Amer J Radiol,* 148:335–340, 1987.
46. O'Callaghan JP, Ulgrich CG, Yuan HA, Keiffer SA: CT of facet distraction in flexion injuries of the thoracolumbar spine: the "naked" facet, *Amer J Radiol,* 134:563–568, 1980.
47. Edelson JG, Nathan H: Stages in the natural history of the vertebral end-plates, *Spine,* 13:21–22, 1988.
48. Lindahl S, Willen J, Nordwall A, Irstam L: The crush cleavage fracture. A new thoracolumbar unstable fracture, *Spine,* 8:559–569, 1983.
49. Scapinelli R, Candiotto S: Spontaneous **remodeling** of the spinal canal after burst fractures of the lower thoracic and lumbar regions, *J Spinal Disorders,* 8:486–493, 1995.
50. Ha KI, Han SH, Chung M, Yung GK: A clinical study of the natural remodeling of burst fractures of the lumbar spine, *Clin Orthop,* 323:210–214, 1996.
51. Chance GQ: Note on a type of flexion fracture of the spine, *Br J Radiol,* 21:452–453, 1948.
52. Wiltse LL: Fatigue fracture: the basic lesion in isthmic spondylolisthesis, *J Bone Joint Surg,* 57A:17–22, 1975.
53. Wiltse LL, Rothman SLG: Lumbar and lumbosacral spondylolisthesis. In Weisel SW, Weinstein JN, Herkowitz, H, et al, editor: *The lumbar spine, ed* 2, Philadelphia, 1996, WB Saunders.
54. Rothman SLG, Glenn WV Jr: CT multiplanar reconstruction in 253 cases of lumbar spondylolysis, *Am J Neuroradiology* 5:81–90, 1984.
55. Rothman SLG, Glenn, WV Jr: *Multiplanar CT of the spine,* Baltimore, 1985, University Park Press.
56. Henales V, Hervas JA, Lopez P, et al: Intervertebral disc herniations (limbus vertebrae) in pediatric patients: report of 15 cases, *Pediatr Rad,* 23:608–610, 1993.
57. Albeck MJ, Madsen FF, Wagner A, Gjerris F: Fracture of the lumbar vertebral ring apophysis imitating disc herniation, *Acta Neurochir,* 113:52–56, 1991.
58. Carette S, Marcoux S, Truchon R, et al: A controlled trial of corticosteroid injections into facet joints for chronic low back pain, *N Engl J Med,* 325:1002–1007, 1992.
59. Carrera GF: Lumbar facet arthrography and injection in low back pain, *Wisconsin Med J,* 78:35–37, 1979.
60. Maravilla KR, Cohen WA: *MRI atlas of the spine,* New York, 1991, Raven Press.
61. Kulkarni MV, McCardle CB, Kopanicky D: Acute spinal cord injury: MR imaging at 1.5T, *Radiology,* 164:837–43, 1987.
62. Chakeres DW, Flickinger F, Bresnahan JC, et al: MR imaging of acute spinal cord injury, *Am J Neuroradiology* 8:5–10, 1987.
63. Fox JL, Wener L, Drennan DC, et al: Central spinal cord injury: magnetic resonance imaging conformation and operative considerations, *Neurosurgery,* 22:340–347, 1988.
64. Hackney DB, Asato R, Joseph P, et al: Hemorrhage and edema in acute spinal cord compression: demonstration by MR imaging, *Radiology,* 61:387–390, 1986.
65. Kalfas I, Wilberger J, Croldberg A, Pvostko ER: Magnetic resonance imaging in acute spinal cord trauma, *Neurosurgery,* 23:295–299, 1988.

66. Mathis JM, Wilson JT, Bernard JW, Zelenik ME: MR imaging of spinal cord avulsion, *Am J Neuroradiology* 9:1232–1233, 1988.
67. Quencer RM: Imaging of spinal cord trauma. In *Catagorial course spine and cord imaging*. Chicago, 1988, American Society of Neuroradiology.
68. Quencer RM, Sheldon JJ, Donovan-Post MJ, et al: MRI of the chronically injured cervical spinal cord, *Amer J Radiol,* 147:125–132, 1986.
69. Cohen WA, Young W, DeCrescito V, et al: Posttraumatic syrinx formation: experimental study, *Am J Neuroradiology* 6:823–827, 1985.
70. Gebarski SS, Maynard FW, Gabrielson TO, et al: Posttruamatic progressive myelopathy: clinical and radiological correlation using MR imaging, delayed CT metrizamide myelography, and intraoperative sonography, *Radiology*, 157:359–385, 1985.
71. Falcone S, Quencer RM, Green BA, et al: Progressive posttraumatic myelomalacic myelopathy: imaging and clinical features, *Am J Neuroradiology* 15:747–754, 1994.
72. Marshall LF, Knowlton S, Garfin SR, et al: Deterioration following spinal cord injury. A multicenter study, *J. Neurosurg,* 66:400–404, 1987.
73. Gundru CR, Heithoff KB: Epidural hematomas of the lumbar spine: 18 surgically confirmed cases, *Radiology,* 87:427–431, 1993.
74. Rothfus WE, Chedid MK, Deeb ZL, et al: MR imaging in diagnosis of spontaneous spinal epidural hematomas, *J. Comput Assist Tomogr,* 11:851–854, 1987.
75. Davis PC, Reisner A, Hudgins PA, et al: Spinal injuries in children: role of MR, *Am J Neuroradiology,* 14:607–617, 1993.
76. Donovan Post MJ, Becerra JL, Madsen PW, et al: Acute spinal subdural hematoma: MR and CT findings with pathologic correlates, *Am J Neuroradiology,* 15:1895–1905, 1996.
77. Cornacchia LG, Abitbol JJ, Heller J, et al: Blunt injuries to the extracranial cerebral vessels associated with spine fractures, *Spine,* 16S:S506–510, 1991.
78. Powell MC, Wilson M, Szypryt P, et al: Prevalence of lumbar disc degeneration observed by magnetic resonance in symptomless women, *Lancet,* 2:1366–1367, 1986.
79. Jensen MC, Brant-Zawadzki MN, Obuchowski N, et al: Magnetic resonance imaging of the lumbar spine in people without back pain, *N Engl J Med,* 331:69–73, 1994.
80. Boden SD, McCowin PR, Davis DO, et al: Abnormal magnetic resonance scans of the cervial spine in asymptomatic subjects, *J Bone Joint Surg,* 72A:1178–1184, 1990.
81. Boden SD, Davis DO, Dina TS, et al: Abnormal magnetic resonance scans of the lumbar spine in asymptomatic subjects, *J Bone Joint Surg,* 72A:403–408, 1990.
82. Teresi LM, Lufkin RB, Reicher MA, et al: Asymptomatic degenerative disk disease and spondylosis of the cervical spine: MR imaging, *Radiology,* 164:83–88, 1987.
83. Videman T, Battie MC, Gill K, et al: Magnetic resonance imaging findings and their relationships in the thoracic and lumbar spine: insites into the etiopathogenesis of spinal degeneration, *Spine,* 20:928–935, 1995.
84. Wood KB, Garvey TA, Gundry C, Heithoff KB: Magnetic resonance imaging of the thoracic spine evaluation of asymptomatic individuals, *J Bone Joint Surg,* 77A:1631–1638, 1995.
85. Boos N, Rieder R, Schade V, et al: The diagnostic accuracy of magnetic resonance imaging, work perception, and psychosocial factors in identifying symptomatic disc herniations, *Spine,* 20:2613–2635, 1995.
86. Ferooznia H, Golimbu CA, Rafii M, et al: *MRI and CT of the musculoskeltal system,* St. Louis, 1992, Mosby–Year Book.
87. Gordon SJ, Yang KH, Mayer PJ, et al: Mechanism of disc rupture a preliminary report, *Spine,* 16:450–456, 1991.
88. Brinckman P, Porter RW: A laboratory model of lumbar disc protrusion, *Spine,* 19:228–235, 1994.
89. Adams MA, Hutton WC, Stott JRR: The resistance of flexion of the lumbar intervertebral joint, *Spine,* 5:245–253, 1980.
90. Markoff KL: Deformation of the thoracolumbar vertebral joints in response to external loads. A biomechanical study using autopsy material, *J Bone Joint Surg,* 54A:511–533, 1972.
91. Brown T, Hansen RJ, Yorra AJ: Some mechanical tests on the lumbosacral spine with particular reference to the intervertebral discs, *J Bone Joint Surg,* 39A:1153–1164, 1957.
92. Perey O: Fracture of the vertebral endplate, *Acta Orthop Scand Suppl,* 25:1–101, 1957.
93. Farfan HF: *Mechanical disorders of the low back,* Philadelphia, 1973, Lea & Febiger.
94. Farfan HF, Cossette JW, Robertson GH, et al: The effects of tortion on the intervertebral joints: the role of tortion in the production of disc degeneration, *J Bone Joint Surg,* 52A:468–497, 1970.
95. Tertti MO, Salminen JJ, Paajenen HEK, et al: Low back pain and disc degeneration in children: a case-control MR imaging study, *Radiology,* 180:503–507, 1991.
96. Varlotta GP, Brown MD, Kelsey JL, Golden AL: Familial predisposition for herniation of a lumbar disc in patients who are less than twenty-one years old, *J Bone Joint Surg,* 73A:124–128, 1991.
97. Schellhaas KP, Pollei SR, Gundry CR, Heithoff KB: Lumbar disc high-intensity zone correlation of magnetic resonance imaging and discography, *Spine,* 21:79–86, 1996.
98. Aprill C, Bogduk N: High intensity zone: a diagnostic sign of painful lumbar disc on magnetic resonance imaging, *Br J Radiol,* 65:361–369, 1992.

99. Komori H, Shinomiya K, Nakai O, et al: The natural history of herniated nucleus pulposus with radiculopathy, *Spine*, 21:225–229, 1996.
100. Komori H: Personal communication re: ref. 99.
101. Saal JA, Saal JS, Herzog RJ: The natural history of lumbar intervertebral disc extrusions treated nonoperatively, *Spine*, 15:683–686, 1990.
102. Bozzao A, Gallucci M, Masciocchi C, et al: Lumbar disc herniation: MR imaging assessment of natural history in patients not treated with surgery, *Radiology*, 185:135–141, 1992.
103. Doita M, Kanatani T, Harada T, Mizuno K: Immunohistologic study of the ruptured intervertebral disc of the lumbar spine, *Spine*, 21:235–241, 1996.
104. Ito T, Yamada M, Ikuta F, et al: Histologic evidence of absorption of sequestration-type herniated disc, *Spine*, 21:230–234, 1996.
105. Modic MT, Ross JS, Obuchowski NA, et al: Contrast-enhanced MR imaging in acute lumbar radiculopathy: a pilot study of the natural history, *Radiology*, 195:429–435, 1995.

5

SOFT TISSUE INJURIES TO THE SPINE FROM ACCELERATION-DECELERATION TRAUMA

Daniel A. Capen

In this nation of 265 million people there are an estimated 190 million vehicles. Other developed nations have proportional numbers of motorized personal and commercial vehicles. As nations emerge from third-world economic conditions, the number of cars, trucks, and buses will continue to grow. One of the results of this trend is surely to be an increase in the number of vehicular accidents. Death from severe trauma remains a primary concern, but lesser trauma is also costly in terms of functional loss and health care cost. Modernization also eventually creates the environment for the added cost of insurance and litigation. The Quebec cohort study[1] cited 70% to 85% of insurance claims were related directly to vehicular whiplash injury.

The single most frequent result of vehicular or, indeed, any type of acceleration-deceleration injury, is the pain producing trauma to the spine. Other chapters in this book deal with the extreme forms of this type of trauma, which results in a grossly unstable spine. Here we explore the etiology, diagnosis, treatment, and results of the soft tissue trauma, so-called whiplash, from vehicular injury. We address the importance of full evaluation, because occasionally severe instability can be misdiagnosed as whiplash.

Research over the past 15 years has brought several modifications in vehicular equipment to enhance safety. The aviation industry served as a laboratory for early whiplash research when naval aviators noted cervical spine problems associated with carrier catapult launches.[2] The extended headrest is the product of that experience. Seatbelt and harnesses have led to a reduction in death and serious trauma but do not insulate against acceleration-deceleration trauma to the spine. It is not clear that airbag appliances will substantially reduce this type of trauma either as these deploy only in frontal collisions. Airbags can create their own injuries.[3,4,5] Front-seated, backward-facing children have received severe trauma from passenger airbags.[4,6] As of publication, the National Traffic Safety Board has recommended that children less than 9 years old do not ride in a seat with an airbag. It is still not clear whether airbags are completely beneficial. Recreational vehicles and offroad vehicles do not really have much in the restraint category of safety equipment, but racing vehicles are extremely well-equipped for driver restraint.

Regardless of safety modifications, it is impossible to completely eliminate the syndrome of whiplash. The speed at which the forces are applied to the cervical and lumbar spine preclude total prevention. The endless permutations of driver and passenger positions at impact also make elimination of all soft tissue, muscle, and disk injury impossible.

NORMAL ANATOMY

To understand the adverse effect of acceleration-deceleration injury, one must fully understand normal adult anatomy. Vertebral column structures that are subjected to forces include anterior and posterior boney elements, disk, facet capsular units, interspinous ligaments, and musculature. The longus colli musculature and the anterior sympathetic chain are close in proximity to the anterior spine. The mechanical relationship of cranial nerves and the upper cords of the brachial plexus may also have forces applied in cervical whiplash.

The symptom complex of protracted pain originates from the rich sensory innervation of all cervical structures. Pain from the injury can emanate from any combination of these structures. The normal anatomy of the calvarium, cerebrospinal fluid (CSF) and brain also must be considered. The normal kinematics of the cervical spine are greatly exceeded in whiplash acceleration-deceleration. Flexion, extension, rotation, and bending motions are all possible in the functioning cervical spine. Trauma to any of the muscle groups of the cervical region can produce symptoms for extended periods. Table 5-1 lists muscle groups responsible for movements of the upper spine.

All muscle groups have variable and overlapping innervation. Even at rest and in sleep there is utilization of these muscle groups. The injury from excess flexion or extension or partial lateral motion, if the head or forces are directed accordingly, causes injury to musculature and support ligaments thereby creating whiplash symptoms. The dynamic research studies using test dummies and primates have clearly shown that forces from vehicle trauma produce motion in the cervical spine that far exceeds normal kinematics.[7,8,9] The cervical symptoms experienced after acceleration-deceleration trauma are the result of injury to normal anatomy. Figure 5-2 shows the general anatomic areas and the normal corresponding root innervation.

CERVICAL STABILITY

The classic work of White and Panjabi[10,11] has clearly defined the criteria for instability of the cervical spine. It is necessary to evaluate for the presence of cervical instability in all cases of vehicular trauma. If there are any symptoms suggestive of neurologic compromise in vehicular trauma or any other high-energy injury, the assumption must be that instability is present. From high-stress trauma, the most severe type of whiplash creates either a compressive-flexion or distractive-flexion injury as described by Allen.[12] These injuries have a high incidence of spinal cord injury (SCI), and the sequelae and treatment are explained in other chapters. Occult instability is always a more difficult diagnosis with potential for cord injury if missed.

At Rancho Los Amigos Spine Injury Center at least one patient per year is admitted with cord injury from vehicular trauma in which the initial evaluation did not detect the injury. Most frequently this is from a cervical whiplash that did not have adequate workup. The initial failure to protect the spine resulted in the cord injury. Fortunately, in the awake and alert patient, partial and recoverable injury is seen more often. Complete quadriplegia in this group is rare, but facet fracture or rotational unilateral facet instability can certainly result in root injury especially if the injury is missed and the patient is dismissed without cervical immobilization.

Initially, the static radiographs may not reveal obvious instability. Multiple trauma may render neck symptoms initially unnoticeable. Cervical muscle spasm may preclude sufficient movement on dynamic (flexion-extension) radiographs to diagnose instability. The recommendation is to perform imaging and to protect the cervical spine until diagnosis can be made. Because of the potentially devastating complication of late cord injury, it is best to overtreat and overstudy rather than miss a significant injury.

Table 5-1. Cervical Spine Musculature

Movement	Muscle
Flexion	Sternomastoid Longus colli Longus capitis Rectus capitis anterior
Extension	Splenius capitis and cervicis Semispinalis capitis and cervicis Longissimus capitis and cervicis Trapezius and interspinalis Rectus capitis posterior—major and minor Obliquus capitis superior
Rotation and bend	Sternomastoid Scalenes Levator scapulae and multifidi Intercostalis and longus colli Rectus capitis lateralis

INCIDENCE OF WHIPLASH

Motor vehicle trauma with a whiplash occurs approximately 1 million times per year in the United States. Other developed nations appear to have proportionally similar statistics. Statistics on vehicle safety suggest that accidents are traffic related. They increase as the number of vehicles increase and as the number of miles driven increase. The percentage of rear-end collisions is 25% to 30% of all vehicle accidents. The Quebec cohort study for 1987 was 70 per 100,000 people receiving compensation for whiplash. Women outnumbered men 1.5 to 1.[1] New Zealand had 13 whiplash injuries per 100,000, and Australia had 106 per 100,000 during 1982 to 1983. Other developed countries have rates in this range as well.[1]

All practitioners see victims of vehicular trauma, and specialists not only treat their long-lasting symptoms but evaluate these patients for frequent litigation. In the evaluation of a patient for injuries sustained in acceleration-deceleration trauma, the examiner must bear in mind that the injuries range from a minor jolt that resolves without medical care, to death. Bucholz showed, however, a high percentage of cervical fracture in fatal injuries.[13] A 24% fracture or fracture dislocation rate in fatal injuries does not translate to no injury if the victim survives. The cervical support and functional anatomic structure is injured on a spectrum roughly related to force applied to the spine.

MECHANISM OF TRAUMA

The mechanism of all vehicle injuries rests upon the theory that bodies in motion will remain in motion while those at rest tend to remain at rest without external forces acting upon them. Energy absorbed by the vehicle and its contents increases as a square of the velocity so that doubling the speed quadruples the energy for any given mass vehicle. While vehicles have some factory-installed safety equipment and support structures that absorb energy, energy is always transmitted to the occupants of the vehicle.

Although it is not expected that the practitioner is a collision expert, it is important in dealing with this trauma to have a basic understanding of what occurs. Whether totally stopped or moving slower than the striking vehicle, the body of the injured person is suddenly thrust forward in relation to the head and neck. The initial forces are applied through the vehicle via the seat. Because the head has no direct support in almost all cases it is extended until it stops or strikes the headrest. This hyperextension force places stress on the anterior muscles, disk annulus, and anterior longitudinal ligament.

The second force occurs when the initial energy is dissipated and the car stops accelerating. This could be from striking an object in front of the vehicle. In this part of the reaction, the head is still unrestrained relative to the body, which is or should be restrained. The hyperflexion moment stresses or injures posterior structures.

Even new vehicles equipped with airbags do not completely eliminate spine injury in vehicle trauma. Blacksin cited early patterns of specific airbag-related injury.[4] Significant injury may still occur in frontal collision with airbags. Deployment usually does not occur in rear-end collision.

In various side collisions, or when the head or trunk is rotated in relation to the direction of force, other lateral structures can be damaged. The history of the trauma provides valuable information. Severy et al. describe well all the forces to the spine in vehicular injury.[14]

It is the higher-speed, higher-energy form of this trauma that often results in severe structural damage to the spine, pelvis, and extremities. Victims often receive spinal cord injury from the instability that is created by such trauma. Lesser speed trauma results in more soft tissue and structural support injury.

Experimental acceleration-deceleration injuries have assisted in providing information regarding spinal trauma. MacNab[2] demonstrated in monkeys that variable tears of sternomastoid and longissimus colli muscles occur. Disk avulsion also occurred in many of the monkeys. Wickstrom demonstrated some brain injury and disk damage as a result of this type of injury.[15] Basic structural damage occurred with experimental injury. Wickstrom's results are noted in Table 5-2.

Liu and associates[7] studied central nervous system (CNS) changes in Rhesus monkeys. Epileptiform activity occurred after whiplash. Heath[16] also was able

Table 5-2. Injury in Experimental Animal Study of Whiplash

Injury Type	Rate of Incidence
Brain damage	32%
Spinal cord damage	5%
Nerve root damage	7%
Cervical ligament tear (C4–C7)	11%
Intervertebral disk injury	2.3%

From Wickstrom JK, Rodriguez RP, Martinez JL, Haines DM-Hypertension and hyperflexion injuries to the head and neck of primates. In Gurdjian ES, Thomas IM, editors: *Neckache and backache*, Springfield, ILL, 1970, Charles C. Thomas, pp 108–117.

to demonstrate a correlation between epileptiform activity and primate behavioral changes. The animal studies serve to provide the clinician with a basis understanding of the exact extent of injury to the spine. The cervical spine is the most susceptible to this type of trauma, but the thoracic and lumbar regions are certainly not exempt from the forces of acceleration-deceleration impact.

Shoulder harnesses in the authors' clinical experience create some shoulder trauma that frequently results in an impingement-like symptom complex. The driver obviously has left-sided pain, while the passenger frequently has right shoulder problems. International studies also document many seat-belt-type injuries for older vehicles, and injury for some back seat passengers can be quite severe.[17–24] The thoracolumbar spine can be involved. Figures 5-1 A and B and 5-2 are clinical radiographs of an 18-year-old rear seat occupant who was discharged from an emergency room and returned within 24 hours with acute pain in the abdomen requiring colostomy. At 6 days postinjury the patient had ligamentous injury at L3-L4. Unsuccessful bracing resulted in the need for surgery after 5 months (Fig. 5-3 A, B). This was a lap-belt injury that was originally thought to be a sprain. Children and adults with any abdominal pain must have not only an appropriate general surgical evaluation but also a complete examination of the spinal column.

CLINICAL PRESENTATION

Acceleration-deceleration injury creates a varied but somewhat consistent group of complaints and physical findings. The direction and force of impact may effect the nature and extent of injury. Vehicle type and the type and use of restraints also directly affects the extent of injury. The contact with airbags also can affect

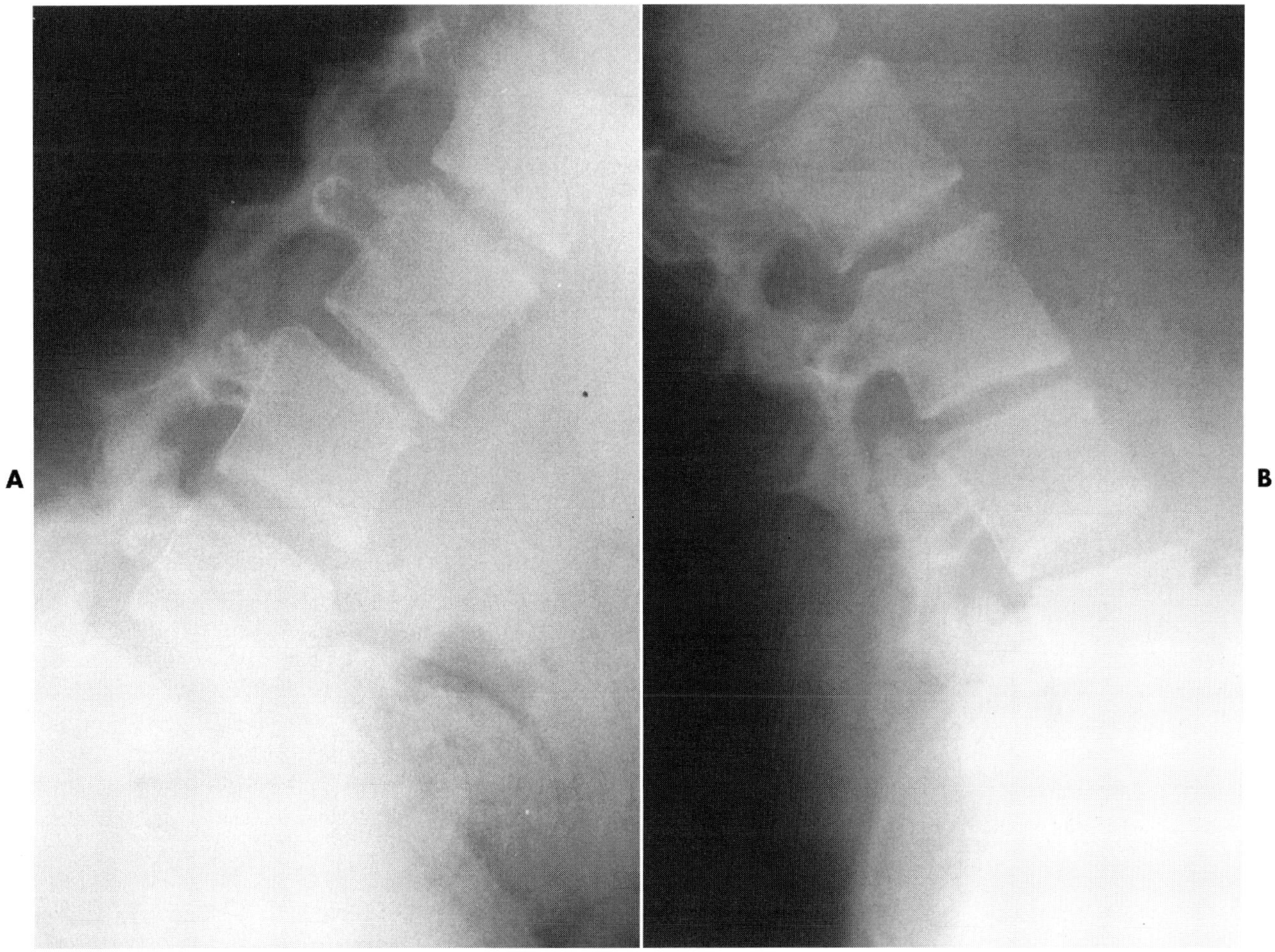

FIGURE 5-1

A, Flexion radiographs 6 days post injury of an 18 year old rear seat occupant who was discharged from an emergency room and returned within 24 hours with an acute abdomen requiring colostomy and at 6 days post injury had this ligamentous injury at L3-4. **1B,** Extension radiographs 6 days post injury.

injury, but insufficient data exists in this area. Most complaints occur early within 24 hours of injury and include neck pain, stiffness and motion loss. Headache is present in a majority of cases because of cervical muscle injury and the intracranial contracoup injury, which accompanies the acceleration-deceleration force. Loss of consciousness and direct head concussion can occur, especially in side and head-on collisions, but the practitioner must be aware that adult brain injury can occur without direct blows to the head.

A frequently confusing picture that frustrates the patient and doctor is the headache and mentation problems that follow a concussion. As can be imagined, loss of memory and difficulty with thought processes are frightening. When the patient is treated with a high degree of skepticism by the doctor, this adds to the psychologic trauma. Some of the complaints are indeed unusual but as Barrée described, hemifacial numbness, unilateral vision disturbance, and auditory symptoms (usually unilateral) are part of a self-limiting but sometimes long-lasting phenomenon.[25] Reassurance and headache relief are often the only treatment. Recognition of potential nonskeletal symptoms is essential when appropriate neurologic consultation may be required. With animal studies in mind, this complex is much more understandable. With many studies documenting the concussion-like effects of the brain injury associated with the hypermotion forces, the practitioner must be prepared to understand and treat these symptoms.

Some of the later symptoms that can develop include low back pain and upper extremity pain that is nonspinal in origin. Shoulder harness injuries can result in impingement syndrome. Although low in incidence, lumbar disk herniation also can occur because of traumatic forces across the lumbar spine, especially in lap

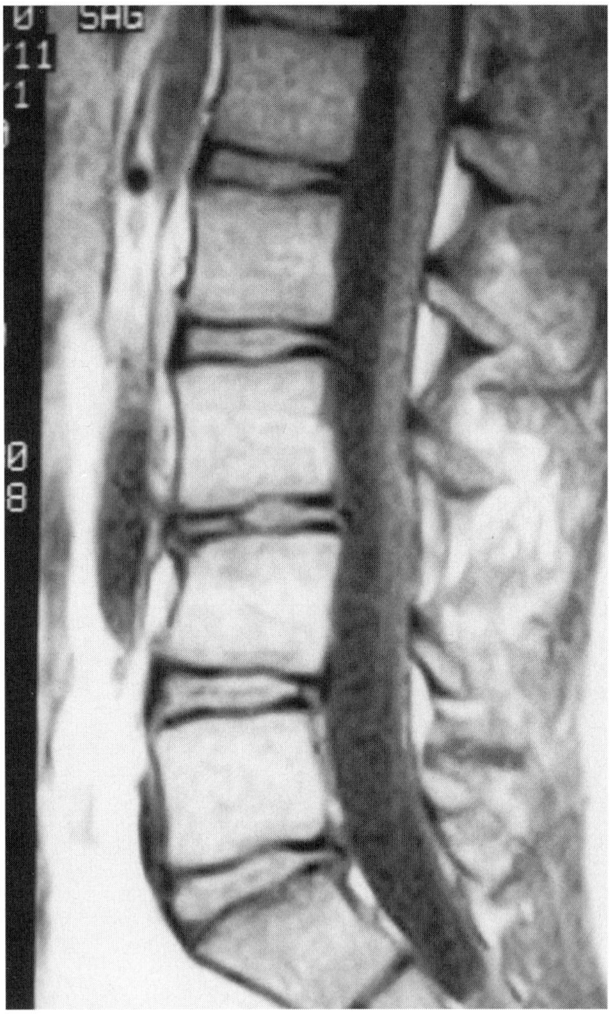

FIGURE 5-2

Sagital view of traumatized area indicating no canal compromise.

belt–only vehicles. Emergency treatment focuses on emergency complaints. The gradual development of additional symptoms is most often the result of the patient noticing the symptoms as severe pains lessen with treatment and as use of the injured parts increases with postaccident activity. In frontal collisions, wrist injury also can occur as a result of tightened grip on the wheel.

The cause of pain has been linked scientifically to several factors. Barnsley from Adelaide, Australia showed cervical zygapophyseal joints to be routinely injured and symptomatic in over half of their study group.[26] In this study destruction of and degeneration of the joints occurred. Muscle tear and hemorrhage are occasionally visible on acute magnetic resonance imaging (MRI). Facet fracture also may occur from the extremes of motion in flexion and extension.

Zygapophyseal trauma is a cause of significant long-term pain.[26,27] Joint capsular injury together with cartilage and joint tears have been demonstrated anatomically. Bogduk elegantly described block techniques to localize the joints involved.[28] The medial nerve branch block can provide information in cases where pain is difficult to pinpoint.

Jonsson et al.[29] found there is clear chronicity in a high percentage of cases. The incidence of surgical injury was 2 in 50 for posterior ligamentous trauma and 8 in 50 for substantial diskogenic pain requiring diskectomy and fusion.

In the primate injury studies of MacNab, the damage in the absence of fracture includes longus colli muscle tears, esophageal hemorrhage, and disk annular injury as demonstrated. Cervical zygapophyseal injury, facet capsular injury, and disk annular injury can occur. Cadaver studies and postmortem examinations also reveal significant trauma to muscles, ligaments, spinal joints, and disks. As with all other types of sport or work trauma, the tearing of these structures can be expected to be symptomatic and treatable when it results from vehicular acceleration-deceleration.

Gay and Abbott described the following: (1) radicular-like pain radiating to the occiput, jaw, shoulders upper anterior chest, and upper extremities in 70% of their patients; (2) cerebral symptoms of irritability, concentration deficit, tension, vertigo headache, and anxiety were present in 60% of the group; (3) low back symptoms were noted in 30% of the group; (4) cervical radiculopathic signs, including reflex, motor, and sensory changes, occurred at least occasionally during treatment in 26% of patients; and (5) accident neurosis including psychologic trauma associated with the social problems and the sudden unexpected nature of the trauma was noted in half the population.[30] Some modification of these symptom complexes has resulted from seat and restrain changes, but my experience in clinical practice is similar to that of Gay and Abbott in terms of clinical presentation. These presenting patterns necessitate treatment.

Temperomandibular joint injury also is described by Weinberg and Lapoint.[31] Sheer stresses applied to the intraarticular disk is cited as the cause for loss of the synchronization of the disk. Clicking and pain are produced and frequently go along with headache and facial pain.

Deans et al. followed 137 patients for 1 to 2 years after an acceleration-deceleration type trauma.[32] In the study group only a small (7%) number had preexisting problems in the cervical region. In 36 of 85 symptomatic cases, the pain lasted for more than 1 year. Obviously this does limit the symptoms to those presenting to a hospital, but a 26% incidence of pain for more than a year does not suggest insignificant injury. Table 5-3 outlines these findings. Permanent symptoms result in many cases, and disability results in a smaller percentage of cases. Nygren found that 10% of patients in rear-end collisions were disabled as were 4% in front- or side impact accidents.[8]

A

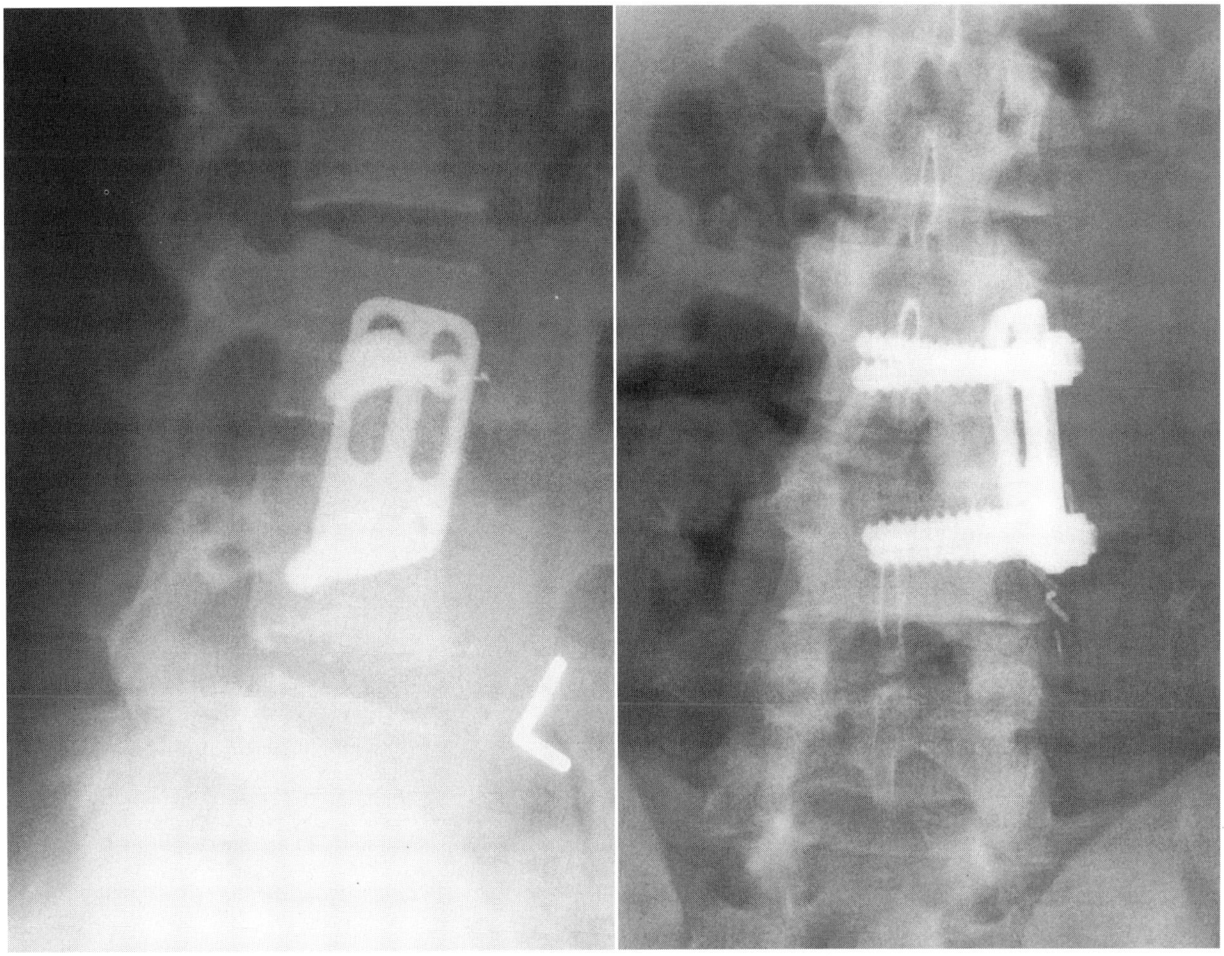

B

FIGURE 5-3

A and **B**, Unsuccessful bracing resulted in the need for surgery at 5 months.

Table 5-3. Dean's Injury Sequelae in 137 Cases

Conditions	Number of Cases	Percent of Cases
Premorbid neck pain	10	7
Pain after accident	85	62
Immediate pain	66	77
Pain after 48 hrs	6	7
Pain at 1 year	36	26

Deans GT, Magarlians JN, Kerr M, Rutherford WH: Neck sprain; a major cause of disability following car accidents, *Injury* 18(1):10–12, 1987.

EARLY DIAGNOSIS AND TREATMENT

The early diagnosis of hyperextension, hyperflexion trauma is based upon the history of injury, the absence of traumatic instability, and the presence of pain, stiffness, early muscle spasm, headache, and some variable radiating symptoms without direct physical evidence of radiculopathy. Some cerebral-type complaints such as memory loss, dizziness, and blurred vision frequently occur.

Radiographic analysis of the spine including adequate occiput C1 views, flexion and extension views, and a good image of C7-T1 are essential. Oblique supine views are also helpful in diagnosing occult fracture or ligament injury.[33] Gas in the disk on flexion-extension radiographs can indicate a disk injury. Pillar views with right and left head rotation can show any facet fracture. This analysis is eloquently described and illustrated in Chapter 4.

In any patient with radicular symptoms, MRI or computed tomography (CT) studies may be required. The literature clearly defines disk herniation with fracture or fracture dislocation of the cervical spine.[34,35] Whiplash, being a lesser form of a similar trauma, produces this injury as well. The Swedish group found nine large disk herniations in 50 patients.[29] Awareness of this clinical syndrome following whiplash is essential. The treating physician must keep in mind that 3% to

8% of auto accident victims develop a diagnosed disk herniation of the cervical or lumbar spine.

When whiplash syndrome has been diagnosed, care must be provided that will focus on restoration of function. Limited use of collars or other cervical supports is imperative. Medication is a potential problem. The physical therapy program should focus on exercise as soon as possible after treatment. Home traction, transcutaneous electrical nerve stimulation (TENS), and other pain relieving devices are ancillary treatments that are preferred over habituating medication and prolonged immobilization. One must always consider prior history of spinal problems and medication when treating vehicular injuries, as the potential for abuse can be greater when the psychologic factors surrounding accident victims are considered. Documentation of the benefit of exercise in the treatment of spinal pain is clear. All groups of soldiers with back pain who were treated with exercise had more rapid return to work.[36]

Cervical exercise has proved to be effective as treatment for cervical musculoligamentous problems. In most circumstances, vehicular trauma is suscipicously embellished by all those other than the injured party. The treating doctor must not enter into any facet of the relationship other than care provider without extremely good reason. The patient has enough difficulty to overcome without loss of the physician as an ally. The doctor must rule out serious trauma and find appropriate treatment remedies. The energy absorbed in vehicular trauma, even at low velocity, is often substantial. Studies on energy show high G loads at low speeds. Little correlation between vehicle damage and injury severity has ever been established. Rather than dismiss people without fracture as neurotic or dishonest, the practitioner must pay heed to the body of evidence concerning whiplash injury. Table 5-4 indicates my preferred treatment protocol.

Table 5-4. Author's Preferred Treatment for Cervical Musculoligamentous Injury*

Time Postinjury	Treatment
First 2 weeks	Medrol dose pack or IM corticosteroids Rest, heat, ice, collar for sleep and riding in car. Some early exercise, TENS, analgesics and muscle relaxers
2 weeks	Start more vigorous exercise Traction-therapy and home Wean analgesics and muscle relaxers Antiinflammatories Reassuring
3–6 months	Home remedies, TENS, home exercises, Mild medications Scan and/or EMG if symptoms longer than 4-6 weeks or earlier if significant radiculopathy.

* Surgery only for clear instability or disk herniation. Consult neurologist for significant head trauma-like symptoms.

Treatment of all symptoms is required. The evaluation of radicular problems is important. When early treatment fails to alleviate pain, the use of imaging becomes necessary, although the published data on scan changes in normal asymptomatic individuals should be considered. If the patient has a symptomatic disk herniation, the surgeon must decide if surgery is necessary. No outcome other than what is anticipated and documented in the literature should be considered. The incidence of lumbar, thoracic, and cervical disk herniation from acceleration-deceleration injury is variably reported as 5% to 7%. Outcomes for these patients are comparable for age and prior history of spinal disorder compared with herniation from other causes in the author's experience.

The notion that a litigation neurosis drives the symptomatology until otherwise shown needs to be dispelled. The state of our knowledge of pain generation in the spine is too great to simply dismiss pain as unfounded or secondary pain. Long-term follow-up series in the United Kingdom and United States all support the fact that the majority of patients resolve symptoms with a combination of time, exercise, and treatment. Approximately 20% to 30% of whiplash victims have symptoms that last beyond 12 months regardless of treatment. Many researchers substantiate the fact that litigation settlement has no effect on resolution of pain despite the older, widely held theory of the "green poultice." Treatment of patients must be provided without prejudice toward any litigation.

LONG-TERM OUTCOME

Most vehicular trauma-related pain is successfully treated and resolved within 6 to 9 months. The rent has positive resolution at 1 year. Several large series suggest that 15% to 30% of the acceleration-deceleration injuries have residual symptoms and pain for years and, indeed, permanently. Conditioning and preaccident spinal health may contribute to persistent pain. Severity of disk and ligament injury in a perpetually mobile anatomic structure is the most likely explanation for chronic pain.

There are several important items in the treatment of whiplash injury (Table 5-5). The first is to avoid

Table 5-5. Checklist for Whiplash Injury

1. Rule out instability
2. Minimize habit-forming medications, braces
3. Emphasize rehabilitation
4. Work-up for joint or disk injury
5. Reassure for central nervous system complaints after appropriate work-up
6. Home remedies in long-term cases
7. Surgery if needed for severe cases
8. Remain aware of potential ancillary injuries

prolonged immobilization if there is no boney or ligamentous instability. The second factor is to avoid the prolonged use of habit-forming medications, the most habit forming being Soma and Vicodin. For a number of reasons these medications, especially when used together create a roadblock to recovery. The third factor in whiplash treatment is the avoidance of prolonged modality-type treatments especially massage and manipulation both of which can be beneficial in early abbreviated courses.

If cost-effective and successful outcome is the goal, exercise rehabilitation and home treatment, such as traction and TENS therapy with tolerated mild analgesics and nonsteroidal antiinflammatory drug (NSAID) therapy, has an extremely high rate of pain reduction and return of function. Expectations of recovery by doctor and patient must be clearly stated and understood early in the treatment course. We have discussed patterns of recovery and the time frames involved, but this cannot be stressed enough as physician and patient expectations, when not met, can be a substantial roadblock in the recovery process. Awareness of some of the ancillary symptoms involving the CNS is important so the patient can be treated rather than mistrusted.

The secondary gain aspects of this kind of spinal trauma has been overemphasized. The literature has served to provide information on long-term follow-up series, which disprove the theory of the "green poultice." Several series also document rather significant late spinal changes consistent with disk injury from acceleration-deceleration trauma.

Development and progress has some detriment with an increased use of motorized transportation. Recreation with emphasis on speed and contact may result in whiplash trauma to the spine. Although often not life threatening, these injuries are responsible for physician visits and for consumption of the health care dollars. The whiplash patient continues to demand skilled diagnosis, management, and support. Treatment goals include spinal cord and neural protection, pain control, and restoration of function. Immediate dismissal of patient's complaints as "litigation neurosis" is a certain recipe for disaster and is very unjust to the patient.

CONCLUSION

In developed and emerging societies, motorized transportation and a sporting sector emphasizing water, land, and air vehicles built to satisfy "the need for speed" will keep health care practitioners busy treating the results of unplanned and sudden stops by these devices. Despite continued improvements in vehicular safety measures, accidents will continue to occur. Not all injuries will result in definitive spine fracture or dislocation, but many will injure support structures sufficiently to require treatment. Hopefully, this chapter has focused on providing a clear method for diagnosis and treatment of the whiplash syndrome, which may not always present as a clear anatomic condition.

REFERENCES

1. Harder S, Veilleux M: The Quebec whiplash-associated disorders cohort study, *Spine*, 20(8S):12S–39S, 1995.
2. MacNab I: The whiplash syndrome, *Orthop Clin North Am* 2:389–403, 1971.
3. Anderson PA, Rivara FP, Maier RV, Drake C: The epidemiology of seatbelt associated injuries, *J Trauma* 31(1):60–67, 1991.
4. Blacksin MF: Patterns of fracture after airbag deployment, *J Trauma* 35(6):840–843, 1993.
5. Traynelis VC, Gold M: Cervical spine injury in an air bag equipped vehicle, *J Spinal Disord* 6(1):60–61, 1993.
6. Drake, C: The epidemiology of seatbelt associated injuries, *J Trauma* 31(1):60–67, 1991.
7. Liu YK, Canoran KB, Heath RG: Subcortical EEG changes in rhesus monkeys following experimental hyperflexion-hyperextension, *Spine* 9:327–329, 1984.
8. Nygren A: Injuries to car occupants: some aspects of the interior safety of cars, *Acta Otolaryngol {Suppl} (Stockh)* 395:1–164, 1984.
9. Rutherford WH, Greenfield AA, Hays HRM: *The medical effects of seatbelt legislation in the U.K.,* London, 1985, HMSD.
10. White AA, Panjabi MM: *Clinical biomechanics of the spine.* Philadelphia, 1978, JB Lippincott.
11. White AA, Southwick WO, Panjabi MM: Clinical instability in the lower cervical spine—a review of past and current concepts, *Spine* 1:15–27, 1976.

12. Allen BA: A mechanistic classification of closed, indirect fractures and dislocations of the lower cervical spine, *Spine* 7(1):1–27, 1982.
13. Bucholz RW, Burkhead WZ, Graham W, Petty C: Occult spine injuries in fatal traffic accidents, *J Trauma* 19:768–771, 1979.
14. Severy D, et al: Controlled automobile rear-end collisons: an investigation of related engineering and medical phenomena, *Can Serv Med J* 11:727, 1955.
15. Wickstrom JK, Rodriguez RP, Martinez JL, Haines DM: Hyperextension and hyperflexion injuries to the head and neck of primates. In Gurdjian ES, Thomas IM, editors: *Neckache and backache.* Springfield, MO. 1970, Thomas.
16. Heath RG: Physiologic basis of emotional expressions evoked potential and mirror focus studies in rhesus monkeys, *Biol Psycho* 15:31, 1972.
17. Epstein BS, Epstein JA, Jones MD: Lapsash three point seat belt fractures of the cervical spine, *Spine* 3:189–93, 1978.
18. Foster JD, Thind IS, Fuller J, Louria DB: Automobile accidents, seatbelts and airbags, *N Engl J Med* 83:715–20, 1986.
19. Girelli GD, Natale R, Manoocchi, MC, Luturen M: Seat belt syndrome, *Radiol Med (Torino)* 86(4):444–450, 1993.
20. Munker H, Langwieder K, Chen E, Well W: Injuries to the cervical spine in automobile accidents, *Versicherungsmedizin* 47(1):26–32, 1995.
21. Arajarvi E, Santavirta S, Tolonen J: Aortic ruptures in seat belt wearers, *J Thorac Cardiovasc Surg* 98:355–361, 1989.
22. Newman KD, Bowman LM, Eichelberger MR, et al: The lap belt complex: intestinal and lumbar spine injury in children, *J Trauma* 30:1133–1134, 1990.
23. Reid AB, Letts RM, Black GB: Pediatric Chance fractures: association with intraabdominal injuries and seatbelt use, *J Trauma* 30:384–391, 1990.
24. Smith W, Kaufer, H: Patterns and mechanism of lumbar injuries associated with lap seat belts, *J Bone Joint Surg {Am}*, 51:239–254, 1969.
25. LaRocca H: Cervical sprain syndrome: diagnoses, treatment, and long-term outcome. In Frymoyer JW, editor: *The adult spine: principles and practice;* New York, 1991 Raven Press.
26. Barnsley L, Lord SM, Wallis BJ, Bogduk N: The prevalence of chronic cervical zygapophyseal joint pain after whiplash, *Spine* 20(1):20–25, 1995.
27. Lord SM, Barnsley, L, Wallis, BJ, Bogduk N: Chronic cervical zygapophysial joint pain after whiplash, *Spine* 21(15):1747–1745, 1996.
28. Bogduk N: Back pain. Zygapophysial blocks and epidural steroids. In Cousins MJ, Bridenbaugh PO, editor: *Neural blockade in clinical anesthesia and management of pain.* Philadelphia, 1988, JB Lippincott.
29. Jonsson H, Cesarini, K, Sahlstedt, B, Raushning, W: Findings and outcome in whiplash type neck distortions, *Spine* 19(24):2733–2743, 1994.
30. Gay J, Abbott K: Common whiplash injuries of the neck. *JAMA* 152:1698, 1953.
31. Weinberg, S, La Pointe H: Cervical extension-flexion injury (whiplash) and internal derangement of the temporomandibular joint, *J Oral Maxillofac Surg* 45:653–656, 1987.
32. Deans GT, Magarlians, JN, Kerr M, Rutherford WH: Neck sprain; a major cause of disability following car accidents, *Injury* 18(1):10–12, 1987.
33. Turetsky DB, Vines FS, Clayman DA, Northup HM: Technique and use of supine oblique views in acute cervical spine trauma, *Ann Emerg Med* 22(4):685–689, 1993.
34. Eismont FJ, Arena MJ, Gren BA: Extrusion of an intervertebral disc associated with traumatic subluxation or dislocation of cervical facets, *J Bone Joint Surg* 73A(10):1555–1560, 1991.
35. Rizzolo, SJ, Piazza MR, Cotler JM, et al: Intervertebral disc injury complicating cervical spine trauma, *Spine* 16(Suppl. 6):S187–S189, 1991.
36. Dettori JR, Bullock SH, Sutlive TG, et al: The effects of spinal flexion and extension exercises and their associated postures in patients with acute low back pain, *Spine* 20:2303–2312, 1995.

6

SPINAL CORD INJURIES FROM MINOR TRAUMA

Mary C. Hume
William C. Neal

The spinal cord is ordinarily well protected by the complex skeletal architecture of the spine. The high energy absorbed during falls from great heights, motor vehicle accidents, and gunshot wounds accounts for the majority of cord injuries. Nonetheless, patients are occasionally stunned (and their clinicians surprised) to find that a catastrophic spinal cord injury (SCI) has occurred as a result of a seemingly minor event: a fall from a step, a stumble, a push, or even a "therapeutic" spine manipulation.

Because these injuries are unexpected, they are often underappreciated or misdiagnosed by the clinicians who are presented with neurologic symptoms or deficits in the face of a relatively innocent history of injury and, often, normal radiographs. Appropriate treatment (including immediate immobilization) may be delayed, with potentially catastrophic consequences.

Spinal cord injury after minor trauma usually occurs in conjunction with underlying abnormalities of the spinal column. Congenitally abnormal bone architecture, ligamentous laxity, acquired bone or soft-tissue abnormalities, or poor bone quality may set the stage for a SCI after minor trauma. In general, these are conditions of childhood or of older adulthood. Rarely does an older child or young adult have a SCI without injury to the spinal canal itself.[1] These injuries also are most frequent in the cervical spine, as the presence of the ribcage and the obliquity of the facet joints gives the thoracic spine much greater inherent stability.

Computerized tomography (CT) and magnetic resonance imaging (MRI) techniques have played an important role in identifying these injuries and understanding their pathophysiology. Clinical suspicion, however, along with awareness of these predisposing medical and orthopedic conditions remain the keys to the initial diagnosis and management of these enigmatic injuries.

INJURIES TO CHILDREN

Approximately 9% of all SCIs occur in children less than 16 years of age, and 19% of these injuries involve no fractures of the spine.[2] While the normally increased laxity of ligaments in children accounts for the spinal segment hypermobility involved in many of these injuries, certain features of normal childhood bony anatomy also contribute to relative instability of the cervical spine.[3] In children less than 10 years of age, the uncinate processes are flat and, therefore, unable to effectively block flexion and rotational forces. In children, the interspinous ligament, posterior joint capsule, and cartilage end plates are elastic and redundant, leading to greater instability.[2]

Many pediatric SCIs result, in part, from developmental or congenital abnormalities of the spinal canal. Many of these "at-risk" conditions can be identified before injury occurs. Developmental or congenital abnormalities can cause spinal segment hypermobility as a result of abnormal ligamentous laxity or abnormal bone architecture. Recognition of the these conditions offers the pediatrician, neurologist, or orthopedist an opportunity to evaluate the spine and prescribe activity restrictions or bracing before neurologic injury occurs as a result of minor childhood trauma.

RADIOLOGIC EVALUATION OF UPPER CERVICAL INSTABILITY

Radiologic evaluation of children at risk for these injuries must address both ligamentous and bone abnormalities. Lateral cervical radiographs in a neutral position allow measurement of the atlas-dens interval (ADI), which indicates instability if greater than 4 mm (3 mm in adults because of greater odontoid ossification). Although flexion views may maximize this interval, these radiographs should be taken with great care after an acute injury.

When atlantoaxial instability is related to odontoid hypermobility, a normal ADI may be present despite cord compromise.[3] Hensinger notes that the space available for the spinal cord (SAC) may be measured on lateral cervical radiographs between the posterior margin of the odontoid and the posterior margin of the foramen magnum or ring of the atlas.[3] Posterior migration of the odontoid is normally limited by both the transverse atlantal ligament and the alar ligaments. With chronic instability, initial displacement of the odontoid into the "safe zone" described by Steel may occur with disruption or laxity of the transverse ligament. Subsequent posterior movement of the odontoid into the cord is resisted only by the relatively weak alar ligaments.

Because childhood cord injuries are so often associated with skeletal abnormalities of the cervical spine, plain radiographs may be difficult to assess. Computed tomography scanning better differentiates the skeletal abnormalities, and MRI scanning, including flexion-extension scanning, may be helpful in evaluating instability and cord compromise.

CHILDHOOD DISORDERS AT RISK FOR CERVICAL INSTABILITY

Upper Respiratory Infections (Grisel's Syndrome). Upper respiratory infections in children, and less frequently in adults, can result in transient atlantoaxial instability. Infection about the neck may spread through the pharyngeovertebral veins to the suboccipital plexus, causing hyperemia with bone resorption and insertional detachment of the ligaments of the upper cervical spine.[5] In this hypermobile state, a twisting force applied to the neck may cause a significant cervical subluxation. A child presenting with painful torticollis with sternocleidomastoid spasm and tenderness over the posterior neck requires a thorough neurologic evaluation and cervical spine radiographs.

Asymmetry of the atlantoaxial joint seen on an open mouth view confirms the diagnosis of subluxation. This must be distinguished from the normal variant of partial anterior subluxation of the second or third vertebra seen on lateral radiographs of many normal children.

Trisomy 21. Trisomy 21, or Down syndrome, is a relatively common (1 in 700 births) syndrome usually caused by chromosomal nondisjunction.[6] Mental retardation, congenital heart disease, and gastrointestinal tract anomalies are often accompanied by orthopedic problems. These reflect a generalized ligamentous hyperlaxity, which can affect the knee (patellar dislocation and genu valgum), the hip (dislocation), the foot (pes planovalgus), and the spine. Atlantoaxial instability occurs in 10% to 20% of those with Down syndrome and may be due both to laxity of the transverse ligament and odontoid hypoplasia or aplasia.[7] Shallower and more horizontal occipitoatlantal articulations allow for excessive cervical extension.[8] Parfenchuck et al. found that 8.5% of patients with Down syndrome had a Powers ratio of less than 0.55, indicating posterior occipitoatlantal hypermobility.[9] Of those with an abnormal Powers ratio, 66% had positive neurologic findings.

Symptoms of spinal cord compromise in these individuals may include neck pain or spasm, changes in bowel or bladder function, increased gait abnormalities, spasticity, or weakness. Because affected individuals with mental retardation may have poor verbal skills, these symptoms and signs may be overlooked by caregivers and clinicians, leading to delayed diagnosis. Lateral flexion and extension radiographs of the cervical spine identify an unstable atlantoaxial articulation, while CT or MRI studies may confirm cord compromise.

Of particular concern is the risk that individuals with trisomy 21 face in sports participation in which head and neck injuries are possible. The ordinarily minor neck injuries seen in contact sports, running or jumping sports, wrestling, diving, gymnastics, or use of a trampoline may lead to SCI when atlantoaxial joint instability is present. As cited by Tachdjian, the Committee on Sports Medicine of the American Academy of Pediatrics has issued the following guidelines related to trisomy 21:[6,10]

1. All children with Down syndrome who wish to participate in sports that could involve head or neck trauma should have lateral view radiographs taken of the cervical region in neutral, flexion, and extension positions before beginning training or competition.
2. A patient should not participate in sports that could result in neck or head trauma if the distance between the odontoid process of the axis and the anterior arch of the atlas is more than 4.5 mm or if the odontoid process is abnormal.
3. It is not necessary to repeat radiographs on patients who have had normal findings. Some physicians may want to screen children with Down syndrome routinely at 5 and 6 years of age for atlantoaxial instability.
4. Children with atlantoaxial subluxation or dislocation and neurologic signs or symptoms should not participate in any strenuous activity.
5. Children with Down syndrome who have no evidence of atlantoaxial instability can participate in all sports.

Individuals with trisomy 21 also require cervical radiographic evaluation prior to undergoing general anesthesia, because intubation may involve significant cervical flexion and extension.

Although Fielding said, "The patient with atlantoaxial instability leads a precarious life" treatment of trisomy 21 patients with recognized atlantoaxial instability is controversial.[12] Minor trauma appears rarely to cause neurologic decline in previously asymptomatic individuals with trisomy 21 and abnormal atlantodens intervals.[7,12,13] The observed high complication rates of upper cervical fusion in these patients (including nonunion, loss of reduction, incomplete reduction, and intraoperative cord injury) argue against prophylactic surgery for asymptomatic individuals.[7] Symptomatic patients may require surgical fusion, with consideration of the occiput.[7]

Klippel-Feil Syndrome. Klippel-Feil syndrome (congenital synostosis of the cervical vertebrae) results from failure of normal segmentation of the mesodermal somites during the third to the eighth weeks of fetal life. Fusions at one or two cervical levels (type II) may be an inherited trait, while the cause of more extensive fusions involving cervical and lower spinal levels (types I and III) is uncertain. Cervical instability may occur as a result of "adaptive hypermobility" in open upper cervical interspaces, and spinal cord injuries have been reported.[14–17]

Ehlers-Danlos Syndrome. The ligamentous hyperlaxity of this syndrome is caused by inherited disorders of collagen metabolism. Atlantoaxial instability and dislocation can occur, in addition to problems of scoliosis and spondylolisthesis.[18]

Rubenstein-Taybi Syndrome. Broadening of the thumb and hallux and severe mental retardation characterize this nonhereditary condition. Cervical spondylolisthesis may also occur, placing the cord at risk for injury.[19]

Mucopolysaccharidoses. Several of these lysosomal storage diseases result in skeletal deformities, which include cranial and cervical dysplasias. Hurler syndrome (mucopolysaccharidosis I), Hunter syndrome (mucopolysaccharidosis II), Morquio syndrome (mucopolysaccharidosis IV), and Maroteaux-Lamy syndrome (mucopolysaccharidosis VI) all share the potential for atlantoaxial instability because of odontoid hypoplasia.[20]

Lesch-Nyhan Syndrome. Lesch-Nyhan syndrome, an inborn error of purine metabolism, is characterized by progressive mental retardation, choreoathetosis, spastic cerebral palsy, and aggressive self-mutilating behavior. In addition to the reported orthopedic complications of gouty arthropathy, Shewell and Thompson have reported two brothers with Lesch-Nyhan syndrome with atlantoaxial instability and progressive cervical cord compromise.[21] Both patients were felt to have type 1 odontoid fractures resulting from minor and unrecognized trauma.

Odontoid Hypoplasia and Os Odontoideum. Although odontoid anomalies causing atlantoaxial instability are frequently associated with the aforementioned syndromes, odontoid hypoplasia and os odointoideum can occur in otherwise normal individuals and may possibly arise from unrecognized trauma in the early years of life. Although many affected individuals are asymptomatic, others may have mechanical or neurologic symptoms. All are probably at increased risk for neurologic loss, although the role of prophylactic surgical fusion remains controversial.

Central Cervical Cord Syndrome. Acute central cervical cord syndrome in children due to minor trauma has been reported and does not seem to be associated with underlying anomalies.[22] Acute compression of the cord due to cervical hyperextension with bulging of the ligamentum flavum combined with possible transient subluxation at the upper cervical levels is thought to be responsible. The cord injury may be caused by localized compression and edema in the cord itself or caused by compression and spasm of the descending anterior spinal artery leading to ischemic cord injury.[23,24] Surgery or halo treatment in many of these pediatric conditions is complicated by underlying bone quality and overall effects of the syndrome. Choice of treatment rests with parents and physician on an individual basis. Basic principles of restoration of alignment and stability are considered along with individual patient needs.

INJURIES IN ADULTS

While SCIs in children predominately involve hypermobility of the upper cervical spine, these injuries in adults can be associated with spinal hypomobility, inflammatory changes, or bone and soft tissue hypertrophy.

ANKYLOSING SPONDYLITIS

When ankylosing spondylitis causes progressive loss of motion in the cervical and thoracic spine, flexion or extension forces tend to be focused on the lower cervical levels.[26] With a fall or other minor trauma, highly unstable fractures and dislocations can occur through bone or calcified ligaments and disk tissue. Because patients with such injuries frequently have chronic complaints of neck or back pain due to their underlying inflammatory disease, symptoms of an acute fracture may go unrecognized. Careful radiographic evaluation is essential after any history of trauma, because the majority of ankylosing spondylitis patients who sustain a spine fracture suffer neurologic loss.[26] The extent of cord injury is variable, but complete quadriplegia or paraplegia frequently results. Because patients with ankylosing spondylitis usually have a fixed cervical kyphotic deformity, immobilization after fracture must maintain this degree of flexion.[25,27] Halo vest immobilization is usually sufficient treatment after fracture, but surgical decompression is indicated if there is neurologic injury or the halo is not well tolerated. Treatment must be prompt, as there is a 27% to 35% mortality rate after fractures in these patients.[25,27,28]

Rheumatoid Arthritis and Psoriatic Spondylitis

Atlantoaxial subluxation has been noted in 25% to 30% of patients with rheumatoid arthritis.[29–32] Instability at lower cervical levels and progressive neuropathy can also occur. Smith reported only 4 of 131 previously asymptomatic patients with radiographic findings of atlantoaxial instability who developed signs of cord compromise after a follow-up interval of many years.[33] Instability primarily reflects erosion of ligament insertions and bone by rheumatoid granulation tissue (pannus). This pannus and the adjacent soft tissue swelling can also compromise the spinal canal. Sudden death caused by atlantoaxial subluxation has been reported, and one Swedish autopsy study suggests that sudden head motion associated with vomiting may have been a precipitating factor in five of seven such patients.[33] Psoriatic spondyloarthropathy may also be accompanied by cervical instability of a similar mechanism.

Patients with these diseases including inflammatory spondylitis are clearly at significant risk for SCI with minimal trauma. Signs and symptoms of cord compromise must be carefully scrutinized and evaluated radiographically. General anesthesia with risks of inadvertent cervical manipulation during intubation and positioning must be preceded by radiologic evaluation. Awake and fiberoptic intubation techniques may be considered. Radiographic criteria for cervical instability are well described, but indications for surgical fusion of unstable levels are based primarily upon symptoms and signs of neurologic progression. Acute SCI usually requires surgical management despite unfortunately high rates of infection, nonunion, and medical complications often related to long-term steroid usage.

Ossification of the Posterior Longitudinal Ligament

Ossification of the posterior longitudinal ligament (OPLL) occurs primarily in people of Japanese descent, affecting 2.4% of the Japanese population.[34] Ossification results in gradual narrowing of the cervical spinal canal, with thoracic involvement less commonly seen. Although a gradually progressive myelopathy is characteristic, acute cord injury may occur with cervical hyperextension. During extension, bulging of the intervertebral disk and buckling of the ligamentum flavum can reduce the canal's sagittal diameter by 50%.[9] Although minor trauma causing acute cord "pinching" with symptoms and signs of neurologic loss dictates prompt imaging studies, surgical decompression of this relatively stable lesion can usually be delayed.

Osteoarthritis

The spondylitic changes of osteoarthritis include loss of disk height, annular and ligamental redundancy, and minor segmental instability. In response to instability, vertebral endplate and facet osteophytes develop, and the ligamentum hypertrophies, further compromising spinal canal volume. Forcible cervical hyperextension in a "slip-and-fall" event can "pinch" the cord between the anterior osteophytes and the posterior ligamentum flavum, causing an acute central cord syndrome. Recovery with conservative treatment of this injury is usually good.

Osteoarthritic patients with cervical kyphosis can sustain cord injuries with minor trauma involving forced neck flexion. In these injuries, anterior osteophytes are thought to acutely impact an already tensioned anterior cord. Recovery of neurologic function in this group of patients is not well documented.

Appropriate management after an acute injury is dictated by the degree of neurologic loss but usually includes immobilization and the administration of oral or intravenous steroids. Greater degrees of neurologic loss, myelopathy, marked radiographic findings, and risk of recurrent injuries may suggest surgical intervention. Surgery with neurologic improvement as the goal usually requires decompression followed by fusion, while prevention of progression may require fusion only. Successful posterior cervical decompression requires the patient to have enough physiologic cervical lordosis to allow the cord to "fall away" from anterior osteophytes. If the cervical spine lacks sufficient lordosis, decompression must be performed anteriorly.

Cervical Manipulation

Therapeutic, as well as unintentional, cervical manipulation occasionally results in spinal cord injury.[35,36,37] Reported complication rates of therapeutic manipulation are 1/40,000 for minor injuries and 1/400,000 for major injuries, which include spinal cord compression, vertebral fractures, and vertebral basilar artery injuries.[36] Of 118 patients reported to have vertebral basilar complications, 21 died and 52 were left with serious deficits.[36]

Acute cervical manipulation can result in vertebral artery spasm or dissection or can cause direct compression of the vertebral artery between the occipital condyle and the arch of C1.[1,38] Vertebral artery occlusion affecting the anterior spinal artery may result in ischemia, edema, necrosis, and a watershed infarct of the cord. Immediate management should include intravenous anticoagulants to prevent propagation of the injury.[37]

REFERENCES

1. Pang D, Wilberger JE: Spinal cord injuries without radiographic abnormalities in children, *J Neurosurg* 57:114–129, 1982.
2. Townsend EH Jr, Rowe ML: Mobility of the upper cervical spine in health and disease, *Pediatric* 10:567, 1952.
3. Hensinger RN: Congenital anomalies of the cervical spine, *Clin Orthop* 264:16–38, 1991.
4. Steel HH: Anatomical and mechanical considerations of the atlantoaxial articulation, *J Bone Joint Surg* 5OA:1481, 1968.
5. Parke WW, Rothman RH, Brown MD: The pharyngovertebral veins; an anatomic rationale for "Grisel's syndrome," *J Bone Joint Surg* 66:568–574, 1984.
6. Tachdjian MO: *Pediatric orthopedics*, ed 2, Philadelphia, 1990, WB Saunders, pp 890–892.
7. Doyle JS, Lauerman WC, Wood KB: Complications and long-term outcome of upper cervical spine arthrodesis in patients with Down syndrome, *Spine* 21(10):1223–1231, 1996.
8. Uno K, Kataoka O, Shiba R: Occipitoatlantal and occipitoaxial hypermobility in Down syndrome, *Spine* 21(12):1430–1434, 1996.
9. Parfenchuck TA, et al: *J Pediatr Orthop* 14(3):304–308, 1994.
10. American Academy of Pediatrics Committee on Sports Medicine: guidelines for Down's syndrome patients active in sports, *News and Comments* 35:8, 1984.
11. Fielding JW: The patient with A-A instability lead a precarious life, *J Bone Joint Surg* 58A:400–407, 1976.
12. Burke SW, et al: Chronic atlantoaxial instability in children, *J Bone Joint Surg* 67:1356–60, 1985.
13. Davidson RG, Atlantoaxial instability in individuals with Down's syndrome: a fresh look at the evidence, *Pediatrics* 81:857–65, 1988.
14. Pizzutillo PD: Risk factors in Klippel-Feil syndrome, *Spine* 19(18):2110–2116, 1994.
15. Sherk HH, Dawoud S: Congenital os odontoideum with Klippel-Feil anomaly and fatal atlantoaxial instability. Report of a case, *Spine* 6:42, 1981.
16. Southwell RB, et al: Klippel-Feil syndrome with cervical compression resulting from cervical subluxation in association with an omo-vertebral bone, *Spine* 5:480, 1980.
17. Strax TE, Baran E: Traumatic quadriplegia associated with Klippel-Feil syndrome, *Arch Phys Med Rehabil* 56:363, 1975.
18. Nagashirna C, et al: Atlantoaxial and atlanto-occipital dislocations; developmental cervical canal stenosis in the Ehlers-Danlos syndrome, *No Shinkei Geka* 9:601, 1981.
19. Tachdjian MO: *Pediatric orthopedics*, ed 2, Philadelphia 1990, WB Saunders, p 865.
20. Kopits SE, et al: Congenital atlantoaxial dislocations in various forms of dwarfism, *J Bone Joint Surg* 54A:1349, 1972.
21. Shewell PC, Thompson AG: Atlantoaxial instability in Lesch-Nyhan syndrome, *Spine* 21(6):757–762, 1996.
22. Chen L, Blaw M: Acute central cervical cord syndrome caused by minor trauma, *J Pediatr* 108(1):96–97, 1986.
23. Schneider RC, Cherry G, Panstek H: The syndrome of acute central cervical spinal cord injury, with special reference to the mechanisms involved in hyperextension injuries of the cervical spine, *J Neurosurg* 11:546–577, 1954.
24. Schneider RC, Grosby EC: Vascular insufficiency of brain stem and spinal cord in spinal trauma, *Neurology* 9:643–656, 1959.
25. Detwiler KN, et al: Management of cervical spine injuries in patients with ankylosing spondylitis, *J Neurosurg* 72(2):210–215, 1990.
26. Hunter T, Dobo H: Spinal fractures complicating ankylosingspondylitis, *Ann Intern Med* 88:546–549, 1978.
27. Kiwerski J, Wieclawek H, Garwaka I: Fractures of the cervical spine in ankylosing spondylitis, *Int Orthop* 8:243–246, 1985.
28. Bernd L, Blasius K, Lukoschek M: Spinal fractures in ankylosing spondylitis, *Z Orthop Ihre Grenzgeb* 130(1):5963, 1992.
29. Conlon PW, Isdale IC, Rose BS: Rheumatoid arthritis of the cervical spine, *Ann Rheum Dis* 25:120–126, 1966.
30. Eulderink F, Meijers KAE: Pathology of the cervical spine in rheumatoid arthritis; a controlled study of 44 spines, *J Pathol* 120:91–108, 1976.
31. Mathews JA: Atlantoaxial stabilization in rheumatoid arthritis, *Ann Rheum Dis* 28:260–265, 1969.
32. Meikle JAK, Wilkinson M: Rheumatoid involvement of the cervical spine, *Ann Rheum Dis* 30:154–161, 1971.
33. Smith PH, Penn RT, Sharp J: Natural history of rheumatoid cervical luxations, *Ann Rheum Dis* 31:431–439, 1972.
34. Kurosa Y, et al: Selecting a surgical method for thoracic myelopathy caused by ossification of the posterior longitudinal ligament, *Spine* 21(12):1458–1466, 1996.

35. Auer RN, Kreck J, Butt JC: Delayed symptoms of death after minor head trauma with occult vertebral artery injury, *J Neurol Neurosurg Psychiatry* 57:500–502, 1994.
36. Hurwitz, et al: Manipulation and mobilization of the cervical spine. A systematic review of the literature, *Spine* 21(15):1746–1760, 1996.
37. Murase S, et al: Vertebral artery injury following mild neck trauma; a report of two cases, *No Skinkei Geka* 22(7):671–2, 1994.
38. Soper JR, Parker GD, Hallinan JM: Vertebral artery dissection diagnosed with CT, *Am J Neuroradiol* 16(4 suppl):952–4, 1995.

7

PATIENT POSITIONING IN SPINAL TRAUMA

Samuel S. Jorgenson
John M. Larsen

Patient positioning for the surgical management of spine trauma offers an extensive challenge to the operating room team. Not only are there a variety of positions and devices for spine procedures, but the potential for spinal instability and neurologic injury exists. The proper management of patients with spine trauma in the operating room requires a true team approach. The surgeon must work closely with the anesthesiologist, nursing personnel, and any other ancillary specialists that are commonly involved in such cases.

Ideal positioning for a surgical procedure is intended to allow the surgeon maximum access to the operative site. A conflict arises, however, because the ideal position for the surgeon and assistant is rarely the ideal position for the patient. The placement of the patient in the operative position also represents a time of substantial risk. With the advent of advanced anesthetic techniques prolonged procedures are now possible. When anesthetized the patient does not experience pain and cannot give feedback to undue stress placed on certain anatomic areas. When pressure or stretch exceeds the physiologic limits of the tissues involved, there is the potential for tissue injury. Attention to detail is required to minimize position related complications and provide the optimal surgical outcome.

Safe surgical positioning requires extensive planning to minimize complications. Because the operating surgeon is the only individual who is fully knowledgeable of both the injury and the desired exposure, he must take responsibility to inform the anesthesiologist and other personnel involved. The procedure must be thought out well in advance, and it is imperative that the surgeon have the appropriate training and experience to anticipate potential problems. Because no patient or injury are exactly the same, there is no "cookbook" approach available, and each procedure must be tailored to each patient's unique needs. The spinal surgeon must be present and direct transfer to the operative position.

Martin, in his textbook on positioning in anesthesia and surgery, provides an excellent review of the various positions utilized for modern surgical procedures.[1] He focuses on positioning from the anesthesiologist's perspective and includes a thorough discussion of the physiologic aspects of anesthesia and the affects of positioning. This chapter specifically focuses on patient positioning in surgery of the traumatic spine. The reader is encouraged to read Dr. Martin's textbook for additional information.[1]

PATIENT TRANSFERRING

The patient transfer may well be the most important aspect of positioning in spinal trauma surgery. In the unstable spine, the potential for neurologic injury exists. The transfer mechanism intensifies the need for teamwork more than any other aspect of the procedure.

Before attempting to transfer the patient from gurney to operating room table, all necessary equipment must be in place and in working order. The head and extremity positions must be thought out well in advance. Adequate padding for the head and extremities should be placed on the operating room table before the transfer to minimize excessive motion and minimize repositioning. Additional operating room personnel should be summoned to the surgical suite in advance and be briefed on the sequence. The spinal apparatus used to facilitate surgery also may create some problems. Certain fracture patterns can exacerbate the fracture or dislocation with change in spinal position. Radiographic confirmation of appropriate position should be done if the spine is unstable. Any change in patient position while under anesthesia should have radiographic evaluation.

Transferring the patient to the supine position from a gurney is a relatively simple maneuver. It is best accomplished with a draw sheet placed underneath the patient's back and buttocks. Operating room personnel grasp the sheet in several positions and maintain constant pressure on the sheet. Slowly, the patient is elevated slightly and moved from the gurney to the operating room table, with care taken to keep the patient's neck and trunk in a neutral position at all times. Commands are given by the individual who controls the patient's head, either the surgeon or the anesthesiologist, as determined beforehand.

Transferring the patient from the supine to the prone position on the operating room table is more difficult and requires additional coordination. Again, all positioning devices should be in place including bolsters and appropriate support for the head. The patient should be placed supine and a draw sheet used to gently slide the patient to the side of the bed toward the operating room table. Assistants are positioned about the patient with at least two on either side, another controlling the feet, and the anesthesiologist or responsible surgeon controlling the head, depending on cervical stability. The arms are best placed along the patient's side to facilitate the rolling maneuver, with the patient rolled over the dependent arm. On the appropriate command, the endotracheal tube is disconnected and the patient is log-rolled, first to the lateral position, and then further to the semiprone position onto the outstretched arms of the receiving individuals. At this point, the patient can be slid further onto the operating room table, again operating room personnel being careful to avoid torsion or undue stress on the torso and cervical spine. The gurney bed should be removed at this time and the endotracheal tube reconnected with ventilation resumed. All venous access lines and electrocardiogram (ECG) leads should be checked before proceeding further. After all assistants are again repositioned, the patient's position is then adjusted to the true prone position. The head and arms are then moved into the desired position and the maneuver is completed.

Patients with known or potential spinal instability offer unique circumstances. Under normal conditions, the anesthesiologist is conveniently positioned at the head of the bed, because he is responsible for the airway. When the cervical spine is unstable, however, it is imperative that the responsible surgeon maintain control of the head at all times during positioning and intubation. The surgeon has the unique advantage of knowing details of the patient's injury and subsequently the limits of safe neck positions. The responsible surgeon must control the head and neck during the maneuver to the prone position. In patients with thoracic or lumbar instability, the surgeon is best served by directly participating in trunk position, while the anesthesiologist resumes his normal role of maintaining control of the head and neck.

A final issue of monitoring neurologic status arises in neurologically unstable patients. When there is cervical instability, the anesthesiologist should perform an awake intubation with proper sedation beforehand. In this situation, the patient can then be transferred to the operating room table while awake, allowing continuous monitoring of neurologic function in the process. This provides the safest method of transferring with instantaneous information allowed during the transfer. Another alternative is to intubate the patient asleep, perform the transfer, and then perform a wake-up test when positioning is complete. This alternative carries the disadvantage of not having continuous access to neurologic function and the possibility of considerable time elapsing before this information is available. Spinal cord monitoring with somatosensory potentials is now often used during spinal procedures and can be helpful during transfers. Because monitoring does not provide continuous feedback of neurologic function, comparing potentials before and after transfer is another alternative. This is not a reliable as performing the transfer with the patient awake. Regardless of the method chosen, the surgeon is responsible for manually controlling the injured area of the spine, placing the head in the desired position upon completion in cervical spine injuries, and checking the neurologic status of the patient when the transfer is complete.

SUPINE POSITION

The supine position is probably the most used position in the operating room. In spinal trauma surgery, the supine position is almost exclusively used for anterior exposure of the cervical spine. Anterior approaches to the thoracolumbar spine are usually performed in the lateral decubitus position. Lumbar approaches may be performed prone or decubitus.

The anterior approach to the cervical spine requires firm support of the head, while allowing flexibility for placement of the head and neck in the desired anatomic position. The Mayfield (OSI) horseshoe device seems ideally suited for this purpose. It is well-padded, adjustable to various head sizes, and can be manipulated to almost any degree of flexion or extension. This device permits simultaneous use of a traction apparatus such as cervical tongs or halter apparatus when desired. Most surgeons prefer to use some type of bolster underneath the patient's shoulders, placed either horizontally or longitudinally, to allow the head to fall back sufficiently and approach the normal amount of cervical lordosis.

Once the head is positioned satisfactorily, great care must be exercised to prevent injury from pressure points. When operating on the cervical spine, the arms are most conveniently placed at the patient's side to allow the surgeon and assistant access to the cervical area. The arms must be well-padded, especially around the elbow and wrist, to avoid nerve palsies. While most conventional operating room tables have a thin layer of cushioning, additional padding should be placed under potential pressure points, such as the buttocks, calves, and feet. The hips and knees are best placed in a slightly flexed position. A rolled towel or other support can be placed under the lumbar spine to maintain lordosis and possibly minimize the incidence of postoperative low back pain.

PRONE POSITION

The majority of spinal surgery is performed with the patient in the prone position. This position is used for the posterior approach to the cervical spine and occiput for both decompression and fusion. The prone position is also used for posterior approach to the thoracic, lumbar, and thoracolumbar junction. Several factors contribute to successful prone positioning including adequate visualization of the surgical site by both the surgeon and the assistant, the avoidance of pressure complications, minimizing blood loss, and maintaining the desired amount of lumbar lordosis.

In 1940, Batson in his classic anatomic work documented an intricate system of sinusoidal channels surrounding the spine throughout its entire length.[2,3] He showed that under normal physiologic conditions, this system drained directly into the superior inferior vena cava through a valveless channel. Most importantly, he showed that this flow can easily be reversed with obstruction or pressure on the caval system. Blood is shunted from the caval system, through the valveless channel, engorging the venous plexus surrounding the spine. This can produce unnecessary blood loss.

Several factors of the prone position can contribute to partial or complete obstruction of the vena cava and engorgement of the spinal plexus veins.[4–8] These include increased thoracic pressure or abdominal pressure created from positioning. Even minimal abdominal pressure causes considerable obstruction of the vena cava and subsequent venous engorgement around the spine. This in turn can lead to uncontrollable venous oozing and a potential compromised surgical result. When the patient is positioned in the prone position, therefore, every effort must be made to minimize chest and abdominal pressure by allowing the abdomen to hang as freely as possible and, subsequently, minimizing the vena cava pressure.

Several prone position devices have evolved over the years and are well documented.[5,9–13] All are intended to minimize abdominal pressure while still maintaining adequate position of the spine with the patient in the prone position. Current techniques include three essential styles of devices. First is the use of longitudinally placed lateral bolsters. This is accomplished either by manually placing bolsters longitudinally on either side of the table, spanning from the chest down to the iliac crest, or with a fixed device such as the Wilson frame. Both of these techniques do allow some reduced abdominal pressure, while maintaining adequate support on the spine (Fig. 7-1).

The second position requires strategically placed bolsters under the chest and pelvis with the abdomen hanging free. A common example of this type of frame is the Relton-Hall, or four-poster frame. This device places pressure on the chest and both iliac crests allowing the entire abdomen to hang free (Fig. 7-2).

The third method is the knee-chest position or one of its many modifications. The Andrews (OSI) frame is the most popular knee-chest positioning device in modern spinal surgery. This device places the patient's torso and thighs at 90 degrees with weight bearing shared between the chest, knees, and buttocks. It offers the advantage of allowing the abdomen to hang freely and creates a slightly kyphotic posture of the lumbar spine, which is desirable in some procedures (Fig. 7-3).

DiStefano and coworkers measured inferior vena caval pressures during anesthesia in patients undergoing spinal surgery on a variety of different devices (Table 7-1).[14] This study illustrates the marked variation in caval pressures with the use of different devices. This data and that of other studies conclusively shows that the laterally placed bolsters, or Wilson frame, have unacceptably high abdominal and vena cava pressures compared to other devices such as the four-poster frame or knee-chest position.[5,11] The last two devices allow minimal abdominal pressure, which results in reduced intraoperative blood loss and better visualization.

When the operative site involves the lumbar spine or thoracolumbar junction, the degree of lumbar lordosis becomes an issue worthy of attention. For purely decompressive procedures such as laminectomies or discectomies, it is often helpful to reverse or at least flatten out the lumbar lordosis to facilitate entrance into the spinal canal. When this position is desired, the knee-chest position and Wilson frame allow for hip flexion and subsequently reduced lordosis. If, on the other hand, fusion is contemplated into the lower lumbar spine or especially the lumbosacral junction, it is imperative to maintain appropriate lumbar lordosis. To prevent a flat-back posture after fusion and subsequent postoperative pain, the lumbar lordosis should be maintained as closely to anatomic as possible. Lumbar lordosis is directly affected by hip position with more lordosis being created with the hips extended and less lordosis with progressive flexion of the hips.[15,16]

LATERAL DECUBITUS POSITION

Trauma of the thoracolumbar spine is being treated anteriorly with increasing frequency. Some fracture patterns, especially with anterior cord compression, are best treated with anterior decompression and subsequent stabilization, effecting the need for spinal exposure through thoracotomy, thoracolumbar approach, or lateral abdominal exposures to the lumbar spine. These approaches are best accomplished in the lateral

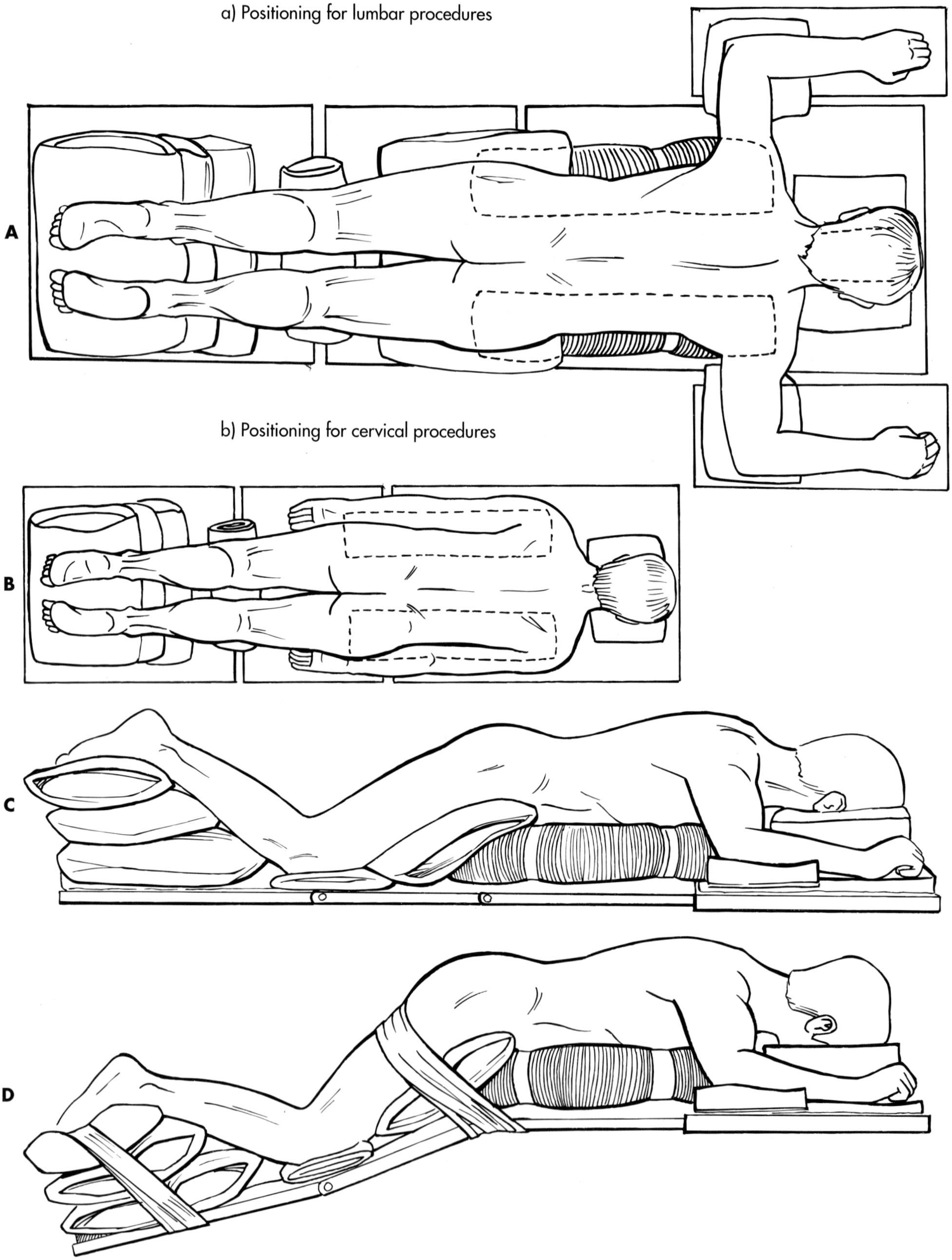

Figure 7-1

Prone position with Bolsters illustrated both with arms tucked and jackknife position.

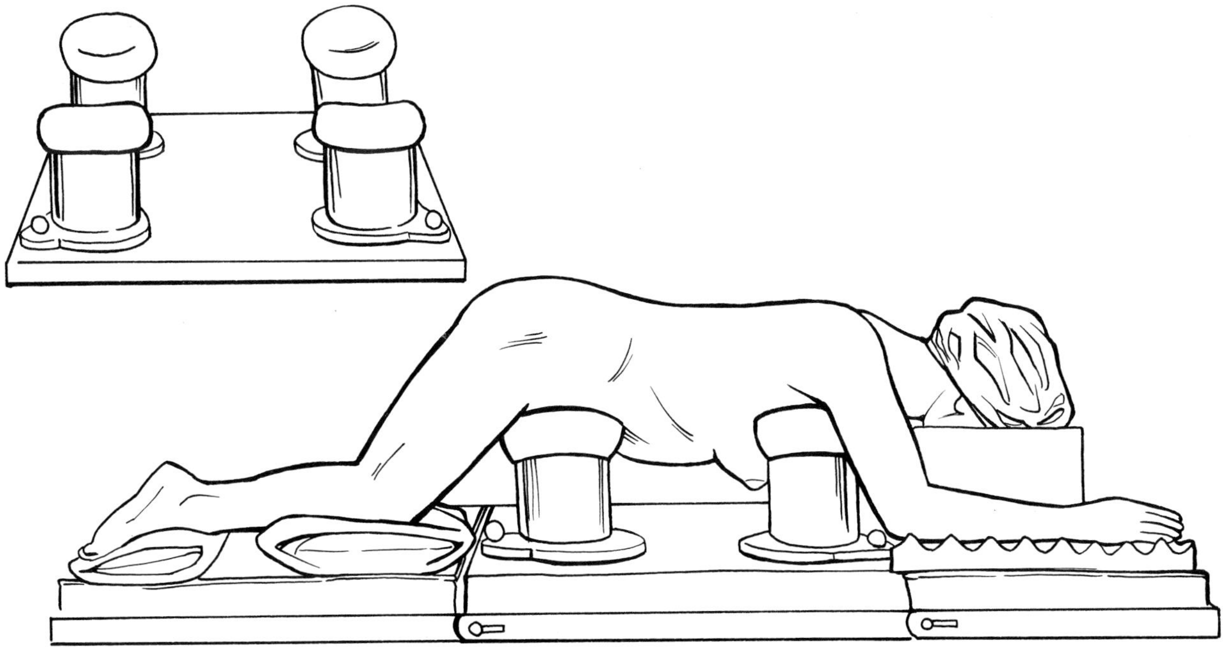

FIGURE 7-2

Four poster frame.

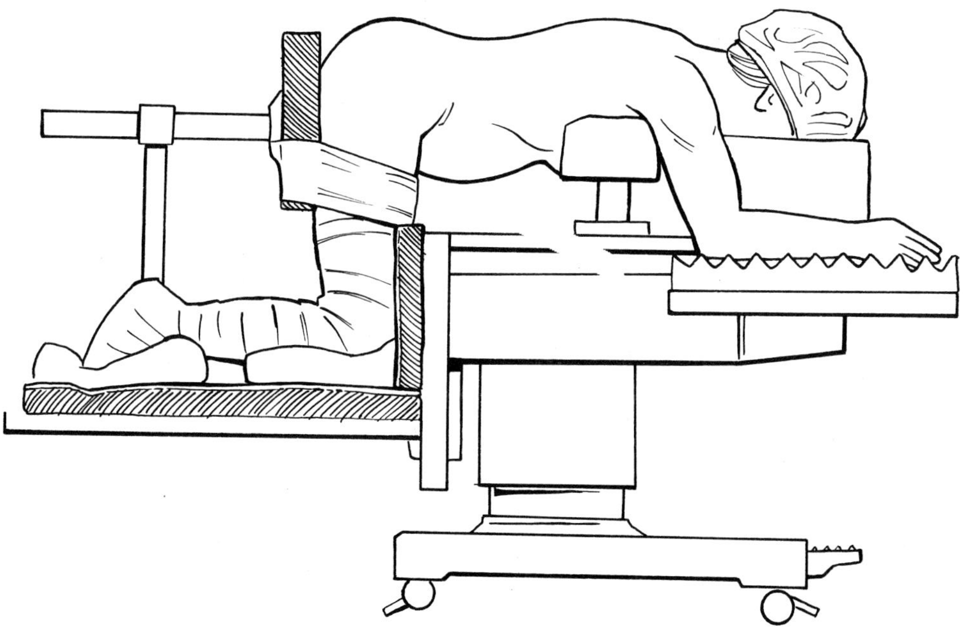

FIGURE 7-3

Knee chest position with Andrews frame.

decubitus position when the anterior aspect of the spine is the site of anatomic interest (Fig. 7-4).

For the majority of anterior spine procedures performed for trauma, the patient is placed in a true lateral position with the back positioned perpendicular to the table. By securing the patient in this position, rotational variations can be achieved by turning the table in the desired direction. The area of injury should be positioned over the break in the table to allow the jackknife position if needed and, of course, if spine stability allows. Once the patient is in the lateral position, the lower hip and knee are flexed slightly with

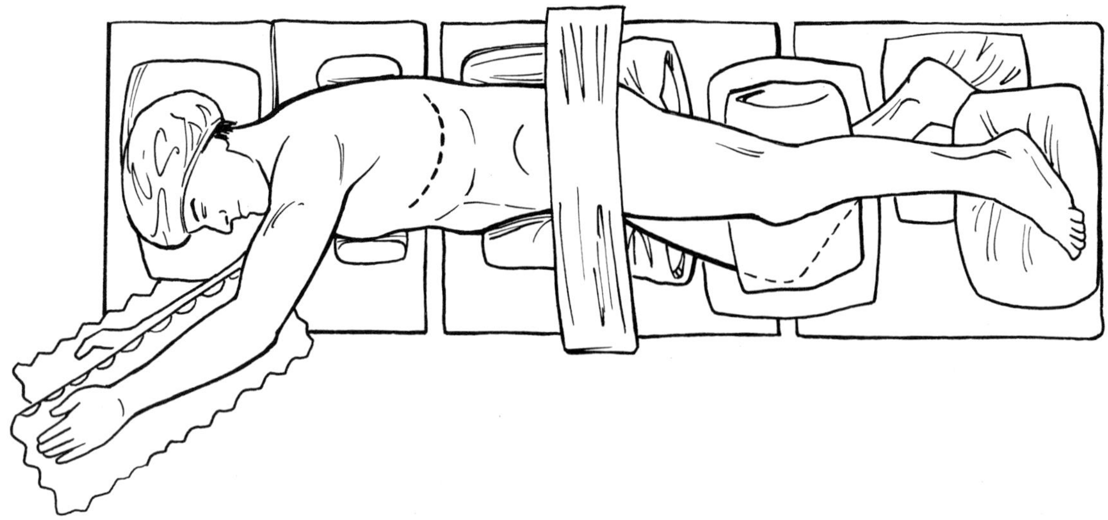

FIGURE 7-4

Lateral decubitus position.

Table 7-1.

Positioning Modes	IVC Pressures (cm H_2O) Average	Range
Prone with bolsters	15.9	8.0–23.5
Wilson frame	10.1	4.0–15.0
Lateral decubitus	11.1	5.4–17.0
Georgia prone	20.7	8.4–39.0
Tuck	9.4	5.8–14.0
Hasting's frame	1.4	−2.0–6.6

From DiStefano DJ, Klein KS, Nixon JE, Andrews ET: Intra-operative analysis of the affects of position and body habitus on surgery of the low back, *Clin Orthop* 99:51, 1974.

the upper hip slightly extended to provide stability. This position also aids in relaxing the abdominal and psoas musculature. The usual care of padding bony prominences on the lower leg become even more important in this position. The lateral aspect of the hip in the area of the trochanter, the lateral aspect of the knee where the peroneal nerve crosses the fibula, and the lateral foot and ankle all require generous padding to prevent nerve palsies. A pillow can then be used between the dependent and upper leg if needed. A small roll such as a rolled towel or cylindrical gel pad is placed just distal to the axilla on the dependent side to minimize compression of the neurovascular structures passing through the axilla. Care should be taken to assure that the pad is positioned well distal to the axilla and stable enough to prevent migration. Any direct pressure on the axilla could affect neurovascular compromise. The dependent arm is placed in a neutral position on an arm board in a slight cephalad position so as to be out of the operative field. The upper arm is most easily placed in an airplane type device that allows flexibility of position. Both arms should be well-padded throughout, and every attempt should be made to provide as neutral a position as possible minimizing excessive stress on shoulders and elbows. Once in position, the torso should be stabilized to prevent motion during the procedure. This can be accomplished by either placing bolsters on the front and back of the pelvis, using a beanbag, placing a wide strip of tape across the trochanteric area and attaching it to either side of the table, or some combination thereof.

COMPLICATIONS

PRONE POSITION

Potential complications of the surgical procedure performed in the prone position begin with patient transfer.[17,18,19] Loss of airway access can easily occur during transfer from the supine to the prone position, even with appropriate planning. Each line must be guarded from entanglement as the patient is turned. Following completion of the turn, the airway and all access lines should be checked to be sure they're in proper working order before progressing with the actual procedure.

With the face dependent, pressure on the facial

structures can lead to injury. Pressure sores to the forehead, cheeks, ears, and chin can occur if pressure is not evenly distributed on an appropriate device. Several devices are available for this including a Mayfield (OSI) horseshoe or several commercial foam pads with cut-outs designed to accommodate the airway. It is imperative to prevent any direct pressure on the eyes in the dependent position. Central retinal artery occlusion has been reported secondary to direct ocular pressure, resulting in permanent blindness.[20–23]

Upper extremity neuropraxia can easily occur to the brachial plexus from excessive abduction of the shoulder. With the elbow placed at 90° on the arm board, the ulnar nerve is extremely vulnerable in the dependent aspect of the elbow. The chance of ulnar neuropathy can be minimized only by generous padding about the elbow.

Pressure to all dependent areas in contact with the table or positioning device requires appropriate padding to prevent injury. Areas of concern are the breasts and nipples, pelvis, and knees, especially in the knee-chest position. The lateral femoral cutaneous nerve can easily be compressed by bolsters or a four-poster frame causing numbness and paresthesias to the anterolateral aspect of the thigh. Patients with pendulous abdomens require extra care to assure there is no unforeseen pressure on the anterior abdominal wall as the abdomen hangs free. Finally, the genitalia need to be inspected to be sure there is no pressure on tissues or traction on the catheter.

Stephens has shown the knee-chest position to diminish predictably the lumbar lordosis.[15] If fusion procedures including rigid segmental internal fixation are performed using the knee-chest position, it is possible to produce flat-back deformity, which may lead to postoperative pain. Careful attention sagittal alignment is necessary to maximize the clinical results of procedures such as these. By using the prone position, such as that accomplished by the Jackson frame, the physiologic lumbar lordosis tends to be maintained. It may be that this position is more appropriate for fusion procedures utilizing internal fixation.

The knee-chest position also deserves special attention because of several rare but catastrophic complications.[24,25] Aschoff reports two cases of lower extremity compartment syndrome after a procedure in the knee-chest position requiring fasciotomy.[24] With the hips and knees flexed 90 degrees, pooling of the venous structures in the dependent position is possible and can lead to compartment syndrome. There is no known practice to avoid this complication, but clinical suspicion is important postoperatively to deal with the problem in a timely manner. Keim[26] reports a patient with acute renal failure as a consequence of myoglobinuria, which subsequently led to acute renal compromise. Finally, venous hypotension in the knee-chest position may lower the clinical suspicion for anterior penetrating injuries to the vena cava. Larsen and coworker reports a case when the anterior annulus was perforated during a posterior discectomy procedure with a minimum of bleeding into the operative field.[29] Low clinical suspicion for a vascular injury was indirectly related to the low vena caval pressures in the knee-chest position. In this particular case, this led to a delay of the diagnosis and eventually resulted in death.

LATERAL DECUBITUS POSITION

Complications of the lateral decubitus position are primarily related to pressure injuries to the head and extremities. Alopecia of the scalp has been described as a consequence of prolonged scalp pressure, which causes occlusive vasculitis. Lawson and coworker noted several patients with permanent alopecia following open heart surgery in the lateral decubitus position. It is believed that frequent head rotation or small changes in position may help prevent this occurrence. Ocular complications have been reported from direct pressure on the dependent eye. Multiple cases of retinal artery thrombosis leading to permanent blindness have been reported.[29,30]

The brachial plexus is at risk as a consequence of either direct compression on the dependent axilla or traction to either the dependent or upward axilla. The mechanism of injury in both of these positions is believed to be secondary to ischemia of the intraneural vasovasorum. These injuries can be minimized by proper placement of the axillary roll and minimizing abduction and forward flexion of the shoulder.

Lower extremity complications are primarily pressure injuries to the skin, tendons, and ligaments of the knee and ankle. Insufficient padding of the common peroneal nerve traversing the fibula distal to the knee can again result in peroneal nerve palsy and postoperative foot dorsiflexion weakness.

Patient positioning for the surgical management of spinal trauma offers an extensive challenge to the operating room team. Safe surgical positioning requires extensive planning and teamwork. Regardless of the operative position chosen, it is the surgeon's responsibility to personally supervise the transfer. In each instance, the surgeon should be physically involved in manually controlling the injured area of the spine.

Regarding the patient with spinal instability, transfers should optimally be performed with the patient awake. If this is impossible, a wakeup test following positioning is necessary. Close radiographic monitoring of changes in fracture position encountered during transfer is essential.

With insightful preoperative planning, good teamwork, and meticulous attention to detail, most complications can be avoided.

REFERENCES

1. Martin JT: *Positioning in anesthesia and surgery*, ed 2, Philadelphia, 1987, WB Saunders.
2. Batson OV: The function of the vertebral veins and their role in the spread of metastases; *Ann Surg* 112:138–149, 1940.
3. Norgore M: Clinical anatomy of the vertebral veins, *Surgery* 17:606–615, 1945.
4. Bostman O, Hyrkas J, Hirvensalo E, et al: Blood loss, operating time, and positioning of the patient in lumbar disc surgery, *Spine* 15(5):360–363, 1990.
5. Callahans R, Brown M: Positioning techniques in spinal surgery, *Clin Orthop* 154:22–26, 1981.
6. McNulty SE, Wiss J, Azad SS, et al: The effect of the prone position on venous pressure and blood loss during lumbar laminectomy, *J Clin Anesth* 4(3):220–225, 1992.
7. Pearce DJ: The role of posture in laminectomy, *Proc R Soc Med* 50:109, 1957.
8. Rollason WN: Anesthesia and the "bloodless field," *Curr Res Anaesth* 32:289, 1953.
9. Alexander JP: Problems associated with the use of the knee-chest position for operations on the lumbar intervertebral discs, *J Bone Joint Surg (Br)* 55(2):279–284, 1973.
10. Eie N, Solgaard T, Kleppe H: The knee-elbow position in lumbar disc surgery: a review of complications, *Spine* 8(8):897–900, 1983.
11. Relton JES, Hall JE: An operation frame for spinal fusion: a new apparatus designed to reduce hemorrhage during operation, *J Bone Joint Surg (BR)* 49B:327, 1967.
12. Smith R, Grambling Z, Volpitto P: Problems related to the prone position for surgical operations, *Anesthesiology* 22:189, 1961.
13. Wayne SJ: A modification of the tuck position for lumbar spine surgery. A fifteen year follow-up study, *Clin Orthop* 184:212–216, 1984.
14. DiStefano DJ, Klein KS, Nixon JE, Andrews ET: Intraoperative analysis of the affects of position and body habitus on surgery of the low back, *Clin Orthop* 99:51, 1974.
15. Stephens GC, Yoo SU, Wilbur R: Comparison of lumbar sagital alignment produced by different operative positions, *Spine* 21(15):1802–1807, 1996.
16. Tan SB, Kozak JA, Dickson JH, et al: Effect of operative position on sagittal alignment of the lumbar spine, *Spine* 19(3):314–318, 1994.
17. Courington FW: The role of posture in anesthesia, *Clin Anesth* 3:24, 1968.
18. Dunn EJ, LeClair WE: How to reduce complications in the treatment of cervical spine trauma—instructional course lectures, 34:155–162, 1985.
19. Garfin SR: *Complications of spine surgery,* Baltimore, 1989, Williams & Wilkins.
20. Mertens E, Smets RM, Sys J, et al: Central retinal artery occlusion after back surgery: a case report, *Bull Soc Belge Ophtalmol* 255:127–131, 1995.
21. Stambough JL, Cheeks ML: Central retinal artery occlusion: a complication of the knee-chest position, *J Spinal Disord* 5(3):363–365, 1992.
22. Walkup HE, Murphy JD: Retinal ischemia during unilateral blindness—a complication occurring during pulmonary resection in the prone position, *J Thoracic Surg* 23:174, 1952.
23. Wolfe SW, Lospinuso MF, Burke SW: Unilateral blindness as a complication of patient positioning for spinal surgery: a case report, *Spine* 17(5):600–605, 1992.
24. Aschoff A, Steiner-Milz H, Steiner HH: Lower limb compartment syndrome following lumbar discectomy in the knee-chest position, *Neurosurg Rev* 13(2):155–159, 1990.
25. Weinlander CM, Coombs DW, Plume SK: Myocardial ischemia due to obstruction of an aortocoronary bypass graft by intraoperative positioning, *Anesth Analg* 64(9):933–936, 1985.
26. Keim HA, Weinstein JD: Acute renal failure—a complication of spine fusion in tuck position, *J Bone Joint Surg* 52A:1248–1250, 1970.
27. Larsen JM, Capen DA, Rimoldi RL, et al: Complications associated with the use of the Andrews operating table. Presented at Rancho Los Amigos MC Research Day, June, 1992, American Back Society Annual Meeting, Dec, 1992, San Francisco, CA, and Advances in Spinal Surgery, Santa Barbara, CA, Jan, 1994.
28. Lawson NW, Mills NL, Ochsner JL: Occipital alopecia following open heart surgery, *J Thorac Cardiovasc Surg* 71:342, 1976.
29. Lincoln JR, Sawyer AP: Complications related to body positions during surgical procedures, *Anesthesiology* 22:800, 1961.
30. Britt BA, Gordon RA: Peripheral nerve injuries associated with anesthesia, *Can Anaesth Soc J* 11:514, 1964.

8

ROLE OF SPINAL CORD MONITORING IN SPINE SURGERY

Robert D. Harbaugh
Robert E. Henry

This chapter explores the role of intraoperative neurophysiologic monitoring during traumatic spine surgery. As there are many and varied neural structures "at risk" during any particular case of spine trauma, broad generalities about monitoring technologies must be drawn. As the technical and advanced physiologic aspects of intraoperative monitoring are beyond the scope of this book, only basic concepts and general principles are addressed. Somewhat analogous to differing surgical styles and techniques, we have focused more on established procedures, which are more readily applied to the majority of spine operations. Unfortunately, intraoperative neurophysiologic monitoring requires more than "off-the-shelf" instrumentation and technique and requires at least a modicum of training and experience. Specific topics are discussed superficially; therefore, the reader must consult reference texts or more detailed sources before employing any outlined technique.[1,2,3]

Intraoperative monitoring is usually performed at the request of the surgeon, as a process to provide "real-time" feedback to assess the status of central and peripheral nervous system structures in jeopardy during operative procedures. As virtually any segment of the neuraxis can be monitored in theory, the surgeon must make specific decisions about which part or components of the nervous system are at greatest risk and how can that risk be assessed effectively with current technology. Within the domain of orthopedic spinal cord trauma, most procedures have the following requirements:

1. Emergency or urgent preparation and execution of intraoperative monitoring (IOM) because of the timeliness of surgery.
2. Simplicity and efficiency of monitoring systems, which can be set up rapidly, be ready at off-hours, and be able to monitor within different operating room environments.
3. Primary monitoring emphasis on threats to the integrity of the spinal cord, nerve root, brainstem, cerebral cortex, etc.

For most purposes, somatosensory evoked potentials (SSEPs) provide a reliable, well-established system for monitoring the integrity of the spinal cord during acute spinal surgery. In addition, acute surgical intervention for trauma generally involves extradural trauma or lesions (e.g., hematoma or bone fragment). This contrasts with other surgical interventions involving intraspinal lesions (e.g., intramedullary neoplasm) in which limits to dissection, risk of vascular compromise, and other operative concerns alter the utility of continuous neurophysiologic monitoring.

More specific technical and physiologic details of spinal cord monitoring are discussed in latter portions of this chapter. Animal models and a large body of observational human data have shown that both SSEP and motor evoked potential (MEP) monitoring is highly sensitive to significant threats to or physiologic impairment of the spinal cord from such insults as external compression, ischemia, distraction, and anatomic distortion.[4,5] If the integrity of the evoked potential pathway is jeopardized during surgery, then an "alarm" is sounded notifying the operative team of this event. Other processes including pharmacologic, systemic, and technical factors may lead to loss or alteration of signal; however, in general, with adequate communication and careful attention to proper technique, highly reliable intraoperative evoked potentials can be obtained. If an alarm sounds during a spinal procedure, the surgical team is notified. If a *reversible* insult to the spinal cord is identified, then in many instances, the surgical team can make major alterations in procedures to correct spinal cord viability.

Although cost-benefit analyses are scarce, conservative estimates suggest that if reversible spinal cord dysfunction is discerned and corrected in as little as 0.25% of operative procedures, then intraoperative neurophysiologic monitoring would be cost-effective.[1,3,6]

Given the absence of morbidity and potential for preventing a costly and devastating neurologic complication, such as paraplegia, the necessity for using continuous intraoperative monitoring is clear. Definitive evidence of the overall impact of electrophysiologic monitoring during spine surgery with respect to outcomes, however, remains largely speculative. Unfortunately, the ethics of performing randomized trials comparing monitored versus unmonitored subjects precludes presumptions of neurophysiologic utility.

Additional factors that may affect the decision to implement intraoperative monitoring include "standards of care" with regard to the medicolegal implications of high-risk patients and the "reassurance" of intact spinal cord function during a given surgical procedure. Such real-time feedback allows for greater confidence in such domains as spinal distraction, decompression, and other manipulative techniques in which cord integrity is threatened. The concept of evoked potentials and their applications in neurophysiology were first promoted by Dawson in the 1950s.[7] Technical limitations, however, precluded their implementation until the late 1970s when efficient analog-to-digital conversion devices and microprocessors were developed, which could handle the immense data flow. The 1980s saw an explosion in the production of integrated systems that could provide efficient monitoring of multiple channels with high user-control interfaces. Further technical developments are refining instrumentation with an emphasis on flexibility and ease-of-use. Currently, intraoperative spinal cord monitoring is based on well-understood principles of neurophysiologic functioning; however, the ability to extract extremely small neurophysiologic information from a literal sea of ambient noise (the operating room) was not practical until the late 1970s. As instrumentation has evolved over the past decade, the number of false-positive and false-negative results has dropped. This is the result of, in part, improved technique and a better understanding of monitored pathways. (A number of early reports of false-negatives were, in part, erroneous, because of misinterpretation of technical aspects of these studies.) In addition, improved shielding and preamplification, coupled with better electrode technology, have provided substantial improvements in the overall technical quality of intraoperative monitoring.

The "science" of intraoperative monitoring matured in the early 1980s.[1] Intraoperative spinal cord monitoring is now considered standard care in many community and referral institutions. Most national organizations that are involved with clinical neurophysiology recognize the importance of intraoperative monitoring and now provide recommended technical guidelines for it.[2]

In addition, regional, national, and international symposia offer "hands-on" experience. Of some interest, expertise in the field of intraoperative monitoring has been provided by specialists and subspecialists from such diverse arenas as audiology, basic clinical neuroscience, anesthesiology, neurosurgery vascular surgery, clinical neurology, pediatric neurology, epileptology, and physiatry and orthopedic surgery. Most electrodiagnostic programs, however, are supervised by neurologists with special training in clinical neurophysiology. (Board subcertification is available for clinical neurophysiology.) A number of orthopedic surgeons have contributed substantially to the widespread use of intraoperative spinal cord monitoring and, in some cases, have provided technical program oversight. Intraoperative monitoring is now regularly covered by a number of journals and is the subject of more than half a dozen textbooks.

ELECTROPHYSIOLOGIC BASIS OF EVOKED POTENTIALS

Evoked potentials refer to neuroelectrical responses "evoked" by stimuli. In theory, any type of stimuli, including taste, smell, and touch, could evoke a response. (The term *evoked response* is considered tautological and the preferred term is *evoked potential*). From a practice standpoint with respect to somatosensory evoked potential monitoring during spinal surgery, however, either direct cord stimulation or, more generally, large fiber, mixed sensory-motor, peripheral nerves are stimulated, and the subsequent afferent volley of sequential potentials are measured "downstream" (beyond the site of operative risk). Specific recording sites are selected based on monitoring strategies as outlined in a later section. Conversely, MEPs imply direct stimulation of motor pathways, either at the cortical or subcortical level with subsequent averaged or unaveraged "responses" being picked up either distal to the surgical site within the spinal cord or, more commonly, at peripheral locations.

In general, the voltages recorded from distal electrodes of an evoked potential (whether it be sensory or motor) are substantially lower than ambient noise or other neural activity. In some settings, this may be many magnitudes lower, and thus the signal-to-noise ratio ultimately depends upon the technical ability of any monitoring system to reliably record an evoked potential. The key concept in the capability of recording small evoked potentials lies in the ability to "signal average." Signal averaging allows for a time-locked neural response to be recorded at a predictable interval after a stimulus has been applied. By repeated averaging of minute electrophysiologic signals, ambient noise and other neurophysiologic activity (e.g., electroencephalogram [EEG]), which is not time-locked and which is *random*, is effectively subtracted out, as their average contribution to many recordings would tend toward zero.[9] The ability to refine the signal-to-noise ratio by increasing the number of responses, however, carries an exponential relationship (directly proportional to the square root of the total number of averaged signals). For example, four times as many responses are needed to reduce the signal-to-noise ratio by half, or nine times as many averages are needed to reduce the ratio by two thirds, and so forth. Thus, a practical limit exists for extracting measurable and reliable evoked potentials.

Evoked potentials are generated by two primary physiologic processes: nerve fiber bundles and nuclei. Nerve fiber bundles convey relatively synchronized action potentials, which in general are recorded as a triphasic "traveling wave" as they pass beneath a referential electrode. In contrast, sensory nuclei are depolarized in a complex fashion without a simple dipole and may manifest anatomic heterogeneity. Hypothesis of evoked potential sources are based on a knowledge of normal animal and human neurophysiology and in both animal and human subjects with disease.[2,3]

Extensive understanding of precise generators for all evoked potential recordings is incomplete, however, Nevertheless, for the purposes of intraoperative monitoring, evoked potentials provide sufficiently accurate and reproducible measures of impairment of the spinal cord so as to be useful to the operative team.[6,10]

TECHNIQUES OF INTRAOPERATIVE SPINAL CORD MONITORING

SOMATOSENSORY EVOKED POTENTIAL

General Principles of Evoked Potential Monitoring. The scope of this chapter remains an overview of intraoperative monitoring for the nontechnologist and nonneurophysiologist. A basic understanding of the common procedures and techniques used, however, is important for all members of the surgical team to understand the capabilities and limitations of intraoperative neurophysiologic monitoring.

Modern neurophysiologic equipment should meet the safety standards outlined by the American Society for Clinical Neurophysiology. For SSEP monitoring standard recording parameters would include the following:[1,2,3]

1. *Stimulation sites.* For structures at risk at or below the seventh cervical level, lower extremity monitoring is advised. Conversely, for structures at risk above the seventh cervical spinal level, the upper extremity (median or ulnar nerve stimulation) may be used. Subdermal needle or silver-tin electrodes applied cutaneously are used for stimulation. Electrical square-wave stimuli are applied at rates of 3 to 8 Hz, with 100 to 300 microsecond stimuli. In general, peripheral stimuli are sufficient to evoke a motor twitch. Most technicians use a stimulation level that exceeds the threshold for a motor twitch by approximately 50% (i.e., 1.5 × motor twitch). Cathodal and anodal electrodes are generally placed approximately 2 to 3 cm apart, directly over the mixed peripheral nerve of choice. In general, the posterior tibial nerve yields the best recordings from the lower extremities, although in selected patients and for other reasons, the peroneal or other nerve may be chosen. For upper extremity stimulation, either the ulnar or median nerves may be stimulated, although, in general, median nerve stimulation, particularly in the awake patient provides more robust SSEPs.
2. *Recording sites.* A variety of recording sites for evoked potentials should be considered in any monitored case. In general, we have favored surface recordings with either cutaneous silver disk electrodes or subdermal needles. This choice allows for quicker, easier, less traumatic and more accessible recordings. A variety of alternative recording electrodes may be used, however, including those applied in intraspinous ligaments, within the vertebral column itself, and in epidural areas. These recording devices, however, must be applied intraoperatively by a surgical team and cannot be used for the entire surgical period. Low linear filters of 1 to 30 Hz and high linear filters of 1500 to 3000 Hz are usually used for somatosensory recordings. Notch (60 Hz rejection) filters are generally used. Artifact rejection systems, stimulus isolation units, and cautery switches are strongly recommended. Intraelectrode impedances must be matched where possible. Proper grounding is imperative, and careful attention to potential "leakage currents" is vital for the patient's safety.
3. *Recording strategies.* In general, we have found the following principles helpful for optimal and "user-friendly" intraoperative somatosensory evoked potential monitoring;
   a. *Redundancy of stimulation and recording sites.* When possible, extra sets of stimulation electrodes and recording electrodes are applied. In addition, recording strategies that use two or more "downstream" recording sites ensure that attenuation or loss of signal is not artifactual and reflects either a pathologic or physiologic change in the monitored structures at risk.
   b. *Monitoring of "upstream" or input evoked potentials.* Recording from proximal large mixed nerves in either the upper or lower extremities is important. Surface sites can easily be

placed over the popliteal fossa or Erb's point to ensure that a perceived loss of evoked potential beyond the operative site is again caused by either pathologic or physiologic changes and not technical failure (such as dislodged stimulating electrodes).

c. *A choice of asynchronous, bilateral stimulation or synchronous, simultaneous bilateral stimulation.* Although hemicord syndromes are rarely reported as a result of spinal cord injury (SCI) during surgical procedures, such nonsurgical observations are extraordinarily rare. Most current instrumentation, however, allows for interleaving asynchronous simultaneous bilateral stimulation in a way that left- and right-sided dorsal column pathways can be stimulated and compared. This also provides a certain degree of redundancy in that separate systems are being monitored contemporaneously. For patients with preexisting neurologic deficit or marginal preoperative evoked potentials, however, bilateral simultaneous stimulation of peripheral structures may be needed for optimal recording. We rely on this alternative strategy in selected circumstances.

4. *Waveform identification.* Recordings are assessed for prominent "early" peak spinal or cortically generated evoked potentials. Absolute latency, amplitude, and symmetry of the evoked response are key indicators of integrity of the somatosensory system.

Technique of Intraoperative Somatosensory Evoked Potential Monitoring. Intraoperative somatosensory evoked potential (IO-SSEP) monitoring remains the mainstay of neurophysiologic monitoring of spinal cord function during surgical procedures for most surgeons and neurophysiologists.[1,3,10] A large body of information has shown that this technology, when technically feasible and performed properly, provides extremely high sensitivity to "significant" cord compromise and, with rare exceptions, can provide the operative surgeon with adequate feedback about the status of the spinal cord during procedures whenever spinal cord integrity may be at risk.[11]

In acute spinal trauma (where baseline studies may not be feasible and arrangements for complex monitoring cannot be made) an expedited team approach to surgery and monitoring is required. We have found SSEPs to be relatively easy to set up, particularly when minimally invasive techniques are use. There are no recognized significant risks to the patient when standard techniques are employed. The IO-SSEP can be generally set up in parallel with other preoperative procedures, such as insertion of intravenous lines, surface site preparations, patient positioning, and early anesthetic intervention. Even in experienced hands, however, a minimum of 30 to 45 minutes of preparation may be needed for a sole electrodiagnostic technologist to apply stimulating and recording devices and obtain initial recordings.

In general, either peroneal or tibial nerve stimulation (for the lower extremities), have been shown in normal human volunteers to provide the most robust spinal and cortically generated evoked responses. In the upper limbs, ulnar or median nerve stimulation has shown similar properties. Recordings can be obtained, however, from virtually any large mixed (sensory motor) nerve (e.g., pudendal or radial). As these other sites have smaller numbers of afferent nerve fibers in general, less well defined and more variable evoked potentials appear in populations of normal volunteers and surgical subjects.

For most studies, we have found posterior tibial nerve stimulation in the leg (ankle) and median or ulnar nerve stimulation in the upper extremity (wrist) to be the most reliable and dependable sites. Substantial variability exists among patients, however, and other sites should be considered in selected persons. As noted, recording locations for somatosensory evoked potentials may be skin, subdermal, intralaminar, interspinous, epidural, or subdural sites. We have generally used surface recordings and primarily used upper cervical or scalp derivations (electrode combinations). No uniform standards apply to all procedures, however, and variability among neurophysiologists precludes consensus.

Monitoring is continuous throughout the surgical period for many reasons, including observation for changes that may occur during initial positioning, establishment of baseline values (and variability), and for assessment of occult cord compromise at any point before, during, or after "critical" surgical maneuvers.

Most neurophysiologists consider an absolute evoked response amplitude reduction of 50% or more in an otherwise stable recording to reflect a potentially significant physiologic or pathologic change in spinal cord function (i.e., "calling an alarm"). In general, such amplitude reductions are commensurably associated with latency prolongation. In general, a latency shift of 10% (generally more than 2–4 ms) or more is considered to represent a significant neurophysiologic change. Experienced neurophysiologists know, however, that for patients with moderate variability in an otherwise uncomplicated procedure, a 50% or more reduction in waveform amplitude may occur transiently; therefore, one must treat each monitored case separately. (With respect to response variability, strict guidelines do not exist for unstable or volatile SSEPs.) Certainly, complete absence of evoked potentials, particularly with two or more trials (when previously demonstrated), merits an alarm.

If repetitive studies show loss or substantial attenuation of the evoked potential, the technologist checks the system integrity and checks if other stimulation sites have recognized evoked potentials *proximal* to the operative field. If technical factors are readily excluded, the technologist looks to the anesthesiologist and to the primary surgeon to announce the alarm. We have found it useful to establish specific roles for each member of the operative team when a neurophysiologic alarm is sounded during an operation. The technologist or neurophysiologist must ensure that technical factors, such as machine malfunctions and inadvertent switching of stimulation or recording channels, have not occurred. The anesthesiologist must determine if recent physiologic changes, such as significant hypotension, hypothermia, or drug use which may affect evoked potential pathways, have occurred. Lastly, the surgeon needs to consider any pathologic process that may be related to current or recent manipulation of neural structures at risk, including positioning, an anticipated distraction or displacement of spinal elements, and other unanticipated processes (e.g., unseen epidural hematoma or vascular injury). An excess of false alarms is far more preferable than a paucity of true alarms.

Unavoidable SCI may occur despite all surgical efforts. Thus, surgical monitoring provides only a measure of neurophysiologic integrity and to that end is valuable in those settings where significant physiologic or reversible surgical processes have occurred or are predicted. In those cases with high risk of *irreversible* detrimental spinal cord effects, the significant loss of evoked potentials is of limited utility and is not unexpected.

Substantial or complete loss of SSEPs, which are not accounted for by technical reasons (and which are presumably based on SCI) and which do not improve during the remainder of the surgical procedure, is highly indicative of substantial neurologic deficit. Conversely, return of IO-SSEP waveforms strongly predicts a good neurologic outcome (as does retention of unchanging evoked potentials throughout the case); however, SCI may obviously occur during spine trauma surgery, and that event can neither be predicted nor avoided. Although accurate data do not exist, a substantial proportion of IO-SSEP waveforms, which are completely lost during spine surgery and which are associated with neurologic impairment, are caused by predictable or unavoidable intraoperative events. As expected, improvement in SSEPs may occur during cord decompression. Finally, from a philosophical perspective, IO-SSEP monitoring carries no outcome guarantee, only the hope of improved results.

In a small but measurable percentage of otherwise "neurologically normal" individuals (depending upon the technique used), readily recorded or reproducible SSEPs *cannot* be obtained. (In trained hands, however, this number may be very small.) Certainly in myelopathic or peripheral nerve disease this percentage is much higher, reflecting the morbidity of the population at hand. Thus, IO-SSEPs cannot be obtained in all patients. Surprisingly, however, following induction of anesthesia with the elimination of muscle artifact, previously unobtainable SSEPs may be recordable in some persons. In cases where intraoperative monitoring is important, therefore, an attempt to obtain SSEPs is reasonable preoperatively and at least during the initial phases of surgery following anesthesia.

Waveform Generation and Nomenclature. The precise details of stimulation and recording site technique, instrumentation analysis, and waveform identification are beyond the scope of this chapter. (Standard textbook and review articles have infarction on these aspects of intraoperative monitoring.[1,2,3,7]) Nevertheless, some familiarity with the interpretive aspects of SSEP monitoring is necessary for implementation by all on the surgical team.

A precise system of identification of evoked potential waveforms has not been established.[9] In general, most authors describe peak waveforms by the designation N or P referring to a peak negative or peak positive waveform. Such identifications, however, would be entirely dependent on the specific relationship of the recording electrodes (i.e., the voltage difference between two points). In general, identified waveforms are stipulated by a capital letter with a subscript number, which refers to an approximate mean (average) absolute latency in milliseconds for that waveform in an awake, control population. Unfortunately, there are no absolute standards in accepted normative groups.

Most evoked potential waveforms are reasonably well established with respect to their neurophysiologic generators.[2,9] Localized generators of important median nerve SSEP waveforms are as follows (specific designations vary among authors):

1. N_9 (sometimes referred to as the Erb's point) refers to a volume-conducted afferent volley in the brachial plexus.
2. N_{11} refers to volume-conducted neural activity in the dorsal root entry zone of the high cervical cord.
3. N_{13} appears to reflect complex afferent volleys and synaptic activity deep in dorsal columns and nuclei at the base of the brainstem.
4. N_{19} or N_{20} activity emanates from early thalamocortical volleys and reflects the first stage of cortical processing, which occurs after the upper limb somatosensory evoked responses arrive in the supratentorial compartment.
5. The P_{22} waveform appears to be derived from association projections.

Subsequent waveforms, which are highly variable and which have unpredictable morphologies, represent "processing" of sensory data.

With respect to peroneal nerve stimulation, certain waveforms have the following putative origins:

1. LP (lumbar potential) appears to originate from conducted activity in the dorsal root entry zones for the lumbosacral nerves, which make up the peroneal nerve.
2. The P_{27} potential appears to be analogous to the median nerve derived N_{20}, in that it reflects thalamocortical activity.
3. Later waveforms the N_{35} potential in particular, appear to represent subsequent secondary or tertiary sensory processing in the association cortex.

For evoked potential monitoring, a robust and readily identified waveform distal to the operative site is used primarily for establishing integrity of the SSEP. Either a high cervical or brainstem signal or a cortically generated evoked potential is used for monitoring purposes. With anesthesia, early operative latency and morphology alterations may be compared to awake, baseline tracings; however, subsequent *changes* in evoked potential recordings are used to delineate disrupted neural function.

For purposes of intraoperative monitoring, the keys for waveform identification and monitoring include:

1. Establishing a baseline, preoperative studies clearly identify reproducible and robust peripheral or "input" potentials, and, similarly, "downstream" recordings are physiologically beyond the operative site of potential cord involvement.
2. Employing techniques that allow for redundancy should one component fail.

In contrast to the diagnostic applications of SSEPs in the outpatient setting, precise waveform morphology, absolute latency, and precise interside asymmetries are not critical *unless* there are observed and reliable changes during the procedure. As mentioned, a 50% reduction of the peak-to-trough amplitude in the initial cervical or cortically recorded evoked potential relevant to the monitored pathway system is criterion for abnormality and suggests change in spinal cord function. This generally correlates with at least a 2 to 4 ms latency or 10% prolongation of the early or initial evoked potential. At such time, the technologist sounds an alarm to the operative team. Two separate trials usually within minutes of each other are recommended to ensure that such changes are not due to sporadic variability, which unfortunately can occur even in stable recording settings. As in any system, however, false alarms occur and, in fact, are desirable. As with any monitoring system, a relatively low threshold for establishing the potential for threats to the integrity of an at-risk neurophysiologic system *is* warranted. False-positive recordings (alarm sounded, but patient awakes with no deficit) occur now in less than 5% to 10% of cases in our experience. Early studies reported much higher frequencies, likely because of less sophisticated instrumentation. False-negative SSEP studies (no alarm, patient awakens with deficit) are reported but are extremely rare (anecdotal reports only with limited population-based data; almost certainly less than 1%). True-negative SSEPs have a greater than 98% to 99% predictive value of good postoperative neurological cord function. The current rate of true-positive studies obviously depends upon the at-risk surgical population but approximates 3% to 15% in most published series, with estimates of significant *reversible* changes accounting for all scenarios, with pharmacologic, physiologic, and surgical likely comprising a substantial portion.[6,10]

The SSEP changes cited above generally occur in one of two settings.

1. An abrupt change in the SSEP, usually appearing over minutes, (assuming it reflects a true physiologic change) suggests an acute compressive or catastrophic effect upon cord function.
2. A slow attenuation or loss of the signal, often occurring over 10 to 30 minutes, suggests the presence of an ischemic injury not directly related to anatomic compression.

For these reasons, we have recommended that monitoring be carried out from "start to finish" in all cases in which the spine is at risk, because the monitored changes may not necessarily occur at the time of highest risk (e.g., distraction or spinal cord manipulation). In addition, we have seen significant and potentially threatening changes in intraoperative evoked potentials during patient positioning at the beginning of surgery and at other times when cord integrity would normally not be in question (e.g., during closing). Some have relied upon concurrent ulnar-nerve SSEPs to assist in monitoring for the possibility of intraoperative ulnar nerve injury secondary to positioning or inadvertent compression during any major spine procedure.

A reasonable summary of potential causes of worrisome SSEP loss, attenuation, or latency prolongation not due to technical factors includes significant global physiologic alterations including hypotension, hypoxemia, and hypothermia and local spinal cord ischemia on the basis of segmental perfusion failure, local compression, and anesthetic effects with potentially many contributions.[2] Surgical times of increased or greater risk include periods of spinal distraction, periods of significant physiologic change as noted above, sublaminar wire insertion or passage, distraction and/or derotation maneuvers, spinal osteotomies, use of certain instruments such as Luque rods or other stabilization frames, ligation of segmental arteries, and pedicle screw insertion. In addition, "active" surgery in and around the spinal cord obviously should be considered as carrying an increased risk of cord injury. Patient risk factors include unstable physiologic status (hypothermia, hypotension, or hypoxemia), significant preexisting kyphosis or congenital scoliosis, neurologic deficits (myelopathic or peripheral neuropathic), and previous spinal traction.

A large body of evidence has been generated over

the past 15 years demonstrating varying effects of anesthetic or other intraoperative pharmacologic agents upon the ability to adequately monitor IO-SSEP or MEP.[2,3] Specifics are complex, and there is no consensus on anesthetic agents. There are, however, several general principles regarding anesthetics and SSEPs.

1. Volatile anesthetics significantly decrease the amplitude of intraoperative spinal cord SSEPs. In general, concentrations of volatile anesthetics should be less than 0.5 maximum allowable concentration (MAC) if noninvasive recording sites are utilized.
2. A "mixed" nitrous/narcotic protocol has proved effective for us, although a variety of authors have reported significant depressant effects of nitrous oxide on SSEPs.
3. Opioids generally decrease SSEP amplitudes minimally.
4. Benzodiazepines tend to decrease SSEP amplitudes with minimal effect upon latencies.
5. Propafol, when provided in relatively low infusion rates without "bolus" administration, is generally associated with retained SSEPs.
6. Etomidate may actually augment the cortically generated somatosensory evoked response.
7. Neuromuscular blockade is encouraged and has no direct effect on the ability to record SSEP waveforms at any level. Neuromuscular blockade tends to reduce background noise generated by muscle and, therefore, is encouraged (as long as electromyographic monitoring is not employed).

The reader is referred to standard reference texts for greater specificity of current recommendations of the appropriate anesthetic choice during intraoperative spinal cord monitoring.[2,3] In general, the principle of multiagent "balanced" anesthesia with avoidance of bolus administration has proved a useful strategy in achieving optimal responses.

WAKE-UP TEST

The "wake-up test" was first reported by Vauzelle, Stagnara, and Jouvinroux in 1973, as a method of intraoperative spinal cord monitoring.[12] They reported a routine, in 124 procedures, of awakening patients intraoperatively following Harrington rod instrumentation. Anesthesia was administered to secure easily partial awakening, and voluntary motor power was tested in the upper and lower extremities. Three case reports were detailed to illustrate the utility of this method. In two cases, there was no lower extremity movement during the wake-up test and, therefore, the instruments were removed. Motor power returned within 5 minutes in one case and within 15 minutes in the other. The rationale is early detection and release of distraction could reverse potential SCI. This test has since been generally referred to as the "Stagnara wake-up test." Many surgeons still consider this to be the "gold standard" of intraoperative spinal cord monitoring. There have been no reported incidences of patients with normal wake-up tests awakening with paraplegia.[2]

The wake-up test is easy to administer, and no extra equipment is required. Various methods of anesthesia may be used, but, in general, a balanced nitrous oxide, narcotic and muscle relaxant sequence is used with goals of sufficient analgesia, amnesia, and minimal gross body motion. First the muscle relaxants are withdrawn. Three to five minutes are allowed for the patient to begin spontaneous respirations. Then the nitrous oxide is turned off, and 100% oxygen is given. The patient is then asked to squeeze a hand or make a fist. Once able to perform this, the patient is then asked to move both feet. Absence of movement or lower extremity weakness indicates spinal cord dysfunction and the need for intervention. In cases involving correction of spinal deformity, for example, this often requires reduction of the correction and repeating the test.[13] Booke et al. reported reversal of a positive wake-up test and SSEP abnormalities following spinal derotation maneuver with Cotrel-Dubousset instrumentation.[14] The patient was hypotensive and anemic at the time of the wake-up test. The SSEPs returned to baseline within 40 minutes of normalization of mean arterial pressure and increased hematocrit following autologous blood transfusion. A second wake-up test showed normal bilateral foot movement and strength. With equivocal spinal cord monitoring changes and mild hypotension, restoration of normal blood pressure often results in normalization of the monitor tracings.[15] A wake-up test "side effect, " which can be advantageous, is the rise in blood pressure and consequent relative increase in spinal cord perfusion, which occurs with awakening from anesthesia.

Before the operation, the patient should be informed about the wake-up test procedure to minimize the potential for adverse psychologic consequences because of remembering the event. Twelve of 150 patients questioned following procedures involving wake-up tests remembered nonpainful awakening.[13] Preoperative rehearsal of specific wake-up test instructions and movements is recommended.

There are several disadvantages to the wake-up test. Although the test can be repeated during a given operation, the test obviously does not offer continuous spinal cord monitoring. The test is not sensitive for nerve root monitoring or sensory pathway monitoring. It can be accomplished only with cooperative patients, which in many cases would exclude, for example, those who are too young, those with developmental delays, or those with cognitive sequela of traumatic brain injuries. Although relatively uncommon, other potential problems include the risk of extubation, dislodging of spinal instrumentation, vascular access lines, eye injuries, air embolism as a result of negative intrathoracic pressure generated with spontaneous breathing (thoracic wounds should be flooded with saline to prevent this), and emotional distress. The test cannot be performed in cervical spine procedures.[2,16]

As experience increases in multimodality motor and sensory spinal cord pathway monitoring, the use of the wake-up test in spinal surgery has begun to decline. In some centers, surgeons no longer perform a wake-up test when intraoperative spinal cord monitoring has remained stable; however, others continue to recommend its use whether or not neuromonitoring changes are appreciated.[2,17]

MOTOR EVOKED POTENTIALS

Somatosensory evoked potential monitoring has remained the standard for intraoperative neuromonitoring. While true false negatives are relatively rare, postoperative neurologic deficits despite normal SSEPs recorded intraoperatively have been reported.[10,18] Such occurrences have sparked increasing interest in development of techniques for monitoring ventral spinal cord function. Over the past 10 to 15 years, multiple techniques for intraoperative monitoring of motor tract functioning have been developed, many of which we describe here. Other techniques for ventral tract functional monitoring under investigation include spinal cord evoked potentials generated by galvanic vestibular stimulation and transcranial sensory evoked potentials recorded from occipital electrodes.[18,19] The ventral spinal cord and motor pathways in the spinal cord receive a different blood supply from that of the dorsal columns, which are monitored by traditionally obtained SSEPs. Selective traumatic or ischemic damage to anterior or anterolateral cord structures, therefore, might go undetected by SSEP.[18,20]

Motor evoked potential monitoring at this point in time is experimental. Advances in technology and increased experience with a variety of techniques, however, render promise for future practical, reliable, and sensitive intraoperative spinal motor pathway monitoring.

The primary descending motor pathway targeted by electrophysiologic monitoring techniques is the corticospinal tract. This travels predominantly from the motor cortex through the posterior limb of the internal capsule, cerebral peduncles, the pons and the lower medulla, where approximately 90% of these fibers cross over to the contralateral, lateral corticospinal tract. Upper motor neurons in the lateral corticospinal tracts then synapse on alpha motor neurons in the ventral horns at targeted segmental levels. Second-order motor neuronal axons then exit the spinal cord through the ventral roots, join the dorsal roots at the level of the intervertebral foramen to form spinal nerves, and then travel peripherally to their target muscles. Ten percent of the axons that did not cross over at the medulla continue descending in the anterior corticospinal tract in the ventral funiculus. Axons from the anterior corticospinal tract cross the midline at targeted segmental levels to synapse on second-order motor neurons in the contralateral ventral horn. Other descending tracts arising from the brainstem include the rubrospinal tract, which travels with the corticospinal tracts, the medial and lateral vestibulospinal tracts, and the reticulospinal tracts, which descend in the ventral funiculus. Major functions of these tracts include motor control, postural maintenance, and modulation of flexor and extensor tone.

Techniques. Motor evoked potentials can be generated using stimulation techniques of essentially two types: cortical stimulation and Spinal cord stimulation. Motor evoked potentials may be recorded at the level of the spinal cord, peripheral nerve, or muscle. Cortical stimulation can be achieved by electrical stimulation or magnetic stimulation.

Transcranial Stimulation. Intraoperative MEP monitoring with transcranial stimulation techniques offer several practical advantages. The technique is not invasive and, therefore, does not introduce any added surgical risk or risk of infection, and with the stimulating equipment outside of the surgical field, continuous monitoring during surgical manipulation is possible.[21]

Electrical stimulation was first introduced in 1980.[22] Brief, high-voltage shocks are applied to the scalp, overlying the motor cortex with cup electrodes or spiral electrodes, stimulating cortical motor neurons or their axons, resulting in corticospinal tract potentials and, ultimately, upper or lower extremity muscles twitches. Selective right or left upper or lower extremity activation can be achieved by careful positioning of the stimulating electrodes over appropriate areas of the motor cortex.[23]

Transcranial magnetic cortical stimulation was first introduced in 1985.[24] A large current pulse of approximately 4,000 A is passed through a wire coil, producing a magnetic field, which then passes through the skull, without attenuation. Cortical and probably subcortical motor neurons are stimulated, resulting in descending motor tract potentials. As with electrical stimulation techniques, upper or lower extremity activation can be achieved by careful positioning of the magnetic coil over the appropriate areas of the motor cortex.[21,25]

There are certain advantages and disadvantages to each technique. Electrical cortical stimulation offers the advantage of relatively less complexity with respect to set up for intraoperative monitoring, and lower equipment cost.[26] Pain associated with electrical stimulation is a disadvantage of this technique in awake subjects; however, this is not an issue intraoperatively, when patients are anesthetized. Transcranial magnetic cortical stimulation is painless, rendering this technique more attractive for evaluation of awake patients in the diagnostic laboratory. A substantial disadvantage of using transcranially elicited MEP for intraoperative monitoring, whether electrically or magnetically induced, is that they are highly sensitive to suppression by most anesthetic agents. Anesthetics have a greater suppressive effect on evoked potentials transmitted through a greater number of synapses.[1,27] The transcranial magnetically elicited, MEP is somewhat more sensitive to anesthetic suppression than the transcranial electrically elicited, motor evoked potential. This may be caused by a preferential excitation of tangentially oriented cortical fibers by magnetic stimulation, leading to transsynaptic activation of the cortical spinal neurons (thus, a greater number of synapses), as opposed to direct excitation of the corticospinal neurons by electrical stimulation.[26] Magnetically generated MEP are also typically more variable, in part because of susceptibility to slight changes in coil position. Recent advances in coil design and magnetic field focusing have resulted in significant improvements in these techniques.[1,21,26]

There are safety factors and relative contraindications to the use of transcranial cortical stimulation, which should be considered when using either of these methods. There is potential for neuronal tissue injury resulting from high-charge densities; therefore, patients with skull fractures or surgical defects, which could result in current shunting, and patients with implanted metallic devices, which may focus current density, should not be monitored with these techniques. Magnetic stimulation may cause dysfunction of implanted electronic devices such as drug pumps or cardiac pacemakers; therefore, patients with these devices also should be excluded. A history of seizure disorder is a relative contraindication, given the possibility of induction of a seizure by repeated electrical stimulation.[1] Potential long-term effects of repeated transcranial cortical stimulation have not yet been determined; however, no permanent adverse effects have been documented.[1]

Myogenic Potentials Obtained with Transcranial Stimulation. Myogenic potentials, or compound motor action potentials (CMAP), are recorded from either surface electrodes or needle electrodes inserted into muscles in the upper and lower extremities. Muscles typically evaluated include the dorsal interosseous or thennar muscles of the hands, dorsal interosseous muscles of the feet, and the tibialis anterior muscles, although a number of other muscles can be monitored.[23,28,29,30] Compound motor action potential recording allows monitoring of multiple motor segments and selective recording from each extremity. Relatively good amplitude responses are obtained; therefore, extensive averaging is not necessary, allowing more rapid feedback of motor tract functioning during surgical manipulations.[21,26] Myogenic MEPs, however, are highly susceptible to suppression by inhalation and intravenous (IV) anesthetic agents and, of course, neuromuscular blocking agents.[21,29,30,31] Anesthesia appears to suppress the MEP transmission within the interneuron pool of the spinal gray matter, or perhaps it acts directly on alpha motor neurons. There is no effect on peripheral conduction or neuromuscular junction.[30] Complete neuromuscular blockade obliterates the CMAP responses. Neuromuscular blockade maintained at 80% to 90% has been found to be optimal using this technique with intraoperative monitoring during spinal operations.[25] Variations, however, in neuromuscular blockade during various stages of surgery can result in difficulties with this technique.[23] Careful monitoring of muscle wave and twitch response to supramaximal peripheral nerve stimulation and neuromuscular blocking agent administration with a constant infusion system can minimize this potential problem.

These factors have contributed to disappointing success rates for reliable CMAP neuromonitoring. Kitagawa et al. reported a 53% overall success rate using an anesthetic protocol of ketamine, fentanyl, nitrous oxide, and oxygen.[25] Manipulation of the anesthetic protocol with reduced fentanyl dosage, however, improved this success rate to 82%. Specific anesthetic protocols have consequently been developed to optimize CMAP recording with transcranial stimulation techniques. In addition to anesthesia manipulation, CMAP responses can be facilitated using paired magnetic stimulation techniques, which result in increased temporal summation of the multiple descending volleys at the spinal level and increases in cortical excitability, improving the response reproducibility and reducing the negative impact of anesthesia.[32]

Spinal Evoked Potentials with Transcranial Stimulation. Spinal cord recordings can be obtained with needle or surface electrodes; however, less artifact is introduced with epidural or subdural recording electrodes. Spinal cord potentials are monitored at two sites, one rostral and one caudal to the spinal segment at risk. The proximal tracing, therefore, provides a "control" for intraoperative comparison with the caudal tracing. The epidural or subdural electrodes may be placed intraoperatively by the surgeon through a laminectomy site or between lamina, or they may be inserted percutaneously at sites above and below the surgical exposure.

Epidural spinal recording of MEP elicited by transcranial cortical stimulation offers several advantages over recording of CMAPs. Anesthetic suppression is significantly less with this method, and the responses are not affected by neuromuscular blockade, allowing for adequate monitoring with full anesthesia and muscle relaxation. The corticospinal volleys recorded are relatively stable. Two types of waves are recorded. Initial D waves are attributed to direct activation of the corticospinal axons, and I waves are attributed to indirect or transsynaptic activation of corticospinal neurons due to stimulation of cortiocortical interneurons.[33] The simple D waves are highly stable within individuals during a constant anesthetic state in the absence of surgical maneuvers, such that amplitude changes of only 20% to 30% have been proposed as warning criteria when evoked by transcranial electrical stimulation.[33] The transcranial magnetic stimulation techniques result in smaller and more variable corticospinal volleys.

Specific warning criteria for MEPs acquired at the spinal cord following transcranial stimulation are not yet well delineated. Sensitivity and specificity for detection of SCI intraoperatively have yet to be determined. Zentner reported intraoperative MEP monitoring in 40 patients with neurosurgical spinal lesions, using transcranial electrical stimulation and epidural recording of spinal cord and cauda equina potentials.[34] All patients were monitored with epidural recording electrodes overlying the cauda equina, and 23 cases were evaluated with bipolar cardiac pacing electrodes placed epidurally overlying the spinal cord above and below the lesion site. Using the criteria of 50% amplitude reduction compared with baseline by the end of operation as defining an abnormal variation, postoperative neurological status of the patients were correlated with MEP results. Spinal cord recording yielded a 65% recordability of potentials intraoperatively, and cauda equina recordability was 82.5%. An overall rate of 23.8% nonrecordable responses was obtained intraoperatively despite maximal stimulation (750 volts). Overall, there was an 85.4% correct correlation of the motor evoked potentials with postoperative neurological status. Similar percentages were noted for cauda equina and spinal cord recording techniques. There were no false negatives. The postoperative motor status deteriorated in 3 of 40 patients. In two of those patients with increased postoperative motor deficits, the MEP amplitudes decreased by more than 50% compared with baseline at the end of operation. The motor evoked potentials were lost intraoperatively in the third patient, who was found postoperatively to have an incomplete tetraparesis. Complete loss of MEPs, therefore, appears to indicate more severe motor tract dysfunction.

Burke reported on simultaneous monitoring of motor and sensory pathways in 120 patients undergoing surgery for scoliosis.[33] Epidural spinal electrodes at the lower cervical and lower thoracic levels recorded descending potentials evoked by transcranial electrical stimulation and ascending volleys elicited by tibial nerve stimulation at the popliteal fossa. Stimulation, recording, and anesthesia techniques were optimized to produce reliable, well-defined sensory and MEP responses in 85% of all cases and in 100% of patients without preoperative clinically detected neurological deficits. Minimal averaging was used, requiring approximately 30 to 75 seconds per trial. Motor evoked potential abnormalities were identified in 12 patients in whom there were also sensory volley changes at the high thoracic recording site; however, motor changes preceded sensory potential deterioration in three patients. Most of the changes occurred during application of correction forces. Warning of these changes resulted in surgical interruption of curve correction and elevation of blood pressure. Complete resolution of MEP abnormalities were noted in nine of the patients and these "substantially" improved in three by the end of the procedure. None of the patients experienced new motor deficits or increased motor deficits postoperatively. No false negatives were reported.

In summary, intraoperative monitoring of MEPs using transcranial stimulation techniques is investigational. A U.S.F.D.A. investigational device exemption is required to use a magnetic stimulator above the foramen magnum.[29] All CMAP responses are highly affected by anesthesia and cannot be obtained with complete neuromuscular blockade. Muscular movement associated with stimulation can be disruptive intraoperatively. Epidural spinal cord recording offers advantages of responses with larger amplitude and less variability, which are significantly less attenuated by anesthesia and can be obtained with full neuromuscular blockade. Clinical trials have yielded some encouraging results with this technique; however, specific warning criteria, sensitivity, and specificity have yet to be determined.

Spinal Cord Stimulation. The spinal cord may be electrically stimulated directly, using subdural or epidural stimulating electrodes, or indirectly, using needle stimulating electrodes placed close to the spinal cord. Epidural electrodes may be placed at the time of surgery at the most rostral aspect of the surgical exposure, or they may be placed percutaneously through a Tuohy needle.[1] Alternatively, needle electrodes may be placed into spinous processes, with the tips located in cancellous bone, close to the anterior cortices of the lamina, or in a disk space.[26] This alternative technique is preferred by some to avoid the increased risk of epidural electrode placement and longer time requirements for set-up.[35,36] Spinal recording is achieved through epidural electrodes placed in the same manner, caudal to the operative site. The rostral and caudal electrodes may then serve as stimulating or recording electrodes, so that both ascending or descending responses can be monitored intraoperative. A recording electrode placed midway between distraction hooks also has been recommended during scoliosis surgery, in light of evidence showing a higher degree of spinal cord evoked potential sensitivity in the middle of the distraction.[37] Well-defined potentials are obtained relatively rapidly with this method. Baba and Kawahara found abnormal spinal cord evoked potentials in more than 80% of 70 patients with proved cervical or thoracic myelopathy, with approximately 10% showing no abnormality, which they attributed to possible technical problems or technique limitations.[38] The descending spinal cord evoked potentials do not necessarily reflect motor tract function. In fact, the descending spinal cord evoked potentials consist primarily of antidromic potentials conducted via dorsal column sensory tracts; therefore, normal responses may be recorded in the setting of anterolateral spinal cord injury.[26,37,39,40]

The concept of neurogenic motor evoked potentials (NMEP) was first introduced by Owen et al. who described a technique for recording of mixed nerve potentials evoked by spinal cord stimulation using needle electrodes positioned near the sciatic nerve at the ischial tuberosity or the popliteal fossa.[17] The evoked potentials consist of a large orthodromic motor response followed by smaller, more unreliable antidromic responses. Owen et al. reported findings from simultaneous monitoring of SSEP and NMEP in 300 cases of spinal surgery.[17] They found that the NEMP were more reliable than cortical SEPs. No false negatives were seen using the criteria of 60% loss amplitude and 10% latency prolongation for the NMEP. During the initial 18 months of testing, 17 false-positive NMEPs were recorded; however, no false-positive NMEPs were reported during the last 14 months of testing. The authors attributed this to an increased understanding of potential methodologic and technical problems, illustrating the importance of neurophysiologic monitoring team experience. Five patients who had undergone surgery for intrathecal or intramedullary tumors awakened with motor paraplegia. In all of these patients, the NMEPs were lost, with preservation of the SEPs. Conversely, two patients who were found to have postoperative sensory deficits demonstrated significant reduction of SSEPs without NMEP changes. Other reports have also suggested that NMEPs are more sensitive to motor tract dysfunction than SEPs and that NMEPs are more sensitive to ischemic change and acute spinal cord compromise compared with spinal cord evoked potentials.[27,41] Anesthesia does not influence the responses substantially. The potentials may be distorted by MEPs resulting from incomplete muscle relaxation, therefore, adequate muscle relaxation must be maintained.[42]

Techniques for evoked potential recording in muscle following spinal cord stimulation were developed to increase the likelihood that monitoring of these responses would reflect purely motor tract functioning.[43] Animal sectioning studies have recently shown that following single stimulation, these responses are obliterated following selective dorsal column ablation and, therefore, appear to travel antidromically down the dorsal columns to activate postsynaptic potentials in the anterior horn.[27] Following stimulation with consecutive paired pulses or train stimulation (up to five pulses), however, the evoked potentials did not change after dorsal column transection and disappeared after ipsilateral, lateral column sectioning. It was thus concluded that myogenic potentials following train spinal cord stimulation represent ipsilateral lateral column function and traverse multiple synapses on their way to target muscles.

Myogenic responses are highly sensitive to anesthetic suppression, particularly when obtained with single stimulation techniques.[27,44] Dual stimulation, however, substantially augments the responses, such that the responses may be reliably obtained, despite IV anesthesia.[27,44] The responses are further augmented by train stimulation, such that responses are obtainable with this method even with inhalation anesthesia.

Mochida et al. reported two true positive cases and no false-positive cases utilizing train spinal cord stimulation and myogenic recording in 25 patients undergoing cervical surgery and 10 patients undergoing thoracic or thoracolumbar surgery.[27] They reported that this technique yielded larger amplitudes than are achieved with NMEP recording, with less interference from operating room "noise." Careful control of muscle relaxation is required to avoid muscle twitches, which could interfere with microsurgical procedures.

SEGMENTAL NEUROPHYSIOLOGIC MONITORING

Spinal operation involving decompression or fusion with instrumentation are associated with considerable risk of nerve root injury.[45–48] Mixed nerve SSEPs are mediated by multiple nerve roots and, therefore, are not sensitive to single nerve root irritation or injury. Highlighting this, radiculopathy with significant weakness and sensory dysfunction following spinal fusion surgery with pedicle screws, despite normal mixed nerve SSEP recordings, have been reported.[48] Pedicle screw placement failures are common.[45–50] Failure rates of 21% and 40% per screw-placement attempt have been reported by experienced surgeons, despite use of radiographic and fluoroscopic guidance.[44,49] Neurologic deficits following pedicle screw instrumentation range from 2% to 7%.[45] Postoperatively, CT scanning can be used to identify pedicle screw malposition in patients with radiculopathic symptoms or signs, and reintervention can then be undertaken as necessary.

Intraoperative detection of nerve root irritation or compromise, however, with immediate appropriate surgical action is obviously preferable.

Intraoperative dermatomal somatosensory evoked potential (DSEP) and motor root monitoring techniques using electromyography (EMG) have been applied with some success in providing surgeons with more sensitive measures of nerve root functioning during cases involving lumbar spondylosis, spinal or foraminal stenosis, spinal instability, spondylolisthesis, degenerative lumbar scoliosis, and cervical radiculopathy associated with disk herniation or spondylosis.[48,51]

Dermatomal SSEP. Dermatomal SSEPs can be useful for spinal cord monitoring in much the same manner as SSEPs; however, single nerve root functioning can be more accurately evaluated by DSEPs than by SEPs.[52] Moreover, multilevel DSEP recording techniques provide information enabling more precise localization of segmental spinal cord dysfunction.[52] Specific dermatomes are stimulated with surface skin electrodes, and cortical responses are recorded with scalp electrodes applied in the same manner as for SEPs. Congruent areas of the dermatomal maps of Foerster, and Keegan and Garrett, have been used to maximize the probability of obtaining evoked responses from a single dermatome.[52–55] As with SSEP monitoring, DSEP responses are sensitive to a number of anesthetic agents, particularly inhalation agents; therefore, a balanced anesthesia technique is used. Despite relatively lower amplitude responses and the consequent need for more extensive averaging compared with SEPs, high recordability of intraoperative DSEP responses are reported.[48]

Warning criteria for intraoperative DSEP monitoring of nerve roots during spinal decompression and fusion surgeries are thus far unclear. A 50% amplitude decrement or 10% latency increase have been proposed as guidelines.[56] However, postoperative root dysfunction corresponding to a 20% amplitude decrement and a 4% latency increase have been reported.[57] Toleikis et al. reported a greater than 50% diminution of amplitude or greater than 10% prolongation of latencies in some patients persisting until the end of the operation without any postoperative neurologic deficits.[48] In that same study, 11 of 80 patients had responses completely disappear intraoperatively, returning to baseline within 3 minutes to 4.5 hours before the end of the operation, with none of these patients demonstrating a corresponding root specific postoperative neurologic deficit (one patient had perineal postoperative numbness, which resolved after several months). Thus, specific indications for surgical corrective maneuvers based upon intraoperative DSEP variations are not yet precisely defined.

In addition to serving as warning criteria for impending neurologic compromise, DSEP monitoring has also been used intraoperatively to evaluate the adequacy of decompression in patients with central or foraminal lumbar stenosis.[55] Improvements in intraoperative wave from latencies or amplitudes paralleling surgical decompression efforts indicate that this technique can provide useful feedback to the surgeon on the adequacy of nerve root decompression. This appears, however, to be less reliable in patients with more chronic symptoms.[58]

Motor Root Monitoring—Electromyography. There are two types of motor root monitoring techniques: mechanically elicited EMG and electrically elicited EMG. Electrically elicited EMG techniques are useful for assessing the functional integrity of a specific nerve root or cauda equina following surgical manipulations, delineating nerve root from scar in complex or reoperation cases, or for confirmation of the correct level of surgery. Direct nerve root or cauda equina stimulation is achieved by the surgeon with a hand-held electrical stimulator.[47] The EMG CMAP recordings are obtained with needle electrodes placed preoperatively into specific upper or lower extremity muscles innervated by the myotomes of interest. Several muscles may be recorded simultaneously. This method may be used in pedicle screw cases as an indicator of pedicle wall integrity following screw placement. The cathode stimulating electrode is placed into the pedicle hole, or the pedicle screw is stimulated. The anode is placed in the surgical field. An intact pedicle wall impedes current flow and nerve root stimulation does not occur at low intensities. Pedicle wall fracture results in decreased impedance and increased current flow, resulting in stimulation of the nerve root and EMG activity; however, a fractured pedicle wall and, therefore, a positive EMG elicited electrically, does not necessarily correlate with postoperative radiculopathy. There has been evidence to suggest that at least 6 mm of pedicle screw breakthrough is associated with a likelihood of neurologic deficit, but penetration of 4 mm or less is generally not associated with postoperative radiculopathy.[45] Mechanically elicited EMG may, therefore, be a more useful tool in this regard, because abnormal responses are elicited only if the nerve root is physically irritated.[45,46,47,52] Characteristic neurotonic discharges are produced by direct compression or tension on ventral nerve roots, which are then displayed in real time. Instantaneous audio feedback is also provided with this technique. Firing patterns are different for brief irritation of nerve roots (burst EMG activity) versus significant or prolonged nerve root compromise (sustained EMG activity). A study of 89 patients undergoing pedicle screw fixation for spinal stenosis, monitored nerve root function with mechanically elicited EMG.[46] Approximately 18% of 476 nerve roots monitored demonstrated abnormal firing intraoperatively. In 98.5% of 66 instances of abnormal firing confirmed by the surgeons to correspond with surgical manipulation, the segmental level correlated exactly with the EMG activity. Beatty et al. reported findings from continuous intraoperative EMG recordings in 120 patients undergoing lumbar laminectomy and 30 patients undergoing cervical surgery for radiculopathy associated with disk herniation or spondylosis.[51] The amplitude and frequency of firing were directly proportional to the degree of nerve root manipulation. Abnormal EMG discharges occurred instantaneously in association with nerve root retraction, touching the nerve root by a transpedicular screw or probe, drilling near a nerve root, or during decompression of the nerve root. In those cases where "presurgical firing" (presumably indicating nerve root compression) was present, cessation of this firing was observed in most cases intraoperatively following decompression and in nearly all cases by 24 hours. These findings illustrate the potential use of mechanically elicited EMG for evaluating the adequacy of decompression.

This method is relatively uncomplicated technically. The responses are not affected by volatile anesthesia, and no patient complications have been reported.[46,51]

SUMMARY

Continuous intraoperative neurophysiologic monitoring during spinal cord surgery has clearly been established as technically feasible, with virtually no morbidity and with very high degrees of sensitivity and specificity in predicting the integrity of the spinal cord and ventral nerve roots during surgical procedures (depending upon technique and monitored system). Potentially reversible spinal cord insults can clearly be announced to the surgeon in "real-time." In general, the operative team does what it can to discover and correct, when possible, processes that may lead to quadra- or paraparesis.

A variety of modalities exist, depending on circumstances (structures at risk), to monitor spinal cord physiology during surgery for traumatic conditions. Currently, we favor "traditional" continuous SSEP monitoring, with or without select segmental electromyographic monitoring of motor roots at risk as the primary monitoring strategy for most trauma cases. To what extent a practitioner wishes to utilize multimodality monitoring embracing combined sensory and motor evoked potentials, with or without segmental monitoring, is dependent on many factors, not the least being resource allocation (instrument capability, technologist and neurophysiologist training and expertise, monetary costs, and overall increase in system complexity).

Intraoperative SSEP monitoring involves established techniques in which stimulation of large mixed peripheral nerve fibers are generally stimulated in the arm or leg with both "upstream" (before operative site) signal processing and "downstream" (beyond operative site) recordings being made. With proper anesthetic technique, robust and easily recorded SSEPs can be obtained in most cases so long as major neurologic deficits are not present preoperatively.

Motor evoked potential techniques continue to remain predominantly investigational at this time and, thus, are not readily available to most practitioners. Concerns regarding the effects of high-current-density electrical stimulation to brain cortex, coupled with marked attenuation of the MEPs by most anesthetic agents has hampered the widespread use of this complementary technology. In addition, patient movement during the application of MEPs makes surgeons reluctant to endorse this technique; however, MEP technology meets or exceeds the high sensitivity of SSEP monitoring.

Motor nerve root monitoring (intraoperative EMG) is robust, simple to establish, and provides sensitive feedback to ventral root irritation and transection. This adjunctive procedure is encouraged when any surgical intervention that might threaten specified motor roots occurs.

Segmental sensory SSEPs (dermatomal SSEPs) have proved to be of limited use because of the presence of substantial intra- and interindividual variability, making them unreliable in general.

The wake-up test remains a viable alternative and backup for assessing spinal cord integrity during virtually any form of spinal cord surgery (except at cervical levels). This offers, however, only a brief window of observation and may miss potential unforeseen complications, which can occur at any time during a particular procedure.

Standards-of-care issues, medicolegal implications, and provision of real-time feedback to the operating team has prompted the proliferation of spinal cord monitoring technology and systems. By providing an alarm for potentially reversible spinal cord impairment, a substantial body of evidence suggests intraoperative neurophysiologic monitoring is a cost-effective adjunct to orthopedic spine surgery for many trauma cases.

REFERENCES

1. Newer MR: *Evoked potential monitoring in the operating room*, New York, 1986, Raven Press.
2. Russell GB, Rodichok LD: *Primer of intraoperative neurophysiologic monitoring*, Newton, MA, 1995, Butterworth-Heinemann.

3. Daube JR, editor: *Clinical neurophysiology*, Philadelphia, 1996, FA Davis.
4. Bennett MH: Effects of compression ischemia and spinal cord evoked potentials, *Exp Neurol*, 80:508–519, 1983.
5. Daube JR: Intraoperative monitoring by evoked potentials for spinal cord surgery, *Prog Electroecephalogr Clin Neurophysiol*, 73:374–377, 1989.
6. Harper CM, Daube JR: Surgical monitoring with evoked potentials: the Mayo Clinic experience. In Desmedt, JE editor: *Neuromonitoring in surgery*, Amsterdam, Elsevier Science Publishers, 1989.
7. Moller AR: Evoked potentials in intraoperative monitoring, Baltimore, 1988, Williams & Wilkins.
8. American Academy of Neurology: Therapeutics and technology assessment subcommittee: intraoperative neurophysiology. *Neurophysiology*, 40:1633–1636, 1990.
9. Misulis KE: *Spehlmann's evoked potential primer: visual, auditory and somatosensory evoked potentials in clinical diagnosis—revised and updated*, Boston, 1996, Butterworth-Heinemann.
10. Fisher RS, Raudzens P, Nunemacher M: Efficacy of intraoperative neurophysiological monitoring, *J Clin Neurophysiol* 12(1):97–109, 1995.
11. Nuwer MR, et al: Somatosensory evoked potential spinal cord monitoring reduces neurologic deficits after scoliosis surgery: results of a large multicenter survey, *Electroencephalogr Clin Neurophysiol* 96:6–11, 1995.
12. Vauzelle C, Stagnara P, Jouvinroux P: Functional monitoring of spinal cord activity during spinal surgery, *Clin Orthop* 1993:173–178, 1973.
13. Hall JE, Levine CR, Sudhir KG: Intraoperative awakening to monitor spinal cord function during Harrington instrumentation and spine fusion, *J Bone Joint Surg* (Am) 60:533–536, 1978.
14. Booke JS, et al: Somatosensory evoked potential monitoring during Cotrel-Dubousset instrumentation, *Spine* 18(4):518–521, 1993.
15. Brown RH, Nash CL: Intraoperative spinal cord monitoring. In Frymoyer JW, editor-in-chief: *The adult spine: principles and practice*, New York, 1991, Raven Press.
16. Gupta B: Anesthesia for the unstable spine. In Menezes AH, Sonntag VK, editors: *Principles of spinal surgery*, vol 1, New York, 1996, McGraw-Hill.
17. Owen JH, et al: The clinical application of neurogenic motor evoked potentials to monitor spinal cord function during surgery, *Spine* 16(8s):385–390, 1991.
18. Hurlbert RJ: Use of sensory-evoked potentials recorded from the human occiput for intraoperative physiologic monitoring of the spinal cord, *Spine* 20(21):2318–2327, 1995.
19. Muto N, et al: Spinal cord monitoring of the ventral funiculus function, *Spine* 20(22):2429–2435, 1995.
20. Levy WJ, et al: Motor evoked potentials from transcranial stimulation of the motor cortex in cats, *Neurosurgery* 15(2):214–227, 1984.
21. Glassman SD, et al: Transcranial magnetic motor evoked potentials in scoliosis surgery, *Orthopedics* 18(10):1017–1023, 1995.
22. Merton PA, Morton HB: Stimulation of the cerebral cortex in the intact human subject, *Nature* 285:227, 1980.
23. Calancie B, et al: Isoflurane-inducted attenuation of motor evoked potentials caused by electrical motor cortex stimulation during surgery, *J Neurosurg* 74:897–904, 1991.
24. Barker AT, et al: Magnetic stimulation of the brain, *J Physiol* 369:3, 1985.
25. Kitagawa H, et al: Magnetic-evoked compound muscle action potential neural monitoring in spine surgery, *Spine* 20(20):2233–2239, 1995.
26. Herdmann J, et al: Spinal cord and nerve root monitoring in spine surgery and related procedures, *Spine* 21(7):879–885, 1996.
27. Mochida, et al: A new method of multi-segment motor pathway monitoring using muscle potentials after trained spinal stimulation, *Spine* 20(20):2240–2246, 1995.
28. Stechison MT: Neurophysiological monitoring in spinal surgery. In Menezes AH, Sonntag VK, editors: *Principles of spinal surgery*, New York, 1996, McGraw-Hill.
29. Taniguchi M, et al: Effects of four intravenous anesthetic agents on motor evoked potentials elicited by magnetic transcranial stimulation, *Neurosurgery* 17(3):407–415, 1993.
30. Jellinek D, et al: Effects of nitrous oxide on motor evoked potentials recorded from skeletal muscle in patients under total anesthesia with intravenously administered Propofol, *Neurosurgery* 29(4):558–562, 1991.
31. Yamada H, et al: The effects of volatile anesthetics on the relative amplitudes and latencies of spinal and muscle potentials evoked by transcranial magnetic stimulation, *Spine* 19(13): 1512–1517, 1994.
32. Inghilleri M, et al: Motor potentials evoked by paired cortical stimuli, *Electroencephalogr Clin Neurophysiol* 77:382–389, 1990.
33. Burke D, et al: Assessment of corticospinal and somatosensory conduction simultaneously during scoliosis surgery, *Electroencephalogr Clin Neurophysiol* 85:388–3396, 1992.
34. Zentner J: Motor evoked potential monitoring during neurosurgical operations on the spinal cord, *Neurosurg Rev* 14:29–36, 1991.
35. Phillips LH: Could neurogenic motor evoked potentials be used to monitor motor and somatosensory pathways during scoliosis surgery? (a reply), *Muscle Nerve* 18(10):12–15, 1995.
36. Phillips LH, Blanco JS, Sussman MD: Direct spinal stimulation for intraoperative monitoring during scoliosis surgery, *Muscle Nerve* 18:319–325, 1995.
37. Dimitrijevich MR, Halter JA: *Atlas of human spinal cord evoked potentials*, Newton, MA, 1995, Butterworth-Heinemann.
38. Baba H, Kawahara N, Spinal cord evoked potential

monitoring in orthopaedic spine surgery. Indimitrijevic MR, Halter JA, editors: *Atlas of human spinal cord evoked potentials*, Newton MA, 1995, Butterworth-Heinemann.
39. Haghighi SS, et al: Monitoring of motor tracts with spinal cord stimulation, *Spine*, 19(13):1518–1524, 1994.
40. Chatrian GE, Berger MS, Wirch Al: Discrepancy between intraoperative SSEP's and postoperative function, *J Neurosurg* 69:450–454, 1988.
41. Mustain WD, Kendig RJ: Dissociation of neurogenic motor and somatosensory evoked potentials, *Spine* 16(7):851–853, 1991.
42. Schwentker MC, et al: Myogenic response distortion of neurogenic motor evoked potential morphology, *Anesthesiology* 83(3):616–619, 1995.
43. Machida M, et al: Monitoring of motor action potentials after stimulation of the spinal cord, *J Bone Joint Surg* (MA) 70:911–918, 1988.
44. Taylor BA, et al: Temporal summation—the key to motor evoked potential spinal cord monitoring in humans, *J Neurol Neurosurg Psych* 56:104–106, 1993.
45. Castro WH, et al: Accuracy of pedicle screw placement in lumbar vertebra, *Spine* 21(11):1320–1324, 1996.
46. Owen JH, et al: The use of mechanically elicited electromyograms to protect nerve roots during surgery for spinal degeneration, *Spine* 19(15):1704–1710, 1994.
47. Hormes JT, Chappuis JL: Monitoring of lumbosacral nerve roots during spinal instrumentation, *Spine* 18(14):2059–2062, 1993.
48. Toleikis JR, et al: The use of dermatomal evoked responses during surgical procedures that use intrapendicular fixation of the lumbosacral spine, *Spine* 18(16):2401–2407, 1993.
49. Weinstein JN, et al: Spinal pedicle fixation: reliability and validity of roentgenogram-based assessment and surgical factors on successful screw placement, *Spine* 13:1012–1018, 1988.
50. Gertzbein S, Robbins S: Accuracy of transpedicular screw placement in vivo, *Spine* 15:11–14, 1990.
51. Beatty RM, et al: Continuous intraoperative electromyographic recording during spinal surgery, *J Neurosurg* 82:401–405, 1995.
52. Slimp JC, et al: Dermatomal somatosensory evoked potentials: cervical, thoracic, and lumbosacral levels, *Electroencephalog Clin Neurophysiol* 84:55–70, 1992.
53. Foerster O: The dermatomes in man, *Brain* 56:1–39, 1933.
54. Keegan JJ, Garrett FD: The segmental distribution of the cutaneous nerves in the limbs of man, *Anat Rec* 102:409–437, 1948.
55. Cohen BA, Major MR, Huizenga BA: Predictability of adequacy of spinal root decompression using evoked potentials, *Spine* 16(82):S379–S384, 1991.
56. Sloan TB, Toleikis JR, Koht A: Evaluation of spinal cord function by means of evoked potentials. In Meyer PR, editor: *Surgery of spine trauma*, New York, 1989, Churchill-Livingston.
57. Cohen BA, Huizenga BA: Dermatomal monitoring for surgical correction of spondylolisthesis, *Spine* 13:1125–1128, 1988.
58. Owen JH, et al: Clinical correlation between degenerative spine disease and dermatomal somatosensory-evoked potentials in humans, *Spine* 16(s):S201–S205, 1991.

9

NONSURGICAL MANAGEMENT OF CERVICAL SPINE INSTABILITY

Russell W. Nelson

Immobilization of the spine and protection of the spinal cord from further injury are the primary goals of both early treatment and emergency care. Over the past 10 years there have been significant advances in the early surgical treatment of cervical spine injuries, which have made surgical fixation easier even on the severely injured patient. These include the ability to do awake posterior fusion with local anesthesia.[1] They also include the improvement of anterior cervical instrumentation and the introduction of lateral mass plating and polycoated thread for posterior cervical fixation.

In spite of the improvement in these surgical techniques, which are discussed in later chapters, there are still many situations in which a patient requires external immobilization to treat a serious spinal cord injury (SCI).

The goals of nonoperative treatment are to immobilize the injured spine in its posttraumatic position or to reduce the deformity and immobilize it in a reduced position. The goal of this chapter is to discuss the different treatments required for specific areas of the cervical spine, including the type of bracing, the length of bracing, and the prognosis for subsequent healing with immobilization.

INITIAL TREATMENT

Initial treatment for a SCI is usually done at the site of the injury. A spine board is essential, and normally sandbags are taped to the side of the board. A rigid cervical collar may be applied in place of sandbags. This should attempt to maintain a neutral alignment and should not hyperextend the neck.

A significant number of cervical spine injuries have had increased permanent neurologic deficit caused by improper handling during transport and initial evaluation. Great care must be taken during this period. Obviously, immobilization should continue until a proper diagnosis is made. Even though at the time of injury it is extremely important to concentrate on the injury site, that is the cervical spine, the complications from ignoring other aspects of the injury can be significant.

Severe bradycardia often accompanies acute quadriplegia because of unopposed vagal output. This can usually be controlled with medication but occasionally requires a transvenous pacemaker.

Severe respiratory distress in any patient is obvious and should be treated immediately; however, in the quadriplegic patient, respiratory distress may occur in a gradual and more subtle manner because of denervation of intercostal musculature. Baseline arterial blood gasses, therefore, should be obtained during the first week following injury, and the patient may require ventilatory assistance. During the first week, respiratory function complications are noted, including atelectasis and pneumonia, and the patient may require respiratory therapy early in treatment.

There are three areas of concern immediately following the injury that can definitely affect the acute care course of treatment, the rehabilitation, and the remainder of the injured patient's life. Appropriate urologic care must be started immediately to avoid over extension of the bladder. Long-term catheterization can permanently shrink the bladder. Range of motion assessment of the joints should be started immediately to prevent joint and muscle contractures. Maintenance of the skin integrity also is essential during this acute phase. It is quite common for Rancho Los Amigos Medical Center and other cord injury centers to receive transfers of quadriplegic patients with severe skin problems, which will limit their rehabilitation for several months.

Deep vein thrombosis is also a relatively frequent phenomenon following SCI. Drug prophylaxis, and intermittent compression stockings are effective in helping to prevent this. Suspicion of deep vein thrombophlebitis must remain high.[2,3,4]

IMMOBILIZATION

Following initial evaluation in the emergency room and determination of an SCI, the patient requires initial immobilization. This can be performed with cervical tongs or halo traction. Halo traction is preferable in this situation as it can be converted to a halo vest if necessary. This allows traction in a standard hospital bed with a mattress to prevent decubiti. A majority of cervical fracture patients can be treated in this manner with log rolling to prevent pressure areas. The multi-traumatized patient with cervical fractures may require a Roto-rest bed, which allows for care of multiple injured areas while maintaining cervical traction and alignment.

NEUROLOGIC EXAMINATION

After initial immobilization of the spine, a complete neurologic examination is necessary. This serves as a basis for predicting neurologic recovery and as an aid in determining treatment options (Table 9-1).

Following initial SCI, the cord often experiences a period of reflex inhibition called "spinal shock." It may last for a few hours up to several months, but 24 to 48 hours is common. It is only after emergence from spinal shock that a diagnosis of a complete SCI can be made based on neurologic examination. This occurs with the return of sacral reflexes in the absence of all function or sensation below the level of injury. The level of injury is determined by describing the lowest normally functional motor level where the corresponding muscles have a fair or better grade and intact sensory unit (see Table 9-1). In a complete injury there is a minimal chance of any neurologic recovery aside from root escape which may occur, producing increased function at one or more neurologic levels directly below the current functional level. There are multiple syndromes of incomplete SCI, and these are discussed fully in Chapter.

Table 9-1. Neurological Motor and Sensory Levels*

Key Muscles for Motor Levels
- C4, diaphragm
- C5, deltoid and/or biceps
- C6, wrist extensions
- C7, triceps
- C8, flexor profundi
- T1, hand intrinsics

Key Sensory Levels
- C1, head
- C2-C3, neck
- C4, anterior chest above level of axillae
- C5, deltoid area, lateral shoulder
- C6, thumb, index finger, and radial forearm
- C7, long finger
- C8, ring and little finger, ulnar forearm
- T1, medial forearm
- T2, medial arm

*Adapted from *Standards for Neurological Classification of Spinal Injury Patients, 1982, American Spinal Injury Association.*

STABILITY OF THE CERVICAL SPINE

After assessing neurologic injury, radiographs are assessed in an attempt to determine initial stability based on the integrity of the spinal column. Initial radiographs should be ordered to include anteroposterior (AP) and lateral radiographs of the entire spine including C7. Normally flexion-extension radiographs are dangerous at this point and should not be performed because of the risk of further neurologic damage. Obvious instability on the plain films occurs with more than 3.5 mm of horizontal displacement of the vertebrae relative to the adjacent vertebrae on resting lateral films or on flexion-extension films, when possible, with more than 11° of angulation compared with either adjacent vertebrae.[5,6,7]

Less obvious ways to identify instability include widening of the disk space, fanning of the spinous processes, disruption of the joints, or evidence of multiple comminuted fractures at one segment.[8] In spite of these guidelines, instability must be assessed on an individual basis.

TYPES OF IMMOBILIZATION

Methods of immobilization vary depending on the severity of the cervical fracture. We find no use at all for the soft cervical collar in any type of injury involving fracture of the neck. It does, however, provide comfort in minor muscle injuries for short periods of time.

The next step is the use of a Philadelphia collar (Fig. 9-1). This provides good immobilization on the neck. A short Philadelphia collar can be used in the upper or midcervical areas. We use a chest extension to provide more stability for lower cervical injuries.

The poster brace consists of the two and four poster braces (Fig. 9-2, 9-3). These braces are much more effective in controlling flexion, especially through the upper cervical area. The chest piece can be extended to help control flexion of the lower cervical region. These do not control lateral bending or rotation well and are not indicated in the early care of unstable fractures.[9,10]

The halo device originally introduced at Rancho Los Amigos Medical Center by Drs. Nickel and Perry provides more rigid fixation of the head and neck.[11,12] It exhibits good control of rotation, lateral bending, and sagittal motions and controls the spine well on flexion and extension. Dr. Nickel did document significant motion and some compressive forces across the device when the patient arise from the supine to upright position and in the midportions of the cervical spine. He reported better control with the halo while using the vests than with the older plaster cast immobilization.[13]

The application of the halo has been well described in various publications and manuals. Because this is an invasive procedure, complications can occur. These have been described in our review of experience at Rancho Los Amigos Medical Center and in the review of Dr. Garfin.[14,15] Care must be taken to monitor pin loosening and infection. Occasionally pins become infected requiring oral antibiotics and changing the infected pin sites.

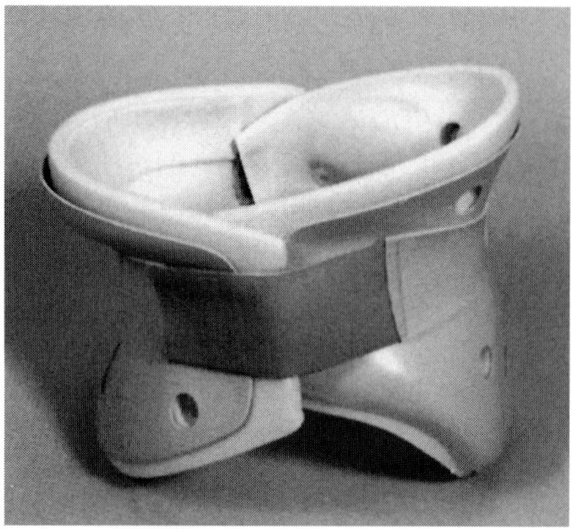

FIGURE 9-1

A Philadelphia collar provides good immobilization of the neck. A short Philadelphia collar can be used in the upper or mid cervical areas. (From Goldberg B, Hsu JD, editors: *Atlas of orthoses and assistive devices,* ed 3, St. Louis, 1997, Mosby-Year Book, p. 254.)

TYPES OF INJURIES

UPPER CERVICAL INJURIES

Occipitoatlantal injury is fairly common and usually fatal.[16] There are rare reports of survival, some with incomplete injuries and neurologic recovery. We have reported the survival of one patient with a complete SCI who subsequently had surgical fusion for stability.[17] The mechanism of this injury is usually hyperextension of the head with distraction force severe enough to

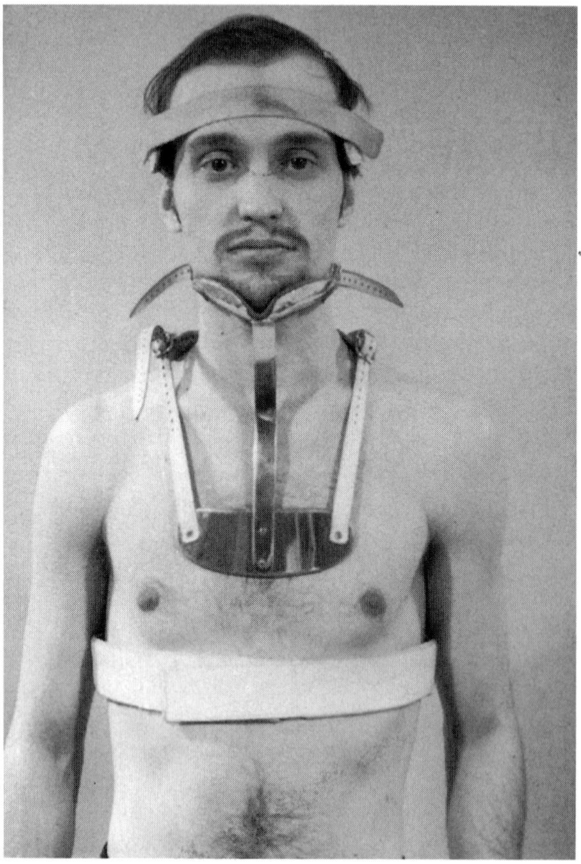

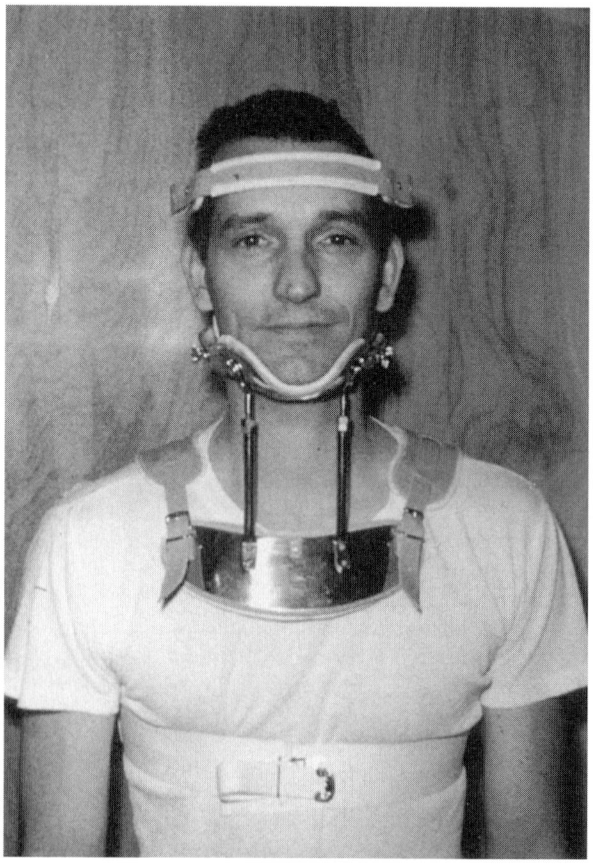

FIGURE 9-2 AND FIGURE 9-3

Two and four poster braces. These braces are effective in controlling flexion, especially through the upper cervical area. (From Goldberg B, Hsu JD, editors: *Atlas of orthoses and assistive devices,* ed 3, St. Louis, 1997, Mosby-Year Book, p. 166.)

separate the spinal column from the cranium. The diagnosis of this fracture is usually made on a lateral radiograph, and the fracture is not amenable to any type of preoperative bracing. It is a surgical lesion that requires bracing postoperatively to stabilize the surgical procedure.

FRACTURES OF THE ATLAS

Fractures of the C1 ring are usually clues to compression forces and are often the result of motor vehicle accidents. Most of these fractures do not cause neurologic damage. They can be identified on lateral radiograph and exhibit soft tissue swelling anteriorly. A plain AP radiograph may show expansion of the lateral masses, but the fracture can best be evaluated fully by computed tomography (CT) scan. Fractures in this area may occur in combination with odontoid fractures and hangman's fractures.

There are three common fracture patterns. The posterior arch fracture is the most common and occurs at the junction of the posterior arch and the lateral mass.[18] This is a relatively stable injury and is usually treated with a Philadelphia-type collar. The second pattern is the burst injury described by Jefferson.[19] This fracture usually produces four fracture lines, two in the anterior and two in the posterior arches with displacement of the lateral masses. If lateral displacement is greater than 7 to 8 mm, this usually represents rupture of the transverse ligament and instability at C1-C2.[20] Fractures with this displacement are considered unstable and are treated with initial halo traction and subsequently a halo vest. Fractures with intact ligaments can be treated with a Philadelphia collar.

The third group of fractures are lateral mass fractures, which are relatively uncommon and are usually not associated with neurologic injury. They are usually treated with a firm Philadelphia collar, and they heal without instability.

ODONTOID FRACTURES

Odontoid fractures are quite common. These are usually high-energy injuries and occur with falls or in automobile accidents. Because of the high energy, neural injury occurs in approximately 25% of the cases. In the elderly these can occur with less energy involved. These fractures are usually identified by open mouth and lateral radiographs. In many cases, reformatted CT scan is the study of choice to describe the odontoid fracture. They also can be identified with AP tomograms.

The classification of these fractures has been described by Anderson and DeAlonzo (Fig. 9-4).[21] Type I fractures are rare and not associated with neurologic injury. They are avulsion fractures of the tip of the odontoid, are considered stable, and can be treated with a Philadelphia collar.

The type II fractures are toward the base of the odontoid. These occur near the attachment of the ligaments. The odontoid often displaces in the direction of the force. This fracture is by far the most difficult to treat in the halo vest.[22] We have treated it with attempted reduction and immobilization in a halo vest. Even with appropriate halo treatment, nonunion rates have been between 30% and 60%.[23] With any sign of failure of this treatment, surgical posterior fusion is then indicated. Type III fractures occur through the body of C2. These fractures can be treated with halo immobilization and have a high rate of union. Usually this fracture can be reduced with gentle traction and held in a halo during the healing period.

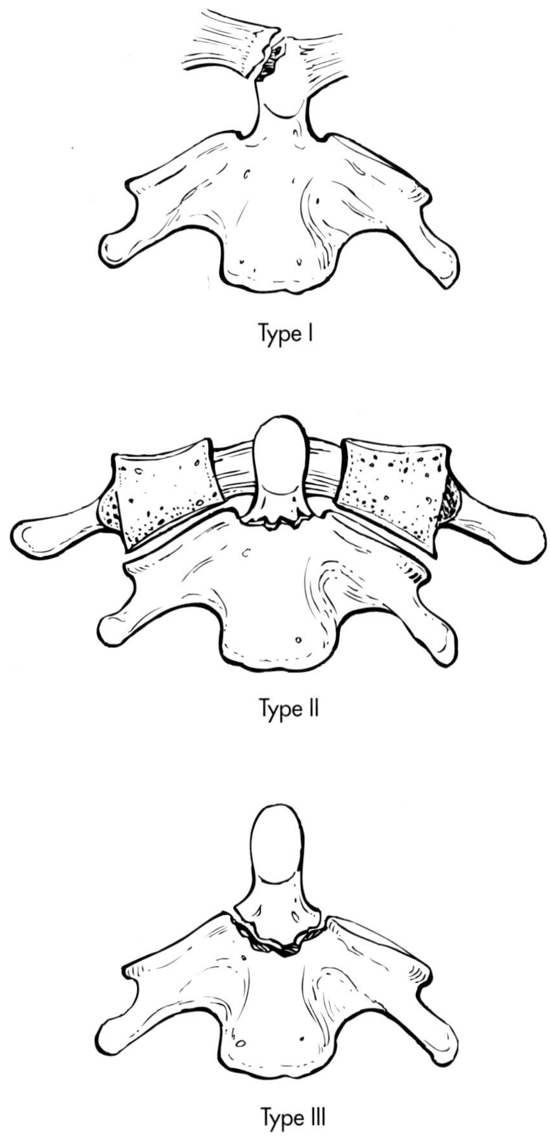

FIGURE 9-4

Classification of odontoid fractures as described by Anderson and DeAlonzo. Type I are avulsion fractures of the alar ligament. Type II are fractures through the waist of the odontoid caudad to the transverse ligament. Type III are fractures into the cancellous body of the axis.

Fractures of the Axis

Traumatic spondylolisthesis of the axis is characterized by the fracture passing downward through the neural arch and pedicles of the axis resulting in displacement of C2 on C3. This fracture has been termed a *Hangman's fracture*. This description was given to an injury caused by hyperextension in which the occiput was driven by extension into the atlas, breaking through the pedicles. The majority of these fractures today occur in diving injuries or automobile accidents, and the majority of these fractures occur without neurologic injury. Usually if neurologic injury occurs, it is fatal as described in the initial Hangman's fracture.

There are three basic fracture patterns.[24] In the type 1 fracture, the pedicles are broken but are not displaced. There is no angulation of C1 on C2, and these are usually well treated without halo but with a poster brace or a Philadelphia collar. This injury normally heals with a period of immobilization and without surgery.

In the type II fracture there is angulation of the C2 vertebrae with pedicle fracture and disruption of the disk space between C2 and C3. This fracture can be treated with reduction by traction and a subsequent halo vest. Reduction attempts usually correct most of the angulation, and the majority of these fractures heal with immobilization.

In type IIB fractures, the type II fracture occurs in combination with a facet dislocation at C2-C3, and, to obtain reduction, this is usually a surgical lesion (Fig. 9-5).

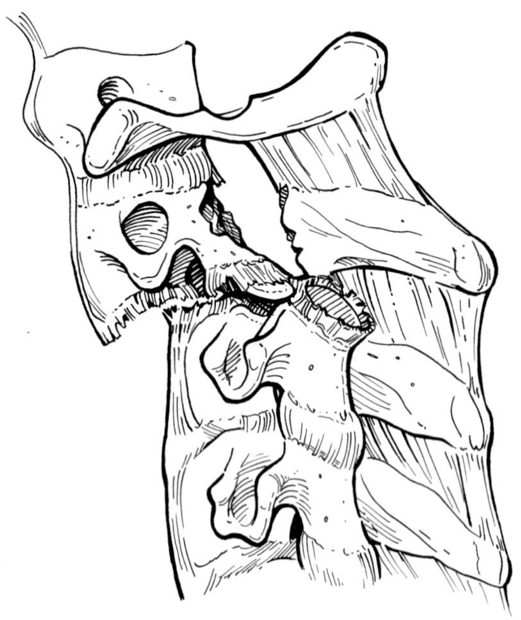

Figure 9-5

Type II Hangman's fracture.

Lower Cervical Fractures and Dislocations

Lower cervical fractures are well described by Allen et al.[25] Following Allen's classification system, we looked at the cervical spine injuries treated at Rancho Los Amigos over the past 10 years in an attempt to determine which of these injuries would respond best to external immobilization and for which injuries immediate surgical treatment may be indicated.[14]

Compressive Flexion Injuries. In first considering the compressive flexion (CF) injuries, Allen described five types of fractures. The compressive flexion stage I and stage II lesions consist of progressive blunting of the anterior margin of the vertebral body. Stage II reveals blunting with obliquity and some loss of the anterior height of the vertebral body. Although there was a significant number of CF I and II fractures producing neurological trauma, these fractures did not show a significant amount of instability with immobilization, and this relates to the fact that there does not appear to be a failure of the posterior ligamentous complex in either of these two injuries.

We felt that Allen's CF III lesion was the transitional lesion of the compressive flexion fractures. In this lesion there was a fracture line passing obliquely from the anterior surface through the endplate of the body. There was minimal displacement of the inferior portion of the body into the neural canal, but in a significant number of these injuries there appears to be some amount of failure of the posterior ligamentous complex. These injuries occur with minimal anterior fracture, and the lesions in our investigation had a 50% rate of postimmobilization instability after halo treatment. In CF IV injury, the fractures through the body combine with mild displacement of the body into the neural canal at the involved motion segment (Fig. 9-6). In the compressive V injury, which is the most severe injury in this classification, bony injury is identical to the CF III and IV along with displacement of the posterior body fragment posteriorly into the neural canal with significant disruption of the lower disk space. Compressive flexion IV and V injuries both exhibit stability after conservative treatment with immobilization in a halo vest. We attributed this stability to the amount of anterior vertebral body injury and disk trauma, and we found high incidence of anterior ankylosis in the lower two fractures where the disk space was obviously disrupted by the shift of the fractured vertebrae posteriorly.

In our review of CF fractures, especially stages III through V, there were a significant number of these fractures with instability at the level above the vertebral fracture. Allen describes this as a corresponding distractive flexion injury above the fracture level. We did see spontaneous ankylosis extending up onto this level in several cases and feel that postimmobilization

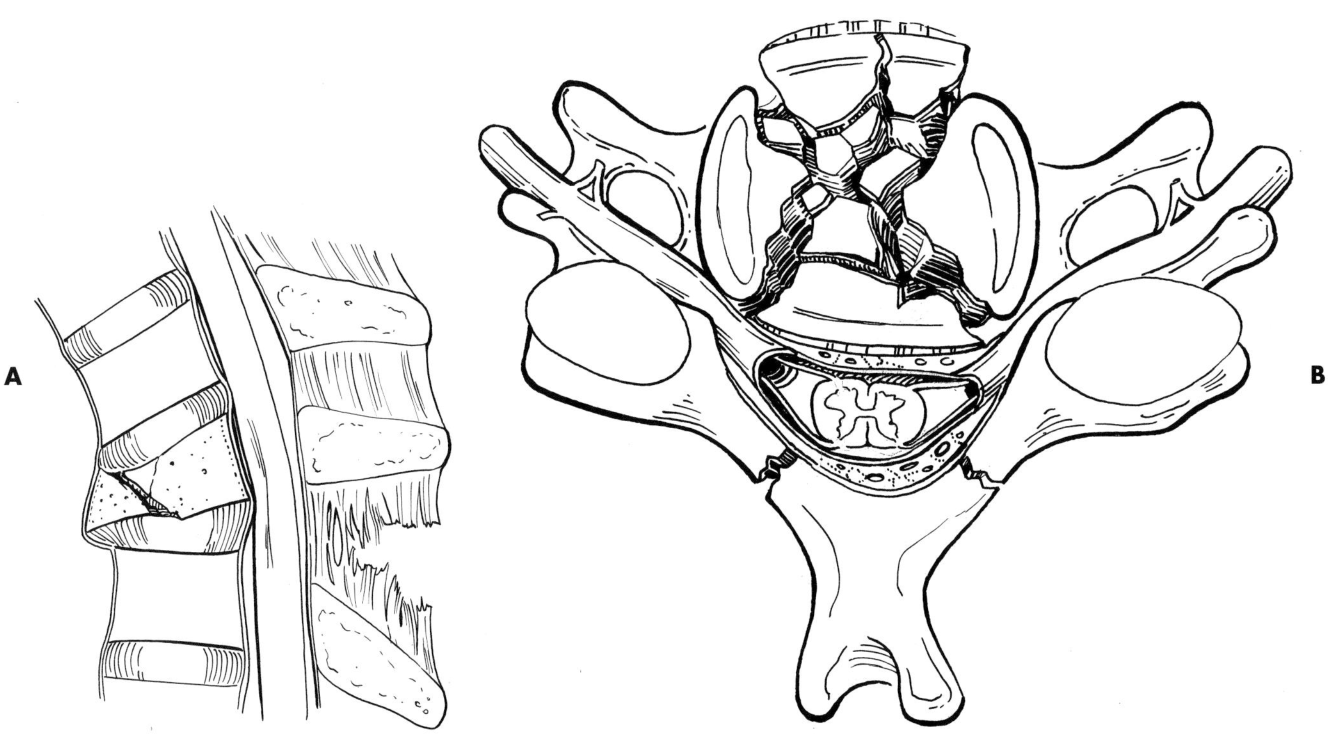

FIGURE 9-6

In compression flexion IV injury, the fractures through the body combine with mild displacement of the body into the neural canal at the involved motion segment.

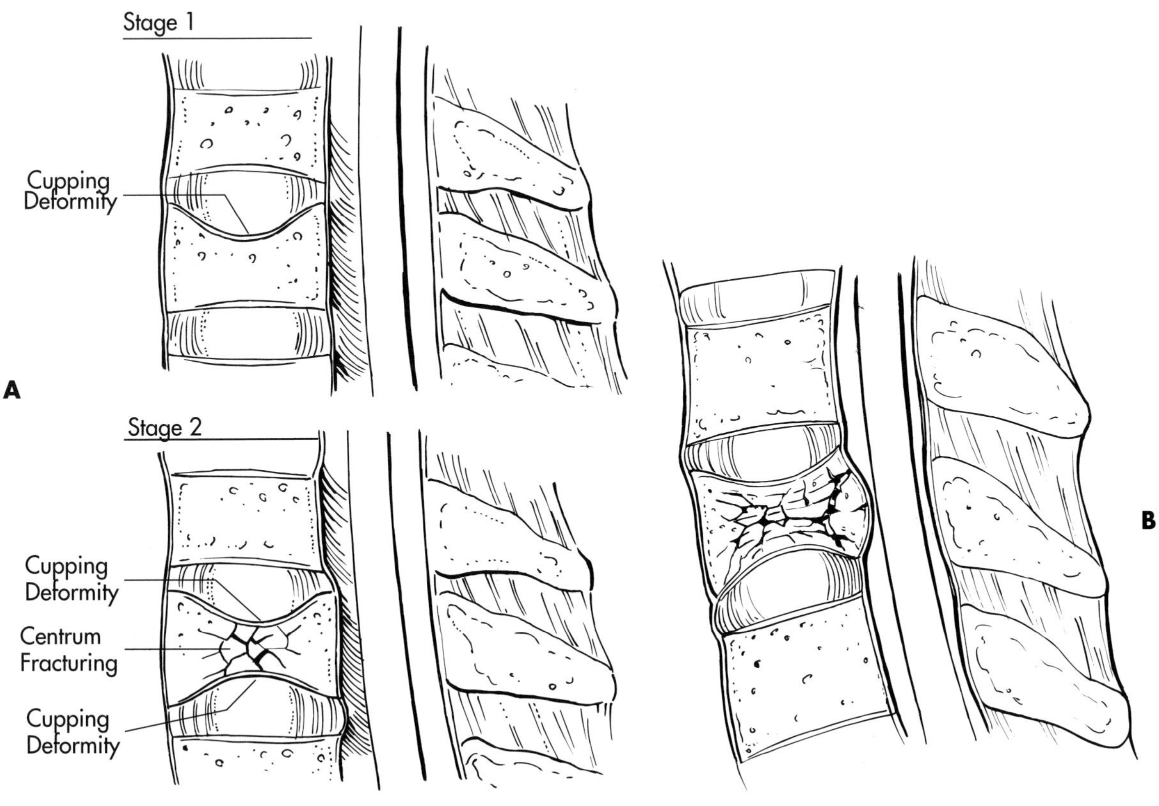

FIGURE 9-7

A, The stage II vertical compression fracture produces fractures through both endplates with a minimal amount of posterior displacement. **B,** In the stage III vertical compression fracture, damage has progressed with pieces of fractures displaced in multiple directions including posteriorly. These fractures can produce significant posterior ligamentous injury at the time of fracture.

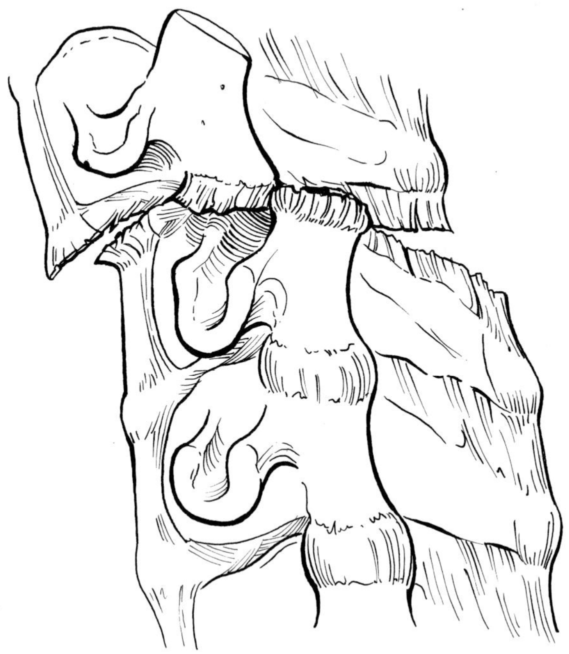

FIGURE 9-8

The distractive flexion, stage III injury is the bilateral facet dislocation with 50% vertebral body displacement.

stability at this level should also be evaluated closely on flexion-extension radiographs.

Vertical Compression Fractures. Vertical compression fractures were previously referred to as burst fractures and are produced by a pure axial load. Allen described three types of vertical compression fractures. Vertical compression stage I fractures are caused by the superior or inferior endplates giving way with cupping of these plates. This is central endplate failure without evidence of posterior ligamentous failure. These fractures were uncommon in our series because they did not produce significant neurologic injury.

The stage II fracture occurs through both endplates with a minimal amount of posterior displacement. In stage III, the vertebral damage progresses from stage II with pieces of fractures displaced in several directions including posteriorly. These fractures can produce significant posterior ligamentous injury at the time of injury.

All of these vertical compression fractures heal quite well with halo immobilization. Traction initially can reduce fragmentation, and the patient can then be placed into a halo vest. Due to the amount of anterior fracture, these fractures readily proceed to anterior ankylosis (Fig. 9-7).

DISTRACTIVE FLEXION

The distractive flexion group is associated with mostly ligamentous injury. The stage I injury is the failure of the posterior ligamentous complex when the facets joints are disrupted and subluxed in flexion and, usually, reduced in extension. This injury can be missed on plain lateral radiographs because of evidence. Usually flexion-extension radiographs are accessory to diagnose this condition. These injuries heal poorly with halo immobilization, and rarely is there enough disk injury anteriorly to produce anterior ankylosis.

The distractive flexion II lesion is the unilateral facet. Surprisingly, this lesion did fairly well with halo although several have been treated without reduction of the facet joint. The nonreduced facet cases all stabilized after halo immobilization. If this injury is reduced and there is not significant joint trauma within the facet joint, there is a significant risk of instability following halo immobilization.

The distractive flexion III injury is the bilateral facet dislocation with 50% vertebral body displacement (Fig. 9-8). When these lesions are treated conservatively, the facet joints are reduced and immobilized. As expected, the posterior ligament heal poorly, and there is not a high percentage of anterior ankylosis.

Distractive flexion IV injuries, which involve full vertebral body anterior displacement, are quite unstable, and if they are reduced, the amount of anterior trauma usually produces anterior ankylosis and stability following a period of halo immobilization.

The other categories of injury described by Dr. Allen are much less common in SCI. The compressive extension injury has two stages. The first is a unilateral vertebral arch fracture with extension. The second is bilateral laminar fracture through the pedicle with extension to the vertebral body and disruption of the disk space. We identified only six of these lesions. Five of them were stage I and were stable with treatment. The stage II injury did slip with halo immobilization and required surgical treatment.

Distractive extension injuries were not identified in our review. They produce central cord injuries but are usually a relatively stable injury and do not require significant immobilization. Lateral flexion injuries are uncommon and do not produce significant instability.

SUMMARY

This chapter has been devoted to discussing conservative treatment options for cervical spine fractures. The author realizes that many of the described fractures can be treated surgically. Often there are associated injuries and medical criteria that would lead one to surgically treat these fractures to mobilize the patient and improve their medical status. Figures 9-9 and 9-10 summarize the usual stable and unstable cervical spine injuries. Obviously, there can be exceptions.

Cervical fractures can be treated with external immobilization and that, with many of these fractures,

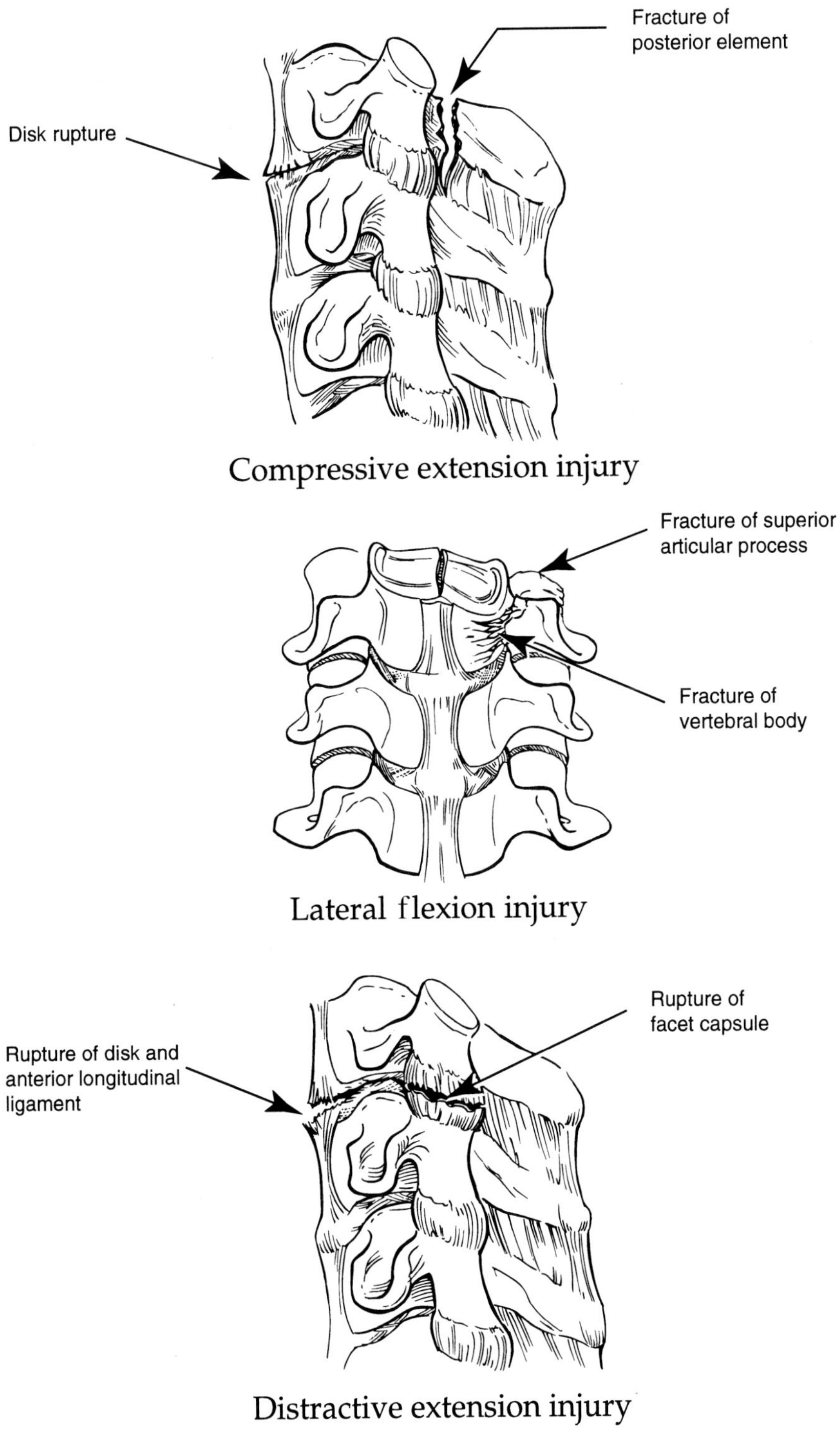

FIGURE 9-9

Stable cervical spine injuries.

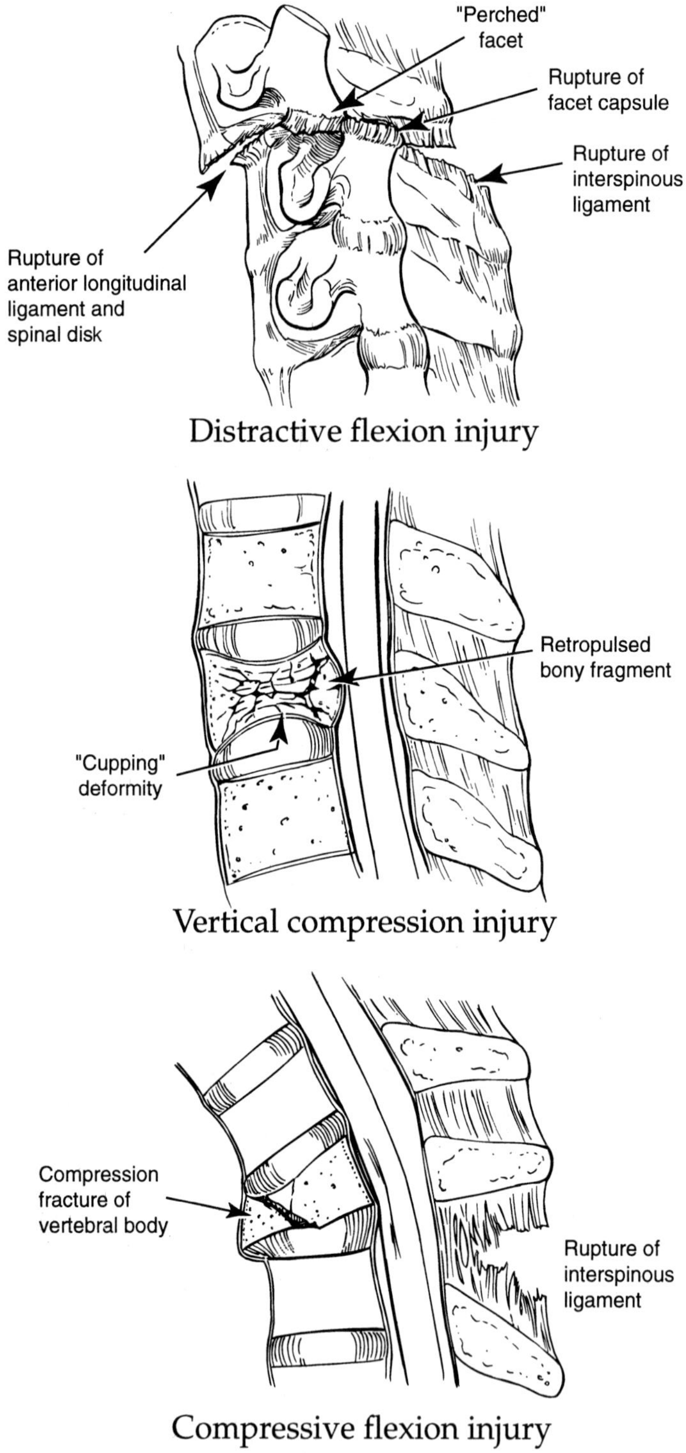

Figure 9-10

Unstable cervical spine injuries.

the physician can expect a satisfactory outcome. These fractures need to be carefully evaluated before a treatment plan can be initiated. The general rule to remember in attempting external immobilization treatment for cervical fractures is the greater the amount of bony injury anteriorly or posteriorly, the better the success rate when the fracture is treated with external immobilization.

REFERENCES

1. Zigler J, et al: Posterior cervical fusion with local anesthesia: the awake patient as the ultimate spinal cord monitor, *Spine* 12:206–208, 1987.
2. Rogers WA: Fractures and dislocations of the cervical spine: an end result study, *J Bone Joint Surg (Am)* 39:34–38, 1957.
3. Mattox KL: The injured patient's injured neck, *Emerg Med* 16(7):24–48, 1984.
4. Soderstrum CA, Brumback RJ: Early care of the patient with a cervical spine injury, *Orthop Clin North Am* 12:3–13, 1986.
5. White AA III, et al: Biomechanical analysis of clinical stability in the cervical spine, *Clin Orthop* 109:85–96, 1975.
6. White AA III, Panjabi MM: Update on the evaluation of instability of the lower cervical spine. In Griffen PP, editor: *Instructional course lectures*, Chicago, 1987, American Academy of Orthopedic Surgeons.
7. White AA III, et al: Spinal stability: evaluation and treatment. In American Academy of Orthopedic Surgeons, editor: *Instructional Course Lectures*, vol 32, St. Louis, 1983, Mosby–Year Book.
8. Shields Cc, Stauffer ES: Late instability in cervical spine fractures secondary to laminectomy, *Clin Orthop* 119:144–147, 1976.
9. Johnson RM, et al: Cervical orthoses: a study comparing their effectiveness and restricting cervical motion in normal subjects, *J Bone Joint Surg (Am)* 59:332–339, 1977.
10. Johnson Rm, Owens Jr, Hart DC, Callahan RA: Cervical orthoses: a guide to their selection and use, *Clin Orthop* 154:34–45, 1981.
11. Nickel VL, Perry J, Garret A, Heppenstall M: The halo, *J Bone Joint Surg* 50A(7):1400–1409, 1968.
12. Perry, J: The halo in spinal abnormalities. Practical factors and avoidance of complications, *Orthop Clin North Am* 3(1):69–80, 1972.
13. Koch Ra, Nickel VL: The halo vest: an evaluation of motion and foces across the neck, *Spine* 3:103–107, 1976.
14. Nelson R, Capen D, Garland D, Waters R: Halovest stabilization of cervical spine fractures and dislocations. A series review and long-term follow-up, Presented at the American Academy of Orthopaedic Surgeons Annual Meeting, Atlanta, 1984.
15. Garfin SR, et al: Complications in the use of the halo fixation device, *J Bone Joint Surg* 68A:320–325, 1986.
16. Dorr LD, Harvey JP: traumatic lesions in fatal acute spinal column injuries, *Clin Orthop* 157:178–190, 1981.
17. Zigler J, et al: Occipito-cervico-thoracic spine fusion in a patient with occipito-cervical dislocation and survival, *Spine* 11:645–646, 1987.
18. Sherk MM, Nicholson JT: Fractures of the atlas, *J Bone Joint Surg (Am)* 52:1017–1020, 1970.
19. Jefferson G: Fracture of the atlas vertebra, *Br J Surg* 7:407–410, 1920.
20. Spence KF Jr: Bursting atlantal fracture associated with rupture of the transverse ligament, *J Bone Joint Surg* 52A:(3)543–549, 1970.
21. Anderson LD, D'Alonzo PT: Odontoid process of the axis, *J Bone Joint Surg* 56A:1663–1674, 1974.
22. Wang GJ, et al: The non-surgical management of odontoid fractures in adults, *Spine* 9(3):229–230, 1984.
23. Levin AM, Edwards CC: Treatment of injuries in the C1-C2 complex, *Ortho Clin North Am* 17(1):31–44, 1986.
24. King AG: Spinal column trauma. In Anderson LD, editor: *Instructional Course Lecture,* St. Louis, 1986, Mosby–Year Book.
25. Allen BL, et al: A mechanistic classification of closed, indirect fractures and dislocations of the lower cervical spine, *Spine* 7:1–27, 1982.

10

SURGICAL MANAGEMENT OF CERVICAL INSTABILITY

Joel A. Finkelstein
Paul A. Anderson

Operative management of cervical spine injury is directed at reducing deformity, decompressing the neural elements, maintaining alignment, and stabilizing the spine while bone fusion occurs.[1] An optimal outcome depends on early recognition, prompt resuscitation of the patient, stabilization of the spine, and prevention of additional neurological injury.[2] Since antiquity, the diagnosis of a crushed vertebra in the neck implied a bad prognosis.[3] Currently, with understanding of the injury and with implementation of established treatment protocols, we can expect recovery to a functional, stable, and pain free cervical spine. Additionally, we can optimize the chance for neurologic recovery in the case of spinal cord injury (SCI).

Ducker et al. demonstrated that rigid immobilization of an injured spinal cord favorably altered the clinical course of that lesion.[4] Surgical management of cervical instability, however, has not been without its detractors. With the advent of modern day instrumentation and techniques, significant improvements have been made in surgical outcomes. The purpose of this chapter is to outline the surgical treatment of specific injury patterns and illustrate our techniques of choice.

ANATOMIC CONSIDERATIONS IN STABILITY

Upper Cervical Spine

Clinical instability of the spine is the loss of the ability under physiologic loads to maintain relationships so that there is neither damage nor subsequent irritation to the spinal cord or nerve roots.[5] The occipitoatlantoaxial complex protects the upper cervical spinal while allowing for a wide range of motion. The occipital condyles are convex projections from the occiput, which articulate with the corresponding concavities in the lateral masses of the atlas. These lateral masses are connected by anterior and posterior arches to form a ring. The odontoid process of C2 projects into this ring behind the anterior atlantal arch. The transverse ligament attaches to the medial side of the lateral masses of C1 and passes behind the odontoid process. This ligament is the primary stabilizer for anterior atlantoaxial translation (Fig. 10-1).[16] The facet articulations of C1-C2 are in the horizontal plane. They aid in rotation and provide lateral column support.

At the occipitoatlantal articulation, the tectorial membrane (the continuation of the posterior longitudinal ligament) passes behind the dens and attaches to the anterior aspect of the foramen magnum. This structure is the primary stabilizer for extension of the occiput on the atlas as well as being a secondary stabilizer for C1-C2 in flexion and extension.[6,7] Flexion at the occiput-C1 joint is limited by impingement of the basion on the anterior arch of the atlas. Axial rotation is limited by the alar ligaments, which are two bands that pass from the tip of the dens to the medial aspect of the occipital condyles (see Fig. 10-1). Dvorak et al. demonstrated their integral role in limiting axial rotation and lateral bending.[8]

Lower Cervical Spine

In the lower cervical spine, both osseous and soft-tissue structures contribute to stability. Vertebral bodies and intervertebral disk provide the ability to withstand axial compression, posterior elements resist tensile loads, and the uncinate processes reduce medial-lateral bending and translation.[9,10] The lateral masses (facet articulations), with their upward inclination angle of 35 to 45°, act to resist anterior translation and rotatory forces.[11] Soft tissue structures, the anterior and posterior longitudinal ligament, ligamentum flavum, facet capsules, nuchal ligament, and interspinous ligaments, resist distractive tensile loading.[12]

INITIAL ASSESSMENT AND DETERMINATION OF STABILITY

Assessment of instability in the acutely traumatized cervical spine begins with a thorough history and

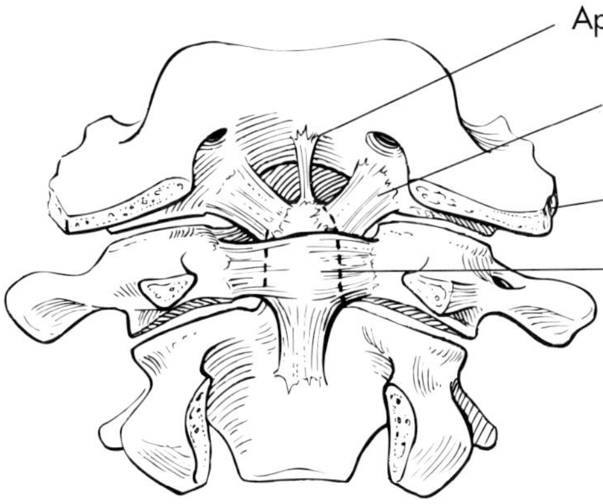

FIGURE 10-1

The internal craniocervical ligaments are depicted after removal of the posterior elements and the tectorial membrane. The strong transverse component of the cruciate ligament (transverse ligament) attaches to the medial side of the lateral masses of C1. The alar ligaments extend obliquely upward and laterally from the lateral aspect of the dens to the medial aspect of the occipital condyles. The apical ligament is a small band from the apex of the dens to the basion.

Table 10-1. Checklist for the Diagnosis of Clinical Instability in the Lower Cervical Spine

Element	Point Value
Anterior element destroyed or unable to function	2
Posterior element destroyed or unable to function	2
Relative sagittal plane translation > 3.5 mm	2
Relative sagittal plane rotation > 11 degrees	2
Positive stretch test	2
Spinal cord damage	2
Root damage	1
Abnormal disk narrowing	1
Dangerous loading anticipated	1
Developmentally narrow spinal canal	1
Total of 5 or more = clinical instability	

physical examination. A complete neurologic examination must be performed including the Glasgow Coma Scale (GCS), examination of the cranial nerves, and spinal cord function. Areas of tenderness and swelling are elicited, and a careful palpation is performed looking for interspinous gaps, which are clues for osseoligamentous disruption. Anteroposterior, lateral, and open mouth odontoid radiographs are obtained. On the lateral radiograph, the entire cervical spine from occiput to the upper endplate of T1 must be visualized.[13] Computed tomography (CT) is indicated when an injury is suspected on plain films or in poorly visualized regions. Magnetic resonance imaging (MRI) is invaluable for evaluation of the spinal cord and the soft tissues. The absence or presence of disk herniation can be assessed, hemorrhage or edema in the soft tissues can be identified, and ligamentous tears and facet capsule disruptions can be visualized from fat suppression techniques[14–17] MRI also permits prognostic assessment of the final outcome for motor function.[18,19]

Based on the information acquired from the clinical and radiographic assessments, a determination can be made regarding the stability of the spine. With varying degrees of bony and ligamentous injury, this determination is often difficult. To aid in the objective assessment of subaxial stability, White and Punjabi have proposed a checklist (Table 10-1). A specific point value is assigned to location of injuries, sagittal plane translation or rotation, cord or root injury, and intervertebral widening or angulation (with the stretch test). Developmental narrowing of the spinal canal and the anticipation of dangerous loading also contribute to their definition of clinical instability. Each element of the checklist is assessed and the total positive values are summated. A score of 5 or greater is suggestive of clinical instability.[5]

The stability of the occipitoatlantoaxial complex is determined primarily by ligamentous structures. Any injury leading to translational or vertical displacement should be considered unstable. Criteria for atlantoaxial instability is discussed in the individual sections on upper cervical spine injuries.

CLASSIFICATION

Classification of any injury is helpful in communication between physicians, in formulating prognosis, and in applying appropriate therapeutic interventions. Neurologic injuries are classified as intact, complete, or incomplete. Syndromes of incomplete SCI include anterior (vibration, proprioception, and light touch are maintained while motor function, pain, and temperature sensation are lost), central (functional loss is greater in the upper limbs than in the lower), and Brown-Sequard (injury to one half of the spinal cord leads to ipsilateral loss of motor function, proprioception, and vibration with contralateral loss of pain and temperature sensation). The neurologic level of injury is the level with at least antigravity motor function.[20]

Classifications of skeletal injury are based on morphology and mechanisms of injury. In the upper cervical spine, because of the unique architecture and articulations of the individual vertebrae, an all encompassing classification system is difficult to achieve. The Orthopedic Trauma Association has developed a comprehensive classification system that covers all areas of the cervical spine; however, we feel that this system has its greatest use in the subaxial region (Table 10-2).[21] Further classification of upper cervical injuries are discussed in the individual sections for each injury type.

Another classification system for subaxial cervical spine injuries with broad use has been the mechanistic classification proposed by Ferguson and Allen.[22] Although not uniformly utilized, it provides useful information in the planning for the surgical and nonsurgical approach to unstable cervical injuries. The injury designation is based on the position of the neck at the time of injury and the dominant mode of the force application. Each injury pattern is graded in terms of the degree of injury; a higher stage is associated with a greater amount of displacement and a greater risk of neurological injury. Six injury phylogenies are recognized: distractive flexion, vertical compression, compressive flexion, compressive extension, distractive extension and lateral flexion.

Limitations of this system are that it may be cumbersome and does not always address the osseous and ligamentous structures injured. In many patients it may be difficult to reliably determine the fracture phylogeny. In the subaxial cervical spine, we recommend the use of the classification system proposed by the Orthopedic Trauma Association as it is more comprehensive and easily reproducible, although other authors in this text clearly rely upon the Allen classification.

Table 10-2. Cervical Spine Trauma Classification of the Orthopedic Trauma Association

51 Upper cervical spine
- 51 A1 Occipital cervical dislocation
  - A1.1 Anterior
  - A1.2 Vertical
  - A1.3 Posterior
- 51 A2 Cervical spine, occipital condyle
  - A2.1 Type 1
  - A2.2 Type 2
  - A2.3 Type 3
- 51 A3 Atlas
  - A3.1 Jefferson
  - A3.2 Lateral mass
  - A3.3 Posterior arch
  - A3.4 Anterior arch
- 51 B1 Cervical spine, transverse ligament
  - B1.1 Rupture mid substance
  - B1.2 Rupture avulsion
- 51 B2 Cervical spine, dens fracture
  - B2.1 Type 1
  - B2.2 Type 2
  - B2.2.2 Type 2a
  - B2.3 Type 3
- 51 C Cervical spine traumatic spondylolisthesis of the axis
  - C1 Type 1
  - C2 Type 2
  - C2.2 Type 2a
  - C3 Type 3

52 Lower cervical spine
- 52 A1.1 Spinous process fracture
  - A1.2 Extension avulsion or teardrop
  - A1.3 Lateral mass fracture without subluxation
  - A1.4 Isolated lamina fracture
  - A1.5 Ligamentous strain
- 52 B1.1 Facet injury
  - B1.1.1 Perched unilateral
  - B1.1.2 Perched bilateral
- 52 B2.2.1 Facet dislocation
  - B2.2.1 Without fracture unilateral
  - B2.2.2 Without fracture bilateral
  - B3.3.1 With displacement unilateral
  - B3.3.2 With displacement bilateral
- 52 C Severe injuries
  - C1.1 Flexion teardrop
  - C2.1 Severe ligamentous injury
  - C3.1 Compression fracture
  - C3.2 Burst fracture

OUTCOME STUDIES: OPERATIVE VERSUS NONOPERATIVE MANAGEMENT

Although it is clear nonoperative treatment is well suited for many situations, careful patient selection is mandatory when considering this for definitive treatment of cervical instability. With the use of the halo vest, Bucholz and Cheung documented an overall failure rate of 15%. For facet subluxation and dislocation, they found loss of reduction to occur in 37% of all patients.[23] Bucci et al. had a 40% incidence of spinal instability following immobilization in a halo orthosis with over half of these subsequently requiring operative stabilization.[24] Purely ligamentous injuries also heal poorly in the halo vest.[25] Chapter 9 on nonsurgical management of cervical injuries by Nelson further describes this problem.

The geriatric population presents a demographic group in which optimal management remains controversial. Hanigan et al., in treating 19 patients over the age of 80 years of age with odontoid fractures, had an in hospital mortality of 36% in those treated with bed rest and a hard collar. Good results were achieved in all five of those patients treated surgically.[26] Pepin et al. also noted that halo vest management in the elderly is poorly tolerated.[27] Bednar et al. have shown that early surgical stabilization of odontoid fractures without neurological deficit can reduce mortality in geriatric patients.[28]

Other retrospective reviews have attempted to assess outcomes of surgical and nonsurgical management of cervical spine instability. Dorr et al. found superior radiologic outcomes from surgery in those patients with injury patterns that they described as anterior subluxations.[29] Patients who underwent surgery had less than 9° of angulation at 3 months after injury, whereas those treated in traction had over 17°. Murphy et al. found no difference in functional outcomes at the end of primary rehabilitation between patients treated surgically and nonsurgically. Their study suggested, however, that with early surgical stabilization there was a shortened overall hospitalization, reduced total hospital costs, and decreased degrees of physical and emotional deconditioning.[30] In a Swedish review of 332 cervical spine fractures treated between the years 1970 and 1980, Ersmark et al. concluded that a collar is sufficient treatment for most undisplaced fractures and that immobilization by a halo vest is an excellent method of treatment for most patients with a displaced fracture. They found the complication rate associated with operative treatment unacceptably high.[31] Graft extrusion and redislocation occurred in 38% of their overall complications. Posthospital treatment and necessity for a disability pension were also higher in the operative group. Munroe also felt that fixation carried a greater mortality and impaired ultimate movement more than conservative treatment.[32]

In the latter two series, anterior interbody fusion was performed without instrumentation. Stauffer and Kelly showed that fracture dislocations of the cervical spine treated by anterior interbody fusion without internal fixation are potentially unstable due to posterior ligamentous disruption. Instability with recurrence of angular deformity occurred in all patients even with postoperative halo immobilization.[33] Kewalramani and Riggins described a 20% incidence of graft extrusion following anterior interbody fusion without instrumentation.[34] Operative disruption of the anterior longitudinal ligament and loss of intervertebral disk further adds to instability.[35,36] The role of anterior cervical plating in addition to strut grafting is now well established.[37,38] Anterior plates provide immediate internal stabilization of the cervical spine and prevent subluxation and graft extrusion until fusion occurs. Ripa et al. noted an incidence of 2% for significant complications related directly to the use of anterior plate and screw fixation; in only 1 of 92 patients was there loss of spinal alignment.[38]

Posterior fixation techniques have had a longer history. Rogers reported the long-term outcome of 37 patients with SCI treated with posterior interspinous wire fixation. Two patients developed nonunion, and one patient had loss of reduction.[39] In a modification to increase rotational stability using a triple wire technique, two series with a total of 172 patients reported a 100% union rate.[40,41] Only two patients required supplemental stabilization with a halo vest.

With the more recent use of lateral mass plates, there have not yet been many long-term outcome studies. Fehlings et al., with a minimum follow-up of 2 years, found a fusion rate of 93%, and in only three patients did instrumentation failure or increased kyphosis necessitate a revision operation.[42] Anderson et al. followed 30 patients prospectively after treatment with posterior cervical reconstruction plates. One patient had loss of correction, and there were no neurovascular injuries.[43]

With the advances made in instrumentation and surgical techniques, earlier outcome studies may have been less probative. Continued outcomes research is required to provide reliable information on surgical technique and instrumentation.

TIMING OF SURGERY

Surgical decompression must be considered in all cases of radiographically demonstrable neurologic compression. Boehler recognized the importance of fracture reduction and realignment of the spine in cord decompression.[44] Breig has shown that residual kyphosis and anterior cord compression creates increased tension on axonal tracts and decreased cord perfusion. These effects were reversed with return to a physiologic alignment.[45,46] Several animal studies have shown an inverse relationship between duration of compression and recovery following SCI.[47,48,49] Although case reports describe significant neurologic recovery following immediate decompression through spinal realignment, well-controlled human studies on the timing of surgical intervention are not available.[50] It is well established, however, that decompression of neural elements performed up to 1 year following injury results in improved neurological function.[51,52] Variables that best predict motor improvement have been shown to be age under 25 years and incomplete injury.[53]

Timing of surgical intervention in acute cervical SCI remains controversial. Marshall et al., in a large multicenter study, noted neurological deterioration in 4 of 26 patients who had an operation within 5-days after a SCI, but in none of the 108 patients who had an operation after the fifth day.[54] In contrast to these results, Levi et al. found no statistically significant difference in the neurological outcome based on timing of operative intervention of patients with incomplete or complete neurological deficits.[55] The authors noted that early surgery simplified patient care and permitted earlier transfer to SCI rehabilitation. Wilberger compared the outcome and perioperative morbidity of spinal stabilization performed early (before 24 hours) and late (after 24 hours) after SCI. There was no difference in the neurological outcome between the two groups, but the late surgery group had a 50% increase in complications of pneumonia, decubuti ulcers, deep vein thrombosis, and pulmonary embolism.[56] Schlegel et al. found that all patients with cervical spine injuries had fewer complications if they underwent surgery within 72 hours regardless of associated injuries.[57]

Given modern day instrumentation and techniques, as well as improvements in radiologic assessment, resuscitation, and anesthesia, the significance of the earlier studies that favor operative intervention on a delayed basis should be reevaluated.

ANESTHETIC CONSIDERATIONS IN CERVICAL SPINE INJURY

The traumatic cervical spine requires special consideration in anesthesia during intubation and positioning. An awake fiber optic nasotracheal intubation is performed and neurologic function then tested. If a posterior approach is to be used, a turning frame should be employed and the neurologic function again assessed. General anesthesia is now induced and a lateral radiograph obtained to ensure satisfactory alignment of the spine.

Use of succinylcholine is contraindicated in patients with acute neurologic injury, as this can cause a sudden release of potassium from the paralyzed muscles and result in cardiac arrest. Hypotension should be avoided and an adequate hematocrit should be maintained at all times to ensure adequate perfusion and oxygenation to the cord. Some inhalational agents (e.g., nitrous oxide) should be avoided, as these alter evoked potential response.[58]

COMPLICATIONS

VERTEBRAL ARTERY INJURY

Vertebral artery injuries have been reported to occur in 0.9% to 46% of patients with cervical spine fractures and dislocations, but clinical consequences are rare.[59,60] Reports in the literature describe vertebrobasilar circulation ischemia after blunt trauma to the cervical spine.[61,62] Bone fragments within the foramen transversarium were found to have a high predictive value for vertebral artery injury (Fig. 10-2).[60] Routine vascular studies for determination of vascular injury are presently not recommended; however, in patients with cervical spine trauma and altered mental status without identifiable head injury, normal vertebral artery flow should be verified.

Iatrogenic injuries to the vertebral artery have been described. Direct trauma from an instrument or dissection carried posterior and lateral to the joints of Luschka may cause arterial injury in the anterior cervical approach.[63] The posterior approach to C1-C2 also poses a risk to the vertebral artery if the dissection is carried more than 1.5 cm from the midline.

Posterior instrumentation may also cause injury to the vertebral artery. The Magerl transarticular facet screw for C1-C2 stabilization may cause injury if oriented too ventral or too lateral (Fig. 10-3). In posterior cervical plating, the vertebral artery is located directly anterior to the valley at the junction of the lamina and facet. Care must be exercised in ensuring the outward orientation of lateral mass screws.

ANTERIOR SURGERY

Complications of anterior cervical decompressions and fusion most commonly are related to the approach. These include dysphagia, esophageal, or pharyngeal perforation and recurrent laryngeal nerve injury.[64,65] It is important that retractors be released frequently during the procedure and that they are placed under the elevated longus colli muscles. In the lower cervical spine, a left-sided approach is advocated as the course of the right recurrent laryngeal nerve is more variable and vulnerable to damage as it crosses from the subclavian artery to the tracheoesophageal groove. Right-handed surgeons may prefer a right-sided approach for easier use of the right hand, particularly with odontoid screw insertion.

The more extensive surgical exposure necessary for plate placement has not been accompanied by higher rates of infection, neurologic, or esophageal injuries.[65,66] Potential complications, however, are associated with instrumentation. Neurologic injury can occur from plating systems that require penetration of the posterior cortex of the vertebral body by the drill bit and screw. Screw backout and plate loosening can cause esophageal perforation. This is of greater risk in the nonrigid plating systems, such as the Orozco and Caspar plates.[66,67]

Postoperative hematoma and retropharyngeal soft tissue swelling may result in tracheal obstruction and respiratory insufficiency, particularly in the complete quadriplegic patient with impaired ventilation. This can be minimized by ensuring meticulous hemostasis and care with retraction at the time of surgery.

Late complications include pseudarthrosis and degenerative changes at adjacent unfused segments. Graft displacement and loss of reduction are much lower than with uninstrumented anterior fusions.[33,34,36,37,38] Nonunion of anterior fusions without significant hardware displacement can be treated with posterior cervical fusion.

POSTERIOR SURGERY

There is generally a lower complication rate from posterior exposures. Injury to the vertebral artery at the C1-C2 level and to the neurovascular structures with subaxial posterior cervical plating present the most significant complications. Seroma and hematoma are somewhat more prevalent with these exposures.

A

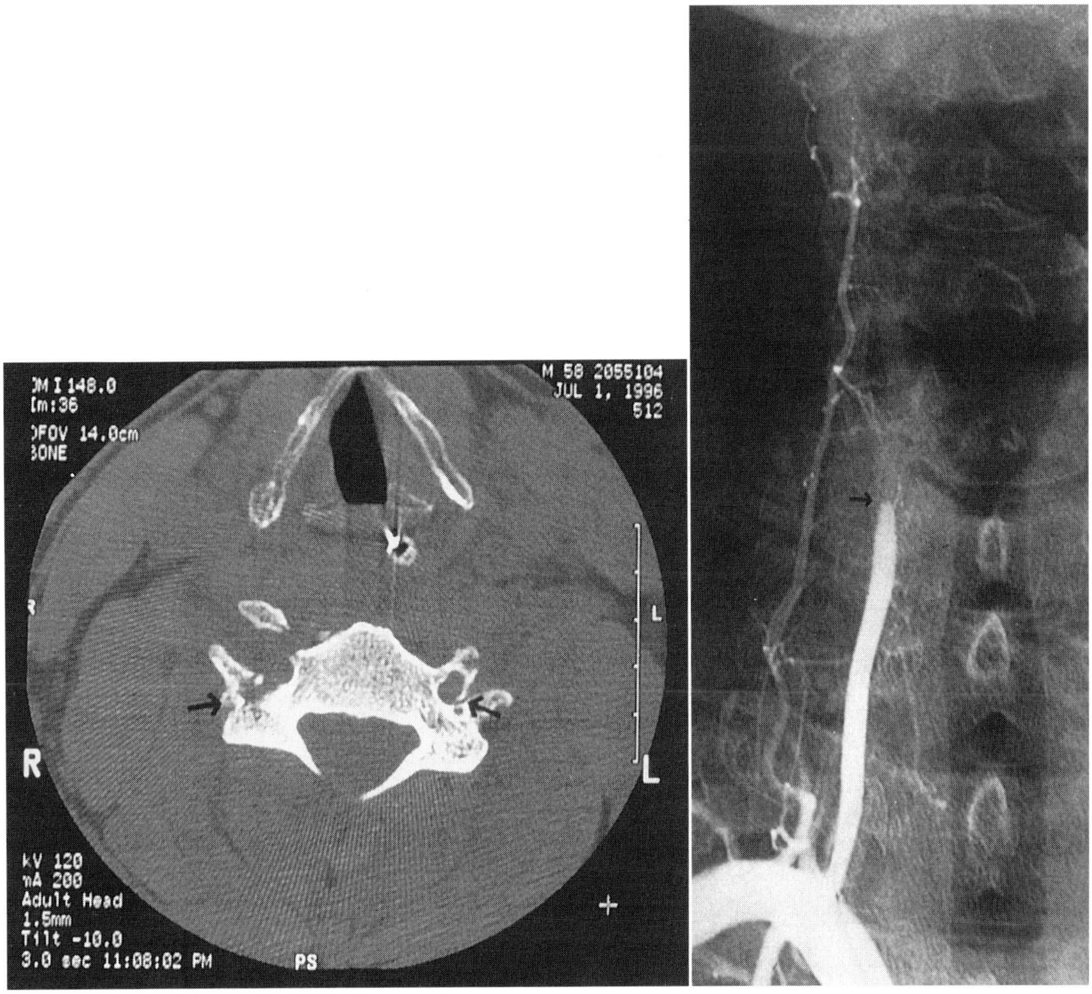

B

FIGURE 10-2

Axial computed tomography (CT) image through C5 from a 56-year-old male who sustained a bilateral facet dislocation. He initially presented with a complete quadriplegia and a normal mental status but rapidly had deterioration in mental status. Bilateral fractures of the foramen transversarium are indicated (*arrows*). Bone fragments are present within the right foramen. CT scan of the head was normal. Following closed reduction using cranial tongs traction, vertebral angiography demonstrated injury to both vertebral arteries. Complete cutoff of dye is illustrated in the right vertebral artery (*arrow*).

BIOMECHANICS OF CERVICAL SPINE FIXATION

UPPER CERVICAL SPINE

Occipital-Cervical Junction. Many techniques for occipitocervical fusion and stabilization have been described. High rates of fusion are reported by many authors with a simple onlay graft technique; however, a long period of bracing is required.[68,69] Internal fixation has been added to increase stability. Autograft and wire fixation was described by Hamblen and a triple wire technique by Wertheim and Bohlman.[70,71] To further increase stability, segmental internal fixation with Luque rods or a steel loop and sublaminar wires have been used.[72,73] More recently screw and plate fixation has been described. This technique avoids the risk of sublaminar wire passage and provides sufficient stability to be used without postoperative halo immobilization.[74,75]

C1-C2 Articulation. Approximately 50% of axial rotation of the cervical spine occurs at the C1-C2 articulation.[76] Instability at this level occurs most commonly as a result of fractures of the odontoid or bursting injuries of the atlas with disruption of the transverse ligament. The goal in the treatment is to reestablish the normal anatomic relationships at the level or the ring of C1 and then to maintain them either through osseosynthesis of the dens or through a solid fusion of C1 and C2.

Biomechanical studies of atlantoaxial arthrodesis techniques have evaluated the Gallie fusion, the Brooks fusion, the Halifax intralaminar clamp, and the Magerl transarticular facet screw fixation. In a study using 15 embalmed cervical spines, Hajek et al. found the Halifax clamp to have significantly greater rotational stiffness when compared with the Brooks construct, which itself demonstrated significantly greater stiffness than the Gallie construct. There was no statistical difference between the translational stiffness of the Brooks and Halifax clamp constructs, but both were significantly greater than the Gallie construct.[77] Grob et al. compared the Gallie construct, Brooks construct, Halifax clamps, and Magerl transarticular facet screw fixation.[78] The Gallie-type fixation was least stable, allowing for a significantly greater range of motion than the other three techniques in flexion and extension, axial rotation, and lateral bending. Stability in flexion and extension was equivalent for the Halifax clamp, the Brooks technique, and the Magerl procedure. The Magerl screw technique, however, provided the most stable construct for lateral bending and axial rotation. The hypothesis proposed for the increased stability using the Magerl technique was the three-point fixation concept of the construct. Hanson et al. also compared the Gallie construct with the Magerl transarticular screw technique. They found the Magerl screw to be stiffer in rotation without permitting anteroposterior translation, but marked anteroposterior translation was noted with the wiring technique.[79]

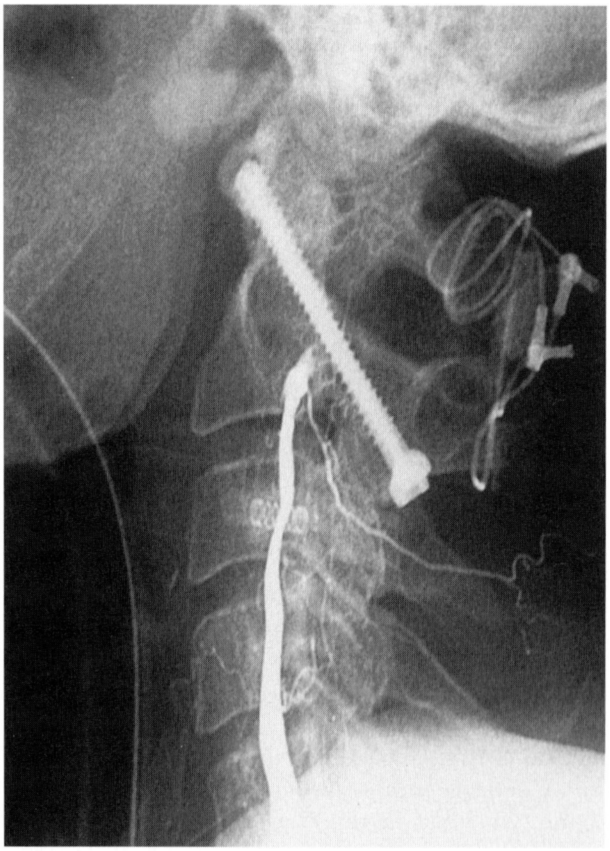

FIGURE 10-3

In this 38-year-old male, after passage of the second threaded guide wire for C1-C2 transarticular screw placement, pulsatile bleeding was encountered. The screw was placed and bleeding controlled. The postoperative vertebral angiogram demonstrates injury to the vertebral artery. Fortunately there was no neurologic sequelae.

Our technique of choice for C1-C2 posterior arthrodesis is the Magerl transarticular screw. This is described later in the chapter.

Odontoid Fractures. Loss of neck motion following posterior C1-C2 fusion led to anterior screw osseosynthesis of odontoid fractures. Graziano et al. compared anterior osseosynthesis of the dens with either one or two 3.5-mm screws to a posterior C1-C2 Brooks sublaminar wiring construct. Bending stiffness was significantly greater with either one or two screws than with the posterior wire technique. There were no significant differences between bending or torsional stiffness for one screw or two screw specimens.[80] Sasso et al. similarly found no difference in stability between a one screw or two screw construct.[81] Doherty et al. have determined that single screw fixation of an odontoid fracture provides stability equal to one half that of the unfractured bone.[82]

The decision to use one or two screws needs to be made on a case-by-case basis. A single screw has proved to provide adequate biomechanical strength; however, two screws provide improved rotational control. A preoperative CT scan should be performed to assess both cross-sectional diameter of the odontoid and bone density. Severe osteopenia is a contraindication to this technique, and a small cross-sectional area necessitates the use of one screw.[83]

LOWER CERVICAL SPINE

Anterior Instrumentation. The anterior cervical approach permits decompression of the ventral aspect of the spinal cord. Restoration of the anterior vertebral column with a strut graft and anterior instrumentation provides immediate internal stabilization of the cervical spine and prevents subluxation and graft extrusion until fusion occurs. Orozco and Caspar plates use 3.5-mm screws that are not rigidly fixed to the plate. Under load, the screws are prone to cantilever bending and can toggle and back out. To lessen this risk, bicortical purchase through both anterior and posterior vertebral body cortices is necessary. Risk of SCI and screw loosening with the inherent threat of esophageal perforation has been previously noted.

To avoid the need for screw engagement through the posterior vertebral cortex and to minimize the risk of screw loosening, the synthes/Morscher cervical spine locking plate (CSLP) incorporates vertebral body screws that rigidly lock to the plate by means of a conical expansion bolt. This bolt inserts into and expands the cross-split head of the vertebral body screw. The screws are angled medially, therefore, increasing pullout resistance (Fig. 10-4).[84] With these design features, bicortical purchase is not necessary. Biomechanical studies have demonstrated no significant difference between the CSLP and the Caspar plate fixed with bicortical screw.[85] Our technique of choice for anterior instrumentation uses the CSLP. This is described in more detail later in this chapter.

Several studies have compared anterior versus posterior implants. Posterior constructs have been shown to be biomechanically superior to anterior implants. Abitbol et al. compared two anterior plates, an interspinous wiring technique and four posterior plates. In flexion the anterior plates allowed significantly greater motion than the posterior implants, while in spinal extension the anterior plates provided the most rigid stabilization.[86]

In a distractive-flexion injury model, Montesano et al. tested the Rogers wiring method versus an anterior cervical plate. The wiring technique was found to provide significantly greater stiffness and strength.[87] Despite in vitro inferior biomechanical results compared with posterior implants, clinical investigations have reported excellent results, and there have been few failures of fixation using anterior cervical plates.[37,38,86,88]

Posterior Instrumentation. Posterior interspinous wire techniques have been the most frequently performed cervical spine stabilization technique. Biomechanically, they increase flexural stiffness to 110% of the normal spine.[89,90] Interspinous wires are less effective in longer fusion constructs, in resisting an extension stress, and in rotationally unstable injuries.[91,92] The addition of the triple wire technique has been shown to add rotational stability to the cervical spine.[40]

Holness et al. has reported on the use of the Halifax interlaminar clamp.[93] Biomechanical testing has shown no advantage of the clamp over interspinous wiring in flexion, extension, or torsional loading.[90,94] This device has several disadvantages. The clamp performs

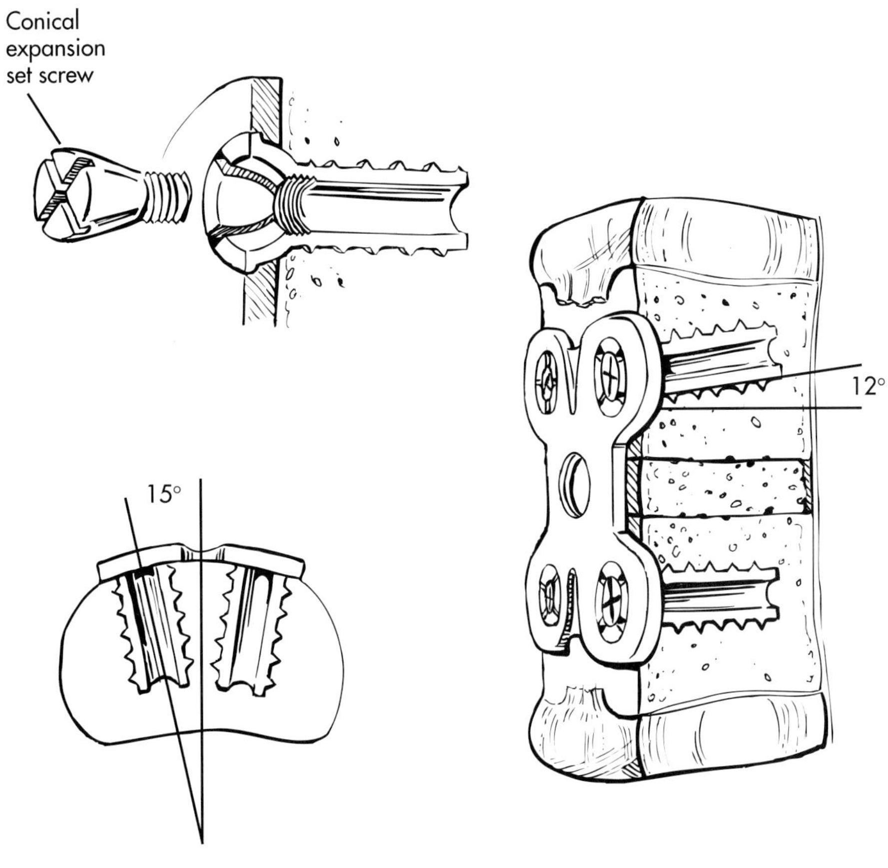

FIGURE 10-4

Anterior decompression and fusion using the AO/cervical spine locking plate. Rigid locking of the screws to the plate is achieved by means of a conical expansion bolt inserted into the head of the 4.0/4.35-mm screw. Medial angulation of the screws also increases pullout resistance. Vertebral body screws have unicortical purchase.

poorly in cyclical loading because of screw back-out. The device is not applicable in the presence of lamina or lateral mass fractures, and multilevel fixation is not possible. The cephalad hook poses neurological risk as it enters the spinal canal, and with clamp overtightening, unrecognized posterior translation of the cranial vertebrae may result.[95]

Posterior cervical plate fixation was developed by Roy-Camille.[91] Biomechanical studies have shown posterior plate systems are stiffer than wire constructs in extension and rotation and are equal to or better than wire constructs in resisting flexion.[89,90,94,96] Gill et al. found that one-third tubular plates with bicortical screw fixation provided the greatest stiffness compared with Rogers wiring and the Halifax clamp.[94]

Screw direction into the lateral mass has been shown to be an important variable in stability of the posterior construct.[97] Two methods of screw placement are used (Fig. 10-5). In the Roy-Camille technique, the screw is placed in the center of the lateral mass and directed in a straight sagittal direction or angled outward 10 to 20 degrees.[97] In the Magerl technique, the screw is placed 1 mm cephalad and medial to the center of the lateral mass, with the screw oriented 20 degrees laterally and parallel to the facet joint (approximately 35 degrees cephalad).[98,99] The Magerl technique demonstrated a

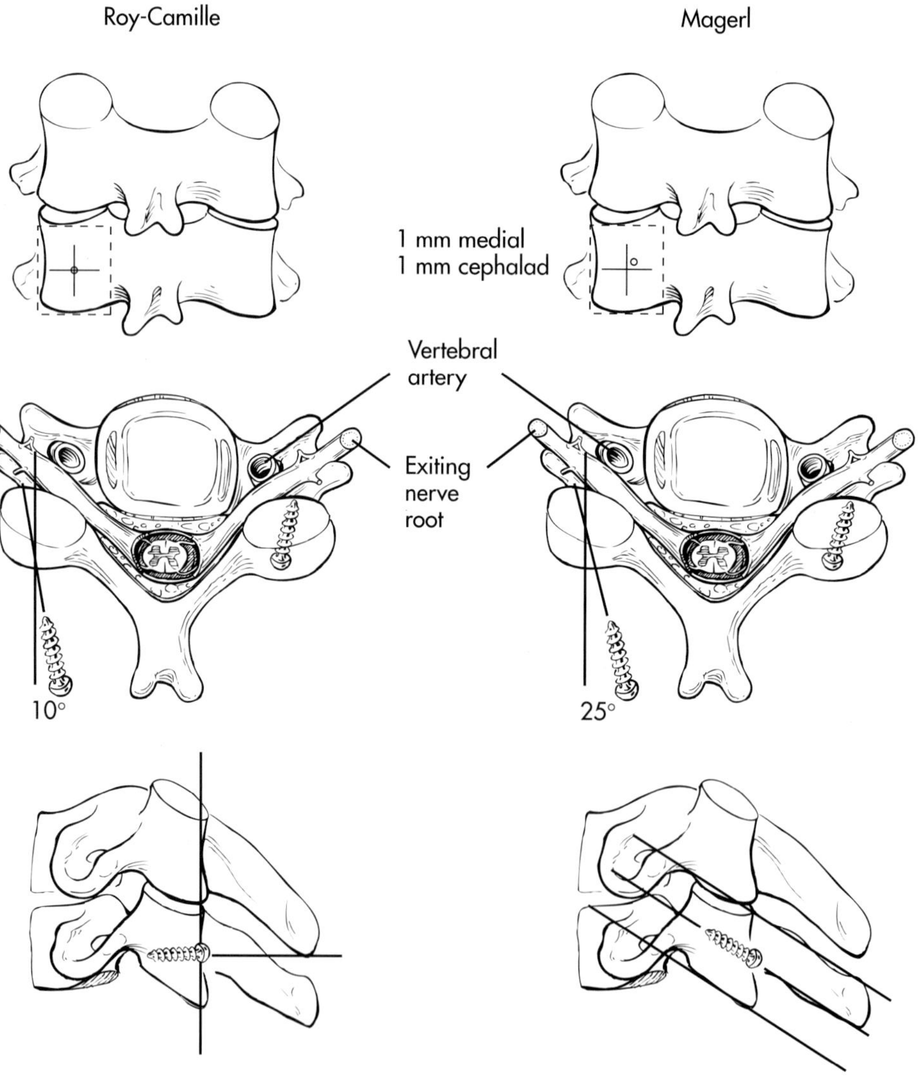

Figure 10-5

Lateral mass placement: Roy-Camille technique of screw insertion (*left*). Starting point is the center of the outlined lateral mass. Screws are directed straight sagittal and outward 10°. Magerl technique of screw insertion (*right*). Screws start 1 mm medial and 1 mm cephalad to the center of the lateral mass and are angulated 20° outward and parallel to the facet joint. In the axial views, the starting point is lateral to the vertebral artery, which is localized posteriorly by the valley at the facet-laminar junction.

higher load to failure, most likely because of the ability to use a longer screw length.[100] In a cadaver study, Heller et al. found that the Magerl technique had a higher risk of injuring the exiting nerve root, and the Roy-Camille technique had a higher risk of penetrating the more caudal motion segment.[101]

Posterior cervical plates or lateral mass plates are indicated for cervical instability associated with posterior element fractures or deficiencies and in multilevel and rotatory instabilities. Lateral mass plates are effective as an alternative to anterior fixation in burst fractures that do not require anterior decompression and for stabilization of three-column cervical injuries.[101,103,104] In addition, this implant has been satisfactory in the treatment of cervicothoracic instability.[105] Lateral mass plating using a Magerl screw orientation is our technique of choice for posterior cervical stabilization. We describe this later in this chapter.

UPPER CERVICAL SPINE INJURIES

OCCIPITAL CONDYLE FRACTURES

Diagnosis. The diagnosis of occipital condyle fracture requires a high index of suspicion. It is commonly associated with closed head injury, and the diagnosis is often made incidentally on head CT scans. Alert patients complain of occipital pain. Neurologic examination should include brainstem and cranial nerve function. In suspected injury, high-resolution CT scan with sagittal and coronal reformations of the occipitocervical region should be obtained.

Classification and Treatment. Occipital condyle fractures have been classified by Anderson and Montesano (Fig. 10-6).[106] Type I are comminuted impaction fractures, which occur as a result of axial loading of the skull onto the atlas. Type II is an occipital condyle fracture, which occurs as part of a basilar skull fracture. The mechanism is a direct blow to the skull. Types I and II are stable injuries and require a cervical orthosis for 6 to 8 weeks. Type III injuries are alar ligament avulsion fractures from the medial aspect of the condyle and may be unstable. If the occipitoatlantal joints are well aligned or if there is only minimal displacement, the treatment is halo vest immobilization for 12 weeks and serial radiographs. If occipitocervical instability is demonstrated by joint diastasis, subluxation, or neurologic findings, the treatment is occipitocervical arthrodesis.

OCCIPITOCERVICAL DISSOCIATION

Diagnosis. A spectrum of injury to the occipitocervical articulation ranges from mild instability to complete dislocation. In extreme cases of bilateral facet dislocations, patients rarely survive the accident because of brainstem injury. The cruciate paralysis of Bell is associated with injury to this region. It is thought to occur secondary to injuries to the pyramidal deccusation at the foramen magnum and C1. Clinically, patients present with a pattern of incomplete SCI consisting of lower cranial nerve palsies and upper extremity weakness.[107,108]

The mechanism of injury involves shear, hyperextension, and distractive forces.[5,109] Significant soft tissue injury involves ligamentous damage to the alar ligaments and tectorial membrane. Massive prevertebral soft tissue swelling occurs in survivors of atlantooccipital dislocations. Diagnostic difficulties arise because the

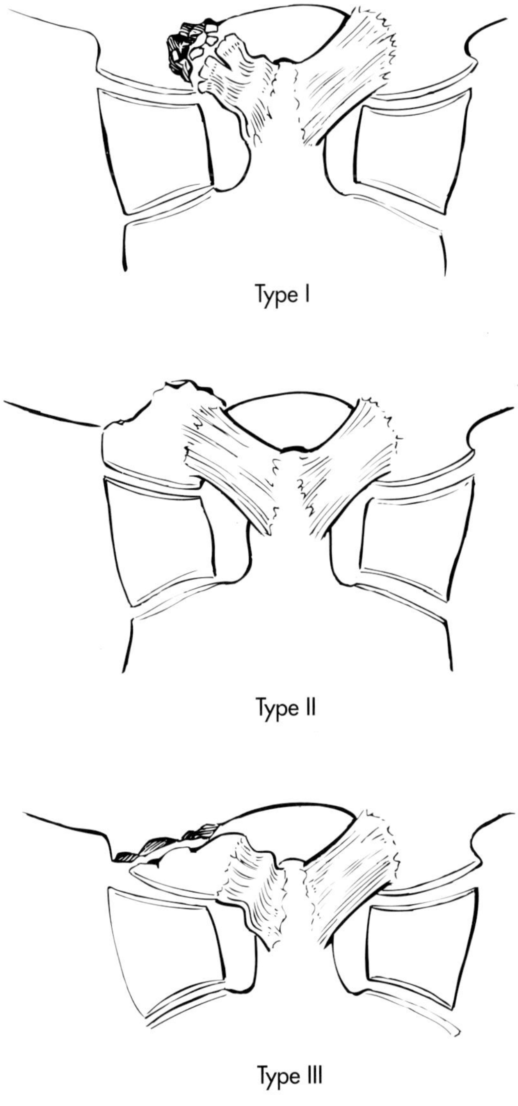

FIGURE 10-6

Classification of occipital condyle fractures. Type I are stable, impacted fractures secondary to axial loading. Type II are basilar skull fractures that involve the occipital condyle. Type III are avulsion fractures of the alar ligaments. These may be associated with occipitocervical instability.

atlantooccipital joints are not visualized on plain radiographs as they lie oblique to the x-ray beam and are obscured by overlying osseous structures.[110]

Several radiographic methods for assessing the craniovertebral relationships have been described. The Powers ratio and the X lines of Lee are often unreliable as they depend on landmarks that are not easily identified on lateral radiographs.[111,112] Harris et al. recently described the rule of twelve. This technique uses the basion-axial interval (BAI), and basion-dens interval (BDI).[113] The BAI is derived from measuring the distance between the basion (the midsagittal point of the anterior margin of the foramen magnum) and the posterior axial line (the rostral extension of the posterior cortex of the axis body). The BDI is the vertical distance between the basion and the dens.[114] In 98% of normal adults the basion is situated within 12 mm anterior to the posterior axial line (PAL). The BDI is less than 12 mm in 95% of uninjured adults (Fig. 10-7). Values in excess of 12 mm for either the BAI or BDI raise suspicion for occipitocervical dissociation. Computed tomography scanning of 1.5-mm thick slices of sagittal and coronal reconstructions should then be obtained. Magnetic resonance imaging is helpful in identifying hematoma and ligamentous disruption.

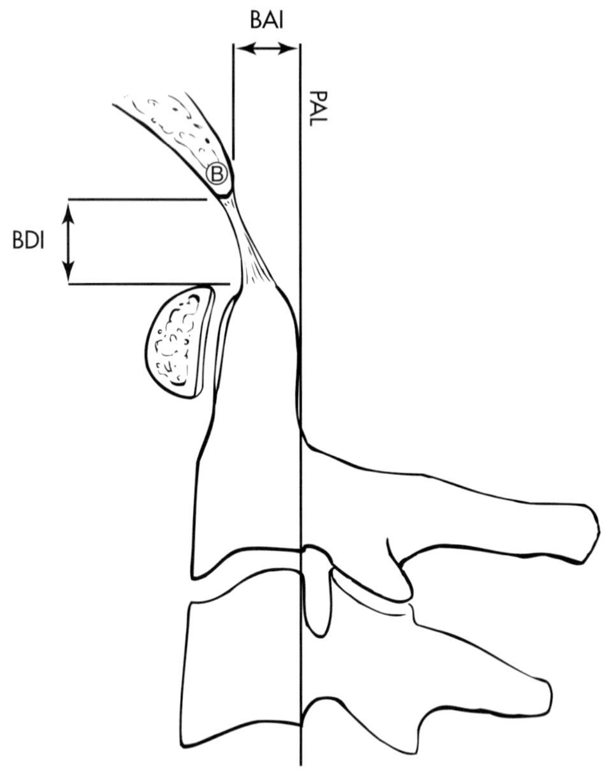

FIGURE 10-7

The rule of twelve for occipitocervical-dissociation. The posterior axial line (PAL) is the rostral extension of the posterior cortex of the axis body. The basion-axial interval (BAI) is the horizontal distance between the basion Ⓑ and the PAL. The basion-dens interval (BDI) is the vertical distance between the basion and the tip of the dens. Values in excess of 12 mm for either the BAI or the BDI suggests of occipitocervical dissociation.

Classification and Treatment. Traynelis et al. have classified occipitocervical injuries as anterior, posterior, and vertical.[115] The use of longitudinal skeletal traction is dangerous as it can result in overdistraction and spinal cord damage.[116] Where gross instability exists, a congruous reduction can be obtained by careful positioning of the head relative to the thorax with strategically placed towels beneath the thorax in anterior dislocations or beneath the occiput in posteriorly displaced injuries. A halo ring and vest should be applied. For vertical displacement, the patient should be sat upright.

The next goal in treatment is the maintenance of long-term stability. These injuries are primarily the result of ligamentous disruption with limited ability for long-term healing. Because of neurological risk associated with loss of reduction, an aggressive surgical approach to treatment is warranted. We recommend posterior occiput to C2 arthrodesis using plate and screw fixation. Our technique of choice for occipitocervical fusion uses posterior screw-plate fixation. Although wire techniques have proved efficacious, rigid internal fixation allows rapid mobilization and maintains reduction without the use of the halo vest (Fig. 10-8).

Technique: Occipitocervical Screw-Plate Fixation Using AO Plates. The patient is carefully turned to the prone position and the halo ring secured to the operating table. Reduction of the occipitocervical junction is evaluated and adjusted if necessary. To reduce vertical displacement, it may be necessary to place the patient in the Trendelenberg position. A midline exposure is carried out from the inion (external occipital protuberance) to C3. The occiput, posterior arch of C1, and the lamina of C2 are subperiostally exposed. The occiput is exposed 5 cm on each side. Distal fixation is generally to the C2 pedicle but occasionally may need to extend to more caudad levels.

Malleable templates are contoured to the occiput and lateral masses of the cervical spine. The AO lateral mass plates or alternatively 3.5-mm reconstruction plates (Synthes) of appropriate length are contoured to match the templates. The C2 pedicle screw, (3.5-mm screw) is drilled and placed first, followed by subaxial lateral mass screws if necessary, and lastly the occipital screws are drilled through the plate. Fixation to the occiput is ideally achieved using two to three 3.2 to 3.5-mm bicortical screws on each side. We have found drilling with a 2-mm diamond air drill to be safe and effective. An understanding of occipital morphology is critical for safe screw application. Drilling above the level of the inion is avoided because of potential injury to the transverse sinus. The maximum bone thickness is found at the level of the inion and is thicker than 8 mm in an area extending laterally 2 cm.[117] Occipital bone becomes progressively thinner towards the foramen magnum. A stop drill avoids intracranial penetration. If cerebral spinal fluid (CSF) is encountered, the hole is bone-waxed and a screw is inserted in the usual way. No persistent CSF leaks have occurred in our experience.[74]

Because plates are placed laterally, the central area on the occiput and the entire width of the arch of the atlas and the C2 lamina are available for arthrodesis. A structural cortical-cancellous graft is shaped to match the occiput and C2 vertebrae closely. A slot is made to straddle the C2 spinous process. The graft is secured with wires or cables looped around the cranial end of the plates or through burr holes placed in the occiput;

A

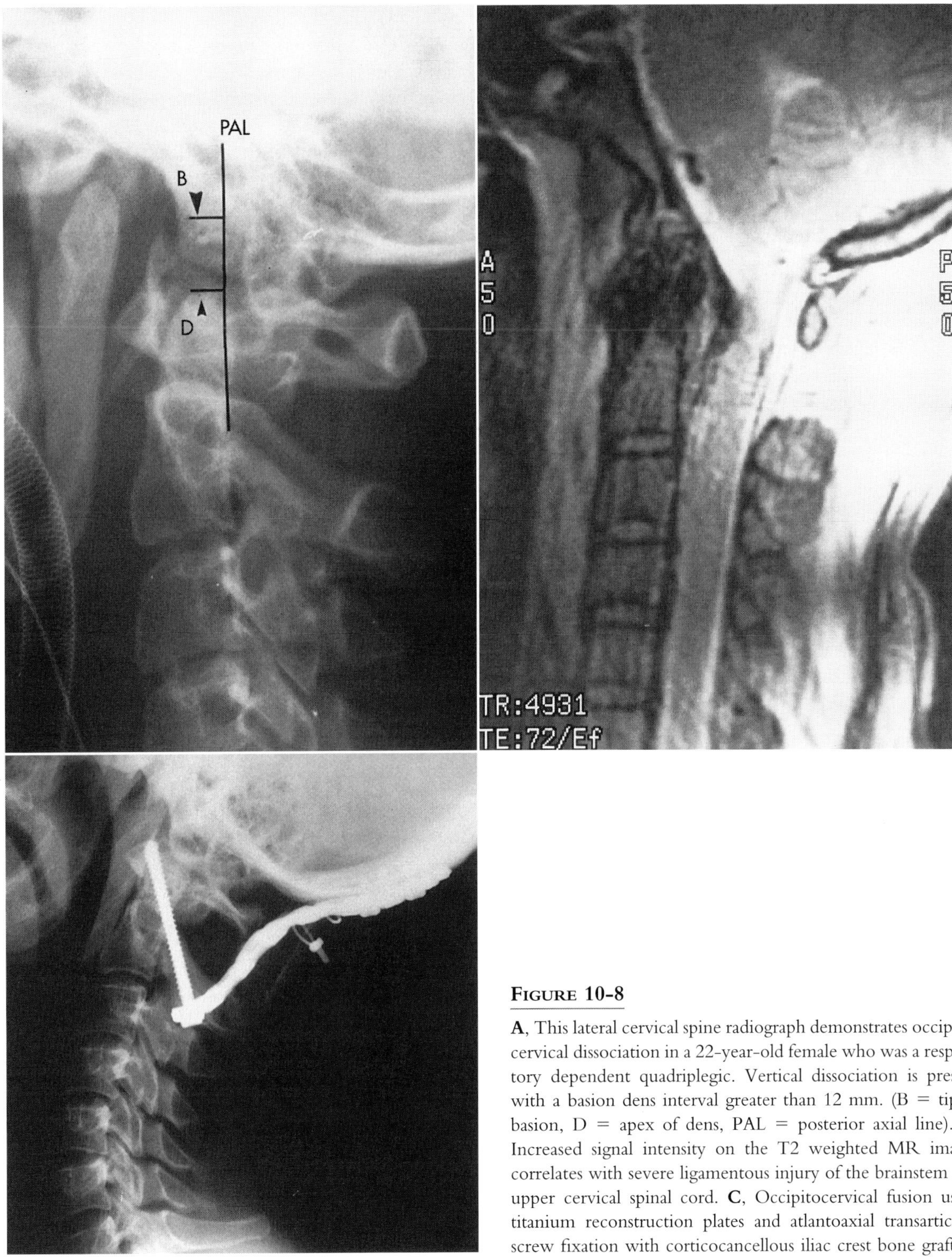

B

C

FIGURE 10-8

A, This lateral cervical spine radiograph demonstrates occipitocervical dissociation in a 22-year-old female who was a respiratory dependent quadriplegic. Vertical dissociation is present with a basion dens interval greater than 12 mm. (B = tip of basion, D = apex of dens, PAL = posterior axial line). **B**, Increased signal intensity on the T2 weighted MR images correlates with severe ligamentous injury of the brainstem and upper cervical spinal cord. **C**, Occipitocervical fusion using titanium reconstruction plates and atlantoaxial transarticular screw fixation with corticocancellous iliac crest bone graft.

caudally a C2 sublaminar wire or cable is used. Supplemental sublaminar wire or cable fixation from C1 to the plate may enhance fixation. A C1-C2 transarticular screw may also be used as an alternative to a C2 pedicle screw. Postoperatively, patients are immobilized in a Minerva orthosis or occasionally halo vest.

Technique: C2 Pedicle Screw Placement. In C2, fixation must be directed medially into the pedicle rather than in the lateral mass. The pedicle axis of C2 lies 20° cephalad to the transverse plane and 30° medial to the sagittal plane.[118] The safest technique for cannulating the C2 pedicle, however, is by direct exposure and palpation of the superior and medial edges of the pedicle.[119] Meticulous dissection and hemostasis using a fine curette and bipolar cautery defines the medial edge of the C2 pedicle. A penfield elevator is then used to identify the medial boundary for screw placement. The starting point in C2 is 5 mm above and just medial to the center of the C2-C3 facet joint. Using an adjustable drill guide, a 2-mm Kirschner wire is sequentially advanced into the pedicle at an angle of 10 to 20 degrees medially and 25 degrees cranially to a depth of 20 to 22 mm (Fig. 10-9). A lateral fluoroscopic image can help to determine the proper cephalad angulation. The drill path from within the pedicle is palpated to ensure that no penetration into the canal has occurred. The pedicle is then tapped with a 3.5-mm tap.

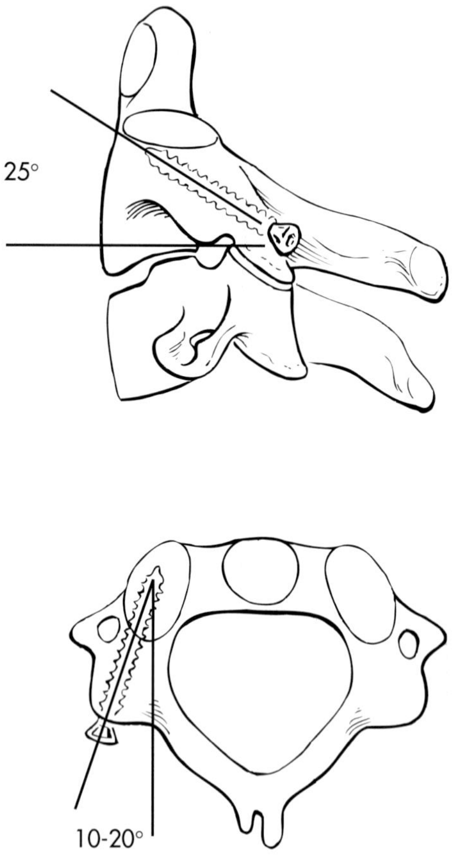

FIGURE 10-9

Orientation of C2 pedicle screw.

INJURIES OF THE ATLAS

Diagnosis. Atlantal fractures represent 3% to 13% of all cervical spine fractures.[120] Motor vehicle accidents and falls account for the majority of injuries. Associated injuries often include closed head injury, scalp lacerations, and, in approximately 50% of cases, other spine fractures, most commonly of the axis.[121,122,123] Neurological deficits are uncommon due to the relatively small proportion of the canal occupied by the cord at this level.[124] Patients present with upper cervical pain, occipital neuralgia, and focal tenderness.

Most injuries to C1 appear on plain radiographs. Standard projections of the C1 ring include the lateral cervical spine and open-mouth odontoid view. On the lateral film, in addition to any obvious bony abnormality, the presence of prevertebral soft-tissue swelling and the atlantodens interval (ADI) should be evaluated. The ADI is the distance between the posterior cortex of the anterior ring of C1 and the anterior cortex of the dens. This should measure less than 3 mm in adults; a greater value suggests rupture of the transverse ligament.

The open-mouth odontoid view is assessed for C1-C2 lateral mass symmetry. Tomograms may be necessary to evaluate better the spatial relationships of the C1 lateral masses to the occipital condyles and to the axis. Outward displacement of the lateral masses of C1 in relation to C2 is indicative of a burst fracture of the atlas (Fig. 10-10).[12] Spence et al. in an anatomic study showed that total displacement of the lateral masses greater than 6.9 mm implied loss of integrity of the transverse ligament.[126] Because of radiographic magnification on the open-mouth odontoid view, Heller et

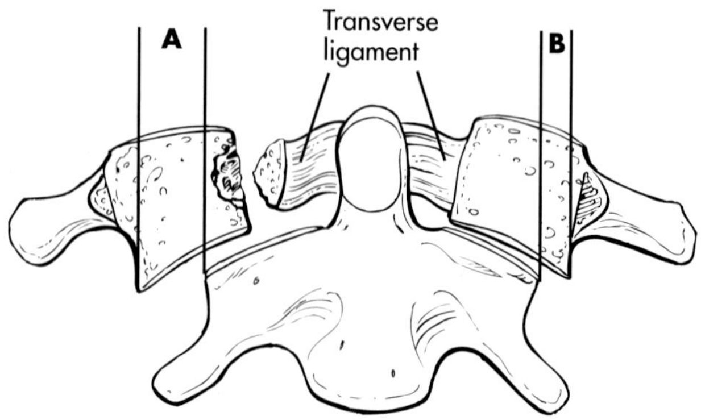

FIGURE 10-10

The distances A and B are the outward displacements of the lateral masses of C1 in relation to C2. If A + B >8.1 mm, this suggests that the transverse ligament is ruptured.

al. have suggested that ligament rupture should not be inferred with a lateral mass overhang less than 8.1 mm (Fig. 10-11).[127]

In the case of an identified or suspected fracture of the atlas, a CT scan with 1.5-mm cuts is indicated to better evaluate the fracture pattern. MRI can be used to evaluate the competence of the transverse ligament but is less useful.

Classification. Fractures of the atlas are classified according to location and stability.[121,122] Hyperextension can cause impingement of the dorsal elements between the occiput and axial pedicles resulting in fracture of the thin posterior arches of C1. These account for nearly two thirds of all atlantal fractures, which are stable injuries.[121]

Anterior arch fractures also can occur secondary to hyperextension. This fracture is produced by an extension moment causing the dens to protrude into the anterior arch. A minimally displaced stable fracture or a displaced unstable "blow-out" fracture of the anterior arch can result.

Lateral bending with an axial load can lead to unilateral lateral mass fractures. These may be unstable if the transverse ligament has been disrupted and can result in progressive lateral displacement of the lateral mass.

Bursting injuries are a result of a compressive load causing the occipital condyles to be driven axially in a caudad direction. Tensile failure of the ring leads to two-, three-, and four-part fractures.[5,121,128] Jefferson originally described the classic four-part fracture with two fracture lines in both the anterior and the posterior arches.[129] More commonly, however, bursting injuries have less than four fractures in the ring.[128] Outward displacement of the lateral masses, the hallmark of this injury, is checked by the transverse ligament.[125] An unstable burst fracture occurs with rupture of this ligament (see Fig. 10-11).

Treatment. Treatment of atlas fractures must take into account the presence of concomitant spinal injuries as these often dictate definitive treatment.[123,124] Minimally displaced fractures of the anterior arch, fractures of the lateral mass, and posterior arch fractures can be treated with a cervical orthosis. Stable burst and displaced lateral mass fractures usually require a cervicothoracic orthosis or halo vest. The open-mouth view is repeated periodically to assure that there is no progressive outward displacement of the lateral masses. At the end of 12 weeks, lateral flexion and extension radiographs are taken to assess stability at C1-C2. Occasionally, nonunions can occur but are rarely painful and usually are not associated with instability.

Treatment of the unstable burst fracture is controversial. Although the fracture is initially unstable, atlantoaxial instability is rarely a long-term problem. For these injuries we recommend initial halo skeletal traction to reduce the distance between the lateral masses. Halo-vest immobilization is maintained with careful monitoring of open-mouth odontoid radiographs. Stability is again checked with flexion and extension radiographs after 12 to 16 weeks. If atlantoaxial instability is present, a delayed posterior C1-C2 fusion is performed. McGuire and Harkey advocate reduction and immediate C1-C2 fixation using Magerl transarticular screws.[130] This has the advantage of anatomic alignment

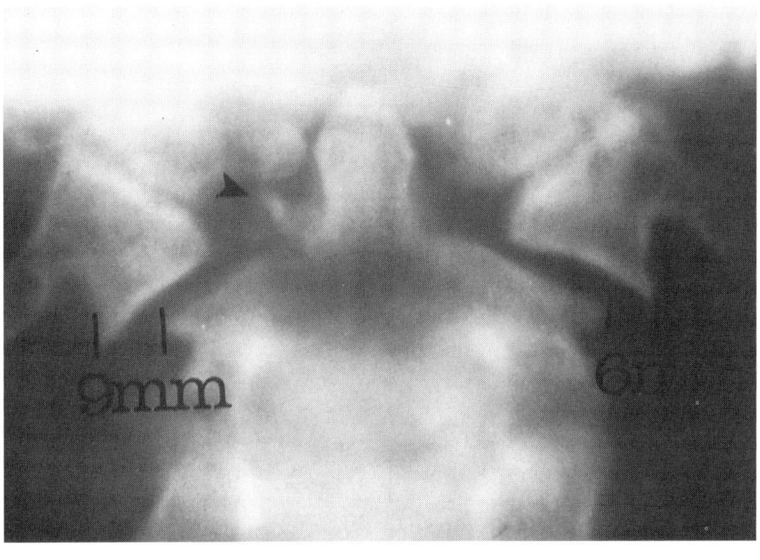

FIGURE 10-11

Burst fracture of C1. The open-mouth odontoid view demonstrates overhand of the C1 lateral masses on C2 measuring 9 mm and 6 mm. Avulsion of the transverse ligament with a piece of bone from the C1 lateral mass is well illustrated (*arrowhead*).

and avoidance of the halo vest but sacrifices atlantoaxial motion.

Anterior blow-out fractures are highly unstable and may be associated with SCI. Traction should be attempted to effect a reduction. If the fracture remains unstable despite halo-vest immobilization, a posterior C1-C2 fusion with Magerl transarticular screws is warranted.

TECHNIQUE: POSTERIOR C1-C2 ARTHRODESIS USING MAGERL TRANSARTICULAR SCREWS

C1-C2 transarticular screws are performed with the patient positioned, prone with the head held in Mayfield tongs or a halo ring. Lateral fluoroscopy is used to check fracture alignment. The lower cervical spine is extended to eliminate the lordosis. At the same time, the atlantooccipital joint is flexed maximally while still maintaining reduction. A posterior midline exposure from the occiput to C3 is performed. The C1-C2 facet joints are dissected and the posterior third joint cartilage is removed with a small cervical curette (Fig. 10-12).

Cancellous bone graft from the posterior iliac crest is packed into the C1-C2 facet joints. The medial wall of the C2 pedicle is dissected with a small blunt probe and clearly identified from within the spinal canal. Long 2.5-mm, terminally threaded guide wires are inserted percutaneously opposite the C7-T1 spinous processes. These are directed to the starting point for screw insertion which is 3 to 5 mm above the C2-C3 joint and just lateral to the medial edge of the C2 pedicle. Under lateral flouroscopic guidance, the guide wire is advanced sagitally and cranially toward the anterior arch of C1. Anatomically, the guide wire crosses the isthmus of the axis and traverses the posterior third of the atlantoaxial joint. After crossing the joint, the guide wire enters the atlas approximately in the midpart of the articular process.[131] Vital structures include the vertebral artery, which lies ventral to the isthmus in C2 and laterally in C1. The structures inside the spinal canal lie medially (Fig. 10-13).

The guide wire is engaged into the anterior arch of C1. Both left- and right-sided guide wires are inserted. The insertion depth is measured, tapping is performed, and 3.5- or 4.0-mm screws usually between 30 and 40 mm are inserted. A small fragment cannulated screw set can make the exchange of the initial drill to screw easier. Depending on direction of instability, partially threaded or fully threaded screws are used to function as a lag screw or positioning screw respectively.

In the event of injury to the vertebral artery during drilling or tapping, the screw should be inserted as this helps effect hemostasis. If the second side has not yet been placed, this screw should not be inserted and a standard C1-C2 posterior wiring technique performed.

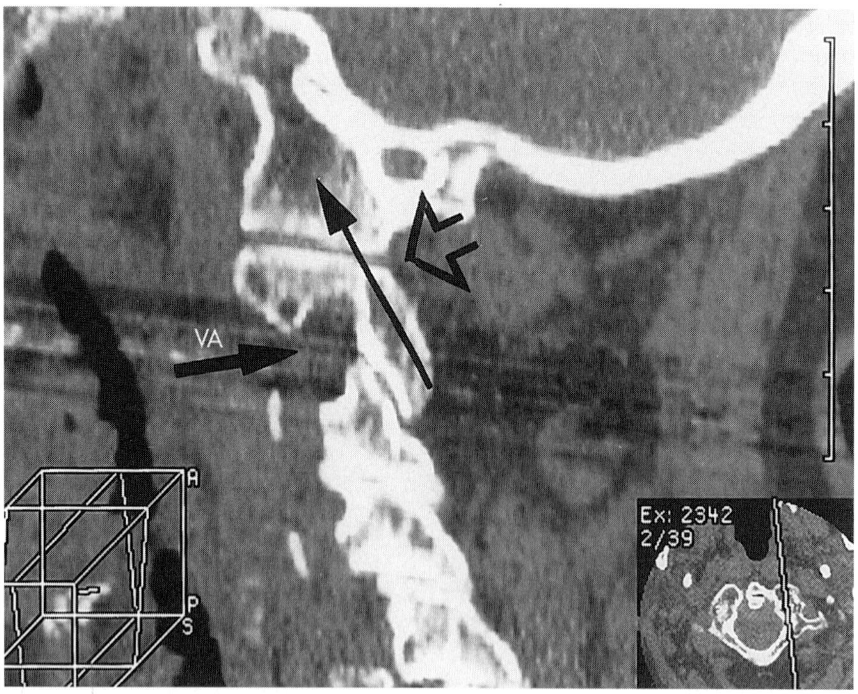

FIGURE 10-12

Computed tomography sagittal reformation of upper cervical spine. The proposed trajectory of the C1-C2 transarticular screw is indicated (*thin arrow*). The position of the vertebral artery within the body of C2 is indicated (*VA*). The ventral position of the vertebral artery to the C1-C2 joint (*open arrow*) is well-visualized.

Postoperatively, a vertebral artery angiogram should be obtained.

The procedure is completed by performing a midline fusion using a corticocancellus bone graft and a Gallie type fusion. In some patients, reduction can be enhanced by use of a sublaminar C1 wire or cable and downward pressure on the C2 spinous process.

ODONTOID FRACTURES

Diagnosis. Odontoid fractures occur in 10% to 15% of all cervical spine injuries.[132,133] In the younger age group, they often occur as a consequence of motor vehicle accidents. In the elderly, a low-velocity fall on the head may cause this fracture. The mechanism of injury can be from forces causing extreme flexion, extension, or rotation.[134,135] Anterior displacement of the odontoid is more common than posterior displacement, suggesting that flexion is a more common cause of fracture than is extension.[136,137]

The alert patient may complain of high cervical pain, which may radiate through the greater occipital nerve to the back of the head. Neurologic injury occurs in 18% to 25% of all cases.[138–141] Fractures are frequently missed, particularly in patients with concomitant head injury or who are intoxicated.[142] Fractures may also be difficult to identify in the osteopenic skeleton of geriatric patients.[143] In the majority of cases, fractures can be identified on either a lateral cervical spine radiograph or open-mouth odontoid view. A CT scan with sagittal and coronal reformations are useful for better understanding of the fracture pattern and for surgical planning.

Classification. Classification of odontoid fractures is based on the level of the fracture. The system of Anderson and D'Alonzo is most widely used. This classification has the greatest clinical applicability and prognostic implications (Fig. 10-14).[136,140]

TYPE I. Type I injuries represent an avulsion fracture of the alar ligament from the dens. The importance of this injury is its potential association with an atlantooccipital dissociation.

TYPE II. Type II injuries are the most common odontoid fractures. These are transverse or oblique fractures through the waist of the odontoid. This fracture occurs in the cortical bone caudad to the transverse ligament and above the cancellous body of the axis. Displacement can be either anterior or posterior. Hadley et al. have described the Type IIa fracture, which includes comminution of either the anterior or posterior cortex.[144]

Type II fractures have the highest incidence of nonunion. Various factors contribute to the poor prognosis associated with these injuries. These are unstable injuries and can cause damage to the vascularity of the dens.[145] The remaining dens is of hard cortical, bone

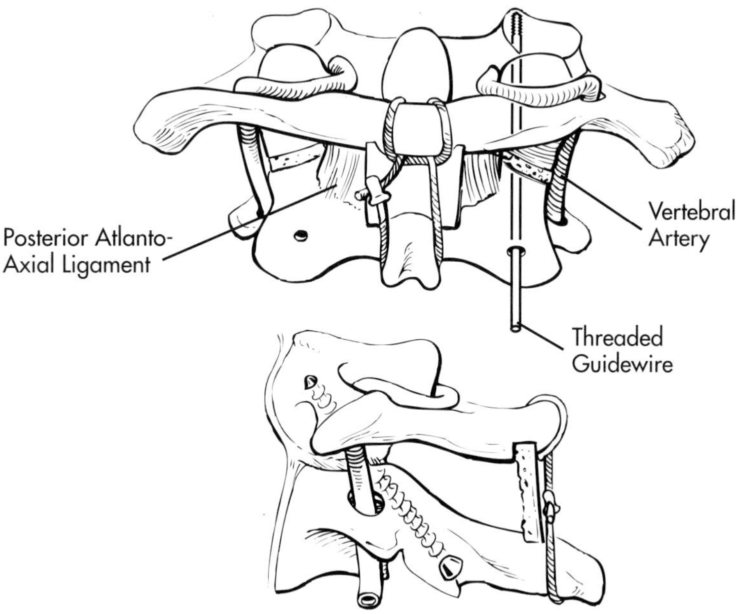

FIGURE 10-13

Magerl screw. The position of the C1-C2 transarticular screw is drawn. The starting point for the guide wire is 3 to 5 mm proximal to the C2-C3 facet joint and directed in a straight sagittal or slight medial orientation. The location of the vertebral artery and the spinal canal are noted. The bone graft and Gallie type fusion using a cable are illustrated.

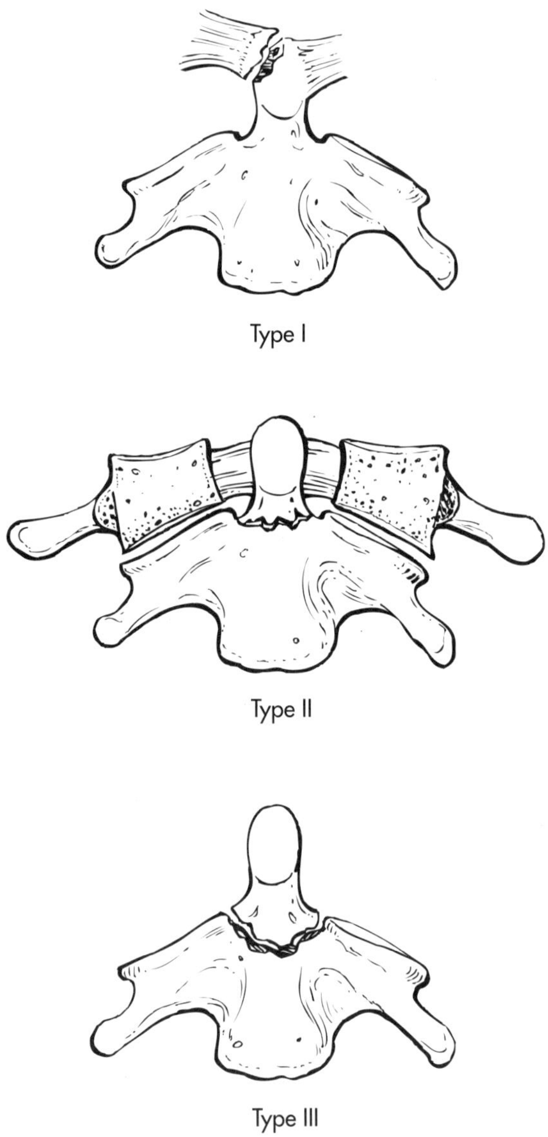

FIGURE 10-14

Dens classification. Classification of odontoid fractures. Type I are avulsion fractures of the alar ligament. Type II are fractures through the waist of the odontoid caudad to the transverse ligament. Type III are fractures into the cancellous body of the axis.

with a small surface area for healing. Other factors have been suggested that may affect union including initial displacement of more than 5 mm, angulation greater than 10°, posterior displacement, type IIa fracture, age over 40, delay in diagnosis, and smoking.[136,139,140,144,146–149] Nonunion in nonsurgically treated patients range from 4% to 68%.[124,139,140,146,150,151]

TYPE III. Type III injuries are fractures into the body of the axis and usually have a well-vascularized, broad cancellous surface area.

Treatment. TYPE I. Isolated type I fractures are stable injuries and treatment is simple immobilization in a hard collar for 6 to 8 weeks.

TYPE II. The treatment for type II fractures remains controversial. These fractures have a significantly poorer prognosis than either type I or type III. For fractures without risk factors for nonunion, patients who can tolerate one are treated in a halo vest for 12 to 16 weeks. During healing, fracture alignment is checked to ensure that reduction is maintained. No more than 20% displacement should be tolerated.[152]

Displaced fractures should be considered for surgical management. Standard treatment is a posterior atlantoaxial arthrodesis using the Gallie or Brooks wiring techniques. This will result in healing in 96% of cases, but requires postoperative halo-vest immobilization.[136] Wiring techniques cannot be used in patients with posterior arch fractures of C1. The Magerl C1-C2 transarticular screw technique is advantageous as it does not require an intact posterior arch, it provides a high fusion rate and has increased rigidity avoiding the need for postoperative halo-vest immobilization (Fig. 10-15).[132,153]

An alternative to posterior arthrodesis is direct anterior osseosynthesis of the dens.[154] Theoretically, this technique preserves atlantoaxial motion; however, Jeanneret et al. have shown that only 50% of normal atlantoaxial motion is maintained after odontoid screw fixation.[155] An 8% to 16% nonunion rate and a major complication rate of 17% to 28% have been reported. These have been attributed in part to poor patient selection.[154,156,157,158] This technique is contraindicated in patients with osteoporosis, nonunion, os odontoideum, or thoracic kyphosis (Fig. 10-16).

TYPE III. Type III fractures are usually stable injuries. These are best treated with fracture reduction using skeletal traction and light weight, followed by halo-vest immobilization for 12 to 16 weeks. Several studies have documented good results and high union rates using the halo-vest, while poorer results have been demonstrated using a less rigid orthosis.[136,146,147,159] Delayed or nonunions of type III odontoid fractures are treated with posterior C1-C2 arthrodeses.

TECHNIQUE: ODONTOID SCREW FIXATION (TWO-SCREW TECHNIQUE)

Odontoid screw fixation is performed with the patient supine and the head held by the Mayfield three-point head clamp. This device is attached to a U-shaped crossbar hence allowing for anteroposterior and lateral C-arm images (Fig. 10-17).[156] A radiolucent bite block further provides unobstructed anteroposterior open-mouth images. Closed reduction of the fracture is performed under image intensification in two planes. The neck is extended as much as possible to accommodate the steep inferior angle of approach necessary for screw insertion.[158]

A right-sided Smith Robinson approach is made over the C5-C6 disk level. Retropharyngeal dissection proceeds cranially exposing the C2-C3 interspace.

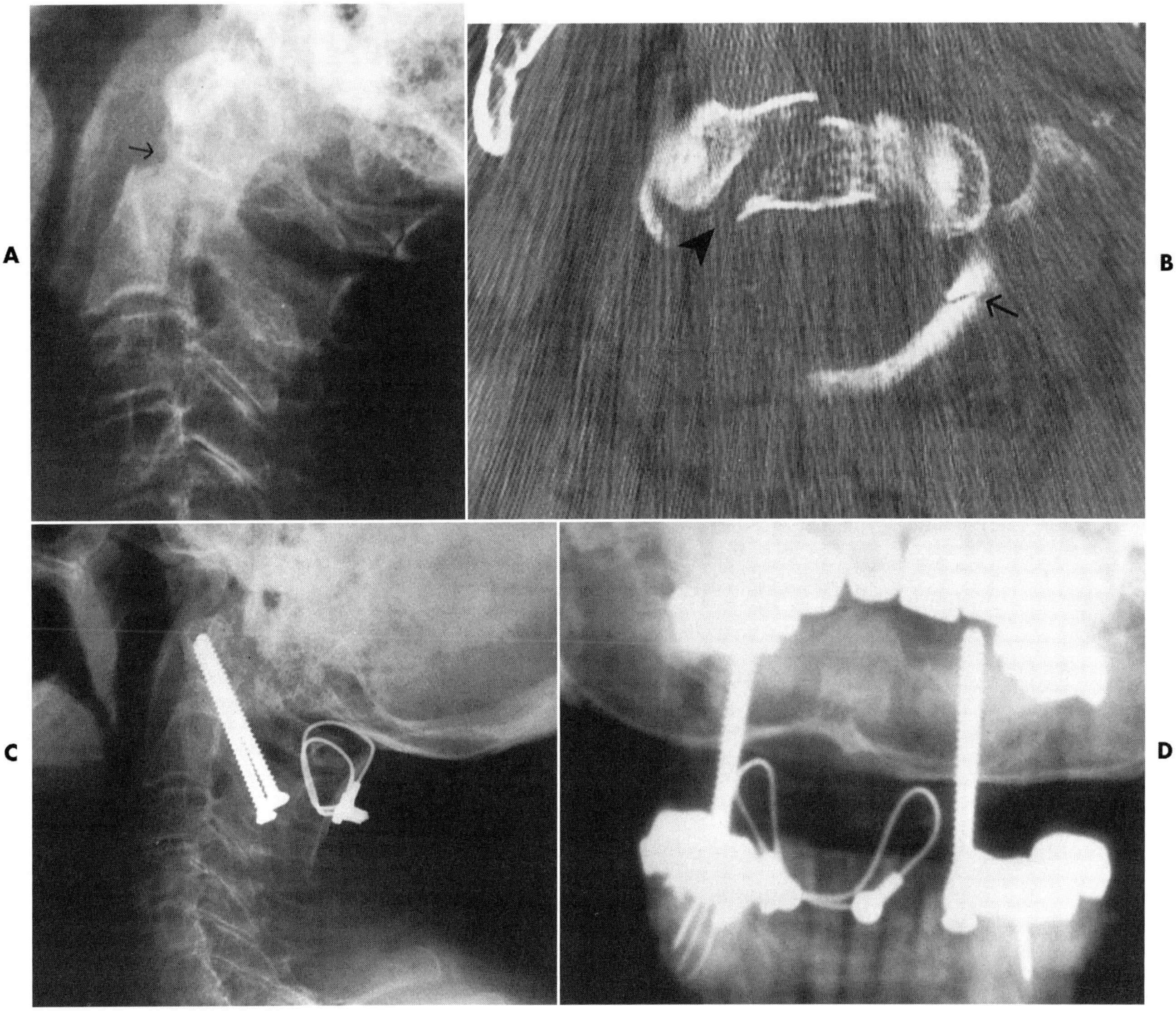

FIGURE 10-15

A, Posteriorly displaced type II odontoid fracture (*arrow*), in a 76-year-old neurologically intact female. Fracture of the posterior arch of C1 is also present. B, Axial CT scan shows fracture at the base of the dens (*arrowhead*) and posterior arch fracture of C1 (*small arrow*). C, Atlantoaxial fusion was performed with Magerl transarticular facet screws supplemented with a Gallie-type fusion using cables and iliac crest bone graft. D, Postoperative open mouth view.

Terminally 1.5-mm threaded guide wires are inserted just under the inferior edge of the body of C2 and 3 to 4 mm lateral to the midline. Left- and right-sided guide wires are oriented in the coronal plane toward the dens tip. Sagittal orientation is toward the posterior apex of the dens. It is often necessary to create a recess at the anterior superior margin of C3 to allow a sufficiently steep angle of inclination. The far dens cortex is just penetrated by the guide wires. Direct measurement of the guide wire insertion depth is made and overdrilling of the axis body is performed. Self-tapping, 3.5-mm cannulated lag screws are inserted over the guide wires. Postoperatively, patients are mobilized in a cervical orthosis for 8 to 10 weeks.

TRAUMATIC SPONDYLOLISTHESIS OF THE AXIS

Diagnosis. Traumatic spondylolisthesis of the axis occurs in approximately 5% to 10% of all cervical spine injuries. There is a high incidence of associated head and facial trauma. Patients present with neck pain and pain with motion. Neurologic deficits are rare as the spinal canal diameter increases with displacement. This fracture is usually well seen on the lateral radiograph of the cervical spine. The term *Hangman's fracture* has been used for this injury because of the similarity in fracture appearance caused by a judicial hanging.[160] However, there are several mechanisms for traumatic spondylolisthesis of the axis, and these account for the variable fracture patterns (Fig. 10-18).

A

B

C

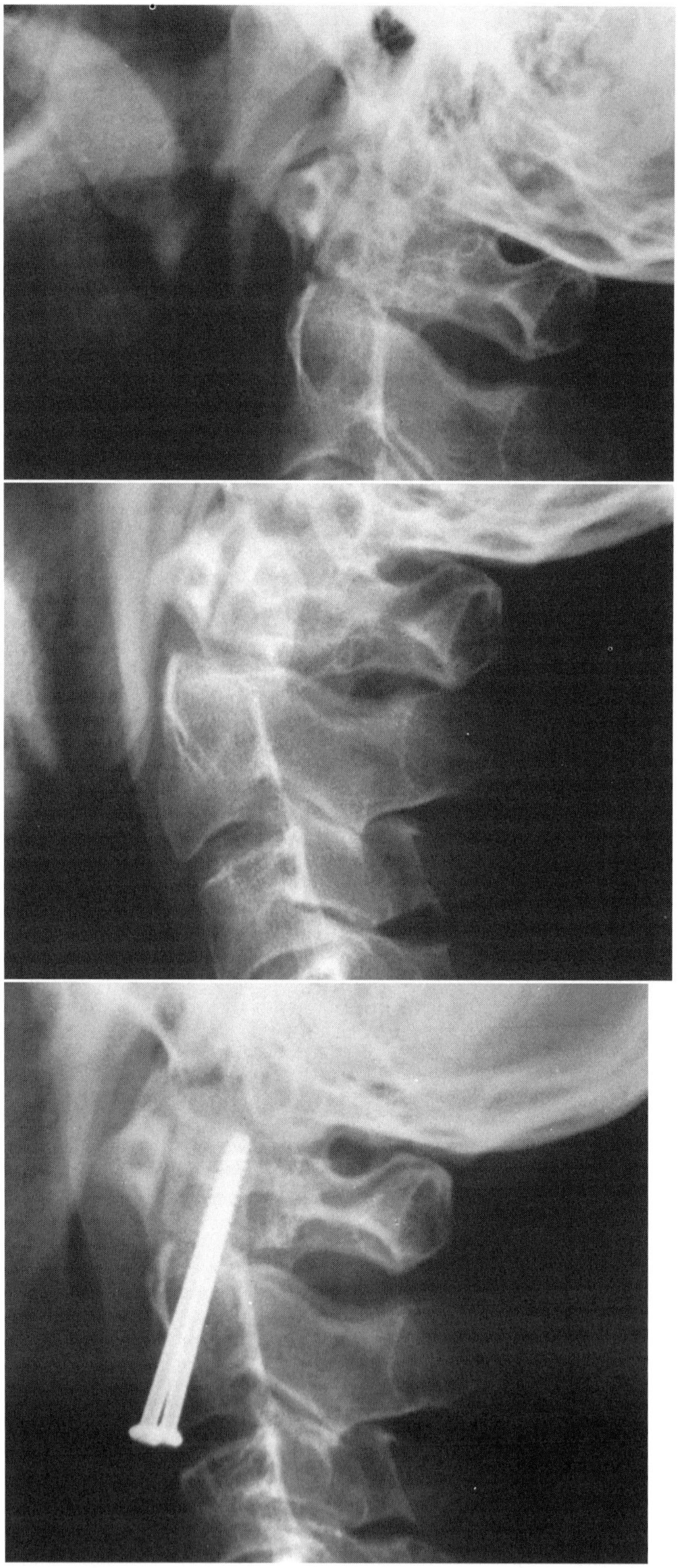

FIGURE 10-16

A, The lateral supine radiograph demonstrates a type II undisplaced odontoid fracture. **B**, Treatment was attempted in a halo vest; however, in an upright position, a stable reduction could not be maintained and posterior translation of the dens is seen. **C**, Postoperative lateral radiograph following anterior dens fixation using two 3.5-mm cannulated screws.

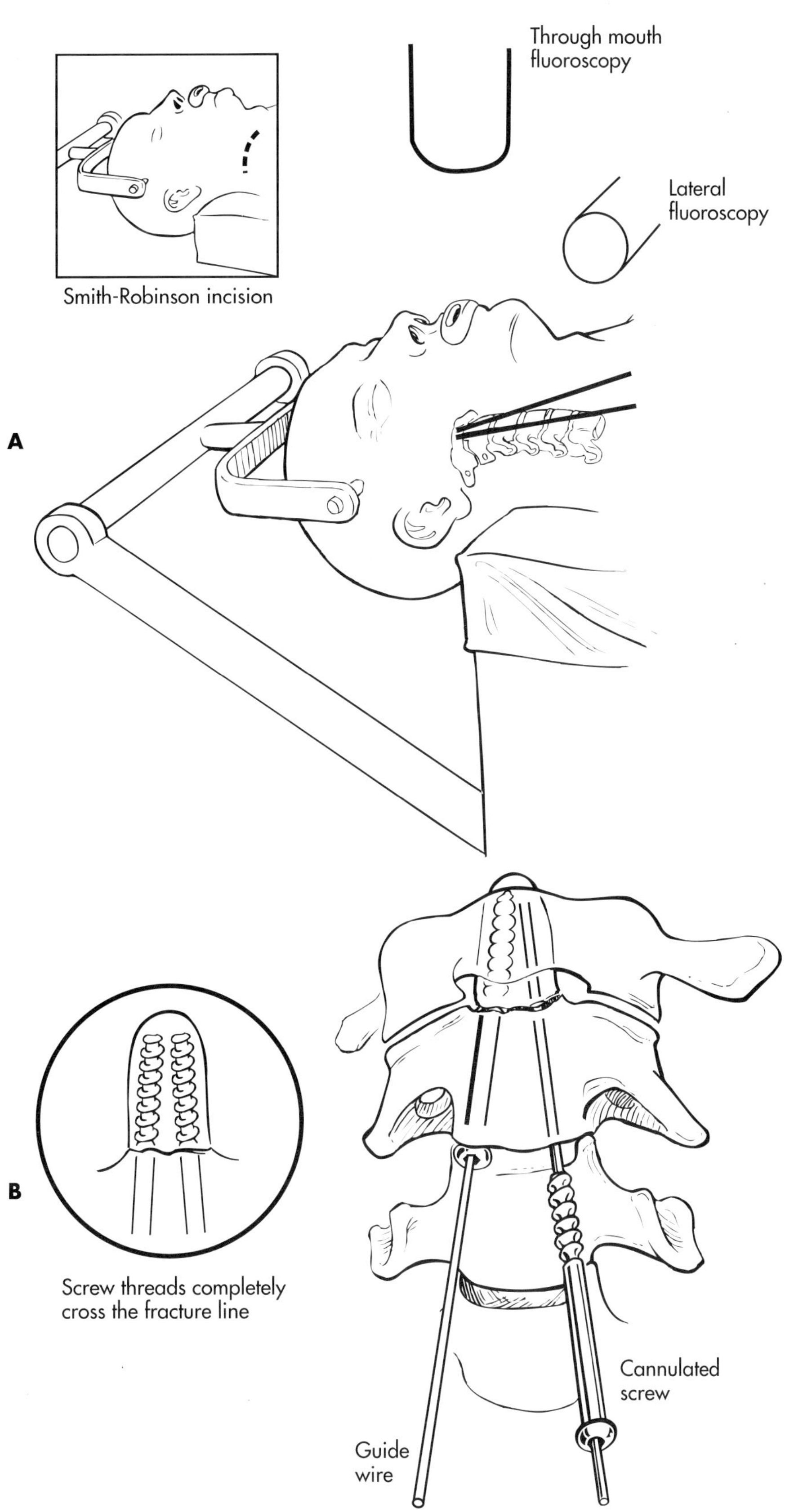

FIGURE 10–17

Odontoid screw fixation. **A**, Patient positioning: High quality AP and lateral C-arm images are facilitated with the use of the Mayfield head clamp attached to a U-shaped crossbar extending from the operating table. A right-sided Smith Robinson incision is performed (*inset*). **B**, Terminally, 1.5-mm threaded guide wires are inserted under the inferior edge of the body of C2 and 3 to 4 mm lateral to the midline. Self-tapping 3.5-mm cannulated lag screws are inserted over the guide wires. Screw threads should completely cross the fracture line (*inset*).

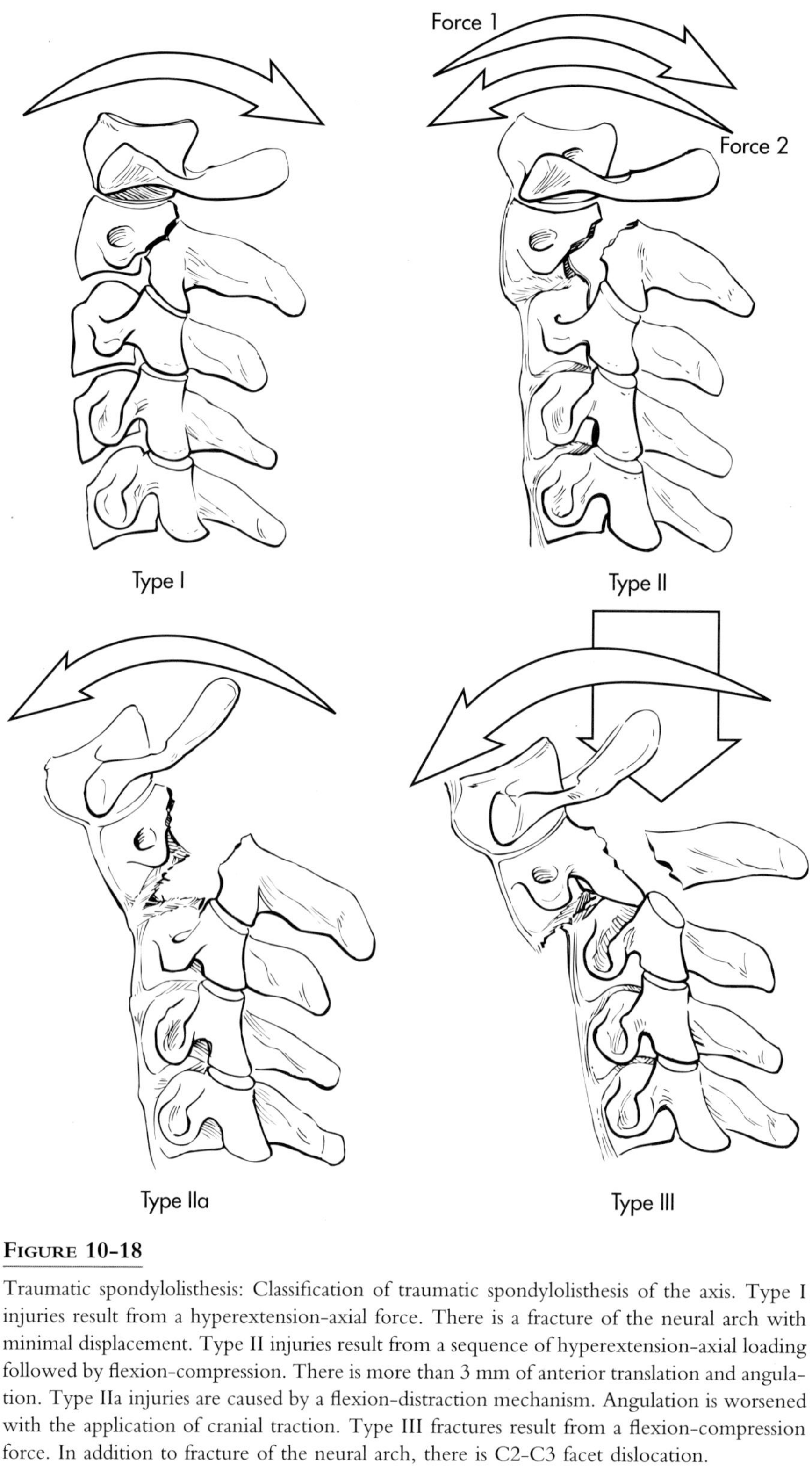

Figure 10-18

Traumatic spondylolisthesis: Classification of traumatic spondylolisthesis of the axis. Type I injuries result from a hyperextension-axial force. There is a fracture of the neural arch with minimal displacement. Type II injuries result from a sequence of hyperextension-axial loading followed by flexion-compression. There is more than 3 mm of anterior translation and angulation. Type IIa injuries are caused by a flexion-distraction mechanism. Angulation is worsened with the application of cranial traction. Type III fractures result from a flexion-compression force. In addition to fracture of the neural arch, there is C2-C3 facet dislocation.

Classification. The classification most widely used is the Levine and Edwards modification of Effendi's system (Fig. 10-19).[161,162] The value in this classification is the association between fracture pattern, mechanism of injury, and resultant instability.

Type I. Type I injuries result from a hyperextension–axial force that fractures the neural arch but is not strong enough to disrupt the C2-C3 discoligamentous structures. There is minimal anterior displacement and the fracture is stable.

TYPE II. The injury mechanism in type II fractures is believed to be a sequence of hyperextension-axial loading followed by flexion-compression. The initial force fractures the neural arch, while the second force causes rupture of the posterior longitudinal ligament and the disk. The anterior longitudinal ligament remains intact. These unstable injuries have more than 3 mm of anterior translation with angulation. Traction does not cause widening of the disk space.

TYPE IIa. Type IIa fractures are created by a flexion-distraction mechanism. These unstable injuries have minimal C2-C3 anterior translation but have significant anterior angulation. Angulatory deformity increases with traction because of widening of the posterior portion of the disk space.

TYPE III. Type III fractures result from a flexion-compression mechanism. An acute flexion moment results in fracture of the lamina or pedicle and a unilateral or bilateral C2-C3 facet dislocation. This injury is unstable and most frequently is associated with neurologic injuries.

Treatment. There is little role for operative management in traumatic spondylolisthesis of the axis.[146,161,163] More than 95% of cases unite by nonoperative means.

Type I injuries are stable and can be treated with a cervical orthosis for 12 weeks. Levine and Edwards suggest confirming the stability by flexion-extension radiographs prior to treatment. We do not recommend this for fear of SCI.[163]

Type II injuries are treated with temporary traction and halo-vest immobilization for 12 to 16 weeks. Type II injuries not stable in a halo vest are at risk for nonunion or malunion. Treatment for symptomatic nonunion is C2-C3 anterior interbody fusion with plate fixation. Posterior instrumentation and fusion is an alternative but requires a C1–C3 arthrodesis and sacrifices an additional motion segment (see Fig. 10-19).[161]

Type IIa injuries are subject to kyphotic angulation with traction. To avoid this deformity it is recommended that immediate halo reduction and immobilization be applied.[163] Instability demonstrated with upright radiographs require anterior or posterior fusion and instrumentation as described above.

Type III fractures with associated C2-C3 facet dislocations cannot be reduced by closed techniques.[163] This injury requires posterior open reduction and fusion. Following facet realignment, isthmus fracture can be treated by three options: (1) Placement of C2 pedicle screws for pars interarticularis fracture stabilization in conjunction with C2-C3 lateral mass plate fixation; (2) C1–C3 arthrodesis without pars fixation; and (3) open reduction of the C2-C3 joint followed by halo-vest immobilization for the ring fractures.

LOWER CERVICAL SPINE INJURIES

TREATMENT OF SPINAL CORD INJURIES

The treatment of SCI caused by fractures and dislocations of the lower cervical spine follows the principles outlined earlier in the chapter. The first priority is protecting the spine from further trauma. Appropriate resuscitation as suggested by the Advanced Trauma Life Supports (ATLS) protocol ensure that cord oxygenation and perfusion are maintained.[164] High-dose methylprednisolone is given for acute SCI within 8 hours of trauma.[165] A loading dose of 30 mg/kg and a maintenance dose of 5.4 mg/kg/hr for 23 hours is administered.

In patients with spinal malalignment, immediate traction reduction should be performed using cranial tongs. The application of Gardner-Wells tongs is simple and fast. Skull fractures and cranial defects pose relative contraindications to their use. Gardner-Wells tongs are inserted in line with the external auditory meatus 1 centimeter above the auricle. The skull pins are symmetrically tightened until the tensionometer indicates sufficient tension (when the plunger backs out 1 mm).[166] Five to ten pounds of weights are applied and a neurologic exam is repeated. The lateral radiograph also is repeated. If reduction has not occurred, the weight is increased by 5 to 10 pounds and the process repeated. Interval radiographs are scrutinized for vertebral alignment and signs of overdistraction. Addition of weight can proceed until either the fracture is reduced or there is an adverse change in neurologic status or signs of overdistraction. If straight axial traction is unsuccessful in effecting a closed reduction, an alteration in the direction of traction and the judicious use of cervical manipulation may succeed in unlocking the facet joints.[167] The use of MRI compatible tongs can facilitate postreduction imaging.

The maximum weight that can safely obtain reduction has been controversial. Historic values for maximum weight application have ranged from 40 pounds to 70% of body weight.[25,168,169] Recent studies however, document the safety and efficacy of very large traction weights (Fig. 10-20).[170,171,172]

Disk Herniation With Unstable Spinal Injuries. The potential for a herniated intervertebral disk in association with acute cervical spine trauma has been well recognized. For all injuries, the incidence of associated disk herniation is from 0.7% without MRI detection to 47% with MRI.[173,174,175] Rizzolo et al. found a 23% incidence of disk injury on MRI in patients presenting with an intact neurologic examination, 36% incidence of disk injury in patients with complete lesions, and 54% incidence in those with incomplete lesions.[15] The clinical importance of herniated disk associated with

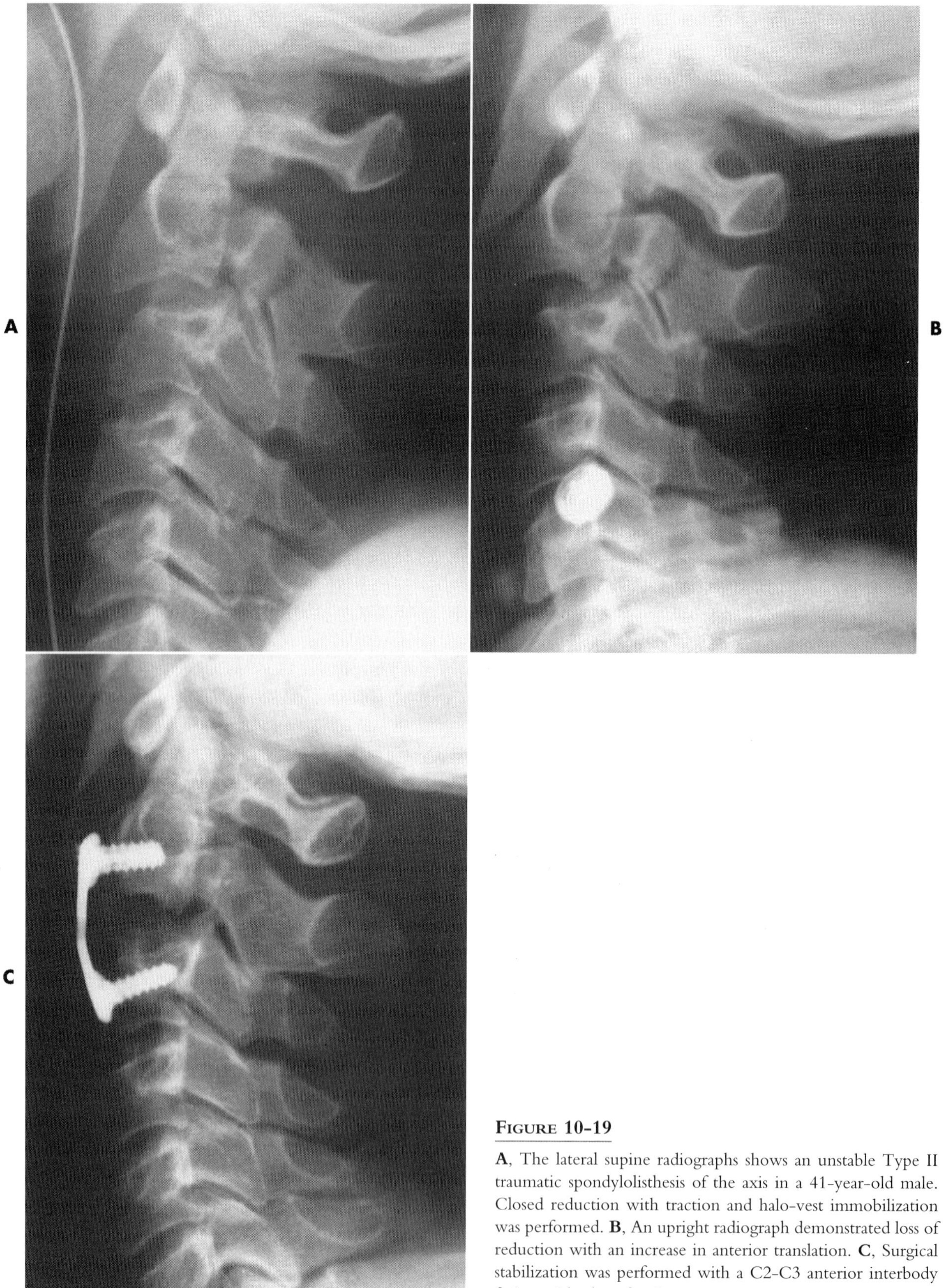

FIGURE 10-19

A, The lateral supine radiographs shows an unstable Type II traumatic spondylolisthesis of the axis in a 41-year-old male. Closed reduction with traction and halo-vest immobilization was performed. **B**, An upright radiograph demonstrated loss of reduction with an increase in anterior translation. **C**, Surgical stabilization was performed with a C2-C3 anterior interbody fusion with place fixation.

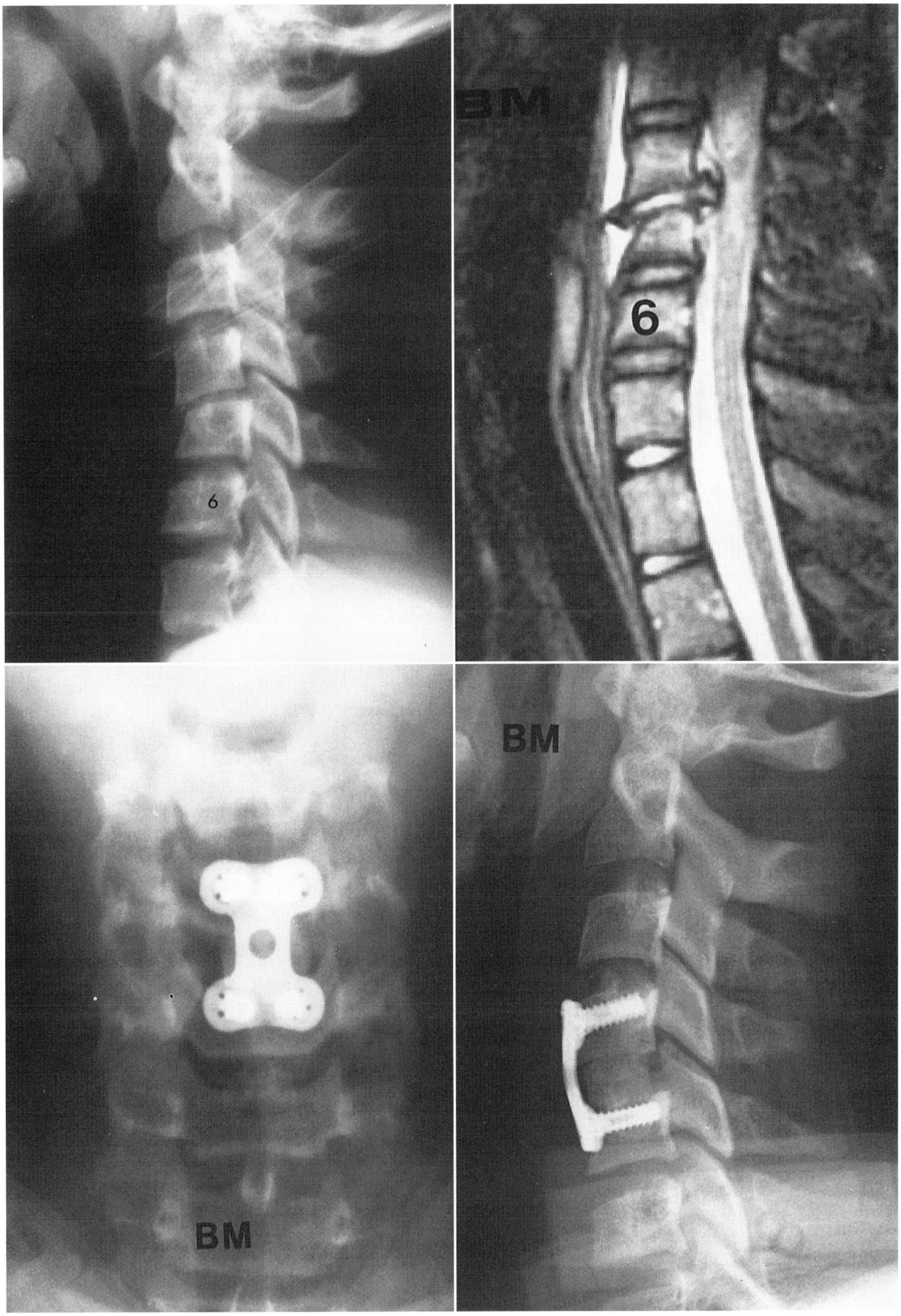

FIGURE 10-20

The lateral cervical spine radiographs of a 29-year-old male who presented with a C4 incomplete quadriplegia from an injury sustained while playing football. There is a focal kyphosis and a narrowed disk space at C4-C5. **B**, The T2-weighted MRI demonstrates a large extruded disk fragment compressing the spinal cord at the C4-C5 level. **C,D**, An emergent anterior discectomy and interbody fusion was performed using iliac crest bone graft and a cervical spine locking plate. The patient recovered to a Frankel D and was independently ambulatory at 6 months.

fractures and dislocations, however, is not always clear. Boden et al. have shown the incidence of MRI-documented cervical disk herniation in a normal population to be approximately 8%.[176] Rizzolo et al. found no correlation in the traumatized spine for the presence of a disk herniation with neurologic outcome.[15]

It remains controversial whether an MRI scan should be obtained prior to an attempted reduction of facet dislocation. Eismont et al. reported six cases of facet dislocation with associated disk herniation. Three of these had increased neurologic deficits after reduction.[177] Robertson and Ryan reported three patients with neurologic deterioration because of disk herniation after reduction of cervical spine dislocation.[178] Doran et al. identified 13 patients with a herniated nucleus pulposus and facet dislocation. Based on their experience, they recommended obtaining an MRI scan prior to any reduction attempt.[14] Others have disagreed with this philosophy and have recommended immediate closed reduction to indirectly decompress the spinal cord and maximize the chance for neurologic recovery.[171,179]

This recommendation is in line with reports in the literature of complete reversal from quadriplegia following rapid spinal realignment.[50,180] We have observed four such cases in patients who underwent reduction of bilateral facet dislocation within 2 hours of trauma and had immediate reversal of their quadriplegia. Support for early decompressive reduction also comes from animal studies.[47,48,181,182] Reduction provides decompression of the blood supply to the spinal cord and minimizes the secondary injury caused by ischemic and hypoxic damage.[183] Delays in obtaining MRI scans can push patients out of this window of opportunity and decrease their chance for neurologic recovery.

From these studies, risk factors can be identified for neurologic worsening due to disk herniation. These include difficult reductions, failure of closed reduction, and abnormal disk space narrowing. Neurologic deterioration is also more likely following an open posterior reduction.

In patients with complete or significantly incomplete neurologic deficits, we place the highest priority in achieving immediate decompression of the spinal cord by reduction of cervical dislocation. An MRI is subsequently obtained, and if spinal cord compression because of disk herniation is present, an anterior diskectomy and interbody fusion with instrumentation is performed. Without evidence of disk herniation, treatment may be performed by either an anterior or posterior stabilizing procedure based on surgeon preference. Patients with minimal or no neurologic deficit should have an MRI prior to attempts at reduction. In the absence of disk herniation, an awake closed reduction is performed as outlined above. In patients with disk herniation, an anterior diskectomy is performed. Following diskectomy, reduction can often be obtained by traction with the patient under general anesthesia or by the use of the Caspar cervical distractor. Spinal cord monitoring should be used during reduction. If reduction is obtained, then an anterior cervical plating and interbody fusion should be performed. If reduction is not obtained, an open reduction through a posterior approach may be required.

HYPERFLEXION INJURY: POSTERIOR LIGAMENTOUS INJURY

Diagnosis. During hyperflexion, tensile forces are created in the posterior ligamentous structures, which causes rupture from posterior to anterior. The spectrum of injury is from mild to severe. In mild injuries, there is a sprain to the posterior ligamentous complex with maintenance of stability. Clinically, patients may have focal tenderness but no neurologic signs or symptoms. Radiographically, there may be slight widening between spinous processes but no kyphosis nor anterior translation. Pure hyperflexion can also result in compression fractures of the vertebral body.[10]

With increased hyperflexion, complete disruption of the posterior osteoligamentous complex may occur. Radiographs may only show subtle abnormalities or even appear normal if the patient is in the supine position. Upright radiographs often expose occult instability by demonstrating focal kyphosis, facet diastasis, or interspinous widening. Although some authors suggest supervised flexion-extension radiographs to assess stability, we do not recommend their use in the acute setting.[184] The presence of paraspinal muscle spasm and pain may only allow a submaximal effort, thereby giving false-negative radiographic examinations.[185] If there is clinical suspicion of posterior ligamentous injury, an MRI with fat suppression techniques is useful.[17] With demonstration of high-intensity signals between spinous processes, patients are treated as having a severe ligamentous injury.

Treatment. Instability can be assessed using the White criteria. Patients with mild ligamentous injuries are stable and have a value less than 5. These injuries are well treated with 6 to 8 weeks of immobilization in a hard collar.

Severe ligamentous injury represents an unstable injury pattern and has poor healing capacity. Nonoperative treatment can lead to loss of reduction, late kyphotic deformity, and pain.[25,185,186,187] Treatment for severe hyperflexion injury is posterior cervical fusion using an interspinous fixation technique or lateral mass plating. Our technique of choice is a one-level fusion using interspinous fixation supplemented with lateral mass plating (Fig. 10-21).

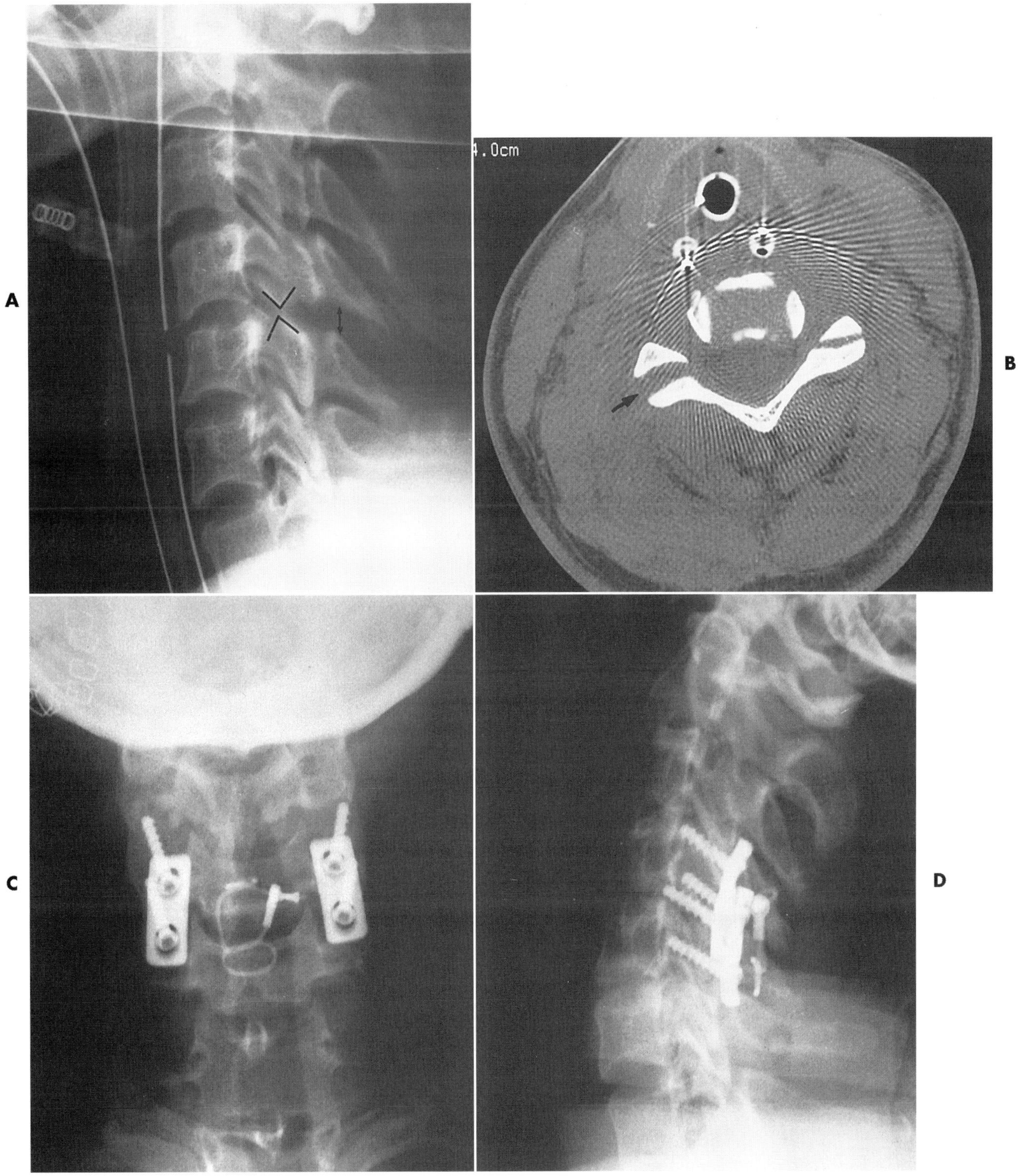

FIGURE 10-21

A, Posterior ligamentous injury. This 26-year-old neurologically intact female was involved in a motor vehicle accident and complained of neck pain in addition to bilateral lower extremity injuries. There is focal kyphosis at the C4-C5 level, interspinous widening and loss of parallelism of the C4-C5 facets. **B**, CT scan shows widening of the right C4-C5 facet joint. **C,D**, Anatomic reduction, posterior stabilization, and a single-level fusion was performed using lateral mass plates, interspinous cable fixation, and iliac crest bone graft.

TECHNIQUE: POSTERIOR CERVICAL FUSION USING LATERAL MASS PLATES AND INTERSPINOUS FIXATION

The patient is in the prone position as described earlier in the chapter. Before skin preparation and draping, a radiograph is taken to assure adequate alignment. Caudally directed traction on the shoulders with tape can provide improved radiographic visualization of the lower cervical spine. Corrections in alignment and traction are made as needed. Intraoperative electrodiagnostic monitoring is recommended.

A midline approach is used with dissection to the lateral edge of the lateral masses without violating the facet capsules at the cephalad and caudad margins of the intended fusion. The intact interspinous ligaments are preserved to minimize the risk of destabilizing adjacent levels.

A Rogers-type interspinous fixation is performed initially to restore the posterior tension band and to obtain a controlled reduction of the subluxated facet joints. Flexible surgical cable is used for this. Cable systems offer better tensioning control, stronger tightening mechanisms, and are less likely to loosen than stainless steel wire. Titanium cables compatible with MRI have sufficient mechanical strength.[188]

In both cranial and caudad vertebrae, 3-mm holes are drilled bilaterally at the base of the spinous processes. The holes are enlarged to accept two passes of the cable. The cable is then passed through the superior spinous process, looped back over top of the spinous process and back through the hole. A second cable is passed through the hole in the caudad spinous process, under the inferior edge and back through the hole. The two cables are connected through their respective eyelets. A tensioning device is used for tightening, and a lateral radiograph is obtained to assure adequate alignment.

The procedure continues with lateral mass fixation. The lateral masses are rectangular in shape and proper screw placement requires clear visualization of the borders. The medial border is the valley at the junction of the lamina and the lateral mass. The vertebral artery is located directly anterior to this (see Fig. 10-5). All screws must start lateral to this valley and angle outward. Screw insertion techniques have been previously described, and we use a modified Magerl technique.

The starting point for screw insertion is 1 mm medial and 1 mm cranial to the center of the facet joint. The screws are oriented in an upward direction parallel to the facet joints and outward 20° (see Fig. 10-5). The initial hole is drilled free hand rather than through the plate. A 2.0-mm K wire is used for drilling and is advanced within an adjustable drill guide with a stop set at 14 mm drilling depth. A 1.1-mm blunt K wire is used to gently probe the hole ensuring that the far cortex has not been penetrated. The adjustable stop drill guide is then lengthened 2 mm and further drilling and probing take place. This process is repeated until a total length of 18 mm or perforation of the far cortex occurs. Bicortical purchase increases construct stiffness; however, it is not necessary for clinical success and increases the risk of neurovascular injury.[94] The near cortex is then tapped with 4.0-mm cancellous bone tap.

Several lateral mass plates are available. The Synthes titanium plates (Synthes) are available with 8- and 12-mm hole spacings. The Axis titanium plates are available in 11-, 13-, and 15-mm hole spacings and have the advantage of variable screw angulation and placement due to the "figure 8" screwhole design. In constructs longer than one motion segment, freehand holes are drilled in the suggested location in the lateral masses of the most cranial and caudad vertebrae. The best fitting template is chosen according to its ability to match these drilled holes and also permit localization of the intervening holes over the intercalary lateral masses. The proper plate is then chosen and bent to approximate the cervical lordosis. Cancellous bone graft is then obtained, the facet joints are burr-decorticated and impacted with graft before plate placement. The endplate holes are then filled using 3.5-mm cancellous screws, which are loosely secured. The plate is then used as a guide for drilling the intercalary screw holes. Screws are tightened in sequential fashion. Occasionally, screw purchase may be suboptimal due to poor bone quality or due to lateral screw cutout. In these situations the interspinous fixation offers an added measure of stability.

Postoperatively, patients may be rapidly mobilized in a hard collar or cervicothoracic brace worn for 8 to 10 weeks. Monthly radiographic follow-up is suggested.

TECHNIQUE: THORACIC PEDICLE SCREW PLACEMENT AND FUSION OF THE CERVICOTHORACIC JUNCTION

The transition from cervical lordosis to thoracic kyphosis poses considerable challenges to posterior instrumentation of the unstable cervicothoracic junction. Lateral mass plating and screw fixation offers the possibility of crossing this region without intrusion of the spinal canal and has been shown to be safe and effective.[189] In the thoracic spine, screws are placed in the pedicles because the transverse processes (which evolve from the lateral masses in the cervical spine), are considerably less strong for fixation purposes.[190]

For thoracic pedicle screw insertion, the starting point is 1 mm inferior to the articular ridge of the superior articular facet and 1 mm lateral to the midfacet line. Screws are directed 7° to 10° medially with a 10° to 20° caudal angulation. Drilling with a 2-mm K wire, blunt probing and plate application is as described above for lateral mass fixation. A final depth of 22 to 24 mm provides adequate screw purchase in the upper thoracic spine.

Unilateral Facet Dislocation

Diagnosis. When rotation is added to hyperflexion, a unilateral facet dislocation may result.[10] These injuries have potential for significant instability. Beatson demonstrated that a single facet could be dislocated only when the interspinous ligament, ligamentum flavum, and ipsilateral joint capsules were disrupted.[191]

The diagnosis of unilateral facet dislocation is often missed.[192,193] Contributing to this is the presence of subtle radiologic abnormalities and a lack of symptoms. Small amounts of subluxation may be present on initial radiographs or the patient may have spontaneously reduced. Radiographic features on the lateral view may show vertebral body displacement of up to 50% and asymmetry of the facets above and below the level of injury.[191,192] The anteroposterior radiograph demonstrates rotation of the spinous process towards the side of the dislocated facet. A CT scan with sagittal reformations is useful in delineating the injury.

Clinically, patients can present with minimal neurologic findings. Radiculopathies are easily overlooked but have been reported to occur in more than 65% of patients.[194,195] Cord injury is less common. Magnetic resonance imaging is helpful in assessing the status of the intervetetebral disk. Associated disk herniations occur in up to 15% of cases.

Three subtypes of unilateral facet dislocations are recognized.

1. *Pure Unilateral Facet Dislocation.* Unilateral facet dislocation without fracture occurs less often than those with fractures. These are difficult to reduce with cranial traction. Once reduced, however, they are more stable than unilateral facet fracture dislocations.
2. *Unilateral Facet Fracture Dislocation.* Unilateral facet fracture dislocations occur in up to 80% of cases.[196] Most commonly the superior facet of the level below is sheared off and less frequently the fracture involves the inferior facet of the cranial vertebra. Due to incompetence of the facet joint, these injuries are usually easy to reduce with light traction but are rotationally unstable.
3. *Fracture Separation of the Lateral Mass.* Fracture separation of the lateral mass results from fracturing of the pedicle and lamina. A free floating lateral mass is created that is separated from its vertebral body and lamina. Because the lateral mass stabilizes both a cranial and caudal level, two motion segments are rendered unstable. This injury is well visualized on CT scan because the fracture lines are perpendicular to the axial cuts of the CT.

Treatment. Closed reduction of these injuries can be achieved in a high percentage of cases. If closed reduction fails, an open reduction is performed. The spinous processes can be manipulated as levers using Kocher clamps or towel clips. A small elevator can be inserted into the dislocated facet joint and levered to attempt to unlock the joint. A last resort involves removing the cranial aspect of the superior facet.

Successful long-term outcome is dependent on anatomic alignment regardless of treatment. Rorabeck et al., in treating unilateral facet dislocation in 26 patients, found that all patients with anatomic reduction were pain free at follow-up, whereas all patients left in an unreduced position had chronic neck and arm pain.[192] Sears and Fazl and Beyer et al. found that halo immobilization was an inadequate method for maintaining an anatomic reduction.[194,197] The latter study also noted that a nonanatomic reduction resulted in cervical translation and frank instability leading to late pain.

1. *Pure Unilateral Facet Dislocations.* Following reduction pure unilateral facet dislocations are usually stable. Nonoperative treatment with a halo vest can be attempted. No loss of reduction should be tolerated because of the high incidence of late pain. A single-level posterior fusion with instrumentation is indicated in this situation. Patients with SCI may be better treated with posterior fusion as the halo vest may interfere with rehabilitation, nursing care, and possibly restrict pulmonary function.
2. *Unilateral Facet Fracture Dislocations.* Unilateral facet fracture dislocations are rotationally unstable. Redisplacement occurs frequently during nonoperative treatment. Operative management is recommended for these injuries. Our technique of choice is lateral mass plating with supplemental interspinous fixation. If a disk herniation is present, an anterior cervical discectomy and fusion is indicated with instrumentation. If foramenal stenosis is present secondary to displaced bone fragments, a posterior foramenotomy in conjunction with a posterior fusion should be performed.
3. *Fracture Separation of the Lateral Mass.* Fracture separation of the lateral mass presents a unique situation in which two motion segments are rendered unstable (Fig. 10-22). This injury is best treated surgically using lateral mass plates and fusing two motion segments.

Bilateral Facet Dislocation

Diagnosis. A distractive flexion force can result in bilateral facet dislocations. The forward translation of the cranial vertebra causes complete rupture of the capsule of the apophyseal joint, the annulus, and the disk.[191,198] The risk for disk herniation associated with bilateral facet dislocation has been discussed. Spinal

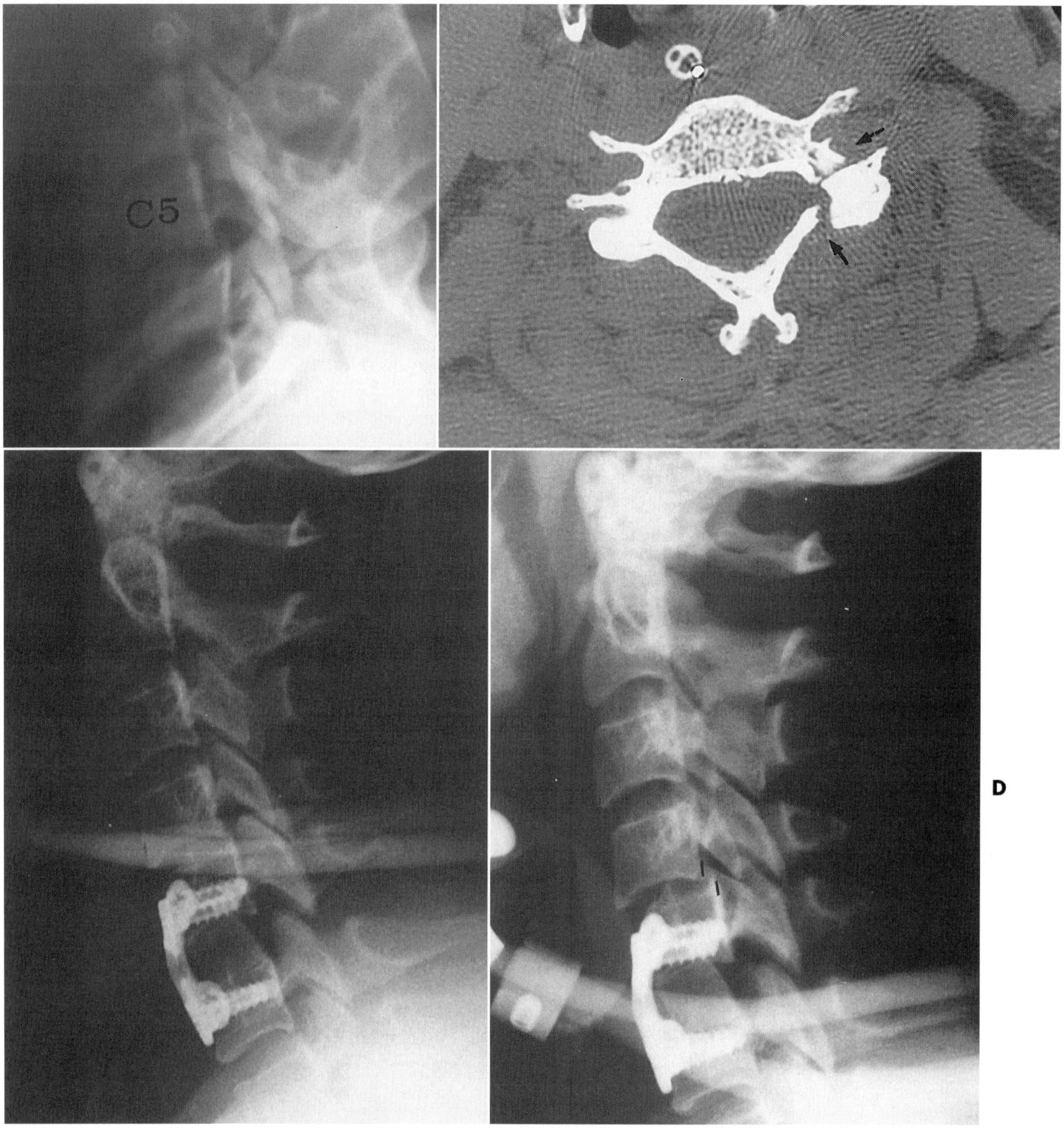

FIGURE 10-22

A, Fracture separation of the lateral mass. The swimmers view lateral radiograph of the cervical spine in this 31-year-old female shows subluxation of C5-C6. She was neurologically intact. **B**, The axial CT scan shows fractures of the left C5 pedicle and lamina (*arrows*). This resulted in a free-floating lateral mass. **C**, Surgical stabilization was performed by a C5-C6 anterior interbody fusion with iliac crest bone graft and a cervical spine locking plate. Postoperatively she wore a Minerva brace. **D**, At 6 weeks she exhibited a positive Lehrmittes sign with tingling into her arms and legs made worse by forward flexion of her head. Repeat radiograph show rotatory subluxation at C4-C5.

cord injury is present in the majority of cases. Radiographically, 50 % or greater of vertebral body translation is present. The potential for vertebral artery occlusion also has been described.

Treatment. Because of the significant instability and ligamentous nature of the injury, most patients should have surgical stabilization. Several important factors are considered in the treatment of patients with bilateral facet dislocations. These include the status of the intervertebral disk, the timing and method of reduction, the possibility of vertebral artery injury, and surgical approach. These have been discussed in detail (Fig. 10-23).

E

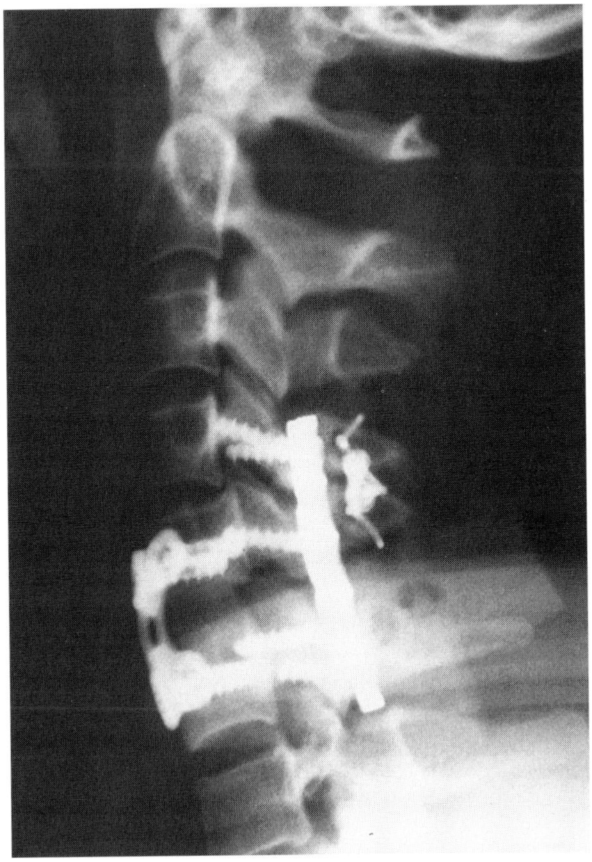

FIGURE 10-22 *continued*

E, A second operative procedure was necessary and a two level posterior stabilization was performed using lateral mass plates and an interspinous wiring technique.

AXIAL LOADING INJURIES

Diagnosis. Axial loading forces result in compression injuries to the vertebral body or posterior elements.[5] The injury pattern depends on the initial head position. With the head neutral, wedge, compression, or burst fractures occur.[199] With the head flexed, fracture of the vertebral body may be combined with tensile failure posteriorly, creating interspinous separation and fractures in the lamina and spinous processes. In bursting injuries, there is comminution of the vertebral body, retropulsion of bone into the spinal canal, and usually a focal kyphotic deformity. Spinal cord injury is usually present.

Treatment. In isolated vertebral body compression injuries, the posterior osseoligamentous complex is intact. These fractures are stable; however, compression fractures associated with posterior ligamentous disruptions are unstable and require restoration of the posterior tension band.

The initial treatment of burst injuries is reduction and realignment using cranial tong traction. In most cases, the posterior and anterior longitudinal ligaments are intact and large traction weights can be safely applied. Indirect spinal canal decompression can often be achieved through traction and realignment. Definitive treatment is then based on fracture stability and neurologic function. Stability is dependent on the integrity of the posterior elements, and the White criteria can be used to help obtain an objective measure.

Nonoperative treatment is indicated if canal decompression can be achieved, fractures do not involve the posterior elements, and alignment can be maintained in a halo vest. With increasing instability, the halo vest can not maintain axial distraction and some loss of reduction occurs.

Surgical stabilization is necessary for unstable fractures and with injury to the posterior osseoligamentous complex. Surgery is also indicated for failure to achieve a satisfactory reduction and decompression by closed means. For single level burst fractures, a vertebral corpectomy with iliac crest strut grafting is performed. With the addition of anterior instrumentation using rigidly locked plates, alignment can be restored and the patient rapidly mobilized (Fig. 10-24). In the presence of multilevel fractures, posterior cervical fusion with lateral mass plates is preferable.[43] In grossly unstable, three-column injuries, a circumferential fusion has been advocated.[200,201] In our experience however, we have found that this is rarely warranted because of the effectiveness of anterior cervical plate stabilization.[37,38,102]

TECHNIQUE: ANTERIOR DECOMPRESSION AND FUSION

The patient is maintained in traction, and an awake nasotracheal intubation is performed. Neurologic status is checked, and the patient is transferred to the operating table and administered a general anesthetic. A small roll is placed behind the shoulders to allow slight neck extension. The shoulders are gently pulled caudally by tape to facilitate intraoperative radiographic visualization. A lateral radiograph is taken to ensure satisfactory alignment. The skin of the anterior neck and of the iliac crest are prepared.

A left-sided Smith Robinson approach is used. A transverse incision from the anterior border of the sternocleidomastoid muscle to the midline and centered over the injured segment is made. The platysma and the superficial layer of the deep cervical fascia are transected using electrocautery. The interval between the sternohyoid muscles medially and the sternocleidomastoid muscle laterally is identified. The middle layer of the deep cervical fascia is released from the sternocleidomastoid. Dissection is deepened bluntly between the trachea and the strap muscles medially and the carotid sheath laterally. A small traversing venous plexus is often encountered and should be coagulated. The prevertebral fascia is identified and divided vertically, exposing the vertebral bodies and intervertebral discs. The longus colli is incised in the midline and

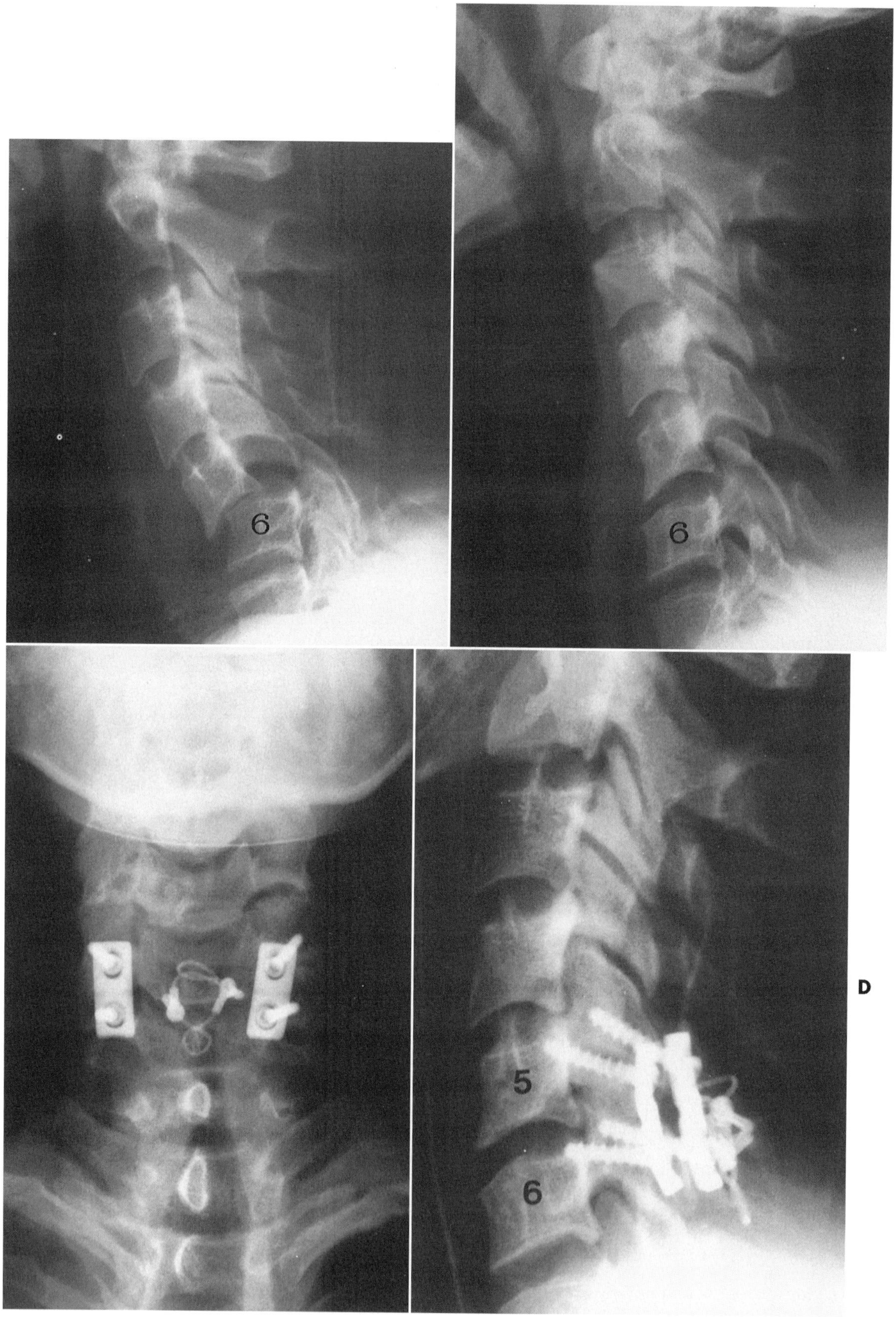

Figure 10-23

A, Bilateral facet dislocation. The lateral cervical spine radiographs is from a 29-year-old male who was thrown from a bull when riding at a rodeo. Bilateral C5-C6 facet dislocation is present. He was hyperreflexic in both lower extremities and had sustained clonus. There was full motor function bilaterally. **B**, Emergent reduction was performed with sequentially increased traction applied by Gardener-Wells tongs. Reduction of the injury was achieved at 65 pounds. The patient remained neurologically intact following reduction. A postreduction MRI did not reveal a traumatic disc herniation. **C,D**, Stabilization of the injured segment was performed with lateral mass plates, interspinous cable fixation, and iliac crest bone graft.

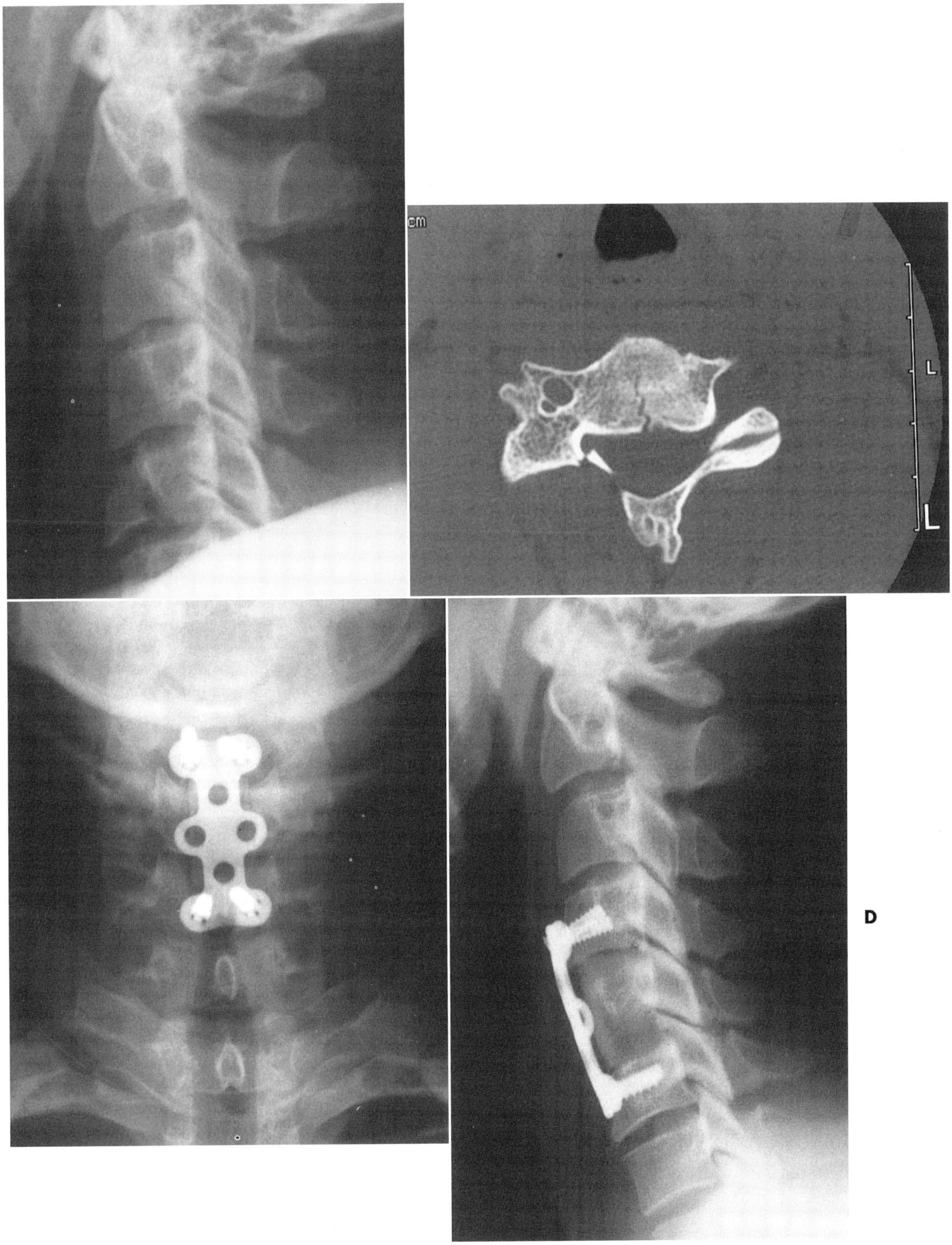

FIGURE 10-24

A, Axial loading injury. The lateral radiograph with 35 pounds traction of a 26-year-old male who sustained a direct axial blow to the head after running into a wall. He fortunately only had signs and symptoms of C6 and C7 radiculopathies. A teardrop burst fracture of C5 is present. **B**, Axial CT scan shows fracture of body and lamina. **C,D**, Stabilization of the injured segment was performed by C5 corpectomy with reconstruction of the anterior column using tricortical iliac crest bone graft and a cervical spine locking plate (Synthes).

reflected laterally safely to the uncovertebral joints. A double bent spinal needle is placed into the disc space for radiologic localization of the level. An operating microscope or loupes and a headlight facilitate visualization for the subsequent decompression.

If diskectomy alone is required, the anterior longitudinal ligament and annulus are incised. The disk and endplates are removed back to the posterior longitudinal ligament using small curettes and pituitary rongeurs. If the posterior longitudinal ligament is ruptured, it should be removed to ensure complete decompression of the neural elements. The neural foramina are palpated with small nerve hooks. An anterior foramenotomy can be performed with 1-mm Kerrison rongeurs or a high-speed burr.

If a corpectomy is indicated, the disks above and below the vertebral body are completely removed. The depth of the vertebral body is best gauged by completing the discectomies to the posterior longitudinal ligament. The vertebral body is removed piecemeal with rongeurs. Care is necessary at all times to maintain orientation to the midline to avoid injury to the vertebral artery. Bony decompression proceeds posteriorly with a high-speed cutting or diamond burr until only a thin shell of bone remains. This is removed with small curettes and 1- or 2-mm Kerrison rongeurs. Lateral decompression is performed safely to the uncovertebral joints. The dura or the posterior longitudinal ligament should bulge convexly, and usually a 12- to 14-mm wide trough is created.

Reconstruction of the spinal column is now performed. The cartilagenous endplates of the cranial and caudal vertebrae are removed and squared with a burr to allow for flush seating of the bone graft. The cortical bony endplate is preserved, and holes are punched into it to encourage revascularization of the graft. The depth and length of the defect are measured. The graft should be several millimeters less in depth than the actual defect to avoid iatrogenic cord compression.

A tricortical iliac crest bone graft is taken and sized accordingly. An oscillating saw should be used for graft harvest. Compared with saw-harvested bone grafts, osteotomy-harvested grafts have a decreased load to failure incidence and an increased incidence of cortical cracking.[202] Fracture propagation in the pelvis also is possible with the use of an osteotome. Care also is necessary to ensure that the bone graft is removed at least 30 mm posterior to the anterior superior iliac crest to minimize the risk of iliac crest fracture.[203,204]

Gentle distraction of the head is exerted during graft insertion. Upon placement, traction is removed and a lateral radiograph is taken. An anterior cervical plate is then applied, as described below. Patients with SCI are monitored in the intensive care unit for 1 to 2 days for signs of respiratory compromise. Postoperatively, patients are immobilized in a cervicothoracic brace for 8 to 12 weeks.

For diskectomy cases, the procedure is identical as outlined for corpectomy except the graft is horseshoe-shaped and is generally 8 to 10 mm in length.

TECHNIQUE: ANTERIOR INSTRUMENTATION USING SYNTHES CERVICAL SPINE LOCKING PLATE

The Synthes cervical spine locking plate allows rigid locking of the screws to the plate.[84] The biomechanical properties of this plate have been described earlier in the chapter. Two diameters of screws are available, 4.0 and 4.35 mm in three screw lengths, 12, 14, and 16 mm. Plates are available in lengths of 24 to 92 mm. All implants are made of titanium and are MRI compatible.

Anterior decompression and fusion have been described. Anterior osteophytes and bony prominences are leveled with a burr to allow proper plate seating. Plate holes should lie over the midpoint of the vertebral bodies and care is exercised to avoid screw placement into the adjacent disks. A lateral radiograph is taken with an appropriately sized plate to ensure ideal position and length. The plate is contoured into slight lordosis. The screw holes are palpated to ensure bone is underlying and then drilled while maintaining plate position. Orientation to the midline must be maintained at all times to prevent injury to the vertebral artery. Drilling uses a set depth 3.0 drill, depending on the desired screw length determined on the preoperative CT scan. The drill guide directs proper screw angulation, which in the cranial holes is 12° cranially and 15° medially. Caudally, the drill is directed orthogonally to the plate and 15° medially. The near cortices are tapped and the screws are inserted. The small conical expansion set screws are inserted, and the construct is checked radiographically. Postoperatively, immobilization is maintained in a hard collar or cervicothoracic orthosis for 8 to 12 weeks. Fusion is checked with flexion-extension radiographs.

HYPEREXTENSION INJURIES

Diagnosis. Extension moments to the cervical spine commonly occur as a result of a fall or a rear-end car collision. Forceful neck flexion may follow. The spectrum of injury can range from the whiplash-associated disorders to a hyperextension dislocation with complete SCI[205,206] The axis of rotation is applied to the lower cervical spine in contrast to traumatic spondylolisthesis of C2. Taylor and Blackwood, and Taylor stressed the importance in suspecting hyperextension injury to the cervical spine in the presence of facial trauma.[207,208]

During forced hyperextension, there is impaction of the posterior arches and compression of the facet joints.[5] Fractures in the posterior elements can occur; however, these are generally stable injuries. With more extreme force, ruptures of the anterior longitudinal ligament and separation of the annulus fibrosus from the associated vertebrae can result.[209] A small avulsion fracture often occurs from the anterior inferior corner of the vertebral body, which may be confused with an osteophyte.[210]

Hyperextension with distraction or shear can cause failure of all three columns of the spine with a transverse fracture through the vertebral body. Spontaneous reduction of dislocation can occur and the residual lesion might show only slight anterior subluxation or widening of the intervertebral disk (Fig. 10-25).[211] An MRI scan shows high intensity signals in the disk and retropharyngeal spaces on T2-weighted images. With more significant force, a grossly unstable traumatic retrolisthesis can result. With the above bony injuries, varying degrees of SCI from transient neurologic deficit to complete quadriplegia may be present.

In patients with cervical spondyolosis or congenitally small canals, significant SCI may be present without radiographic abnormalities.[212] Spinal cord compression can occur anteriorly from bulging disks and osteophytes, and posteriorly from infolding of the ligamentum flavum.[213] The clinical picture of a central cord syndrome may be seen or more variable incomplete spinal cord syndromes may be present.[211,212] An MRI scan may be helpful in assessing the severity of SCI and can provide some prognostic information for the return of motor function.[19] Generally the prognosis is good for the lower extremities and for sacral return of function, but there is often poor return of hand function.[214,215]

Treatment. The initial treatment of SCI from hyperextension injury is gentle tong traction with the head in neutral position. Neck extension is avoided. In addition to stabilizing the spine, traction prevents further injury, may reduce malalignment, and lengthens the

A

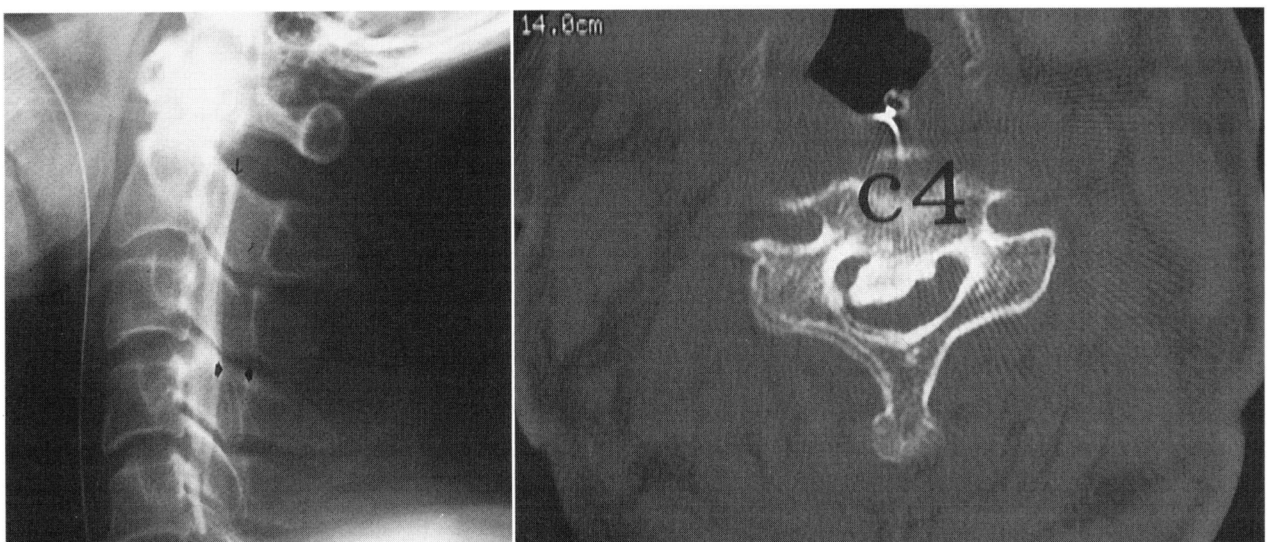

B

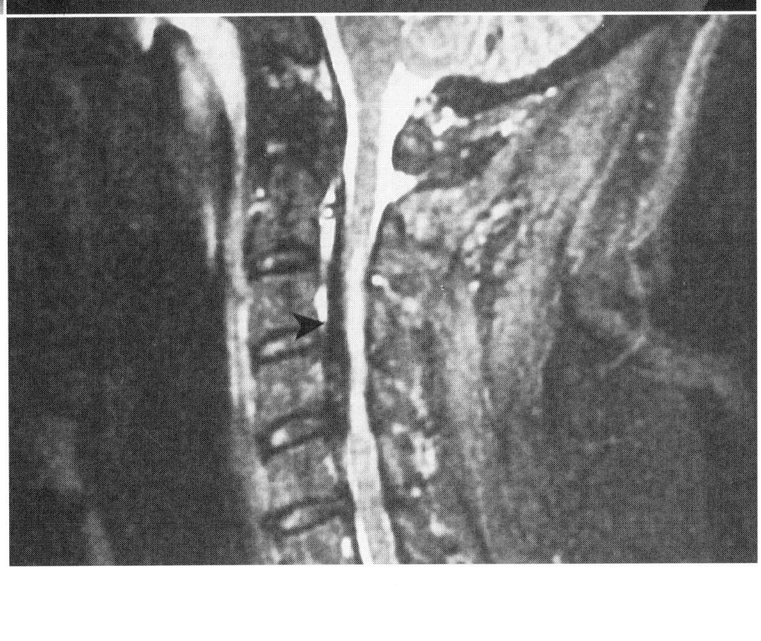

C

FIGURE 10-25

Hyperextension injury. **A** The lateral radiograph of a 44-year-old Japanese woman who was involved in a low-speed motor vehicle accident. She presented with a complete C3 tetraplegia. Ossification of the posterior longitudinal ligament gives the appearance of a cervical myelogram (*small arrow*). The congenitally small anteriposterior diameter of the spinal canal is shown (*large arrows*). **B**, A noncontrast axial CT scan at C4 shows the large ossified ligament occupying 40% of the volume of the canal. **C**, The sagittal MRI shows the ossified posterior longitudinal ligament (*arrow*) and the severe cord contusion. The patient was treated with a short period of traction and a hard collar.

spinal column. Increasing spinal column length may pull the ligamentum flavum out of the spinal canal, thereby indirectly decompressing the spinal cord. In grossly unstable injuries associated with shear or distraction, excess traction must be avoided. With injuries in which stability is in question, a carefully administered traction test can be useful in planning further management.

Definitive treatment is based on imaging studies, stability, and the progress of neurologic recovery. In stable injuries and with neurologic improvement, patients are mobilized in 3 to 5 days in a hard collar. Upright radiographs are obtained to assure alignment. Patients who are not improving, have unstable fractures, or have reached a neurologic plateau are candidates for surgical decompression and stabilization. An MRI or CT myelogram is indicated to assess ongoing compression. Earlier investigators have recommended conservative treatment of central cord injury without radiologic abnormality.[212,213] More recent studies have suggested that surgical decompression may offer improved motor recovery once a neurologic plateau has been reached.[216] We prefer to perform decompression at 4 to 6 weeks.

The approach to decompression is dependent on the site and extent of cord compression. In most cases with less than three levels of anterior disk or osteophyte involvement, anterior decompression and strut grafting with instrumentation is indicated. Posterior decompression may be performed if the spine has maintained its lordosis and compression is localized posteriorly. Additionally, posterior decompression may be indicated where more than three levels of anteroposterior compression is present. In the presence of cervical lordosis, a multilevel laminectomy allows the dura to displace posteriorly therefore, providing some ventral decompression.[217] In all traumatic cases, posterior decompression is performed with a concurrent posterior fusion and instrumentation.[218]

Technique: Foramenotomy

Prior to surgery, radiologic investigations should be assessed for foramenal compression caused by displaced facet fractures or disk herniations. If present, a posterior foramenotomy can be performed at the time of posterior fusion.

Patients are in the prone position on a turning frame in Gardner-Wells traction. Alignment of the spine is checked radiographically. Subperiosteal exposure is carried out to the far lateral edge of the facets. The use of loupe magnification and a headlight facilitates visualization.

After level localization, foramenotomy is performed by dissecting free the lateral insertion of the ligamentum flavum with a 3-0 cervical curette. To facilitate exposure, a limited laminotomy is performed using 2-mm Kerrison rongeurs or a high-speed drill removing the caudal portion of the cranial lamina. The ligamentum flavum is partially removed along its lateral border to expose the lateral edge of the dura and the origin of the exiting nerve root. Foramenotomy is performed with 2-mm Kerrison rongeurs or a high-speed drill to resect the medial halves of the cranial inferior articular process and the caudal superior articular process. Biomechanically, up to 50% of a unilateral facet and 25 % of bilateral facets can be removed without development of instability.[219,220] The decompression is completed with small curved cervical curettes and with removal of any loose fragments within the neuroforamen. Small nerve hooks are passed out the foramen to assure lateral decompression. Laminectomy may be indicated, and posterior fusion with lateral mass plates are then performed.

Technique: Posterior Decompression—Laminectomy

Patients are in the prone position on a turning frame in Gardner-Wells traction. Hyperextension of the neck should be avoided. Alignment of the spine is checked radiographically. Subperiosteal exposure is carried out to the far lateral edge of the facets. The use of loupe magnification and a headlight facilitates visualization.

After level localization, cranial and caudal to the level to be decompressed, the interspinous ligaments and ligamentum flavum are divided. Laminectomy is performed by cutting bilateral longitudinal channels at the junctions of the laminae and lateral masses using a high-speed air drill. As the anterior cortex of the lamina is approached, the burr is changed to a diamond tip. If needed, 1-mm Kerrison rongeurs may be used to complete the laminotomy. It is best to avoid inserting anything larger beneath the laminae, and great care should be exercised in avoiding downward pressure on or beneath the laminae.

Once the channels have been completed, the laminae en bloc are grasped and displaced upwards. Beginning from the caudal direction, the laminae are teased away as to unroof the canal. Residual ligaments can be divided with scissors. Any residual compression laterally is removed with Kerrison rongeurs.

A slight modification to this technique is required in the presence of depressed laminar fractures as these may be associated with torn or entrapped dural and neural tissues.[221] After exposure of the margins of the lamina, the ligamentum flavum insertion is removed sharply. Any downward pressure on the depressed segment is avoided. Elevation of the depressed segment can be performed with small angled cervical curettes. Careful attention is paid to any dural adherence. Remaining jagged fracture ends should be smoothened with Kerrison rongeurs. The dura should be carefully inspected and repaired as indicated.

Following laminectomy for trauma, a posterior lateral mass fusion is routinely performed.

SUMMARY

Injuries to the cervical spine are associated with significant morbidity and mortality. Improvements in prehospitalization, emergency, and rehabilitative care have resulted in a better prognosis for many patients. Nonoperative management can be successful in the treatment of many injuries. In unstable injuries, newer surgical techniques provide rigid fixation and allow rapid patient mobilization without the use of a halo vest. Success using these techniques requires a thorough understanding of the patient's fracture pattern, the regional anatomy, and the implants biomechanical properties. With this understanding and the collaborative efforts of the orthopedic surgeon, the neurosurgeon, and SCI and rehabilitation services, optimal functional outcomes can be expected.

REFERENCES

1. Slone RM, McEnery KW, Bridwell KH, Montgomery WJ: Fixation techniques and instrumentation used in the cervical spine, *Radiol Clin North Am* 33:213, 1995.
2. Slucky AV, Eismont FJ: Treatment of acute injury of the cervical spine; *J Bone Joint Surg* 76A:1882, 1994.
3. Husein MK: An ancient Egyptian treatise on traumatology 2800 B.C. *J Bone Joint Surg* 31B:309, 1949.
4. Ducker TB, Saleman M, Daniell HB: Experimental cord trauma, III: therapeutic effect of immobilization and pharmacologic agents, *Surg Neurol* 10:71, 1978.
5. White AA III, Panjabi MM: The problem of clinical instability in the human spine: a systematic approach. White AA Panjabi MM, editors: *Clinical Biomechanics of the Spine* ed 2, Philadelphia, 1990, JB Lippincott.
6. Fielding JW, et al: Tears of the transverse ligament of the atlas. A clinical and biomechanical study, *J Bone Joint Surg* 56A:1683, 1974.
7. Werne S: Studies in spontaneous atlas dislocation, *Acta Scand Orthop* Suppl 23:1, 1957.
8. Dvorak J, et al: CT-functional diagnostics of the rotatory instability of upper cervical spine: I. An experimental study on cadavers, *Spine* 12:197, 1987.
9. White AA, Southwick WO, Panjabi MM: Clinical instability of the lower cervical spine. A review of past and current concepts, *Spine* 1:15, 1976.
10. Roaf R: A Study of the mechanics of spinal injuries, *J Bone Joint Surg* 42B:810, 1960.
11. Louis RP: Spinal stability as defined by the three column spine concept, *Anat Clin* 7:33, 1985.
12. Holdsworth FW: Fractures, dislocations and fracture dislocations of the spine, *J Bone Joint Surg (Br)* 45:6, 1963.
13. MacDonald RL, et al: Diagnosis of cervical spine injury in motor vehicle crash victims: how many X-rays are enough? *J Trauma* 30:392, 1990.
14. Doran SE, et al: Magnetic resonance image documentation of coexistent traumatic locked facets of the cervical spine and disc herniation, *J Neurosurg* 79:341, 1993.
15. Rizzolo SJ, et al: Intervertebral disc injury complicating cervical spine trauma, *Spine* 16:S187, 1991.
16. Goldberg AL, et al: The impact of magnetic resonance on the diagnostic evaluation of acute cervicothoracic spinal trauma, *Skeletal Radiol* 17:89, 1988.
17. Tien RD: Fat-suppression MR imaging in neuroradiology: Techniques and clinical application, *Am J Radiology* 158:369, 1992.
18. Flanders AE, et al: Acute cervical spine trauma: correlation of MR imaging findings with degree of neurologic deficit, *Radiology* 177:25, 1990.
19. Schaefer DM, et al: Prognostic significance of magnetic resonance imaging in the acute phase of cervical spinal cord injury, *J Neurosurg* 76:218, 1992.
20. American Spinal Injury Association and International Medical Society of Paraplegia: *Standard for neurologic and functional classification of spinal cord injury*, Atlanta, rev ed, 1992, American Spinal Injury Association.
21. Orthopedic Trauma Association: Comprehensive classification of fractures, Supplement to *J Orthop Trauma*, 1995.
22. Allen BL, et al: A mechanistic classification of closed, indirect fractures and dislocations of the lower cervical spine, *Spine* 7:1, 1982.
23. Bucholz RD, Cheung C: Halo vest versus spinal fusion for cervical injury: evidence form an outcome study, *J Neurosurg* 70:884, 1989.
24. Bucci MN, et al: Management of posttraumatic cervical spine instability: operative fusion versus halo vest immobilization: analysis of 49 cases, *J Trauma* 28:1001, 1988.
25. Bohlman HH: Acute fractures and dislocations of the cervical spine: an analysis of three hundred hospitalized patients and review of the literature, *J Bone Joint Surg* 61A:1119, 1979.
26. Hanigan WC, et al: Odontoid fractures in elderly patients, *J Neurosurg* 78:32, 1993.
27. Pepin JW, Bourne RB, Hawkins RJ: Odontoid fracture, with special reference to the elderly patient, *Clin Orthop* 193:178, 1985.
28. Bednar DA, Parikh J, Hummel J: Management of type II odontoid process fractures in geriatric patients; a

prospective study of sequential cohorts with attention to survivorship, *J Spinal Disord* 8:166, 1995.

29. Dorr LD, Harvey JP, Nickel VL: Clinical review of the early stability of spine injuries, *Spine* 7:545, 1982.
30. Murphy KP, et al: Cervical fractures and spinal cord injury: outcome of surgical and nonsurgical management, *Mayo Clin Proc* 65:949, 1990.
31. Ersmark H, Dalen N, Kalen R: Cervical spine injuries: a follow-up of 332 patients, *Paraplegia* 28:25, 1990.
32. Munroe D: The role of fusion or wiring in the treatment of acute traumatic instability, *Paraplegia* 3:97, 1965.
33. Stauffer ES, Kelly EG: Fracture-dislocations of the cervical spine: instability and recurrent deformity following treatment by anterior interbody fusion, *J Bone Joint Surg* 59A:45, 1977.
34. Kewalramani LS, Riggins RS: Complications of anterior spondylodesis for traumatic lesions of the cervical spine, *Spine* 2:25, 1977.
35. Van Peteghem PK, Schweigel JF: The fractured cervical spine rendered unstable by anterior cervical fusion, *J Trauma* 19:110, 1979.
36. Flynn TB: Neurologic complications of anterior cervical interbody fusion, *Spine* 7:536, 1982.
37. Aebi M, Zuber K, Marchesi D: Treatment of cervical spine injuries with anterior plating: indications, techniques, and results, *Spine* 16:S38, 1991.
38. Ripa DR, et al: Series of ninety-two traumatic cervical spine injuries stabilized with anterior ASIF plate fusion technique, *Spine* 16:S46, 1991.
39. Rogers WA: Fractures and dislocations of the cervical spine: an end-result study, *J Bone Joint Surg* 39A:341, 1957.
40. McAfee PC, Bohlmann HH, Wilson WL: The triple wire fixation technique for stabilization of acute cervical fracture dislocations: a biomechanical analysis, *Ortho Trans* 9:142, 1985.
41. Weiland DJ, McAfee PC: Posterior cervical fusion with triple wire strut graft technique: one hundred consecutive patients, *J Spin Dis* 4:15, 1991.
42. Fehlings MG, Cooper PR, Errico TJ: Posterior plates in the management of cervical instability: long-term results in 44 patients, *J Neurosurg* 81:341, 1994.
43. Anderson PA, et al: Posterior cervical arthrodesis with AO reconstruction plates and bone graft, *Spine* 16:S72, 1991.
44. Boehler L: *The treatment of fractures,* ed 4 (Eng). Baltimore, 1935, W Wood.
45. Breig A: The therapeutic possibilities of surgical bioengineering in incomplete spinal cord lesions, *Paraplegia* 9:173, 1972.
46. Breig A, El-Hade F: Biomechanics of the cervical spinal cord. Relief of contact pressure on and overstretching of the spinal cord, *Acta Radiol (Diag)* 4:602, 1966.
47. Delamarter RB, Sherman J, Carr JB: Pathophysiology of spinal cord injury. Recovery after immediate and delayed decompression, *J Bone Joint Surg* 77A:1042, 1995.
48. Delamarter RB, Sherman J, Carr JB: Cauda equina syndrome: neurologic recovery following immediate, early, or late decompression, *Spine* 16:1022, 1991.
49. Dolan EJ, Tator CH, Endrenyi L: The value of decompression for acute spinal cord compression injury, *J Neurosurg* 53:749, 1980.
50. Brunette DD, Rockswold GL: Neurologic recovery following rapid spinal realignment for complete cervical spinal cord injury, *J Trauma* 27:445, 1987.
51. Bohlman HH, Anderson PA: Anterior decompression and arthrodesis of the cervical spine: Long term motor improvement. Part 1—Improvement in incomplete traumatic quadriparesis, *J Bone Joint Surg* 74A:671, 1992.
52. Anderson PA, Bohlman HH: Anterior decompression and arthrodesis of the cervical spine: long-term motor improvement. Part II—Improvement in complete traumatic quadriplegia, *J Bone Joint Surg* 74A:683, 1992.
53. Duh MS, et al: The effectiveness of surgery on the treatment of acute spinal cord injury and its relation to pharmacological treatment, *Neurosurgery* 35:240, 1994.
54. Marshall LF, et al: Deterioration following spinal cord injury. A multicenter study, *J Neurosurg* 66:400, 1987.
55. Levi L, et al: Anterior decompression in cervical spine trauma: does the timing of surgery affect the outcome, *Neurosurgery* 29:216, 1991.
56. Wilberger JE: Diagnosis and management of spinal cord trauma, *J Neurotrauma* 8:S21, 1991.
57. Schlegel J, et al: Timing of surgical decompression and fixation of acute spinal fractures, *J Orthop Trauma* 10:323, 1996.
58. McPherson RW, et al: Effects of enflurane, isoflurane, and nitrous oxide on somatosensory evoked potentials during fentanyl anesthesia, *Anesthesiology* 62:626, 1985.
59. Parent AD, et al: Lateral cervical spine dislocation and vertebral artery injury, *Neurosurgery* 31:501, 1992.
60. Willis BK, et al: The incidence of vertebral artery injury after midcervical spine fracture or subluxation, *Neurosurgery* 34:435, 1994.
61. Bivens D, et al: Recovery from post-traumatic locked-in syndrome with basilar artery occlusion, *Surg Neurol* 16:230, 1981.
62. Rae-Grant AD, et al: Post traumatic extracranial vertebral artery dissection with locked-in syndrome: a case with MRI documentation and unusually favorable outcome, *J Neurol Neurosurg Psychiatry* 52:1191, 1989.
63. Cosgrove GR, Theron J: Vertebral arteriovenous fistula following anterior cervical spine surgery. Report of two cases, *J Neurosurg* 66:297, 1987.
64. Newhouse KE, et al: Esophageal perforation following anterior cervical spine surgery, *Spine* 14:1051, 1989.
65. Bassett T, Zdeblick TA: Complications of cervical spine instrumentation, *Tech Orthop* 9:8, 1994.

66. Caspar W, Barbier DD, Klara PM: Anterior cervical fusion and Caspar plate stabilization for cervical trauma, *Neurosurgery* 25:491, 1989.
67. Orozco DR, Llovet TJ: Osteosintesis en las fracturas de raquis cervical. Nota de technica, *Rev Ortop Traumatol* 14:285, 1970.
68. Elia M, Mazzara JT, Fielding JW: Onlay technique for occipitocervical fusion, *Clin Orthop* 280:170, 1992.
69. Newman P, Sweeman R: Occipital cervical fusion, *J Bone Joint Surg* 51B:423, 1969.
70. Hamblen DL: Occipitocervical fusion: indications technique and results, *J Bone Joint Surg* 49B:33, 1967.
71. Wertheim SB, Bohlman HH: Occipitocervical fusion: Indications, technique and long-term results in thirteen patients, *J Bone Joint Surg* 69A:833, 1987.
72. Ransford AO, et al: Craniocervical instability treated by contoured loop fixation, *J Bone Joint Surg* 68B:173, 1986.
73. Itoh T, et al: Occipitocervical fusion reinforced by Luque's segmental spinal instrumentation for rheumatoid diseases, *Spine* 13:1234, 1988.
74. Smith MD, Anderson P Grady MS: Occipitocervical arthrodesis using contoured plate fixation. An early report on a versatile fixation technique, *Spine* 18:1984, 1993.
75. Sasso RC, et al: Occipitocervical fusion with posterior plate and screw instrumentation. A long-term follow-up study, *Spine* 19:2364, 1994.
76. Penning L: Normal movements of the cervical spine, *Am J Radiol* 130:317, 1979.
77. Hajek PD, et al: Biomechanical study of C1-C2 posterior arthrodesis techniques, *Spine* 18:173, 1993.
78. Grob D, et al: Biomechanical evaluation of four different posterior atlantoaxial fixation techniques, *Spine* 17:480, 1992.
79. Hanson PB, et al: Anatomic and biomechanical assessment of transarticular screw fixation for atlantoaxial instability, *Spine* 16:1141, 1991.
80. Graziano G, et al: A comparative study of fixation techniques for type II fractures of odontoid process, *Spine* 18:2383, 1993.
81. Sasso RC, Heggeness MH, Doherty BJ: Biomechanics of odontoid fracture fixation: comparison of one and two screw techniques, *Spine* 18:1950, 1993.
82. Doherty BJ, Heggeness MH, Esses SI: A biomechanical study of odontoid fractures and fracture fixation, *Spine* 18:178, 1993.
83. Heller JG, et al: Quantitative internal dens morphology, *Spine* 17:861, 1992.
84. Morscher E, et al: Die vordere verplattung der halswirbelsaeule mit dem hohlschrauben-plattensystem aus titanium, *Chirurg* 57:702, 1986.
85. Traynelis VC, et al: Biomechanical comparison of anterior Caspar plate and three-level posterior fixation techniques in a human cadaveric model, *J Neurosurg* 79:96, 1993.
86. Abitbol JJ, et al: A biomechanical analysis of modern anterior and posterior cervical stabilization techniques. Presented at the Cervical Spine Research Society, Palm Desert, 1992.
87. Montesano PX, et al: Biomechanics of cervical spine internal fixation, *Spine* 16:S10, 1991.
88. Garvey TA, Eismont FJ, Roberti LF: Anterior decompression, structural bone grafting, and Caspar plate stabilization for unstable spine fractures and dislocations, *Spine* 17:S431, 1992.
89. Coe JD, et al: Biomechanical evaluation of cervical spinal stabilization methods in human cadaveric model, *Spine* 14:1122, 1989.
90. Sutterlin III CE, et al: A biomechanical evaluation of cervical spinal stabilization of cervical spinal stabilization methods in a bovine model: static and cyclical loading, *Spine* 13:795, 1988.
91. Roy-Camille R, Saillant G, Mazel C: *Internal fixation of the unstable cervical spine by a posterior osteosynthesis with plates and screws. The Cervical Spine Research Society,* ed 2, Philadelphia, 1989, JB Lippincott.
92. Garfin SR, Moore MR, Marshall LF: A modified technique for cervical facet fusions, *Clin Orthop* 230:149, 1988.
93. Holness RP, et al: Poterior stabilization with an interlaminar clamp in cervical injuries: technical notes and review of the long term experience with the method, *Neurosurgery* 14:318, 1984.
94. Gill K, et al: Posterior plating of the cervical spine: a biomechanical comparison of different posterior fusion techniques, *Spine* 13:813, 1988.
95. Statham P, O'Sullivan M, Russell T: The Halifax interlaminar clamp for posterior cervical fusion: initial experience in the United Kingdom, *Neurosurgery* 32:396, 1993.
96. Ulrich C, et al: Comparative study of the stability of anterior and posterior cervical spine fixation procedures, *Arch Orthop Trauma Surg* 106:226, 1987.
97. Errico T, et al: Pull out strength comparison of two methods of orienting screw insertion in the lateral masses of the bovine cervical spine, *J Spinal Disord* 5:459, 1992.
98. Jeanneret B, Magerl F, Haterward E: Posterior stabilization of the cervical spine with hook plates, *Spine* 16:56, 1991.
99. Grob D, Hagerl F: Dorsal spondylodesis of the cervical spine using a hooked plate, *Orthopade* 16:55, 1987.
100. Montesano PX, Jauch E, Jonsson H: Anatomic and biomechanical study of posterior cervical spine plate arthrodesis: an evaluation of two different techniques of screw placement, *J Spinal Disord* 5:301, 1992.
101. Heller JG, et al: Anatomic comparison of the Roy-Camille and Magerl techniques for screw placement in the lower cervical spine, *Spine* 16:S552, 1991.
102. Brodky DS, et al: Anterior versus posterior stabilization of cervical spine fractures in spinal cord injured patients. Presented at the American Academy of

Orthopedic Surgeons 64th Annual Meeting, San Francisco, Feb 1997.
103. Anderson PA, et al: Posterior cervical arthrodesis with AO reconstruction plates and bone graft, *Spine* 16:S72, 1991.
104. Grady MS, Anderson PA: Subaxial lateral mass plates in the cervical spine, *Techn Neurosurg* 1:123, 1995.
105. Chapman JR, et al: Posterior instrumentation of the unstable cervicothoracic spine, *J Neurosurg* 84:552, 1996.
106. Anderson PA, Montesano PX: Morphology and treatment of occipital condyle fractures, *Spine* 13:731, 1988.
107. Dickman CA, et al: Curciate paralysis of injuries to the cervicomedullary junction, *J Neurosurg* 73:850, 1990.
108. Ladouceur D, Veilleux M, Levesque RY: Cruciate paralysis secondary to C1 on C2 fracture-dislocation, *Spine* 17:1383, 1991.
109. Bucholz RW, Burkhead WZ: The pathologic anatomy of fatal atlanto-occipital dislocations, *J Bone Joint Surg* 61A:248, 1979.
110. Wholey MH, Bruwer AJ, Hillier LB: The lateral roentgenogram of the neck (with comments on the atlanto-odontoid-basion relationship), *Radiology* 71:350, 1958.
111. Powers B, et al: Traumatic anterior atlanto-occipital dislocation, *Neurosurgery* 4:12, 1979.
112. Lee C. Evaluation of traumatic atlantooccipital dislocations, *AJNR* 8:19, 1987.
113. Harris JH Jr., et al: Radiologic diagnosis of traumatic occipitovertebral dissociation: 2. Comparison of three methods of detecting occipitovertebral relationships on lateral radiographs of supine subjects, *Am J Radiol* 162:887, 1994.
114. Harris JH Jr., Carson GC, Wagner LK: Radiologic diagnosis of traumatic occipitovertebral dissociation: 1. Normal occipitovertebral relationships on lateral radiographs of supine subjects, *Am J Radiol* 162:881, 1994.
115. Traynelis VC, et al: Traumatic atlanto-occipital dislocation: case Report, *J Neurosurg* 65:863, 1988.
116. Cone W, Nicholoson JT: The treatment of fracture-dislocations of the cervical vertebrae by skeletal traction and fusion, *J Bone Joint Surg* 19A:584, 1937.
117. Ebraheim NA, et al: An anatomic study of the thickness of the occipital bone: implications for occipitocervical instrumentation, *Spine* 15:1725, 1996.
118. Xu R, et al: Morphology of the second cervical vertebra and the posterior projection of the C2 pedicle axis, *Spine* 20:259, 1995.
119. Ebraheim N, et al: Anatomic consideration of C2 pedicle screw placement, *Spine* 21:691, 1996.
120. Hadley MN, et al: Acute traumatic atlas fractures: management and long term outcome, *Neurosurgery* 23:31, 1988.
121. Sherk HH, Nicholson JT: Fractures of the atlas, *J Bone Joint Surg* 52A:1017, 1970.
122. Landells CD, Van Peteghem PK: Fractures of the atlas: classification, treatment and morbidity, *Spine* 13:450, 1988.
123. Levine AM, Edwards CC: Fractures of the atlas, *J Bone Joint Surg* 73A:680, 1991.
124. Levine AM, Edwards CC: Treatment of injuries in the C1-C2 complex, *Orthop Clin North Am* 17:31, 1986.
125. Schlicke LH, Callahan RA: A rational approach to burst fractures of the atlas, *Clin Orthop* 154:18, 1981.
126. Spence KF, Dedser D, Sell KW: Bursting atlantal fracture associated with rupture of the transverse ligament, *J Bone Joint Surg* 52A:543, 1970.
127. Heller JG, Viroslav S, Hudson T: Jefferson fractures: the role of magnification artifact in assessing transverse ligament integrity, *J Spinal Disord* 6:392, 1993.
128. Hays MB, Alker GJ Jr: Fractures of the atlas vertebra; the two-part burst fracture of Jefferson, *Spine* 13:601, 1988.
129. Jefferson G: Fracture of the atlas vertebra, report of four cases, and a review of those previously recorded, *Br J Surg* 7:407, 1920.
130. McGuire RA, Harkey HL: Primary treatment of unstable Jefferson's fractures, *J Spinal Disord* 8:233, 1995.
131. Grob D, et al: Atlanto-axial fusion with transarticular screw fixation, *J Bone Joint Surg* 73B:972, 1991.
132. Sherk HH: Fractures of the atlas and odontoid process, *Orthop Clin North Am* 9:973, 1978.
133. Husby J, Sorensen KH: Fracture of the odontoid process of the axis, *Acta Orthop Scand* 45:182, 1974.
134. Mouradian WH, et al: Fractures of the odontoid: a laboratory and clinical study of mechanism, *Orthop Clin North Am* 9:985, 1978.
135. Blockey NJ, Purser DW: Fractures of the odontoid process of the axis, *J Bone Joint Surg* 38B:794, 1956.
136. Clark CR, White AA: Fractures of the dens: a multicenter study, *J Bone Joint Surg* 67:1340, 1985.
137. Anderson LD, Clark CR: Fractures of the odontoid process of the axis. In *The cervical spine,* Philadelphia, 1989, JB Lippincott.
138. Pepin JW, Bourne RB, Hawkins RJ: Odontoid fractures, with special reference to the elderly patient, *Clin Orthop* 193:178, 1985.
139. Apuzzo MLJ, et al: Acute fractures of the odontoid process: an analysis of forty-five cases, *J Neurosurg* 48:85, 1978.
140. Anderson LD, D'Alonzo RT: Fractures of the odontoid process of the axis, *J Bone Joint Surg* 56A:1663, 1974.
141. Funk EJ, Wells RE: Injuries of the cervical spine in football, *Clin Orthop* 109:50, 1975.
142. Paradis GR, Janes JM: Posttraumatic atlantoaxial instability: the fate of the odontoid process fracture in 46 cases, *J Trauma* 13:359, 1973.
143. Ryan MD, Taylor TKF: Odontoid fractures in the elderly, *J Spinal Disord* 6:397, 1993.
144. Hadley MN, et al: Axis fractures: new subtype of acute odontoid fracture (type IIa), *Neurosurg* 22:67, 1988.

145. Southwick WO: Current concepts review: Management of fractures of the dens (odontoid process), *J Bone Joint Surg* 62A:482, 1980.
146. Hadley MN, Browner CM, Sonntag VKH: Axis fractures: a comprehensive review of management and treatment in 107 cases, *Neurosurg* 17:281, 1985.
147. Lind B, Nordall A, Sihlbom H: Odontoid fracture treated with halo-vest, *Spine* 12:173, 1987.
148. Brown CW, Orme TJ, Richardson HD: The rate of pseudarthrosis (surgical nonunion) in patients who are smokers and patients who are nonsmokers: a comparison study, *Spine* 11:942, 1986.
149. Lau G, et al: The effect of cigarette smoking on fracture healing: an animal model, *Clin Res* 37:132, 1989.
150. Schatzker J, Rorabeck CH, Waddell JP: Fractures of the dens (odontoid process). An analysis of 37 cases, *J Bone Joint Surg* 53B:392, 1971.
151. Amyes EW, Anderson FM: Fractur of the odontoid process: report of sixty-three cases, *Arch Surg* 72:377, 1956.
152. Ryan MD, Taylor TKF: Odontoid fracture, *J Bone Joint Surg* 64B:416, 1982.
153. Jeanneret B, Magerl F: Primary posterior fusion C1-2 in odontoid fractures: indication, technique, and results of transarticular screw fixation, *J Spinal Disord* 5:464, 1992.
154. Bohler J: Anterior stabilization for acute fractures and non-unions of the dens, *J Bone Joint Surg* 64A:18, 1982.
155. Jeanneret B, et al: Atlantoaxial mobility after screw fixation of the odontoid: a computed tomographic study, *J Spinal Disord* 4:203, 1991.
156. Montesano PA, et al: Odontoid fractures treated by anterior odontoid screw fixation, *Spine* 16:S33, 1991.
157. Aebi M, Etter C, Coscia M: Fractures of the odontoid process: treatment with anterior screw fixation, *Spine* 14:1065, 1989.
158. Etter C, et al: Direct anterior fixation of dens fractures with a cannulated screw system, *Spine* 16:S25, 1991.
159. Schweigel JF: Management of the fractured odontoid with halo-thoracic bracing, *Spine* 12:838, 1987.
160. Francis WR, et al: Traumatic spondylolisthesis of the axis, *J Bone Joint Surg* 63B:313, 1981.
161. Effendi B, et al: Fractures of the ring of the axis: a classification based on the analysis of 131 cases, *J Bone Joint Surg* 63B:319, 1981.
162. Levine AM, Edwards CC: The management of traumatic spondylolisthesis of the axis, *J Bone Joint Surg* 67A:217, 1985.
163. Levine AM, Edwards CC: Traumatic lesions of the atlantoaxial complex, *Clin Orthop* 239:53, 1989.
164. Committee on Trauma: *Advanced Trauma Life Support, Program for Physicians 1993,* Chicago, 1993, American College of Surgeons.
165. Bracken MB, et al: A randomized controlled trial of methylprednisolone or naloxone in the treatment of acute spinal cord injury: results of the Second National Acute Spinal Cord Injury Study, *N Engl J Med* 322:1405, 1990.
166. Gardner WJ: The principle of spring loaded points for cervical traction, *J Neurosurg* 39:543, 1973.
167. Cotler HB, et al: Closed reduction of cervical spine dislocations, *Clin Orthop* 214:185, 1987.
168. Crutchfield WG: Skeletal traction for dislocations of the cervical spine: a report of a case, *South Surgeon* 2:156, 1933.
169. Sabiston CP, et al: Closed reductions of dislocations of the lower cervical sine, *J Trauma* 28:832, 1988.
170. Lee AS, MacLean, Newton DA: Rapid traction for reduction of cervical spine dislocations, *J Bone Joint Surg* 76B:352, 1994.
171. Star AM, et al: Immediate closed reduction of cervical spine dislocations using traction, *Spine* 15:1068, 1990.
172. Cotler JM, et al: Closed reduction of traumatic cervical spine dislocation using traction weights up to 140 pounds, *Spine* 18:386, 1993.
173. Apple DF Jr, McDonald AP, Smith RA: Identification of herniated nucleus pulposis in spinal cord injury, *Paraplegia* 25:78, 1987.
174. Pratt ES, Green DA, Spengler DM: Herniated intervertebral discs associated with unstable spinal injuries, *Spine* 15:662, 1990.
175. Schaefer DM, et al: Magnetic resonance imaging of acute cervical spine trauma: correlation with severity of neurologic injury, *Spine* 14:1090, 1989.
176. Boden SD, et al: Abnormal magnetic-resonance scans of the cervical spine in asymptomatic subjects, *J Bone Joint Surg* 72A:1178, 1990.
177. Eismont FJ, Arena MJ, Green BA: Extrusion of an intervertebral disc associated with traumatic subluxation or dislocation of cervical facets, *J Bone Joint Surg* 73A:1555, 1991.
178. Robertson PA, Ryan MD: Neurological deterioration after reduction of cervical subluxation: mechanical compression by disc tissue, *J Bone Joint Surg* 74B:224, 1992.
179. Knightly JJ, et al: Neurosurgical forum, *J Neurosurg* 80:952, 1994.
180. Hadley MN, et al: Facet fracture-dislocation injuries of the cervical spine, *Neurosurgery* 30:661, 1992.
181. Rivlin AS, Tator CH: Effect of duration of acute spinal cord compression in a new acute cord injury model in the rat, *Surg Neurol* 10:39, 1978.
182. Assenmacher DR, Ducker TB: Experimental traumatic paraplegia, *J Bone Joint Surg* 53A:671, 1971.
183. Tator CH, Fehlings MG: Review of the secondary injury theory of acute spinal cord trauma with emphasis on vascular mechanisms, *J Neurosurg* 75:15, 1991.
184. Fazl M, et al: Posttraumatic ligamentous disruption of the cervical spine, an easily overlooked diagnosis: presentation of three cases, *Neurosurgery* 26:674, 1990.
185. Webb JK, et al: Hidden flexion injury of the cervical spine, *J Bone Joint Surg* 58B:322, 1976.

186. Whitehill R, Richman JA, Glaser JA: Failure of immobilization of the cervical spine by halo-vest, *J Bone Joint Surg* 68:326, 1986.
187. Glaser JA, et al: Complications associated with the halo vest, *J Neurosurg* 65:762, 1986.
188. Songer MN, et al: The use of sublaminar cables to replace Luque wires, *Spine* 16:S418, 1991.
189. Chapman JR, Anderson PA: Posterior plate fixation of the cervicothoracic junction, *Tech Orthoped* 9:80, 1994.
190. Chapman JR, et al: Posterior instrumentation of the unstable cervico-thoracic, Spine. *J Neurosurg* 84:552, 1996.
191. Beatson TR: Fractures and dislocations of the cervical spine, *J Bone Joint Surg* 45B:21, 1963.
192. Rorabeck CH, et al: Unilateral facet dislocation of the cervical spine. An analysis of the results of treatment in 26 patients, *Spine* 12:23, 1987.
193. Braakman R, Vinken PJ: Unilateral facet interlocking in the lower cervical spine, *J Bone Joint Surg* 49B:249, 1967.
194. Beyer CA, Cabanela ME, Berquist TH: Unilateral facet dislocations and fracture-dislocations of the cervical spine, *J Bone Joint Surg* 73B:977, 1991.
195. Roy-Camille R, Mazel G, Edourard B: Luxations et luxations fractures. In Roy-Camille R, editor: *Rachis cervical inferieur,* Masson, 1988.
196. Levine AM: Facet injuries in the cervical spine. In *Disorders of the cervical spine,* Baltimore, 1992, Williams & Wilkins.
197. Sears W, Fazl M: Prediction of stability of cervical spine fracture managed in the halo vest and indications for surgical intervention, *J Neurosurg* 72:426, 1990.
198. Bauze RJ, Ardran GM: Experimental production of forward dislocation in the human cervical spine, *J Bone Joint Surg* 60B:239, 1978.
199. Shono Y, McAfee PC, Cunningham BW: The pathomechanics of compression injuries in the cervical spine, *Spine* 18:2009, 1993.
200. McNamare MJ, Devito DP, Spengler DM: Circumferential fusion for the management of acue cervical spine trauma, *J Spinal Disord* 4:467, 1991.
201. Cybulski GR, et al: Complications in three-column cervical spine injuries requiring anterior-posterior stabilization, *Spine* 17:253, 1992.
202. Jones AAM, et al: Iliac crest bone graft osteotome versus saw, *Spine* 18:2048, 1993.
203. Hu R, Hearn T, Yang J: Bone graft harvest site as a determinant of iliac crest strength, *Clin Orthop* 310:252, 1995.
204. Hu R, Bohlman HH: Fracture at the iliac bone graft harvest site after fusion of the spine, *Clin Orthop* 309:208, 1994.
205. Spitzer WO, et al: Scientific monograph of the Quebec task force on whiplash-associated disorders: redefining "whiplash" and its management, *Spine* 8S:10S, 1995.
206. Harris JH, Yeakley JW: Hyperextension-dislocation of the cervical spine, *J Bone Joint Surg* 74B:567, 1992.
207. Taylor AR, Blackwood W: Paraplegia in hyperextension cervical injuries with normal radiographic appearances, *J Bone Joint Surg* 30B:245, 1948.
208. Taylor AR: The mechanism of injury to the spinal cord in the neck with out damage to the vertebral column, *J Bone Joint Surg* 33B:543, 1951.
209. Macnab I: Acceleration injuries of the cervical spine, *J Bone Joint Surg* 46A:1797, 1964.
210. Forsyth HF: Extension injuries of the cervical spine, *J Bone Joint Surg* 436A:1792, 1964.
211. Marar BC: Hyperextension injuries of the cervical spine. The pathogenesis of damage to the spinal cord, *J Bone Joint Surg* 56A:1655, 1974.
212. Schneider RC, Knighton R: Chronic neurological sequelae of acute trauma to the spine and spinal cord. The syndrome of chronic injury to the cervical spinal cord in the region of the central canal, *J Bone Joint Surg* 41A:905, 1959.
213. Taylor AR, Blackwood W: Paraplegia in hyperextension cervical injuries with normal radiographic appearances, *J Bone Joint Surg* 30B:245, 1948.
214. Schneider RC, Cherry EC, Pantek H: Syndrome of acute central cervical spinal cord injury with special reference to mechanisms involved in hyperextension injuries of cervical spine, *J Neurosurg* 11:546, 1954.
215. Merriam WF, et al: A reappraisal of acute traumatic central cord syndrome, *J Bone Joint Surg* 68B:708, 1986.
216. Bose B, et al: Reanalysis of central cervical cord injury management, *Neurosurgery* 15:367, 1984.
217. Epstein JA: The surgical management of cervical spinal stenosis, spondylosis, and myeloradiculopathy by means of the posterior approach, *Spine* 13:864, 1988.
218. Capen DA, Nelson RW, Zigler JE: Decompressive laminectomy in cervical spine trauma: a review of early and late complications, *Contemp Orthop* 17:21, 1987.
219. Raynor RB, Pugh J, Shapiro I: Cervical facetectomy and its effect on spine strength, *J Neurosurg* 64:278, 1985.
220. Zdeblick TA, et al: Cervical stability after foraminotomy: a biomechanical in vitro analysis, *J Bone Joint Surg* 74:22, 1992.
221. Cammisa Jr FP, Eismont FJ, Green BA: Dural laceration occurring with burst fractures and associated laminar fractures, *J Bone Joint Surg* 71A:1044, 1989.

11

SURGICAL AND NONSURGICAL TREATMENT OF VERTEBRAL FRACTURES TO THE UPPER THORACIC SPINE

Reynold L. Rimoldi

The principle indications for surgical treatment of all spinal fractures are to decompress a partial neurologic injury and to stabilize an unstable motion segment. The vast majority of scientific literature focuses on these principles as they apply to the thoracolumbar and cervical areas. There is a paucity of information on fractures of the upper thoracic spine.

The upper thoracic spine is defined by the area from T1 to T10. Below the T10 level, the orientation of the vertebral facet joints resemble those of the lumbar spine. This is secondary to the orientation of the facet joints being in the coronal plane. At the T11 and T12 levels the facets are more sagitally oriented like those of the lumbar spine.[1] Historically, fractures of the upper thoracic spine have been grouped with fractures occurring at the thoracolumbar junction.[2–15]

These two regions, however, are anatomically unique because of the dissimilar neurologic and osseous components. The upper thoracic area is stiffer and, therefore, a greater amount of energy is required to produce fractures or dislocations in this area. The narrow spinal canal leads to an increased frequency of associated neurologic injuries with fractures in this area.[1,16,17] Fractures occurring in this region are uncommon. Sixteen percent of all spinal fractures involve the upper thoracic spine.[18,19]

The supporting structures associated with the upper thoracic spine account for this area having the fewest fractures of all the spinal motion segments. Anatomic variations need to be considered when evaluating the upper thoracic spine for surgical stabilization. Kyphosis is present in this area unlike that of the cervical and lumbar regions. The presence of the rib cage and sternum accords an inherent stability to this region. It is apparent, therefore, that fewer surgical procedures are necessary to achieve stability related to fractures in the thoracic spine. Panjabi and White have stated that clinical instability is the loss of the ability of the spine under physiologic loads to maintain relationships between vertebrae.[20] The presence of the surrounding rib cage and sternum make the two-column theory of instability as proposed by Holdsworth and the three-column theory of Denis inaccurate in predicting spinal stability.[3,21] Dafner et al., however, have proposed radiographic criteria to determine instability that is more useful when evaluating the upper thoracic spine.[22] When two or more of the five following radiographic signs are present the injury is considered unstable: translational displacement of adjacent vertebra, widening of the interspinous distance, perched or dislocated facet joints, increased interpeduncular distance, and disruption of the posterior vertebral body line.

The thoracic spine consists of 12 vertebral bodies. This is the only portion of the spine that exhibits a natural kyphotic curve. This curve develops in utero and is maintained throughout life. The load-bearing axis is in the anterior column of the thoracic spine. The anterior-posterior dimension of the thoracic vertebral bodies increases as one progresses in a cephalad to caudad direction. The vertical height of the thoracic vertebral bodies is approximately 3 mm less anteriorly than posteriorly. This accounts for the kyphosis exhibited in this area.

The vertebral foramen has the smallest volume in the thoracic spine. The supporting ribs articulate with each vertebral body at two places. In the upper thoracic spine the ribs articulate with their respective transverse processes and at the more cephalad disk space. Below T9 the ribs articulate at the level of the pedicle and the transverse processes of their respective vertebral body. The rib cage in the thoracic spine restricts motion and adds stiffness. This is most true in extension and to a lesser degree in flexion and lateral rotation. The ribs provide strength and absorb energy during traumatic events. The spine in this area is stiffer when subjected to translational and torsional forces.[6,20,23]

The compressive forces that lead to failure in the spinal column are increased by a factor of four in the thoracic spine secondary to the presence of the rib cage.[23–25] Clinical situations in which the ribs are fractured or disassociated from their respective vertebra should lead one to suspect the existence of an unstable spine. The pedicles are of smaller dimension than those of the lumbar spine, and they do not angle lateral to medial as one views their course from posterior to anterior as in the lumbar spine. The transverse processes are shorter but wider when the thoracic spine is compared to the lumbar spine. The facet joints lie in the coronal plane, while the facets are sagittally oriented in the lumbar spine. The orientation of the facet joints serve to resist translation in the anterior-posterior direction. Intervertebral disks exhibit different dimensions in the thoracic spine. The height of the disk is decreased, but the annulus fibrosis is thicker; therefore, these structures are less elastic and more effective in limiting rotation.[1] These observations account for the infrequency with which fractures occur in this area and corresponds with the clinical observation that most fractures in the upper thoracic spine are secondary to extremes of flexion and vertical compression. These anatomical variances are important when considering internal fixation devices for stabilization.

The small pedicular dimensions and the close proximity of the spinal cord make interpedicular fixation more difficult in the thoracic spine. The consequence of spinal cord injury (SCI) if the pedicle is missed medially can be catastrophic; therefore, segmental spinal instrumentation via the hook rod technique remains the most popular type of posterior instrumentation in the thoracic spine. The hooks can be fixed to the pedicle, the transverse process or under the lamina to accomplish stabilization of the thoracic spine. The most popular anterior constructs include screw plate systems or screw rod systems that allow for stable fixation with compression loads being generated across structural bone grafts.

The last decade has seen a change in the etiology of SCIs. Historically, fractures to the vertebral column have been a result of high-speed motor vehicular trauma. As our society has become a more violent place to live, the number of SCIs secondary to gunshot wounds has increased at an alarming rate in the larger metropolitan areas. From 1981 to 1991, the incidence of fractures due to motor vehicular trauma has decreased from 42% to 28%, whereas, those due to civilian gunshot wounds have increased from 25% to 52%.[26]

PREOPERATIVE EVALUATION

Before deciding on proper treatment options for upper thoracic spine fractures a thorough initial evaluation and general assessment is necessary. Life-saving measures are attended to at the scene. Patients with suspected injuries to the thoracic spine frequently have associated multiple traumatic injuries to the chest and abdomen.[13,17,27,28] The clinician must evaluate and treat an obstructed airway, hypovolemic shock and chest injuries. Eight percent of all patients with spinal fractures exhibit an associated spinal fracture that is separated from the parent fracture by a minimum of three motion segments.[29] All patients, therefore, are assumed to have neck injuries and should be immobilized until lateral radiographs have cleared the cervical spine.

After a general physical examination to assess all organ systems, a careful spinal evaluation is mandatory. The evaluation of the thoracic spine begins with a thorough inspection for contusions, ecchymosis, and lacerations about the chest area. Palpation determines widening or rotational malalignment of the thoracic spinous processes. Palpation of the rib cage and sternum may reveal sources of tenderness consistent with a fracture. A detailed neurologic examination is imperative. Neurologic evaluation includes sensory, motor, and reflex testing. A sensory examination should include an evaluation of all dermatomes and the perineal area for evidence of sacral sparing. The medial aspect of the upper arm, the nipple line, and the umbilicus constitutes the T1, T4, and T10 dermatomes, respectively. The motor examination includes the intrinsic muscles of the hand, which receive innervation from the T1 level. All patients should have a rectal examination to determine voluntary sphincter control as a sign of sacral sparing. A bulbocavernosus reflex is observed to determine the end of spinal shock, usually at 24 to 48 hours after injury. This reflex involves the lower sacral nerve roots. In all thoracic fractures, its presence is of great prognostic value. If there is no neurologic function distal to the injured motion segment along with the presence of the bulbocavernous reflex, this connotates a complete SCI. Return of neurologic function in this scenario is negligible.

The bulbocavernosus reflex is performed by placing a digit into the patient's rectum feeling for involuntary rectal contractions while the other hand is used to gently squeeze the glans penis or clitoris. This constitutes a positive bulbocavernosus test and alerts the examiner that an accurate assessment of spinal cord integrity can be made.

Lower extremity reflexes that are hyperactive suggest SCI. One observes for lower extremity clonus. Up going toes determined by a Babinski test is another sign of SCI.

Once a SCI has been diagnosed intravenous corticosteroids should be administered. Patients with neurologic injuries exhibit significant improvement in both motor and sensory function if methylprednisolone is begun within 8 hours of injury.[30] The treatment should be continued for 24 hours.

DIAGNOSTIC IMAGING

Imaging modalities should be recommended in a thoughtful process to avoid unnecessary tests that may delay treatment. Plane radiographs are often the only tests needed for the evaluation of upper thoracic spine fractures in neurologically intact patients. The fractures included in this group are minimally displaced anterior or lateral compression injuries. Anterior-posterior and lateral projections are required to determine the mechanism of injury in the majority of cases. Oblique views are of greater importance when evaluating cervical and lumbar spine injuries. They are not as helpful when evaluating bony injuries to the thoracic spine because the overlying osseous structures make interpretation difficult. Oblique views are not as useful in evaluating flexion, extension, and lateral compression injuries, which are the principle mechanisms of injury to the upper thoracic spine.[16]

More significant fractures with associated neurologic injuries require further studies. Although plane radiographs determine basic fracture anatomy, computer tomography (CT) is necessary to outline bony detail and document sources of spinal canal compromise. Magnetic resonance imaging (MRI) is usually not indicated in cases involving bony fractures. An MRI scan does not provide the cortical bone detail that is necessary in evaluating thoracic vertebral fractures. This test is reserved for injuries in which neurologic injury can not be explained on the basis of plane radiographs. The anatomy of the surrounding rib cage and sternum must be scrutinized to determine fracture stability. Fractures of the ribs and sternum are difficult to evaluate on radiographs that are centered on the thoracic spine. Rib-detail radiographs are necessary to evaluate rib cage integrity. Plane or CT is necessary to evaluate suspected sternal injuries.

Fractures involving the most cephalad portion of the thoracic spine can be difficult to evaluate with standard radiographs. A swimmer's view can be helpful. Detailed evaluation can be made with plane or CT.

TREATMENT

The majority of fractures to the upper thoracic spine can be adequately treated without operative intervention. Thoracic fractures associated with complete SCI are less likely to require operative intervention compared to incomplete SCI or fractures in the cervical or lumbar areas. This is because of the inherent stability provided by the surrounding skeletal structures. Thoracic spine fractures with associated incomplete spinal cord lesions with documented canal compromise or instability are treated with surgical methods.

Compression fractures in the absence of multiple rib fractures are stable injuries. These injuries without associated neurologic compromise heal rapidly with minimal tendency toward progressive deformity. Symptomatic treatment consisting of a short period of bed rest (1–2 days), followed by immobilization in a cast or brace for a minimum of 6 weeks is appropriate. Hospitalization is not required for the treatment of these fractures.

The volume of the spinal canal is smaller in the thoracic spine.[1,16,17] Low energy fractures, therefore, are more likely to be associated with neurologic compromise in this area. Many of these fractures have inherent stability because of the surrounding structural support; therefore, surgical intervention is not required. Imaging modalities must be scrutinized for two reasons: (1) to exclude sternal and rib injuries, which would render these fractures unstable, and (2) to reveal sources of compression in patients with incomplete neurologic injuries. These two scenarios require surgical intervention. Once fracture stability is confirmed, even when there is a complete neurologic injury, operative treatment is not indicated. These patients are best treated in a SCI rehabilitation program. Transfer from a primary care facility should be expedited once the patient is stable.

Although cast and brace immobilization is not always necessary in the treatment of stable fractures to the upper thoracic spine, they can provide comfort by immobilizing the vertebral column. Cast or brace immobilization may be detrimental in some circumstances. Stable injuries with insensate skin can break down rapidly with snug fitting casts or braces. These orthotic devices can also limit rehabilitation in patients with thoracic fractures and significant SCI.[29] Hip flexion is limited by the use of these braces making activities such as self-dressing and transferring to and from a wheelchair more difficult to master.

There are three types of thoracic orthoses which can be used with upper thoracic spine fractures. Thoracic corsets provide minimal control of motion and are most appropriate for minor traumatic compression fractures and fatigue fractures in patients with osteoporosis. The Jewett and Taylor braces provide intermediate control of spinal motion and are appropriate for fractures that exhibit greater than 33% compromise of the anterior and middle columns but are still judged stable by diagnostic imaging criteria. The Risser jacket and body cast are the most effective at limiting spinal motion and can be considered for unstable injuries in patients that can not tolerate surgical intervention.

SURGICAL DECISION-MAKING

When the decision has been made to treat these fractures with surgery, the timing of the procedure is the next issue to be resolved. Many of these patients have life-threatening injuries. The most frequent are closed-head injuries, long-bone fractures of the extremities, chest injuries, and abdominal visceral injuries.[2,13,17,27,28] These require treatment prior to addressing the thoracic spine. Although the timing of surgical intervention, whether it be to decompress or stabilize, has been debated. The rapidity of the definitive surgery may prevent hospital complications. These complications include atelectesis, pneumonia, vein thrombosis, skin breakdown, and urinary infections. Surgical treatment should be performed within the first week of injury in patients with thoracic spine fractures. Urgent operative treatment is indicated in the face of progressive neurologic compromise in a patient with an incomplete neurologic injury.

The vast majority of fractures from T1 to T10 that require decompression are properly treated through an anterior approach. Cases in which upper thoracic spine fractures are associated with rib or sternal fractures are considered unstable necessitating operative treatment. In these cases the anterior or posterior approach is appropriate.

The use of spinal cord monitoring has been widely advocated in procedures of decompression or stabilization of the thoracic spine. This is secondary to the possibility of neurologic deterioration during decompression or stabilization procedures that require reduction forces. If there is any question pertaining to spinal cord integrity during surgery in patients with incomplete neurologic lesions, a wake-up test remains the gold standard and should be performed.

GUNSHOT WOUNDS

Civilian gunshot wounds are now the principle cause of SCI in large metropolitan areas; therefore, these injuries deserve special mention. Recent studies have shown that penetrating missile injuries have displaced motor vehicle accidents as the number one cause of catastrophic SCI (Fig. 11-1).[26] The damage caused by a projectile is proportional to the mass but more importantly to the square of the projectile's velocity. In other words, doubling the mass of the missile doubles its destructive effect; however, doubling the velocity increases the destructive effect by a factor of four.[31,32,33] Because velocity is the more important factor governing tissue damage, gunshot wounds are routinely classified based on velocity. Low-velocity gunshot wounds are those in which the projectile's velocity is less than 2000 ft/sec. Most hand guns are in this category. High-velocity gunshot wounds are those in which the projectile travels at velocities greater than 2000 ft/sec. Military and assault weapons are in this category.

There are two principle mechanisms by which projectiles cause tissue damage once the victim is struck. The first is by direct trauma as the bullet passes through physiologic tissue. The second is by indirect shock waves to the immediate adjacent tissue.

The Rancho Los Amigos Medical Center study shows that gunshot wounds in the upper thoracic spine highly outweigh fractures as a source of SCI.[34] There is limited information on spinal stability relative to gunshot wounds. Studies have shown that the vast majority of gunshot wounds involving the vertebral column result in stable injuries irrespective of the neurologic consequences.[35] The few cases resulting in spinal instability were wounds that involved damage to both pedicles or facet joints of the same vertebra or motion segment, respectively. All of the cases resulting

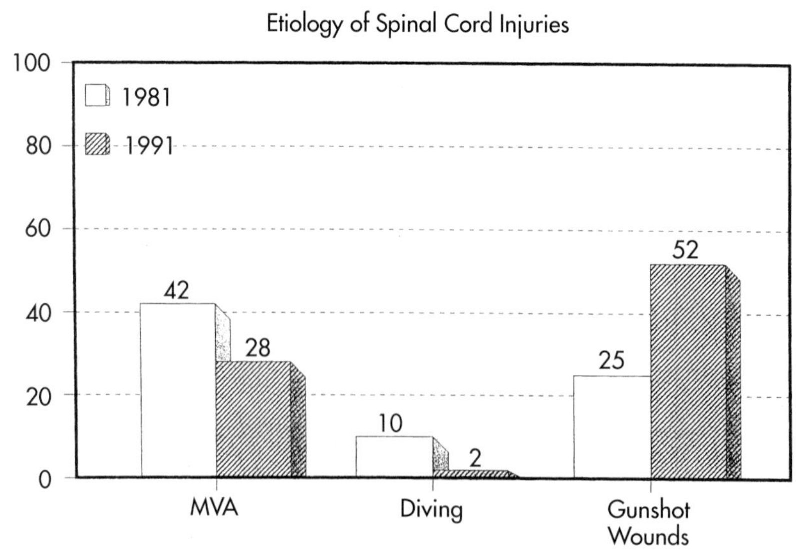

FIGURE 11-1

A, Multiple gunshot wounds to thoracic spine with projectile fragment in the spinal canal. **B,** CT scan demonstrating spinal canal violation.

in instability occurred in the cervical or lumbar spine.[34] The presence of the rib cage and sternum as supporting structures to the thoracic spine serve as a hindrance to instability from gunshot wounds. This includes those missile injuries that cause fractures of both pedicles or both facet joints in the thoracic spine.

Gunshot wounds to the spine with associated neurologic deficits usually result in complete SCI.[36] If the missile is located within the spinal canal and the patient has a complete SCI, there is no benefit to removing the bullet (Fig. 11-2). Controversy continues to exist regarding the treatment of incomplete SCI secondary to gunshot wounds in which the bullet lies within the spinal canal. The Rancho study showed that in patients who sustained gunshot wounds between T1 and T11 with incomplete SCI did improve following bullet removal. The results, however, were not statistically significant when compared with a similar population in which the bullet was left in situ.[36] These patients also had improvement. There was no significant difference in motor return in these two populations. This suggests that when a missile lies within the spinal canal in the region of the thoracic spine there is no need to remove the bullet. At the thoracolumbar junction the results of two similar populations indicated that bullets should be removed in patients with incomplete injuries. Regarding the cervical spine, it seems reasonable to remove all bullets within the spinal canal regardless of neurologic injury. This is because in the cervical region root escape allows a significant increase in functional ability when compared with the thoracic spine.

Recent studies have shown that low velocity gun shot wounds penetrating the abdominal viscera and resulting in SCI do not require removal to prevent infection.[37] Lead toxicity secondary to missile injuries to the spine is extremely rare thus removal is not indicated in these cases.[38,39]

A

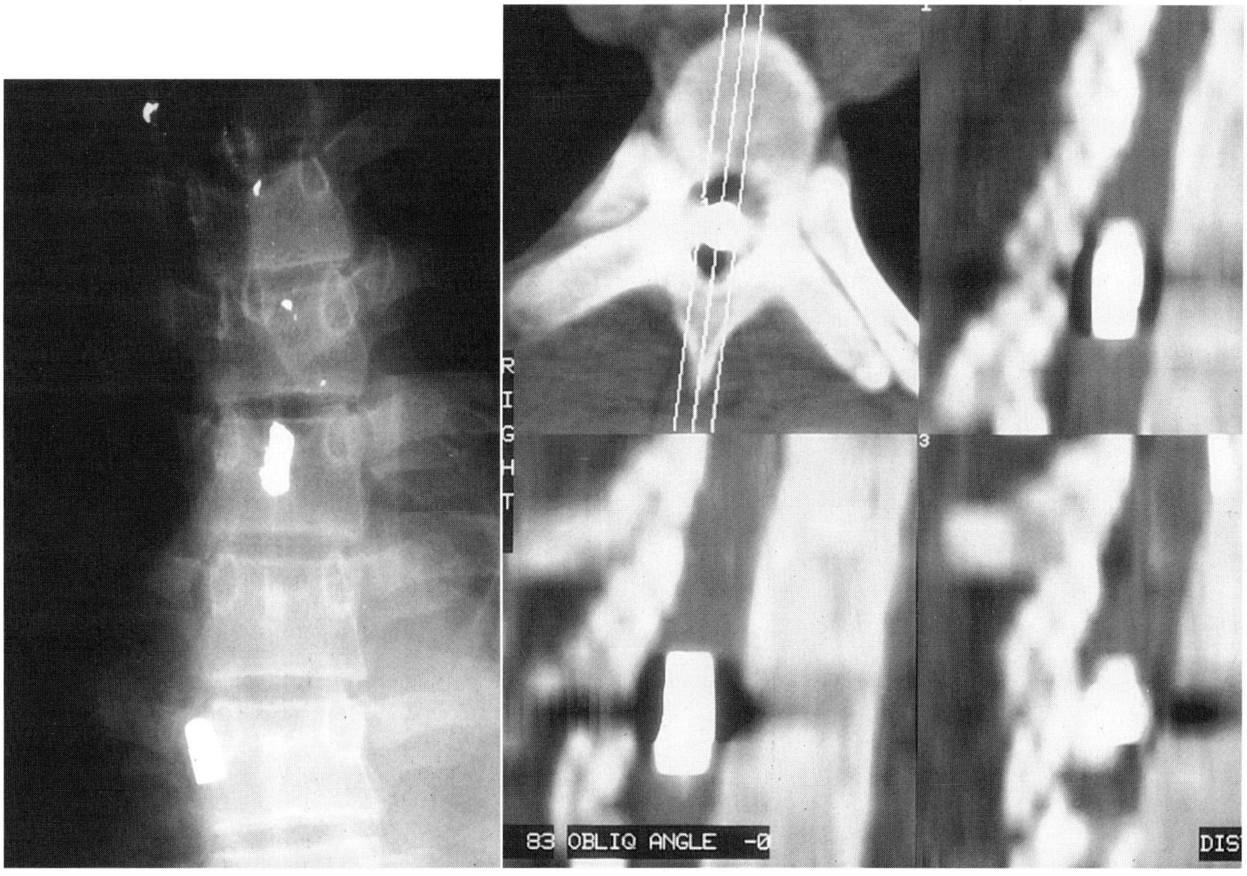

B

FIGURE 11-2

Computed tomography (CT) scan demonstrating spinal canal violation.

SURGICAL APPROACHES

The debate over which surgical approach is the most appropriate for upper thoracic fractures (T1–T4) with spinal canal compromise continues (Table 11-1). Fractures occurring in the upper thoracic vertebra, T1–T4, present a unique problem in the decision making process. This is due to the close proximity of the great vessels as well as the overlying sternum and clavicle. There are many approaches described for this area of the thoracic spine. When the decision has been made to decompress these most cephalad thoracic vertebra, a choice between the extension of the Smith-Robinson (anterior cervical), supraclavicular, transaxillary, and the third rib resection transthoracic approach has to be made. The supraclavicular approach may require resection of the sternoclavicular area. Below the level of the fourth thoracic vertebra, the transthoracic approach is the principle technique providing anterior access.

Recently, advocates of anterior procedures have used minimally invasive thoracoscopic techniques to perform decompression and anterior stabilization of the thoracic spine. There is a costotransversectomy extrapleural approach, which provides anterior lateral exposure, and the standard posterior approach. Cases requiring decompression should be approached through an anterior technique. This route directly addresses the pathology and allows for adequate placement of rigid fixation to reconstruct the anterior and middle columns of the thoracic spine. Furthermore, the anterior approach permits fusion of a minimum number of motion segments. Cases requiring stabilization alone are most easily approached posteriorly. This includes fractures associated with rib and sternal injuries in patients who are complete paraplegics.

ANTERIOR APPROACHES TO THE CERVICAL THORACIC JUNCTION—SMITH-ROBINSON EXTENSION

The extension of the Smith-Robinson approach is indicated for the exposure of the first and second thoracic vertebra.[40] It allows for anterior decompression for spinal canal compromise. It cannot be used for decompression or instrumentation at the third thoracic vertebra.[41,42] One should consider another approach to the upper thoracic spine in patients with short stout necks. These patients require a variant of the supraclavicular approach and may require an osteotomy of the manubrium and proximal clavicle to achieve adequate exposure of the second thoracic vertebra.

This anterior approach is straightforward. This approach is medial to the sternocleidomastoid muscle and the carotid sheath.[41,42] The patient is placed in the supine position on the operating table. A longitudinal roll is placed between the scapulae. This facilities extension of the cervical spine and allows greater exposure. Placement of an esophageal stethoscope allows for definitive location of the esophagus later in the approach. A decision is now made whether to approach the cervical thoracic junction from the right or left side. Proponents of the right-sided approach cite the possibility of an injury to the thoracic duct when making a left-sided approach. The thoracic duct enters the venous blood flow at the junction of the left subclavian an left internal jugular veins. It is in the vicinity of the cervical thoracic junction in a left-sided approach. A fatty meal the evening before surgery may help in identifying this structure. Attempts should be made to isolate this structure. If it is injured, a chylothorax may ensue. The thoracic duct should be double ligated if injured. Proponents of the left-sided approach cite the more dangerous location of the recurrent laryngeal

Table 11-1. Anterior Surgical Approaches

Approach	Indication	Levels
Cervical extension	Anterior decompression Anterior stabilization	T1–T2
Supraclavicular	Anterior decompression Anterior stabilization	T1–T3
Transaxillary	Anterior decompression Anterior stabilization	T1–T4
Third rib resection Transthoracic approach	Anterior decompression Anterior stabilization	T1–T4
Transthoracic approach	Anterior decompression Anterior stabilization	T5–T10
Thorascopic	Anterior decompression Anterior stabilization	T5–T10
Costrotransversectomy	Anterior decompression	T4–T10

nerve on the right side. Damage to the recurrent laryngeal nerve manifests itself clinically by producing hoarseness secondary to vocal cord dysfunction. The nerve on the right side courses lateral to medial over the lower cervical spine (C6-C7 area). On the left side the nerve lies in the more protected area between the trachea and the esophagus. Once the decision has been made to approach the cervical thoracic junction from the right or left side, the head is turned to the opposite side of the intended approach.

The intervertebral disks above and below the vertebral body in question are isolated. Complete removal of these disks is executed before performing the vertebrectomy. Small angled curettes now readily pass posterior to the thoracic vertebral body at its cephalad and caudad levels. A high-speed burr rapidly removes the anterior 75% of the vertebral body. Two mm Kerisson rongeurs are used to complete the decompression. Autogenous bone graft is contoured to fit into key holes channeled in the bodies above and below the decompression. Internal fixation in the way of an anterior spinal plate also can be applied to increase stability.

SUPRACLAVICULAR APPROACH

If inadequate exposure for the upper thoracic spine is apparent, the surgeon should change to a supraclavicular approach.[41,42] This is done by dividing the sternocleidomastoid at the sternoclavicular origin. The external jugular vein has a variable course and may have to be taken at this time. Care should be taken to avoid damaging the underlying internal jugular vein. The omohyoid muscle is divided which reveals the carotid sheath. The route to the upper thoracic spine is posterior and lateral to the sheath as it is retracted medially. The anterior scalene muscle with the overlying phrenic nerve is now visible. The phrenic nerve courses lateral to medial as one progresses in a more caudad direction. The phrenic nerve is gently retracted medially. The anterior scalene muscle can now be safely divided. Posterior to this muscle lies the prevertebral (Sibson's) fascia. The upper thoracic spine is apparent in the midline and the pleural cavity is lateral. Incision of the prevertebral fascia at the level of the transverse processes of the upper thoracic spine allows the surgeon to retract the visceral pleura inferiorly. Dissection now proceeds to expose the second and third rib heads. The surgeon is now prepared to perform an anterior decompression of the upper thoracic spine. For further details on thoracic vertebrectomy, see the section "Transthoracic Approach."

TRANSAXILLARY APPROACH

Yet another approach to the upper thoracic spine is the transaxillary approach, which provides good access to the first through fourth thoracic vertebra. This approach is advantageous in that no major muscle groups require division during the procedure; therefore, patients are able to recover rapidly. The approach is difficult in obese patients. Postoperative neuralgia occurs in 3% of cases.[42]

The patient is positioned in the right or left lateral decubitus position. The extremity is well padded and abducted exposing the axilla. A 10-cm transverse incision is made at the base of the axillary hair line. The subcutaneous fat is divided in line with the incision. Take care not to undermine the soft tissues at this level. This leads to a high preponderance of seromas that may result in wound dehiscence and/or infection. The pectoralis major muscle is identified and isolated in the anterior half of the wound. It is divided with electrocautery. Locate the chest wall and mobilize the soft tissues in a cephalad direction. This is an avascular plane. The first rib is palpated within the arch of the second rib at the apex of the chest cavity. Counting in a caudad direction, the third rib is identified. The intercostal brachial nerve, which is seen exiting from the second intercostal space, is located. This sensory nerve innervates the medial aspect of the upper arm. It should be segmentally resected to avoid postoperative neuralgia, which occurs in 3% of cases.[42]

As was described for the third rib resection transthoracic approach, it is the third rib that is the gateway for gaining exposure to the upper thoracic spine. The third rib is identified and exposed using electrocautery as well as Alexander and Doyen elevators. The rib is removed with bone cutters. The thorax is entered by incising the parietal pleura in the bed of the resected third rib. Care is taken not to damage the lung. A rib spreader is used to facilitate exposure. The lung may be packed with moist laparotomy pads to increase visualization. The parietal pleura can now be seen on the anterior aspect of the upper thoracic vertebral bodies. Intercostal vessels are located at the midpoint of the thoracic vertebral bodies. These vessels are mobilized with right angle clamps and ligated with silk sutures or vascular clips. They can now safely be divided. Care should be taken not to divide these vessels in close proximity to the aorta. If this is done and the ligature inadvertently comes off, repair may be difficult. Confirmation of the vertebral level of interest is documented by counting the ribs or radiography. Anterior decompression can now be performed. For details on vertebral body decompression, refer to the section "Transthoracic Approach."

TRANSTHORACIC APPROACH

The third rib resection transthoracic approach to the upper thoracic vertebral bodies is indicated for anterior decompression and stabilization of the first through the fourth thoracic vertebra. This is the most common anterior approach to the upper thoracic spine.[41,42] Kyphosis may allow extension of this approach to the lower cervical level. Removal of the third rib enlarges the operative area and provides visualization and bone graft material when a complete vertebrectomy is indicated.

General anesthesia is induced with the use of a double-lumen endotracheal tube. The patient is placed in the right lateral decubitus position. Entry to the left chest cavity is preferred because in the event of vascular injury, the aorta is readily mobilized and easier to repair than the venous structures on the opposite side. The skin is incised along the medial caudal border of the scapula under the axilla to the sternocostal junction of the third rib. The trapezius, latissimus dorsi, rhomboid, and serratus muscles are dissected with electrocautery to minimize bleeding.

The third rib is mobilized and removed from the costal cartilage anteriorly to the rib angle posterolaterally. The left lung is deflated. Intercostal vessels (segmental vessels) are mobilized and tied as needed. A vertebrectomy is performed by first identifying the correct level. This is facilitated by remembering that the respective rib inserts at the disk space above the respective vertebral body. For example, the third rib inserts posteriorly at the T2-T3 disk space. If one is in doubt intraoperative radiographs are necessary. Next the caudal level of the vertebral body pedicle is located. This is properly done by removing the head of the rib and inserting a nerve hook or small angled curette gently into the nerve root foramen. The posterior extent of the vertebra is now apparent allowing for rapid removal of the anterior and middle columns. Please see the "transthoracic approach" section for further details regarding thoracic vertebrectomy. The disk space above and below are completely debrided, which completes the anterior decompression. Bone graft and rigid fixation now complete the procedure.

THIRD RIB RESECTION TRANSTHORACIC APPROACH

The indications for the transthoracic approach are anterior decompression and stabilization of the fourth through the tenth thoracic vertebral bodies.[41,42] Proper rib resection is imperative. If the surgeon desires to remove an entire vertebral body, the rib cephalad to the body in question should be removed. This allows for a direct in line view of vertebral pathology rather than an angled view, which would make decompression of the spinal canal difficult. If exposure of the disk space only is necessary, then remove the rib that leads to that disk, for example, the T5 rib for the T4-T5 disk.

A double lumen endotracheal tube is place. The patient is placed in the right lateral decubitus position. The chest is centered over the break in the table. The table is extended to facilitate rib separation during this approach. The skin is incised from the sternocostal junction anteriorly to the lateral border of the paraspinous muscles posteriorly. The surgeon counts the ribs from a caudad to cephalad direction. Electrocautery is used to dissect the outer periosteum off the rib. Elevators are used to free the medial surface of the rib from the underlying pleura. Care must be taken to avoid damaging the intercostal vessels and nerves on the inferior aspect of the rib in question. Cut the rib as far posteriorly as possible. This is approximately midway between the costotransverse joint and the rib angle. Remove the anterior aspect of the rib and the sternocostal junction. The rib is saved to use for a source of autogenous bone graft. The posterior cut edge is carefully smoothed with a rongeur, and bone wax is added to prevent bleeding. Incision of the underlying parietal pleura opens the chest cavity. Self-retaining rib retractors are used to develop the interspace. The lung is deflated.

Careful placement of retractors can further mobilize the lung medially. The thoracic spine is easily palpated underneath the parietal pleura. The parietal pleura is elevated off of the thoracic disk space. This area is avascular. The pleura is mobilized in a caudad or cephalad direction with Metzenbaum scissors. Care should be taken to mobilize the segmental vessels, which lie in the middle of the thoracic bodies and are parallel to the disk space. These are mobilized with right-angle clamps and double ligated with silk ties. The rib head is removed. This exposes the cephalad disk space. For example, the T5 rib head exposes the T4-T5 disk space. The inferior aspect of the rib head marks the superior aspect of the vertebral pedicle. The superior and inferior aspects of the pedicle can be demarcated with a nerve hook or a number 4 Pennfield dissector. The surgeon now has access to the posterior aspect of the vertebral body. Malleable retractors are placed between the thoracic aorta and the anterior longitudinal ligament of the thoracic spine. An aggressive pneumatic burr is used to perform a rapid vertebrectomy of the anterior 75% of the vertebral body. A less aggressive diamond burr or curved curettes and Kerrison rongeurs complete the decompression. Epidural bleeding may be encountered. This is controlled with bipolar electrocautery, thrombin-soaked gelfoam, or avitene. Care is taken to completely remove the intervertebral disk above and below the debrided vertebral body. The rib is fashioned to bridge from the body above to the body below. This is accomplished by troughing the next caudad and cephalad vertebral body. Once the bone graft is in place, the decision to stabilize the spine using internal fixation can be easily performed.

The preferred way to perform anterior stabilization is through the use of screw plate or screw rod systems (e.g., Kaneda device or Z plate).

THORASCOPIC APPROACH

Although video-assisted thoracic surgery was described nearly a century ago, its application in the treatment of thoracic spine fractures has only recently become popular.[43,44,45] The indications for the use of thorascopic techniques include fracture decompression and stabilization. This technique allows access to the thoracic spine from the second to the twelfth thoracic level. There is a significant learning curve that accompanies the use of this new technique. Preoperative planning is mandatory and patients should be consulted on the possibility of converting this minimally invasive procedure to an open technique if problems arise. These problems include inadequate visualization because of equipment failure or increased bleeding, injury to the great vessels or lungs, and the inability to adequately decompress or stabilize the thoracic spine.

The use of a larger room is advisable because of the amount of equipment necessary to perform this procedure successfully. Equipment includes the fluoroscope, video module, ventilator, and the surgical instruments. The use of somatosensory evoked potentials is also recommended.

Patients are placed in the lateral decubitus position. It is important that the patient is placed directly lateral, and this position is maintained throughout the procedure. This allows the surgeon to maintain three-dimensional orientation about the thoracic spine. Intraoperative fluoroscopy is necessary to confirm specific vertebral levels. Anesthesia should be induced with the use of a double lumen endotracheal tube. Lung deflation facilitates visualization during thorascopic procedures.

The initial portal should always be placed between the 6th and 7th ribs in the midaxillary line. This allows for clear visualization that is not impeded by the diaphragm. Care should be taken when portals are made inferior to the 7th rib. This is because, when the lung is deflated, the diaphragm elevates placing intraabdominal contents at risk when portals are made below the 7th rib. Additional portals should not be placed in close proximity to the initial one. This causes difficulty when attempting to triangulate instruments in thoracic spine decompression. The so-called reverse "L" pattern described by McAfee is useful when making subsequent portals.[43] Two additional portals are made in the midaxillary line usually two interspaces above and two interspaces below the 6th interspace. The final portal is located at the posterior axillary line superiorly to retract the lung or inferiorly to retract the diaphragm. Once all portals are in place, the correct level is located by counting the ribs in a cephalad to caudad direction. Fluoroscopic confirmation is also recommended. The rib head corresponding to the thoracic vertebral body is removed. This exposes the cephalad disk space and the pedicle. Removal of the pedicle is now accomplished with the use of endoscopic instruments. The posterior vertebral body can now be excised under direct visualization. Anterior stabilization is possible but difficult via the thorascopic approach. Staged posterior stabilization can be performed in these cases. Postoperatively, a chest tube is placed in one of the portals. It can be removed on the second postoperative day.

McAfee et al. have reported on complications in a multicentered study.[43] The common complications are intercostal neuralgia and atelectasis. Blood loss greater than 2400 ml has occurred in a small number of patients undergoing vertebrectomy. Puncture of the hemidiaphragm was reported in one patient. Inadvertent durotomy also has been reported.

ANTERIOR LATERAL APPROACH (COSTOTRANSVERSECTOMY)

This approach is indicated in patients who exhibit significant obstructive or restrictive pulmonary disease and require an approach that does not violate the chest cavity. Costotransversectomy provides such an approach. Access to the anterior lateral and posterior elements of the entire thoracic spine is possible. The exposure of the anterior vertebral body is limited and if complete decompression is required, the transthoracic approach is preferred. Although this approach can be entirely extrapleural, entry into the chest cavity also is possible to afford greater visualization.

The patient is placed in the lateral decubitus position. The rib to be removed is determined by the level of the fracture. A longitudinal incision is made midway between the medial border of the scapula and the spinous processes of the thoracic vertebral bodies. This incision is centered over the rib corresponding to the level of pathology. The thoracolumbar fascia inferiorly or the trapezius and rhomboid muscles superiorly are divided with electrocautery. The medial border of the latissimus dorsi muscle also is cut. The paravertebral muscles are retracted to expose the ribs and the transverse processes of the thoracic spine. The costotransverse joints are located. The rib is subperiosteally dissected with electrocautery and periosteal elevators. Cut the rib 8 cm lateral to the costotransverse joint. The ligaments securing this joint are transsected and the dissection proceeds to the costovertebral joint. The ligaments securing the costovertebral joint are cut, and the rib is removed completely. Care should be taken to make sure that the anterior rib periosteum is completely free before removing the remaining rib. If this is not performed meticulously, the pleura can be disrupted and the chest cavity entered. The approach may be enlarged by removing adjacent ribs. In this case ligation of intercostal vessels is necessary. The transverse process is removed revealing the intervertebral foramen, which is located at the caudal level of the transverse process. Proceed medially following the intercostal nerve into the foramen. The posterior aspect of the vertebral body is now apparent along with the pedicle and lamina. Kerrison rongeurs can be used to perform an anterior lateral decompression.

Posterior Approach

The posterior approach to the thoracic spine is common and straightforward. It allows exposure of all thoracic vertebrae. The posterior approach is primarily indicated to provide stabilization and only to decompress the spinal cord if the source of compression involves the posterior elements.

Intraoperative radiographs confirm the correct level. Decompressive laminectomy, if indicated, can now be performed. Do not decompress posteriorly when diagnostic imaging demonstrates anterior compression. This does not improve neurologic outcome and may further destabilize the spinal motion segment.

Stabilization is best accomplished with the use of a hook rod system that allows the spine to be segmentally instrumented. The literature on fusion levels of fractures at the thoracolumbar region is extensive. The thoracic spine requires stabilization two levels above and two levels below the unstable vertebra. The surgeon need not worry about loss of motion segments in the more rigid thoracic area.

Once the spine is adequately exposed, preparation of the fusion levels can begin. Cephalad directed hook sites consist of pedicle hooks. These are prepared by exposing the coronally oriented facet joints. This is done by excising the inferior margin of the facet with a quarter-inch osteotome. Exposure of the superior facet cartilage is apparent. Pedicle hook trials are introduced in a cephalad direction and engage the pedicle inferiorly. A gentle medial-lateral translational force assures that the pedicle is engaged. Caudally directed hook sites are easily placed around the transverse processes. Do not confuse the ribs for the transverse processes. The remaining free facets are exposed in a similar fashion as described for pedicle hook placement. Currets are used to remove the facet cartilage. Autogenous bone graft is packed into the debrided facet joints. Additional grafts can be placed over decorticated lamina and transverse processes.

POSTOPERATIVE MANAGEMENT

Once decompression and stabilization of the thoracic spine has been achieved, postoperative care and rehabilitation begins. In the absence of neurologic injury, routine care consists of strict monitoring of intake and output. On the first postoperative day, the patient is allowed to be up in a chair and assisted ambulation is begun. This improves pulmonary function and limits skin breakdown. Prophylactic antibiotics are administered for 24 to 48 hours postoperatively. First-generation cephalosporins provide the best coverage for the most common infecting organisms.[46,47] Blood collection drains are discontinued on the second postoperative day. The hemoglobin level is monitored for the first 3 days after surgical intervention. All patients should have indwelling foley catheters. The foley is discontinued when the patient can safely transfer and ambulate. Nasogastric tubes are necessary to prevent the development of an ileus, which is common after trauma to the spinal cord. The nasogastric tube is discontinued when abdominal bowel sounds are auscultated, usually by the third postoperative day. Gastric pH is monitored, and antacids are administered when the nasogastric tube is in place to prevent the development of a stress ulcer. Electrolytes are monitored when the nasogastric tube is in place. Discharge to home is anticipated by the fourth or fifth postoperative day.

Patients who have undergone a transthoracic approach require the placement of chest tubes. These are kept to suction for 1 to 2 days and then converted to water seal. Chest tubes are routinely discontinued on the third postoperative day.

Patients with neurologic injuries require more extensive rehabilitation. Once the acute postoperative period is over, transfer to a facility dedicated to the rehabilitation of spinal cord–injured patients is highly recommended. Skin care is vital. These patients are log rolled every 2 hours to relieve pressure areas. This is done to prevent skin breakdown and decubitus ulcer formation. The most common areas for the development of skin breakdown in thoracic paraplegics are over the sacrum and trochanteric regions. The presence of an SCI often necessitates the initiation and instruction of a bowel and bladder program. The Foley catheter can be discontinued within the first week after surgery and self-catheterization every 4 to 6 hours is begun. The interval is adjusted based on urine volumes. Ideal postcatheterization volume is between 400 and 700 ml. Oral fluid restriction can be helpful in achieving longer catheterization intervals. A bowel program is integrated within the first week after surgery. This consists of a high fiber diet, stool softeners, and digital stimulation on a daily basis. The patient with a catastrophic SCI requires comprehensive rehabilitation. The expedient treatment of the initial traumatic injury allows for the rapid placement in a SCI facility.

BLOOD LOSS DURING SURGERY

Blood loss during spinal surgery can be extensive. Minimizing intraoperative blood loss is accomplished through comprehensive preoperative planning and meticulous surgical technique. Blood loss can be affected by a variety of factors, such as the type of approach, whether it be anterior or posterior, bleeding disorders, patient positioning, anesthesia factors, and medications. The preoperative evaluation should include a complete history to screen for bleeding disorders. If the bleeding history is questionable, a partial thromboplastin time, prothrombin time, and platelet count are indicated. A positive bleeding history requires specific tests for hemophilia (factor VIII and IX) in addition to the above tests. Many medications can increase bleeding and should be stopped prior to embarking on spinal surgery (Table 11-2).

Proper positioning during surgery may be the principle factor in decreasing blood loss.[48] Batson showed that obstruction of the inferior vena cava diverted blood flow into the vertebral epidural plexus.[49,50] Patients undergoing posterior approaches should be positioned with the abdomen free of pressure.[51] This limits the pressure on the inferior vena cava limiting blood loss through the surgical incision.

Hypotensive anesthesia is an invaluable tool in reducing intraoperative blood loss. It has been used extensively to reduce blood loss by 34 to 55% during spine surgery.[52–57] We define hypotensive anesthesia as that which maintains the mean arterial pressure between 40 and 70 mm Hg.

The availability of hemostatic agents can reduce intraoperative and postoperative blood loss. Substances such as bone wax, gel foam, surgicel, thrombin, and avitene can be applied to bone or soft tissue areas in which bleeding is difficult to control.

Table 11-2. Drugs That Can Affect Bleeding

1. Aspirin*
2. Dipyndamole*
3. Indomethacin*
4. Pheynylbutazone*
5. Ibuprofen, naproxen, and other NSAIDs*
6. Propranolol and other beta-blocking agents
7. Verapamil, diltiazem, and other calcium channel blockers
8. Penicillin and derivatives, cephalosporins, generally in high doses*
9. Nitrofurantoin*
10. Glyceryl guaiacolate
11. Nitroprusside
12. Furosemide
13. Clofibrale*
14. Dextran*
15. Diethylstilbesterol*
16. Penicillamine*
17. Promethazine and other antihistamines*
18. Glucocorticoids
19. Ethanol

From Hardaway RM, Adams WH: Blood clotting problems in acute care, 14–15:128–207, Acute Care 1988–89. Reproduced with permission of S. Karger AG, Basel.

* These drugs may prolong the bleeding time and therefore may contribute to bleeding.

PREVENTION OF INTRAOPERATIVE NEUROLOGIC COMPROMISE

The most disconcerting event that can occur during spinal surgery is that of inadvertent neurologic compromise. The mechanisms of spinal cord compromise during surgery include direct contusions of the spinal cord, malposition of bone grafts or implants, traction injuries from overcorrection, and the rarest, vascular compromise due to the ligation of main feeder branches to the spinal cord.

Prevention of these mechanisms are centered around proper visualization and instrument handling. Poor visualization can result in direct contusion of the neural elements. Visualization is kept at an optimal level by assuring good lighting, maintaining proper exposure, and controlling hemostasis. High-speed instruments should be used with care near the neurologic structures. Aggressive burrs should be changed to less aggressive diamond burrs as one approaches neural elements. These instruments should be used with two-hand control. One hand should rest against the patient to assure steadiness and prevent sudden movements. Spine instruments should be checked for sharpness. Sharp instruments require less force and, in the event of spinal cord contusion, cause less damage. Spinal monitoring is standard for these surgical procedures.

DURAL INJURY

Although dural tears can occur during both anterior and posterior operations on the upper thoracic spine, they are almost always avoidable. Adequate exposure and lighting is important in preventing inadvertent dural tears. If a tear occurs, a water tight closure with a 4-0 neurolon or silk suture should avoid long-term morbidity. Patients should be well hydrated postoperatively and remain at bed rest for 48 hours. If a dural tear is unrecognized at the time of surgery but manifests itself later by localized swelling or drainage of clear fluid from the wound, antibiotics should be started and reexploration and direct repair should be considered. At times, a leak occurs through an anterior approach and direct repair is not possible. These cases require the placement of an intrathecal catheter as described by Kitchel and Eismont.[58]

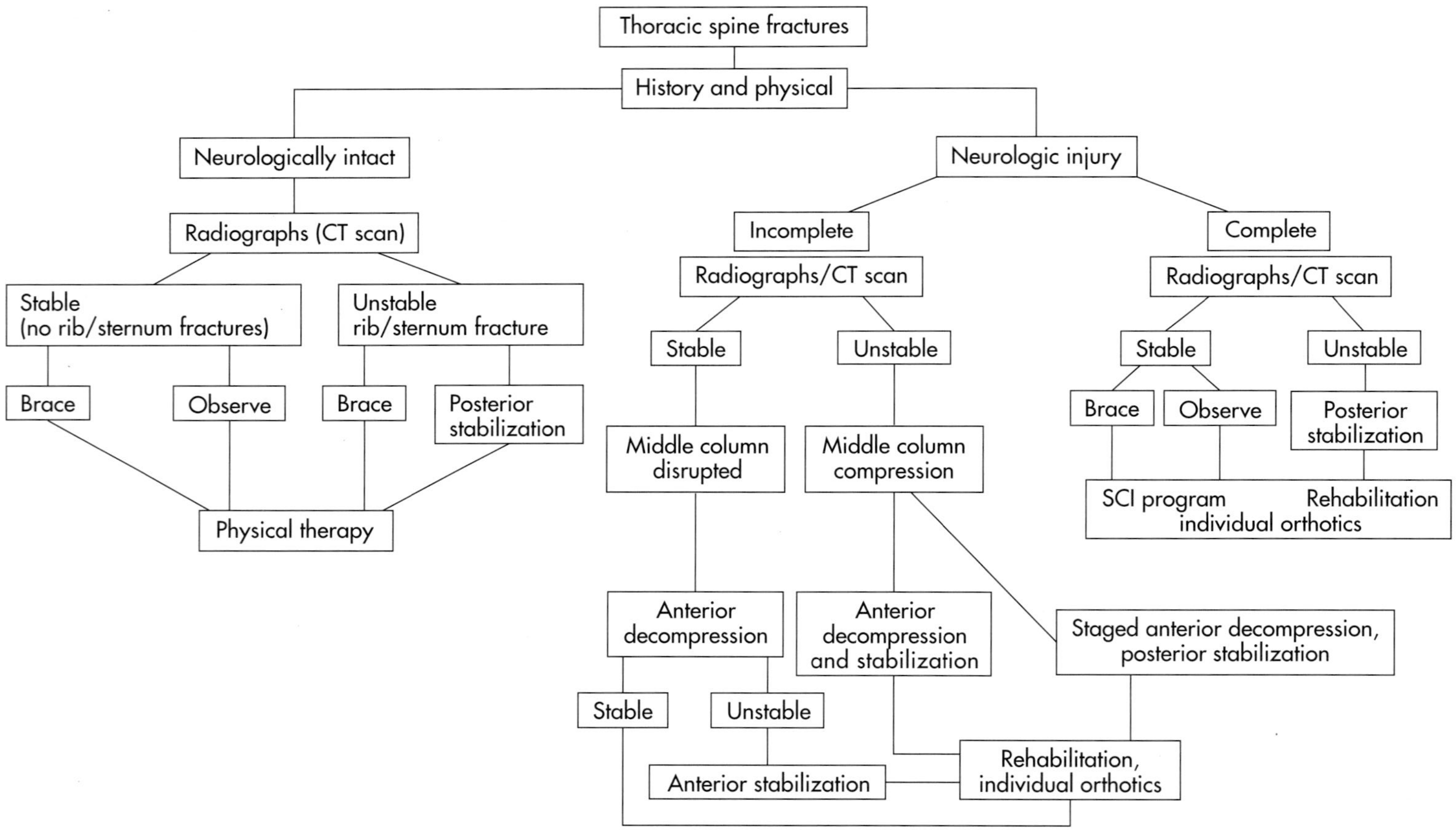

FIGURE 11-3

Suggested algorithm for thoracic spine fracture treatment.

SUMMARY

Fractures of the upper thoracic spine are rare and different criteria exist for determining instability when compared with fractures of the cervical and thoracolumbar regions. Radiographic criteria have been presented to aid the clinician in determining instability. Many of these fractures may be treated nonoperatively because of the inherent stability provided by the sternum and rib cage. Decompression should be performed in patients with incomplete SCIs. Decompressive procedures are usually accomplished through an anterior approach, but stabilization can be done anteriorly or posteriorly. The surgeon must adhere to proper patient positioning and operative technique to avoid the numerous complications associated with the treatment of upper thoracic spine fractures. An algorithm for diagnosis and treatment of thoracic spine fractures appears in Figure 11-3.

REFERENCES

1. Maiman DJ, Pintar FA: Anatomy and clinical biomechanics of the thoracic spine, *Clin Neurosurg* 38:296–324, 1992.
2. Nicoll EA: Fractures of the dorso-lumbar spine, *J Bone Joint Surg* 31B:376–394, 1949.
3. Holdsworth F: Fractures, dislocations, and fracture dislocations of the spine, *J Bone Joint Surg* 52A, 1534–1551, 1970.
4. Holdsworth FW: Fractures, dislocations and fracture dislocation of the spine, *J Bone Joint Surg* 45B, 6–20, 1963.
5. Bedbrook GM: Stability of spinal fractures and fracture dislocation, *Paraplegia* 9:23–32, 1971.
6. Bohlman HH: Treatment of fractures and dislocations of the thoracic and lumbar spine, *J Bone Joint Surg* 67A:165–169, 1985.
7. Bradford DS, et al: Surgical stabilization of fracture and fracture-dislocation of the thoracic spine, *Spine* 2:185–196, 1977.
8. Bryant CE, Sullivan JA: Management of thoracic and lumbar spine fractures with Harrington distraction rods supplemented with segmental wiring, *Spine* 8:532–537, 1983.
9. Burke DC, Murray DD: The management of thoracic and thoraclumbar injuries of the spine and neurological involvement, *J Bone Joint Surg* 58B, 72–78, 1976.
10. Dickson BH, Harrington PR, Erwin WO: Results of reduction and stabilization of the severely fractured thoracic and lumbar spine, *J Bone Joint Surg* 60A, 799–805, 1978.
11. Flexch JR, Leider LL, Erickson DL, et al: Harrington instruments and spine fusion for unstable fractures and fracture-dislocations of the thoracic and lumbar spine, *J Bone Joint Surg* 59A, 143–153, 1977.
12. Gertzbein SD, Offierski C: Complete fracture dislocation of the thoracic spine without spinal cord injury, *J Bone Joint Surg* 61A, 449–451, 1979.
13. Griffith HB, Gleave JRW, Taylor RG: Changing patterns of fracture in the dorsal and lumbar spine, *Br Med J* 1:891–894, 1966.
14. Nash CL, et al: The unstable thoracic compression fracture, *Spine* 2:261–265, 1977.
15. Sureff J, et al: Treatment of patients with unstable fractures of the thoracic and lumbar spine, *Acta Orthop Scan* 53:369–381, 1982.
16. Bohlman HH: Traumatic fractures of the upper thoracic spine with paralysis, *J Bone Joint Surg* 56A, 1299, 1974.
17. Clark K: Management of thoracic spinal injuries. In Youmans JR, editor: *Neurological surgery*, vol 4, Philadelphia, 1982,
18. Meyer PR: Fractures of the thoracic spine. T1 to T10. In Meyer PR, editors: *Surgery of spine trauma*, New York, 1989, Churchill Livingstone.
19. Hanley EN, Eskay MZ: Thoracic spine fractures, *Orthopedics* 12(5):689–696, 1989.
20. White AA III, Panjabi MM: *Clinical biomechanics of the spine*, Philadelphia, 1978, J B Lippincott.
21. Denis F: The three column spine and its significance in the classification of acute thoracolumbar spinal injuries, *Spine* 8:817–831, 1983.
22. Daffner RH, et al: The radiologic assessment of post-traumatic vertebral stability, *Skeletal Radiol* 19:103–108, 1990.
23. El-Khoury GY, Whitten CG: Trauma to the upper thoracic spine. Anatomy, biomechanics and unique imaging features, *Am J Radiol* 160:95–102, 1993.
24. Andriacchi T, et al: A model for studies of mechanical interactions between the human spine and rib cage, *J Biomech* 7:497–507, 1974.
25. Scher A: Associated sternal and spinal fractures, *S Afr Med J* 64:98–100, 1983.
26. Capen DA, et al: Etiology of spinal cord injuries: significant changes over ten years, *Ortho Trans*, vol. 17, No. 4, p. 1035.
27. Wolfe WG: Traumatic aneurysms of the aorta. In Sabiston DC, (editor). *Davis-Christopher's textbook of surgery*. vol 2, Philadelphia, 1978, WB Saunders, pp. 1890–1896.
28. Capen DA, et al: Non-operative management of upper thoracic spine fractures, *Orthoped Rev* 23(10):818–821, 1994.
29. Rimoldi RL, et al: The effect of surgical intervention on rehabilitation time in patients with thoracolumbar and lumbar spinal cord injuries, *Spine* 17:1443–1449, 1992.

30. Bracken MB, et al: A randomized, controlled trial of methylprednisolone or naloxone in the treatment of acute spinal cord injury: results of the second national acute spinal cord injury study, *N Engl J Med* 322:1405–1411, 1990.
31. de Muth WE Jr: Bullet velocity and design as determinants of wounding capability: an experimental study, *J Trauma* 6(2):222–232, 1966.
32. de Muth WE Jr: Bullet velocity as applied to military rifle wounding capacity, *J Trauma* 9(1):27–38, 1969.
33. Hopkinson DA, Marshall TK: Firearm injuries, *Br J Surg* 54(5):344–353, 1967.
34. Davis HW, Rosen C, Zigler JE: *The effect of gunshot wounds on stability of the thoracolumbar spine in paraplegia. Rancho proceedings* Downey, 1990, Rancho Los Amigos Medical Center.
35. Meyer PR: Symposium: management of fractures of the thoracolumbar spine, *Contemp Orthop* 16:57–86, 1988.
36. Waters RL, Atkins RH: Profiles of neurologic injury and recovery following gunshot wound to the spine, *Clin Orthop* 267:1421, 1991.
37. Raffi RP, Waters RL, Atkins RH: Gunshot wounds to the spine associated with a perforated viscus, *Spine* 14:808–811, 1989.
38. Dillman RO, Crumb CK, Lidsky MJ: Lead poisoning from a gunshot wound. Report of a case and review of the literature, *Am J Med* 66:509–514, 1979.
39. Switz DM, Elmorshidy ME, Deyerle WM: Bullets, joints, and lead intoxication. A remarkable and instructive case, *Arch Intern Med* 136:939–941, 1976.
40. Riley L: Surgical approaches to the anterior structures to the cervical spine, *Clin Orthop* 91:10–20, 1973.
41. Watkins RG: Cervical, thoracic and lumbar complications—anterior approach. In Garfin SR, editor: *Complications of spine surgery*, Baltimore, 1989, Williams & Wilkins.
42. Watkins RG: *Surgical approaches to the spine*, New York, 1983, Springer-Verlag.
43. McAfee PC, et al: Anterior thoracic corpectomy for spinal cord decompression performed endoscopically, Unpublished data (Minimally invasive approach to the spine course), 1996.
44. Regan JJ, McAfee PC, Mack MJ: *Atlas of endoscopic spine surgery*, St Louis, 1995, Quality Medical Publishing.
45. Parker, LM, et al: Minimally invasive surgical techniques to treat spine infections, *Orthop Clin North Am* 27(1):183–199, 1996.
46. Rubenstein E, et al: Perioperative prophylactic cephazolin in spine surgery, *J Bone Joint Surg* 76B:99–102, 1994.
47. Rimoldi, RL, Haye W: The use of antibiotics for wound prophylaxis in spinal surgery, *Orthop Clin North Am* 27(1):47–52, 1996.
48. DiStefano VJ, et al: Intra-operative analysis of the effects of position and body habitus on surgery of the low back, *Clin Orthop* 99:51, 1974.
49. Batson OJ: The function of the vertebral views and their role in the spread of metastases, *An Surg* 112:138–149, 1940.
50. Norgore M: Clinical anatomy of the vertebral views, *Surgery* 17:606–615, 1945.
51. Relton JES, Hall JE: An operation frame for spinal fusion: a new apparatus designed to reduce haemorrhage during operation, *J Bone Joint Surg* 49B:327, 1967.
52. Grundy BL, Nash CL, Brown RH: Arterial pressure manipulation alters spinal cord function during correction of scoliosis, *Anesthesiology* 54:249, 1981.
53. Khambatta Hi, et al: Hypotensive anesthesia for spinal fusion with sodium nitroprusside, *Spine* 3:171–174, 1978.
54. Lawhon M, et al: Controlled hypotensive anesthesia during spinal surgery. A retrospective study, *Spine* 9:450–453, 1984.
55. Malcolm-Smith, N, McMaster M: The use of induced hypotension to control bleeding during posterior fusion for scoliosis, *J Bone Joint Surg* 65(B):255–258, 1983.
56. Matras H: The use fibrin sealant in oral and maxillofacial surgery, *J Oral Maxilofac Surg* 40:617–622, 1982.
57. Messmer K: Hemodilution, *Surg Clin North Am* 55:659–578, 1975.
58. Kitchel SH, Eismont FJ, Green BA: Closed subarachnoid drainage for management of cerebrospinal fluid leakage after an operation on the spine, *J Bone Joint Surg* 71A(7):984–987, 1989.

12

NONSURGICAL AND SURGICAL MANAGEMENT OF FRACTURES AT THE THORACOLUMBAR JUNCTION

Alexander R. Vaccaro
Christopher P. Silveri
Richard A. Balderston

There are three distinct anatomic regions of the thoracolumbar spine. The thoracolumbar junction, consisting of the T11 to L2 vertebrae, acts as a transitional zone between the stable thoracic spine (T1–T11) and the flexible lumbar spine (L2–L5). The addition of the ribs in the thoracic spine, with their attachment anteriorly to the sternum, provide the majority of stability to this region. As with any structure that transmits applied forces, the potential for injury or failure is accented at the transitional zone (T11–L2) between rigid (thoracic spine) and nonrigid (lumbar) coupled segments.

The sagittal contour of the thoracolumbar spine results in a balanced posture with the occiput coming to lie in a vertical plane over the lumbosacral junction. This is possible through balance of a kyphotic thoracic spine (average 20° to 40°) and a lordotic lumbar spine (40° to 60°). As a result of this sagittal profile, when an axial load is imparted to the spine, it is transmitted primarily by the anterior elements of the thoracic spine and the posterior elements of the lumbar spine. In addition to the changes in sagittal alignment of the thoracolumbar spine, the morphology of the posterior vertebral elements (facet joints), undergo a gradual transition from the upper thoracic to lower lumbar spine. In the upper thoracic spine, the facets are aligned primarily in the coronal plane similar to those of the cervical spine. The facet orientation gradually changes to a more vertical posture as one moves in a caudal direction associated with a gradual rotation in the transverse plane to its final sagittal alignment in the lumbar spine. The coronal facet orientation in the thoracic spine allows for rotation in this region with restriction of flexion and extension, while the converse is true because of facet alignment in the lumbar spine. Panjabi,[1] in the textbook *Biomechanics of the Spine*, has shown that as a result of changes in both facet morphology and sagittal alignment there is an increase in torsional stiffness between T7 and L4 with the peak stiffness concentrated at the T12 and L1 levels.

FRACTURE MANAGEMENT

The goals of spinal fracture treatment are to obtain a stable, pain-free spine and prevent or limit the degree of neurological compromise. Treatment for stable thoracolumbar junction spinal fractures continues to be nonoperative care with early ambulation. Indications for surgery revolve around the presence and degree of neurologic deterioration and the severity of bony and ligamentous disruption incurred at the time of injury. The purpose of this review is to assist physicians in selecting the best treatment for a thoracolumbar junction fracture in specific patients. These recommendations are based on published fracture classification systems, including mechanisms of injury and extent of spinal cord compression. In addition, recommendations reflect a review of the clinical effectiveness of various treatment options, based on clinical and radiographic analyses and complication rates.

HISTORICAL PERSPECTIVE

Originally nonoperative treatment methods were the standard.[2] Postural reduction for spinal fractures was first suggested by Hippocrates and then Malgaigne.[3] Closed reduction for vertebral injuries was originally emphasized by Sir Ludwig Guttman in the 1920s.[4,5,6] Frankel, Bedbrook, and others began to concur with the notion of postural reduction for spinal fractures.[7,4,8] Unfortunately, the use of nonoperative treatment for certain fractures and spinal cord compressions yielded poor results, encouraging the need for better treatment regimens. In a 1977 study, Soreff reported a 23% incidence of excessive gibbus, scoliosis, and vertebral degeneration in patients treated nonoperatively.[9] Advances in anesthesia, radiology, and surgical techniques encouraged the use of more aggressive methods of treatment of these spinal fractures. By the early 1980s, it was reported that surgical fixation gave better control of spinal deformity, allowed earlier rehabilitation, and decreased hospital stays over nonoperative care.[10]

RADIOGRAPHIC ANALYSIS

The initial radiographic examination of a patient with a suspected thoracolumbar junction spinal injury should be an anteroposterior (AP) and lateral radiograph of the involved vertebral bodies.[11] The sensitivity of radiograph in delineating the degree of bony and soft tissue pathology is limited as simple compression fractures may be differentiated from burst-type injuries in only 54% of cases.[12] Further clarification of the degree of injury may require the use of tomography, computed tomography (CT) scanning, or magnetic resonance imaging (MRI) of the levels of injury.

Computed tomography scanning is useful to evaluate the integrity of the middle (posterior vertebral body) and posterior columns (posterior elements) of the vertebral body. The degree of facet subluxation is easily visualized as in the case of a naked facet sign after a fracture dislocation.

Magnetic resonance imaging is useful when visualization of the nonbony elements of the spinal column is necessary. Subtle ligamentous injuries inferred by the presence of tissue edema may be detected (i.e., the interspinous and anterior [ALL] and posterior longitudinal ligaments [PLL] as well as the presence of extrinsic cord compression from a disk extrusion, epidural hematoma, or invagination of the ligamentum flavum. Emory and coworkers found a 90% sensitivity and 100% specificity in the detection of torn posterior spinal ligaments with T2-weighted MRI sequences.[13] A "black-stripe sign" indicating a disruption of the PLL or supraspinous ligament and a bright signal within the substance of the interspinous space reliably represented ligamentous injury. An MRI scan is especially useful to rule out significant ligamentous or soft-tissue pathology in spinal cord injury (SCI) patients without evidence of radiographic abnormalities (SCIWORA). Sagittal MRI images, similar to reconstructed CT cuts, clearly allows visualization of upper thoracic injuries, which are easily obscured with plain radiography by overlying soft tissue and bony elements. Magnetic resonance technology delineates the degree of neural destruction by demonstrating spinal cord edema, hemorrhage, and neural transection.

Myelography is rarely used today after spinal trauma but may be selected in addition to CT scanning if MRI is not available to evaluate for extrinsic neural compression in the setting of a neural deficit. Myelography is also useful in the postoperative period after spinal instrumentation for fracture stabilization to evaluate the degree of residual thecal sac compression from intracanal debris or possibly hook impingement.[14,15]

Intraoperative spinal sonography (ISS) is another infrequently used imaging technique that allows detection of intracanal bone fragments after attempted indirect reduction with posterior spinal instrumentation.[16,17,18]

CLASSIFICATION SYSTEMS

An acceptable classification system of thoracolumbar injuries should be simple, logical, and easily accepted facilitating communication between caregivers and making research more efficient. The classification system should encompass the morphometry and mechanism of the injury, the severity of forces involved, an understanding of compromised neural and nonneural structures, and an inference to stability, all directing the caregiver to a logical treatment regime.[19,20,21] A summation of the more popular classification systems commonly used are listed in Tables 12-1 to 12-4.

It becomes self-evident from reviewing various classification systems that authors have classified thoracolumbar fractures according to morphology, mechanism of injury, or a combination of these factors in addition to injury severity in a complex and nonuser friendly fashion.[22–26] To complicate matters further, various authors use similar terminology to describe different fracture patterns adding further confusion to poorly understood subject matter. For example, the Denis flexion-distraction injury describes a tension failure to the posterior, middle, and anterior column with the axis of rotation anterior to the ALL. This is similar to the Chance fracture description of McAfee and the distraction-flexion injury of Ferguson and Allen.

A guiding light of all classification systems should be the emphasis on injury stability, which in turn should dictate treatment options determined specifically by fracture subtype.

SPINAL STABILITY

A compelling determination to make following an injury to the thoracolumbar junction is whether or not the spine is stable.[28] A precise determination of spinal stability is at best arbitrary due to lack of accurate knowledge regarding the mechanism of injury, the precise morphometry of the bony and soft tissue anatomy following trauma, a knowledge of normal spinal biomechanics related to the contributions to stability of the various spinal elements, and the degree of residual neurologic compromise. Early or acute instability may result in injury to the neural structures, whereas late instability may have consequences related to progressive deformity and chronic pain. An accurate description of stability would logically dictate an appropriate

Table 12-1. The Denis Classification System for Spinal Fractures

	Columns				
Type of Fracture	**Anterior**	**Middle**	**Posterior**	**Mechanism**	**Injury**
Compression					
Type A—anterior	Compression	None	None or distraction	Anterior flexion	
Type B—lateral	Compression	None	None or distraction	Lateral flexion	
Burst					
Type A	Compression	Compression	None	Axial load	Fracture of both endplates
Type B	Compression	Compression	None	Axial load and flexion	Fracture of superior endplate
Type C	Compression	Compression	None	Axial load and flexion	Fracture of inferior endplate
Type D	Compression	Compression	None	Axial load and rotation	Burst rotation
Type E	Compression	Compression	None	Axial load and lateral flexion	Burst lateral flexion
Seatbelt	None or compression	Distraction	Distraction	Flexion distraction	
Fracture dislocation					
Type A—flexion rotation	Compression/ rotation	Tension/ rotation	Tension/ rotation	Flexion rotation	
Type B–shear	Shear	Shear	Shear	Shear	
Type C–flexion-distraction	None or compression	Tension	Tension	Flexion distraction	

From Denis F: The three-column spine and its significance in the classification of the acute thoracolumbar spinal injurier, *Spine* 8:817–831, 1983.

Table 12-2. The McAfee Classification System

	Columns			
Type of Fracture	**Anterior**	**Middle**	**Posterior**	**Mechanism**
Wedge compression	Compression	None	None	Forward flexion
Stable burst	Compression	Compression	None	Compressive load
Unstable burst	Compression	Compression	Compression, lateral flexion, rotation	Compression, lateral flexion, rotation
Chance	Tension	Tension	Tension	Horizontal avulsion
Flexion-distraction	Compression	Tension	Tension	Flexion-distraction
Translational	Shear	Shear	Shear	Shear

Modified from McAfee PC, et al: The value of computed tomography in thoracolumbar fractures, *J Bone Joint Surg* 65A:461–473, 1983.

Table 12-3. The Ferguson and Allen Classification System for Spinal Fractures

	Columns		
Type of Fracture	**Anterior**	**Middle**	**Posterior**
Compressive flexion			
Type I	Compression	None	None
Type II	Compression	None	Tension
Type III	Compression	Blown out*	Tension
Distractive flexion	Tension	Tension	Tension
Lateral flexion			
Type I	Unilateral compression	Unilateral compression	None
Type II	Unilateral compression	Unilateral compression	Ipsilateral compression/ contralateral tension
Translational	Shear	Shear	Shear
Torsional flexion	Compression/rotation	Disrupted	Tension/rotation
Vertical compression	Compression	Bony compression	Bony involvement
Distractive-extension	Tension		Compression

From Ferguson RL, Allen BL Jr: A mechanistic classification of thoracolumbar spine fractures, *Clin Orthop* 189:77–88, 1984.
*Blown out—Evidence of middle column bone rotated into the neural canal between pedicles.

Table 12-4. The Dall and Stauffer Classification System for Thoracolumbar Junction Fractures and Neurologic Recovery

Fracture Subtype	**Degree of Kyphosis**	**Level of Maximal Canal Compromise**	**Neurologic Recovery**
Type I	>15°	Ligamentum flavum	>90%
Type II	>15°	Bone encircling canal	>90%
Type III	≤15°	Bone encircling canal	<50%
Type IV	≤15°	Ligamentum flavum	Variable

From Dall BE, Stauffer ES: Neurologic injury and recovery patterns in burst fractures at the T12 or L1 motion segment, *Clin Orthop* 233:171–176, 1988.

therapeutic regime. White and Panjabi defined instability as "the loss of the ability of the spine under physiologic loads to maintain its pattern of displacement so that there is no initial or additional neurologic deficit, no major deformity, and no incapacitating pain."[1] In an attempt to develop an applicable clinical algorithm regarding the determination of spinal stability, White and Panjabi proposed a clinical checklist following cadaveric biomechanical studies, which evaluated the degree of bony and soft tissue disruption as well as the neurologic status of the patient after injury (Table 12-5).

This checklist is based on the premise that with sequential loss of integrity of individual bony and soft tissue structures, the spine moves along a continuum toward eventual pathologic instability at which point further destabilization would result in pain or neurologic compromise.

Through retrospective analysis of radiographic and clinical outcomes, investigators have attempted to correlate the presenting degree of radiographic spinal deformity and neurologic examination with the potential for progressive bony deformity and neurologic compromise. Nicoll and Holdsworth believed that the most important factor for spinal stability was the integrity of the posterior ligamentous complex, including the supraspinous and interspinous ligaments, the facet joint capsule, and the ligamentum flavum.[29,30] Bedbrook believed that the anterior disk and vertebral body were the major sources of the spine's stability, not the posterior ligament complex.[7,31] From these two differing opinions came the two-column theory of spinal

Table 12-5. Determination of Thoracolumbar Instability

Element	Point Value*
Anterior elements destroyed or unable to function	2
Posterior elements destroyed or unable to function	2
Disruption of costovertebral articulations	1
Radiographic criteria	
Sagittal plane displacement >2.5 mm	2
Relative sagittal plane angulation >5°	2
Spinal cord or cauda equina damage	2
Dangerous loading anticipated	1

From White AA, Punjabi MM: *Clinical biomechanics of the spine*, ed 4, Philadelphia, 1990, JB Lippincott.
*Total of 5 or more unstable.

stability, which views the spine as having an anterior weight bearing column of vertebral bodies and disks with a posterior neural arch column resisting tension.[24,32] It was originally believed that destruction of either column would lead to an unstable spinal injury. In 1983, Denis proposed the three-column model of the spine previously described to more fully explain the wide diversity and results of spinal injuries.[22,33] Denis believed that injury to two out of three of these columns led to an unstable situation—an assertion subsequently supported in various biomechanical studies.[33] McAfee, also in 1983, supported the three-column concept of Denis but believed that certain two-column injuries such as a burst fracture with intact, posterior, bony and soft-tissue structures were stable mechanically.[34]

Other investigators have again correlated the degree of initial radiographic deformity with eventual functional and radiographic outcome to infer the degree or potential for spinal instability. Injuries involving the anterior vertebral body as a result of a compression force with an intact middle column are generally stable unless there is evidence of ligamentous disruption posteriorly due to tension failure, which may occur with greater than 50% loss of anterior vertebral body height.[35] Significant loss of posterior ligamentous integrity with the potential for progressive gibbus formation and late chronic pain in the setting of a compression fracture has also been experienced with patients who present with a kyphotic deformity of 30° or more.[36] Burst fractures (failure of anterior and middle column in compression) with significant disruption of the posterior bony or ligamentous structures is considered unstable especially if associated with loss of anterior vertebral height of greater than 50% or a kyphotic angulation greater than 25° to 30°.[36] The typical greenstick lamina fracture of the anterior laimina cortex is not considered a significant disruption of the posterior elements. Flexion-distraction injuries with tension failure of the posterior, middle, and possibly the anterior spinal column are considered unstable especially if the injury involves primarily the soft tissues, which heal poorly in the adult or if it occurs at the unstable transitional zone of the thoracolumbar junction between the rigid thoracic spine and mobile lumbar spine.[36]

TREATMENT OPTIONS

NONOPERATIVE

Patients without a Neurologic Deficit. Nonoperative treatment may be considered when there is sufficient posttraumatic spinal stability and when limited chance exists for progressive kyphosis and neurologic compromise to develop.[37,38] Nonoperative care provides for spinal stability through bracing or casting and allows for early rehabilitation and ambulation of the patient. The presence of spinal instability does not always require surgical treatment.[39] Prolonged bed rest or carefully supervised early ambulation with effective immobilization in some patients may be able to achieve the same degree of spinal stability as that achieved by spinal surgery.[40]

MINOR FRACTURES. Transverse process, spinous process, and articular process fractures resulting from direct trauma or severe muscular contractions may be treated symptomatically with or without a brace for comfort. Diligence in evaluating for occult instability or associated injuries must be undertaken to avoid under treatment. Before allowing full activity, dynamic flexion and extension radiographs should be obtained to rule out any significant injury. An acute isolated fracture of the pars interarticularis should be immobilized in a well-molded, total contact thoracolumbosacral (TLSO) orthosis.

COMPRESSION FRACTURES. One-column stable injuries such as a compression fracture can be treated with external immobilization such as plaster casts or orthotics (e.g., TLSO), which apply a force vector directly opposite to the traumatic force. Thoracolumbar braces should be designed to provide a three-point pressure force to resist flexion forces.[41] Injuries at the thoracolumbar junction require a TLSO for approximately 12 to 16 weeks. Severe compression fractures with attenuation of the posterior ligamentous complex may be treated nonoperatively as outlined above, especially in cases of mild kyphosis (<25° to 30°) and loss of anterior vertebral height of less than 50%.

BURST FRACTURES. Thoracolumbar junction burst fractures without evidence of significant posterior

Box 1. Treatment of Thoracolumbar Junction Spinal Injuries

Nonoperative Treatment	
No Neurologic Deficit	*Neurologic Deficit*
Sufficient Spinal stability	Sufficient spinal stability
Limited chance for progressive kyphosis and neurologic compromise	Lack of significant neural compression
Bedrest-limited	
Brace/cast wear	

Examples

1) *Minor Fractures*
2) *Compression Fractures*
   - Kyphosis <25–30°
   - Loss anterior vertebral height <50%
3) *Burst Fractures*
   - Kyphosis <30°
   - Loss anterior vertebral height <50%
4) *Flexion Distraction Injuries*
   - Bony involvement only - stable

column disruption, such as an initial sagittal kyphotic angle greater than 30°, loss of greater than 50% of anterior vertebral height or subluxation of the posterior facet joints, or widening of the interspinous process distance may be treated effectively nonoperatively with early ambulation and a total contact extension TLSO or body cast for 12 to 24 weeks. Cantor and Eismont evaluated 18 patients with fractures at the thoracolumbar junction at an average follow-up of 19 months after being treated in this manner.[42] No patient underwent a postural reduction. The average sagittal kyphosis angle at follow up was 20° (range of 9 to 31°) compared with 19° at initial presentation with all patients reporting minimal or no pain or restrictions in activities of daily living. Ninety-five percent of patients reported a satisfactory work score and no patient developed a neurologic deficit during their treatment period. Fracture morphology or deformity did not correlate with symptoms at follow-up.

Weinstein reported one of the few long-term follow-up studies on patients treated nonoperatively for thoracolumbar burst fractures in general not specifically localized to the thoracolumbar junction.[43] Seventy-eight percent of patients at initial follow-up were without a neurologic compromise and no patient developed a significant deterioration in their neurologic status at an average follow-up of 20.2 years. Eighty-eight percent of patients overall were able to return to their usual activities with only minimal discomfort and only 4 out of 42 patients experienced incapacitating pain secondary to a progressive deformity. The average sagittal kyphosis at follow-up averaged 26.4° in flexion and 16.8° in extension with the degree of kyphosis not correlating with pain or function at the patients last evaluation. Following this retrospective review, Mumford and Weinstein reviewed 41 patients retrospectively with a thoracolumbar burst fracture (78% type B) without evidence of a presenting neurologic deficit treated nonoperatively.[3] At the time of injury canal compromise averaged 37% (range 16%–69%), loss of vertebral height averaged 38.5% (range 6%–76%) and sagittal kyphosis averaged 16° (range 0° to 47°). At an average follow-up of 2 years, only one patient developed a neurologic deficit requiring surgery, and 66% of patients reported an excellent or good outcome concerning pain and function. Ninety percent of patients had a satisfactory work status related to their spinal injury. Sagittal kyphosis progressed an average of only 4° while canal compromise because of bony remodeling improved an average of 23%. The authors noted no correlation between the initial radiographic deformity and eventual outcome.

It appears that thoracolumbar junction burst fractures without significant compromise to the posterior column, that is, initial kyphosis angle less than 30 degrees, the absence of facet subluxation or spreading of the interspinous process distance, or less than 50% loss of anterior vertebral body height may be managed successfully with a well-molded orthosis or cast. Residual canal compromise or sagittal deformity at follow-up in the majority of reports has not correlated with subjective pain scores, work ability, or a patient's functional status. This has been supported by the series of Nicoll, McAfee, Mumford, and Weinstein.[3,25,43,44] Additionally, symptomatic posttraumatic spinal stenosis caused by retained intracanal fragments is an infrequent finding in the majority of nonoperatively treated patients.[45] It appears from a review of the literature that bony deformity, inclusive of sagittal alignment and anterior vertebral height, progresses marginally with nonoperative care. It is clear from the study of Gertzbein reviewing more than 1,019 spinal fractures in the multicenter spine fracture study for the Scoliosis Research Society that a residual kyphosis of 30° or more is associated with an increased incidence of back discomfort.[46] It is not clear as to which patients will progress to this degree of deformity. Indirect inference from the previous radiographic findings suggesting posterior column deficiency may be used to justify more aggressive treatment in this fracture group; although, as is seen in the previous review not all patients with evidence of posterior column attenuation develop a progressive deformity, and if they do, not all patients are symptomatic. Unfortunately, later surgical decompression and stabilization in instances of symptomatic posttraumatic thoracolumbar deformities is complex and is associated with a high incidence of posttreatment complications.

Disabling back pain may be a reflection of progressive degenerative changes developing over time as a result of the initial injury or a manifestation of residual foraminal stenosis, segmental instability, or sagittal deformity. Residual pain, although minor, is frequently reported at follow-up in nonoperatively treated patients. Mumford reported a 93% incidence of residual back (76%) and leg discomfort at follow-up, the majority of which was considered mild.[3] A similar incidence was reported by Weinstein (90%).[43] Nicoll reported a residual back discomfort at follow in 59% of patients with 40% of patients complaining of pain at their fracture site.[25] A definite shortcoming of nonoperative care in this patient population is the increased duration of bed rest and hospitalization time compared with surgically treated patients. Mumford's study, published in 1993, reported an average duration of bed rest of 31 days (range of 7–68 days) and an average duration of hospitalization of 29 days (range of 2–61 days). They recommended an average of 4 weeks of bed rest followed by 12 weeks of bracing in the treatment of these fractures.

Flexion Distraction Injuries. Flexion distraction injuries involving tension failure of the posterior, middle, and possibly the anterior bony columns may be treated in a hyperextension orthosis or cast for 12 to 24 weeks. At the completion of immobilization, dynamic flexion, and extension plain radiographs should be obtained to access for residual instability. Tension injuries violating the disk or intervertebral ligaments heal unpredictably and should be stabilized surgically.

Patients With a Neurologic Deficit. The literature is confused as to the most optimum treatment regimen in selected patients with spinal injuries and neurologic deficits. Reduction of fracture displacement and maintenance of vertebral body stability are the most important factors to consider in treating this subgroup of patients. These goals may be achieved by nonoperative treatment, but surgical treatment must be strongly considered if spinal stability or progressive neurologic deterioration is present. Many authors argue as to the precise causative factors for a patient's neurologic compromise relating it with various weighted emphasis to the initial force of impact or residual canal deformity and neural compression. While selected studies support the correlation between residual canal compromise and neurologic status, others support no relationship and postulate the cause for neurologic changes are related to the initial forces involved at the time of injury.[47,46,48] In the multicenter spine fracture study supported by the Scoliosis Research Society, only a weak relationship was determined between canal compromise and neurologic status including bowel and bladder function.[46] Hashimoto on the other hand noted an increased risk of neurologic deterioration in patients with greater than 35% canal compromise at T11-T12, 45% canal compromise at L1, and greater than 55% canal compromise at L2 and below.[48] Confusing matters further are reports citing no obvious relationship between functional outcome at follow-up and operative decompression.[49–52] Although it is well supported than significant canal remodeling is possible after thoracolumbar burst injuries, especially in younger patients, such remodeling with bony reabsorption is reported less frequently with greater than 50% canal compromise and evidence of deficiency of the posterior longitudinal ligament.[53,54,55] Radiographically (CT evaluation) it appears that lateral canal margins resorb preferentially possibly because of the pulsations of the anterior internal longitudinal venous plexus leaving behind a heart-shaped canal with a midsagittal spike of bone.[3,56]

Weinstein's retrospective long-term follow-up reported a 17% improvement in neurologic function in neurologically impaired patients without any worsening in patients treated nonoperatively.[43] Unfortunately, a comparative matched group of patients with similar motor deficits were not available to evaluate neurologic improvement in surgically treated patients. Less optimistic results have been reported by other authors in patients with a neurologic deficit who were treated nonoperatively. Willen et al. reported on 54 patients treated nonsurgically with T12 and L1 burst fractures of which the majority had significant neurological impairment.[57] Patients with certain fracture subtypes such as Denis type B, D, and E burst fractures faired poorly with nonoperative treatment as a result of persistent intractable pain, neurologic impairment, and radiographic signs of instability. Six patients required a delayed decompression and stabilization procedure, with 12 patients reporting severe pain with radiculitis. These authors noted a marked progression in the patients gibbus deformity with early mobilization and found those patients with greater than 50% canal compromise had no significant bony resorption at follow-up. They concluded that predictors of poor outcome in nonoperative-treated patients with thoracolumbar Burst fractures included loss of anterior vertebral height of greater than 50%, narrowing of the spinal canal greater than 50%, and any evidence of rotational malalignment.

Nonoperative treatment protocols may be effective in certain fracture subtypes of the thoracolumbar junction not at risk for progressive deformity as few patients develop significant neurologic deterioration, and the majority of incomplete lesions improve at least one Frankel grade. To date, no controlled prospective analysis has been performed comparing surgical decompression and stabilization with nonoperative care in neurologically impaired patients with obvious neural compression. Surgical care in this patient group may significantly improve functional outcome although this has not been definitively proved. Retrospectively, surgical stabilization shortens in-hospital stays and rehabilitation times although it has not conclusively improved long-term neurologic function or improved subjective pain profiles in patients without significant gibbus deformities (over 30 degrees) at follow-up.

BOX 2. OPERATIVE TREATMENT

No Neurologic Deficit	Neurologic Deficit
Lack of sufficient spinal stability	Similar to no neurologic deficit

Consider anterior approach with or without posterior approach depending on location of neural compression

Examples

1) *Compression Fracture*
   - -Loss of anterior vertebral height ×50%
   - -Kyphosis ×25–30°
   - -Subluxation posterior facets
   - -Widening posterior interspinous ligaments
2) *Burst Fractures*
   - -Similar to compression fractures
3) *Flexion Distraction Injuries*
   - -Ligamentous disruption
   - -Unstable bony involvement
4) *Fracture Dislocation*
   - -All types
5) *Distraction Extension Injuries*
   - -All types

OPERATIVE TREATMENT

Patients Without a Neurologic Deficit.

COMPRESSION FRACTURES. Surgical stabilization may benefit patients with a thoracolumbar junction compression fracture with loss of anterior vertebral height greater than 50% or initial kyphosis of greater than 25 to 30 degrees due to evidence of posterior ligamentous disruption and the potential for late pain and deformity. A four-hook, two-rod distraction system utilizing three- or four-point fixation is usually satisfactory. The more neutral orientation in both the coronal and sagittal plane of the thoracolumbar junction allows the application of short segment distractive forces to regain lost vertebral height without altering significantly spinal posture. This may be accomplished with a hook-rod construct posteriorly with down going hooks one or two levels below the injury level to two to three levels above the injury level depending on the fixation system utilized. A compression system may be used also because of the intact integrity of the middle column. The potential for retropulsion of an intervertebral disk must be considered with this mode of treatment. A lateral flexion injury at risk for progression may be treated with a distraction force (hooks, pedicle screws, rods) on the side of injury and a compression force on the contralateral side for adequate stability. The order of fixation is determined by the localized sagittal alignment at the level of injury to prevent unnecessary lordosis or kyphosis.

BURST FRACTURES. Although not uniformly agreed upon, some authors believe that patients with burst type injuries without neurologic sequelae benefit more with surgical rather than nonsurgical treatment.

Denis reported that surgical stabilization was superior over nonoperative treatment in all burst fracture subtypes after retrospectively reviewing 52 patients without evidence of a neurologic deficit.[58] Of the 39 patients treated nonoperatively, six experienced neurologic weakening during follow-up with 25% of patients not returning to full-time employment. Of the 13 patients treated surgically, all returned to their previous level of work, unless there were unrelated disability factors, which prevented employment. Surgical treatment as suggested by Denis for all patients with thoracolumbar burst fractures, regardless of neurologic injury, has not been supported in the literature. A common denominator in all well-designed studies is that those patients with evidence of anterior and middle column disruption with significant compromise to the posterior column, that is, kyphosis greater than 30 degrees, subluxation of the posterior facets, increase in the interspinous process distance, or loss of greater than 50% of anterior vertebral height may benefit from a posterior surgical stabilization procedure. Nonoperative treatment in this patient subgroup may lead to progressive spinal instability, late pain, and the possibility of neurologic embarrassment.

A posterior surgical approach utilizing distraction rod-hook instrumentation with three- or four-point fixation is usually adequate in stabilizing these injuries in the setting of intact posterior elements. The length of fusion levels is determined by the instrumentation system chosen and the region of the spine. Distraction is responsible for the majority of deformity correction. Combined with lordosing force, optimal sagittal alignment is obtained. A pedicle screw–based system may be utilized at the thoracolumbar junction to avoid immobilization of unnecessary spinal segments. Short segment pedicle instrumentation theoretically have several advantages including the ability to localize the levels of arthrodesis to one level cephalad and one level caudal to the injured vertebral segment, the ability to manipulate instrumented vertebral levels by means of three-column bony fixation, avoidance of canal penetration by surgical hardware, and the lack of dependence on the posterior lamina elements for fixation. Unfortunately, several authors have reported an early high failure rate of short segment pedicle screw configurations without reconstruction of the anterior column. These complications have included a progressive loss of sagittal alignment over time and a high screw breakage rate with associated pseudoarthrosis. Carl in 1992 reported on 38 patients who underwent posterior pedicle screw stabilization and fusion for unstable thoracolumbar and lumbar spine fractures.[59] At an average follow up of 2 years, there was an average loss of 6 degrees of kyphosis following the operative correction. Nine patients had broken hardware with fractures at the thoracolumbar junction.

McLain in 1993 reported on the early follow-up of 52 patients with thoracolumbar fractures treated with posterior pedicle screw instrumentation.[60] Nineteen patients in their study underwent short-segment pedicle fixation. At 6 months postoperatively, 10 of these 19 patients experienced significant loss of sagittal alignment with hardware failure contributing to loss of vertebral alignment in seven patients. The experience of the Thomas Jefferson University Spinal Cord Injury Center of the Delaware Valley attests to similar results with short-segment pedicle screw instrumentation. In unpublished data, 35 patients underwent short-segment pedicle instrumentation for thoracolumbar burst fractures followed for an average of 16 months.[61] All patients were noted to have complete restoration of vertebral height at the completion of their operations, and all were immobilized in a body cast in extension for approximately 3 months during fracture and fusion healing. At follow-up, 10 patients had an increase in sagittal kyphosis of greater than 10 degrees from their postsurgical alignment with 10 out of 148 pedicle screws either bending or broken (Fig. 12-1). Loss of vertebral alignment occurred in 47% of patients and was attributed to screw bending, breakage, or pedicle screw cutout through the cancellous vertebral body. If pedicle screw fixation is chosen, we recommend postoperative hyperextension cast treatment with a thigh extension followed by early instrument removal (around 18 months to avoid the possibility of inevitable hardware fatigue).

FLEXION-DISTRACTION INJURIES. Adult patients with flexion-distraction injuries with disruption through the interspinous ligaments, posterior longitudinal ligament, or disk space heal these injuries slowly and unpredictably and benefit from surgical stabilization.[62] A posterior compression system immobilizing the level above and below the injury usually is sufficient to insure stability. Caution in the use of this reduction maneuver must be exercised if the middle column is comminuted because of retropulsion of bone or if the posterior facets are incompetent, preventing controlled anatomic reduction. If the axis of rotation involves the anterior column with compression failure in this region, a distraction hook-rod, screw construct may be used to apply tension to the anterior longitudinal ligament with care not to overdistract the middle (i.e., incompetent PLL) or posterior columns.

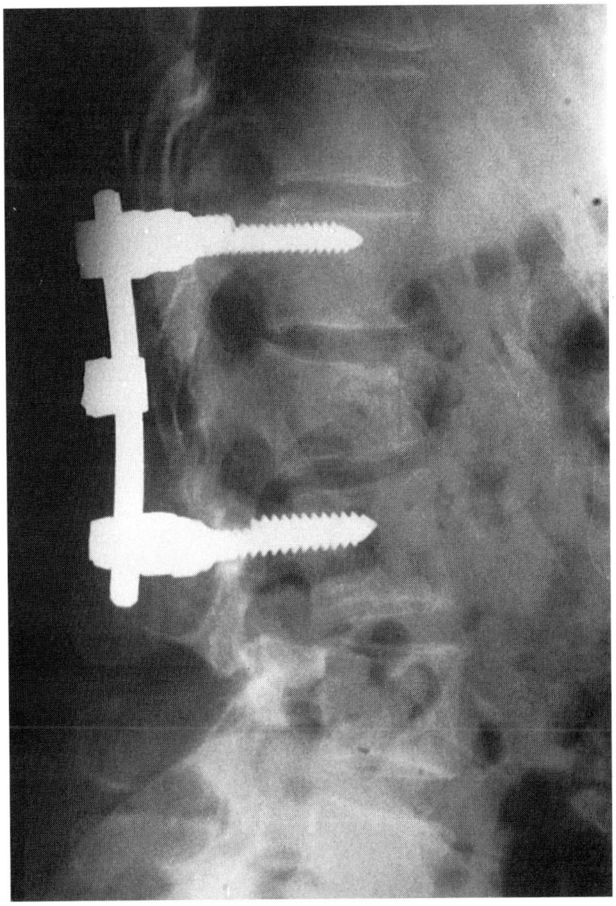

FIGURE 12-1

A lateral plain radiograph illustrating breakage of both the cephalad and caudal pedicle screws at 6-month follow-up after short segment pedicle fixation for an L1 burst fracture.

FRACTURE DISLOCATION. Any evidence of a posterior facet fracture dislocation, rotational instability, or a translational shear injury in the absence of a neurologic deficit is in need of a posterior segmental stabilization procedure to prevent further vertebral displacement and the potential for neurologic compromise.[63] An awake intubation followed by awake patient positioning is mandatory to allow the patient to assist voluntarily in splinting the unstable spinal lesion and to access neurologic status before induction of anesthesia at the completion of positioning. In flexion compression or flexion rotational injuries with an intact posterior longitudinal ligament, a distraction instrumentation system is used. A central tension band construct consisting of a doubled 16-gauge wire or a limited hook-rod claw configuration between the involved vertebral bodies may prevent over distraction in cases of suspected anterior longitudinal ligament attenuation. Various vector forces using universal hook-rod systems may be employed to enable anatomic fracture reduction in complete dislocations or severely unstable shear type injuries. Once reduction is complete, a neutralization construct consisting of multiple claws or pedicle screw fixation may be completed to prevent future fracture displacement.

DISTRACTION-EXTENSION INJURIES. Distraction-extension injuries fortunately are rare but are potentially devastating in terms of significant neurologic compromise (Fig. 12-2). These are usually seen in patients with metabolic or inflammatory bone disease, such as, ankylosing spondylitis or diffuse idiopathic skeletal hyperostosis, and a preexisting skeletal deformity, such as, excessive kyphosis. Great care must be taken in attempting to recreate the preinjury spinal alignment with flexion of the upper torso. Supine positioning may exacerbate the distraction-extension deformity and result in neurologic impairment. Once reduced, segmental internal fixation without an attempt to alter the preinjury sagittal alignment may be performed.

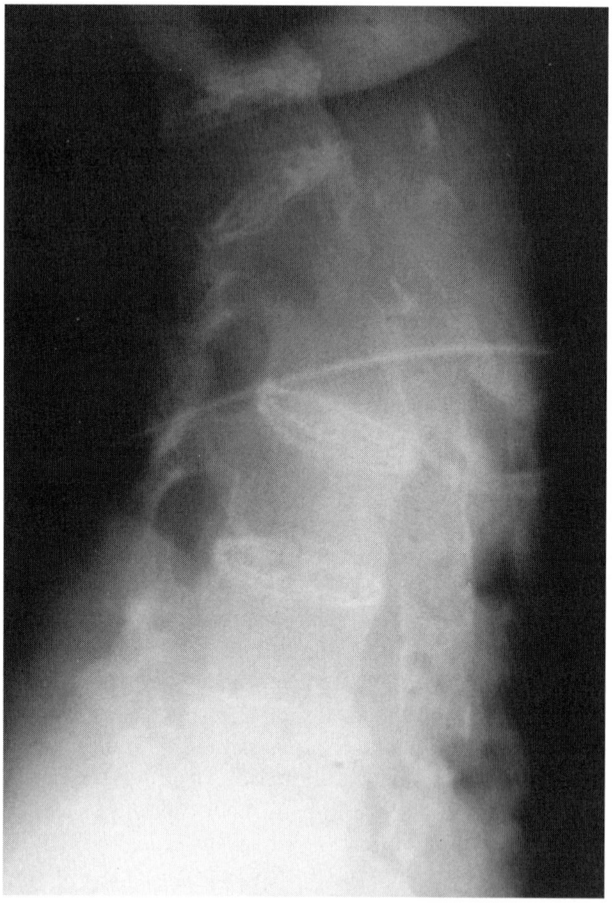

FIGURE 12-2

Distraction extension injury at the thoracolumbar junction in a patient with ankylosing spondylitis.

Rarely, if ever, is an anterior decompressive procedure necessary in the neurologically intact patient with an unstable spinal fracture. A later anterior decompression may be performed if evidence of neurologic deterioration develops in the face of significant anterior thecal sac impingement.

Patients With a Neurologic Deficit. The goals of surgical treatment in the patient with a thoracolumbar spinal fracture and a neurologic deficit include the restoration of spinal alignment and stability and the alleviation of neural compression.[64,65] The literature is unclear as to the precise benefit of acute surgical decompression over nonoperative treatment in a patient with documented neural compression and a neurologic deficit.[66,67] Operative and nonoperative treatment modalities may result in an improvement in neurologic function in both complete and incomplete SCI as bony stability ensues.[68] The rate and quality of neurologic improvement may be better with surgical decompression, but this has not been proved in a controlled prospective fashion. In Gertzbein's review of 1,019 spinal fracture patients for the Scoliosis Research Society, surgically treated patients had a greater improvement in neurologic function than nonsurgically treated patients, although the rate of improvement was not statistically significant.[46] In those patients who deteriorated neurologically after admission, surgically treated patients had a greater improvement neurologically at follow-up than those treated nonsurgically. Emergent surgical decompression is recommended for patients with documented neural compression and a progressive neurologic deficit or for patients with an incomplete SCI and an irreducible spinal dislocation.

The literature is clear on the fact that surgery shortens the in-hospital stay and rehabilitation time of neurologically deficient patients.[69,70,71] Surgery is also effective in improving the neurologic status of patients once neurologic improvement has reached its plateau as late as 2 or more years after the traumatic event.[72–79] Surgical decompression may be beneficial in the setting of a complete SCI especially at the thoracolumbar junction to gain function of important individual nerve roots to improve a patients overall quality of life.

BURST FRACTURES. Burst fractures with an incomplete neurologic deficit at the thoracolumbar junction should undergo direct decompression of all compromised neural elements followed by graft and instrument reconstruction (Fig. 12-3 A,B).[80] A limited posterior compression construct, consisting of hooks or pedicle screws and rods, following anterior strut graft reconstruction of the corpectomized level is a common means of treating this injury (Fig. 12-4). The bone graft, preferably autogenous iliac crest, may span from the superior endplate of the vertebral body above the injured level to the inferior endplate of the vertebral body below the level of injury. Sutton et al. retrospectively reviewed the experience of the Thomas Jefferson University Spinal Cord Injury Center with this form of vertebral reconstruction in 30 patients following anterior decompression for a thoracolumbar burst fracture.[81] The average preoperative sagittal kyphosis at the fracture level measured 17.9° with an average loss of vertebral height of 49.9%. Immediately, postoperatively sagittal angulation improved an average of 19° to a final lordotic angle of 1 degree with an improvement of vertebral height of 74%. At an average follow-up of 24 months, all patients had a solid arthrodesis radiographically with a final loss of 3° of sagittal alignment at follow-up. An alternative means of stabilization is with anterior plate fixation following graft application between the inferior endplate of the cephalad vertebral body and the superior endplate of the caudal vertebral body (Fig. 12-5). This may potentially avoid a subsequent posterior stabilization procedure. In neurologically impaired patients with evidence of a lamina fracture on a preoperative CT scan, the possibility of entrapped neural elements within the fracture fragments noted in 50% of such cases must be considered and an appropriate posterior decompression followed by dural repair if necessary should be undertaken.[82] The initial exposure should be centered over the level above and below the fractured lamina to avoid injury to vulnerable entrapped neural elements lying outside of the protective posterior elements.

FRACTURE DISLOCATIONS. Unstable fracture dislocations with evidence of rotational instability or unstable shear translational injuries in the setting of an incomplete neurologic deficit, usually require a combination posterior-anterior procedure to accomplish spinal alignment and adequate neural decompression. Shear injuries fortunately are uncommon at the thoracolumbar junction and consist of disruption of all three spinal columns usually associated with a severe neurologic deficit. A posterior exposure with instrumentation (hook-rod, pedicle screws, wires) applying the necessary vector forces to reduce the spinal elements is undertaken followed by an assessment of residual neural compression by either intraoperative sonography or myelography or postoperative myelography

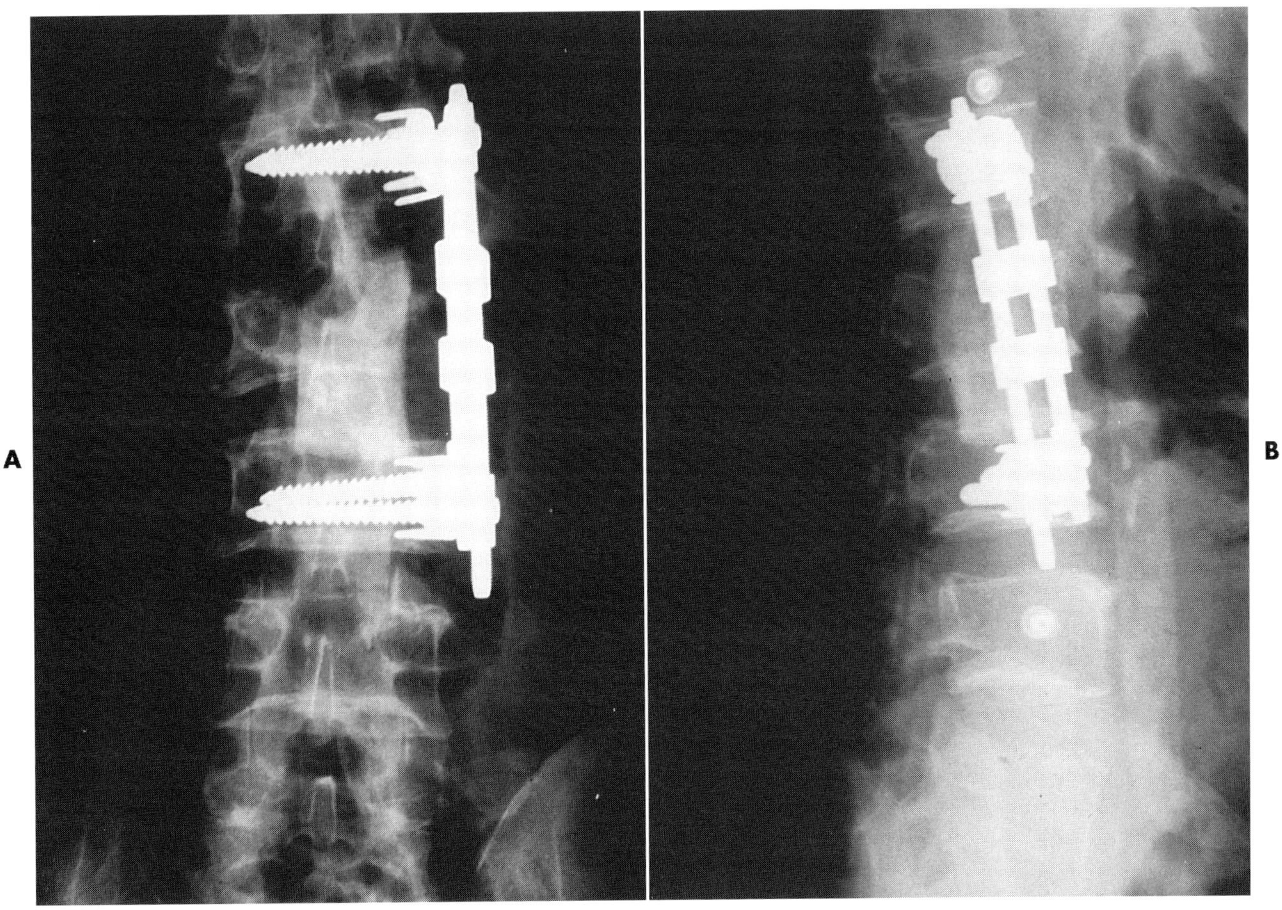

FIGURE 12-3

A, B An anterior tricortical graft reconstruction with Kaneda anterior instrumentation following decompression of an L2 burst fracture.

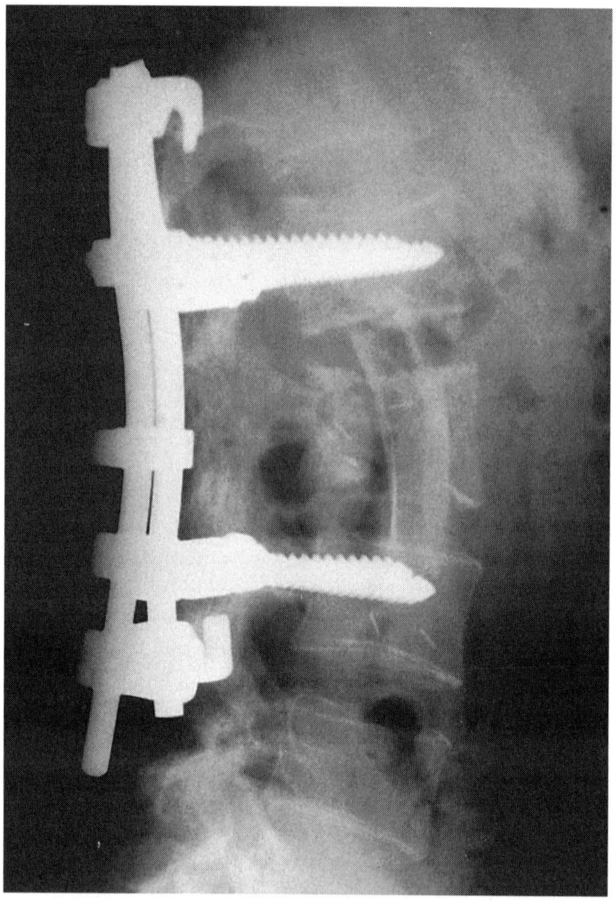

FIGURE 12-4

An posterior short segment pedicle screw stabilization following an L1 to L3 anterior iliac crest bone grafting procedure for an L2 burst fracture.

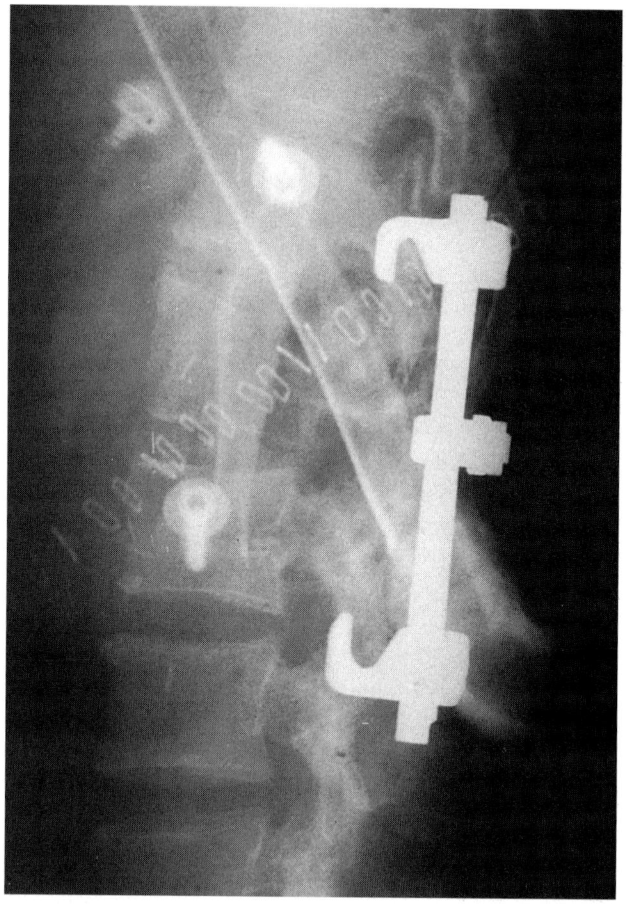

FIGURE 12-5

An anterior tricortical iliac strut graft reconstruction with posterior hook rod compression instrumentation following decompression of a T12 burst fracture.

and/or CT (Fig. 12-6 A,B). Residual bony and soft tissue compression, if present, is then removed preferably by an anterior exposure.

REHABILITATION

Early patient mobilization is paramount in the care of the spinal injury patient who is treated surgically or nonsurgically. In patients with evidence of a SCI, early passive motion exercises prevent joint contractures and facilitate a patient's participation in activities of daily living including personal hygeine, transfer, and feeding. Bowel and bladder training and the selected use of orthotics in low level SCI patients decreases the level of dependency and, therefore, financial burden on external resources.

DISCUSSION

Appropriate treatment of thoracolumbar junction spinal fractures varies with the type of fracture, the degree of neural deficit if any, and the level of the spinal fracture. Operative and nonoperative treatment can both give effective results if appropriate patients are selected. The goal of treatment is to maximize a patient's level of independence without risk of developing a spinal deformity and subsequent neurologic deficit. Nonoperative treatment is appropriate for stable spine injuries with the use of a total contact TLSO or cast immobilization. Surgical treatment is indicated for unstable spinal fractures with or without neurological deficit. Early surgical intervention is appropriate for fractures associated with progressive neurologic deterioration. The main goals in the surgical treatment of spinal fractures are to maximize neurologic recovery, to achieve and maintain anatomic reduction, and to provide a stable spine for early patient rehabilitation. The optimum instrumentation system depends on the fracture type, the vertebral level, its mechanism of causation, and the experience of the surgeon. Spinal surgeons must remain aware of the many complications associated with surgical treatment of thoracolumbar fractures and the various instrumentation systems used

A 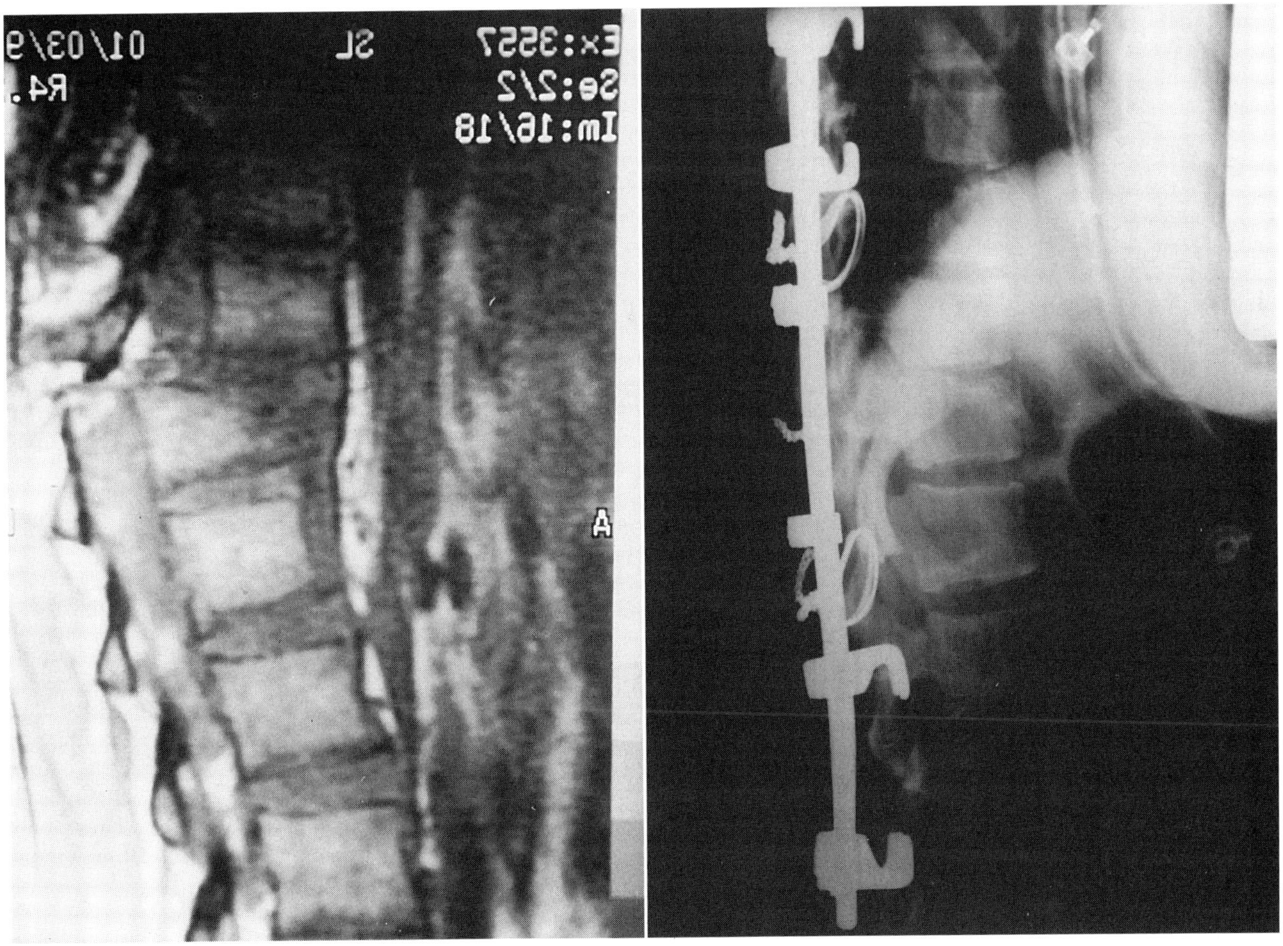 B

FIGURE 12-6

A, A T12-L1 fracture dislocation in a patient with a complete spinal cord injury. **B,** Following a posterior thoracolumbar stabilization procedure, the patient was found to have a patent canal by intraoperative sonography.

to maintain fracture reduction and spinal stability. Only with well-controlled prospective studies will the optimum treatment regimen, that is, operative versus nonoperative, be clarified in specific fracture patterns.

REFERENCES

1. White AA, Panjabi MM: *Clinical biomechanics of the spine*, ed 4, Philadelphia, 1990, JB Lippincott.
2. Davis AG: Fractures of the spine, *J Bone Joint Surg* 11:133–156, 1929.
3. Mumford J, et al: Thoracolumbar burst fractures: the clinical efficacy and outcome of nonoperative management, *Spine* 18:955–970, 1993.
4. Frankel HL, et al: The value of the postural reduction in the initial management of closed injuries of the spine with paraplegia and tetraplegia, *Paraplegia* 31:179–192, 1969.
5. Guttman L: History of the National Spinal Injuries Centre, Stoke Manderville Hospital, Aylesburg, *Paraplegia* 5:115–126, 1967.
6. Guttman L: Surgical aspects of the treatment of traumatic paraplegia. *J Bone Joint Surg*, 31B:399–403, 1949.
7. Bedbrook GM: Treatment of thoracolumbar dislocation and fractures with paraplegia, *Clin Orthop* 112:27–43, 1975.
8. Guttman L: Initial treatment of traumatic paraplegia, *Proc R Soc Med* 47:1103–1121, 1954.
9. Soreff J: *Assessment of the late results of traumatic compression fractures of the thoracolumbar vertebral bodies,* Stockholm, 1977, Karolinska Hospital.
10. Convery FR, Minteer MA, Smith RN: Fracture dislocations of the dorsal lumbar spine: acute operative stabilization by Harrington instrumentation, *Spine* 3(2):160–166, 1978.
11. Chapman JR, Anderson PA: Thoracolumbar spine fractures with neurologic deficit, *Orthop Clin North Am* 25(4):595–612, 1994.

12. Ballock RT, et al: Can burst fractures be predicted from plain radiographs? *J Bone Joint Surg* 74B:147–150, 1992.
13. Emery SE, et al: Magnetic resonance imaging of post-traumatic spinal ligament injury, *J Spinal Dis* 2:229–233, 1989.
14. Eismont FJ, Garfin SR, Abitbol JJ: Thoracic and upper lumbar spine injuries. In Browner BD, et al, editors: *Skeletal trauma,* vol 1, Philadelphia, 1992, W.B. Saunders.
15. Grimes PF, Vaccaro AR, Garfin SR: Treatment complications of thoracolumbar spine trauma. Seminars in spine surgery, 7:141–151, 1995.
16. Eismont FJ, et al: The role of intraoperative ultrasonography in the treatment of thoracic and lumbar spine fractures, *Spine* 9(8):788–795, 1984.
17. Garfin SR, et al: Confirmation of the posteriolateral technique to decompress and fuse thoracolumbar spine burst fractures, *Spine* 10:218–228, 1985.
18. Vincent KA, Benson DR, McGahan JP: Intraoperative ultrasonography for reduction of thoracolumbar burst fractures, *Spine* 14:387–390, 1989.
19. Bucholz RW, Gill K: Classification of injuries to the thoracolumbar spine, *Orthop Clin North Am* 17:67–73, 1986.
20. Kornberg M, Rechtine GR: Common fractures of the thoracic and lumbar spine, *Orthop Rev* XI:67–75, 1982.
21. Willen J, Lindahl S, Irstam L: Unstable thoracolumbar fractures, *Spine* 9:214–219, 1984.
22. Denis F: The three-column spine and its significance in the classification of acute thoracolumbar spinal injuries, *Spine* 8:817–831, 1983.
23. Denis F: Updated classification of thoracolumbar fractures, *Orthop Trans* 6:8, 1982.
24. Kelly RP, Whitesides TE: Treatment of lumbodorsal fracture-dislocations, *Ann Surg* 167:705–717, 1968.
25. Nicoll EA: Fractures of the dorso-lumbar spine, *J Bone Joint Surg* 31B:376–394, 1949.
26. Ferguson RL, Allen BL Jr: A mechanistic classification of thoracolumbar spine fractures, *Clin Orthop* 189:77–88, 1984.
27. Chance GQ: Note on a type of flexion fracture of the spine, *Br J Radiol* 21:452–453, 1948.
28. Dorr LD, Harvey JF Jr, Nick JL: Clinical review of the early stability of spine injuries, *Spine* 7:545–550, 1982.
29. Holdsworth FW: Fractures, dislocations, and fracture dislocations of the spine, *J Bone Joint Surg* 52A(8):1534–1551, 1970.
30. Holdsworth FW, Hardy AG: Early treatment of paraplegia from fractures of the thoracolumbar spine, *J Bone Joint Surg* 35B:540–550, 1953.
31. Bedbrook GM: Spinal injuries with tetraplegia and paraplegia, *J Bone Joint Surg* 61B:267–284, 1979.
32. Whitesides TE Jr, Ali Shah SG: On the management of unstable fractures of the thoracolumbar spine: rationale for use of anterior decompression and fusion and posterior stabilization, *Spine* 1:99–107, 1976.
33. Haher TR, et al: The contribution of the three columns of the spine to spinal stability: a biomechanical model, *Paraplegia* 27:432–439, 1989.
34. McAfee PC, et al: The value of computed tomography in thoracolumbar fractures, *J Bone Joint Surg* 65A:461–473, 1983.
35. Hallowell JP, Maiman DJ: Management of thoracolumbar spine trauma. In Rea GL, Miller CA, editors: Current evaluation and management of spinal trauma, Park Ridge, IL, 1993, American Association of Neurological Surgeons.
36. Rea GL, Zerick WR: Clinical review. The treatment of thoracolumbar fractures: one point of view, *J Spinal Dis* 8:368–382, 1995.
37. Bayley JC: The nonsurgical treatment of spinal injuries, *Sem Spine Surg* 7:98–102, 1995.
38. Chan DPK, Seng NK, Kaan KT: Nonoperative treatment in burst fractures of the lumbar spine (L2–L5) without neurologic deficits, *Spine* 18:320–325, 1993.
39. Gumley G, Taylor TKF, Ryan MD: Distraction fractures of the lumbar spine, *J Bone Joint Surg* 64B:520–525, 1982.
40. Davies WE, Morris JH, Hill V: An analysis of conservative (non-surgical) management of thoracolumbar fractures and fracture-dislocations with neural damage, *J Bone Joint Surg* 62A(8):1324–1328, 1980.
41. Fredrickson BE, Yuan HA: Nonoperative treatment of the spine: external immobilization. In Browner BD, et al, editors: *Skeletal trauma,* vol 1, Philadelphia, 1992, WB Saunders.
42. Cantor JB, et al: Nonoperative management of stable thoracolumbar burst fractures with early ambulation and bracing, *Spine* 18:971–976, 1993.
43. Weinstein JN, Collalto P, Lehmann TR: Thoracolumbar "burst" fractures treated conservatively: a long-term follow up, *Spine* 12:33–38, 1988.
44. McAfee PC, Bohlmann HH, Yuan HA: Anterior decompression of traumatic thoracolumbar fractures with incomplete neurological deficit using a retroperitoneal approach, *J Bone Joint Surg* 67A:89–104, 1985.
45. McEvoy RD, Bradford DS: The management of burst fractures of the thoracic and lumbar spine. Experience in 53 patients, *Spine* 10:631–637, 1985.
46. Gertzbein SD: Scoliosis Research Society. Multicenter spine fracture study. *Spine* 17:528–540, 1992.
47. Dall BE, Stauffer ES: Neurologic injury and recovery patterns in burst fractures at the T12 or L1 motion segment, *Clin Orthop* 233:171–176, 1988.
48. Heiden JS, et al: Penetrating gunshot wounds of the cervical spine in civilians. Review of 38 cases, *J Neurosurg* 42:575–579, 1975.
49. Durward QJ, Schweigel JF, Harrison P: Management of fractures of the thoracolumbar and lumbar spine, *Neurosurgery* 8:555–561, 1981.
50. Herndon WA, Galloway D: Neurologic return versus cross-sectional canal area in incomplete thoracolumbar spinal cord injuries, *J Trauma* 28:680–683, 1988.
51. Lemons VR, Wagner FC, Montesano PX: Manage-

ment of thoracolumbar fractures with accompanying neurological injury, *Neurosurgery* 30:667–671, 1992.

52. Wiberg J, Hague HN: Neurological outcome after surgery for thoracic and lumbar spine injuries, *Acta Neurochir* 91:106–112, 1988.
53. Fidler M: Remodeling of the spinal canal after burst fracture, *J Bone Joint Surg* 70B:730–732, 1988.
54. Johnson R, et al: Spinal canal remodeling after thoracolumbar fractures with intraspinal bone fragments, *Acta Orthop Scand* 62:125–127, 1991.
55. Willen JAG, Gaekwad UH, Kakulas BA: Burst fractures in the thoracic and lumbar spine: a clinico-neuropathologic analysis, *Spine* 12:1316–1323, 1989.
56. Edwards CC, et al: The fate of retropulsed bone following vertebral body fractures, *Orthop Trans* 13:19, 1989.
57. Willen J, et al: The natural history of burst fractures at the thoracolumbar junction, *J Spinal Disord* 3:39–46, 1990.
58. Denis F, et al: Acute thoracolumbar burst fracture in the absence of a neurologic deficit: a comparison between operative and nonoperative treatment, *Clin Orthop* 189:142–149, 1984.
59. Carl AL, Tromanhauser SG, Roger DJ: Pedicle screw instrumentation for thoracolumbar burst fractures and fracture dislocations, *Spine* 17:317–324, 1992.
60. McLain RF, Sparling E, Benson DR: Early failure of short-segment pedicle instrumentation for thoracolumbar fractures, *J Bone Joint Surg* 75A:162–167, 1993.
61. Allardyce TJ, et al: Early outcome of short segment pedicle fixation for thoracolumbar and lumbar burst fractures. Presented at the American Academy Orthopaedic Surgeons, Atlanta, February, 1996.
62. Gertzbein SD, Court-Brown CM: Flexion distraction injuries of the lumbar spine, *Clin Orthop* 227:52–60, 1988.
63. Denis F, Burkus JK: Shear fracture-dislocations of the thoracic and lumbar spine associated with forceful hyperextension (lumberjack paraplegia), *Spine* 17:156–161, 1992.
64. Jelsma RK, et al: Surgical treatment of thoracolumbar fractures, *Surg Neurol* 18:156–166, 1982.
65. Jodoin A, et al: Unstable fractures of the thoracolumbar spine: a ten year experience at Sacre-Coeur Hospital, *J Trauma* 25:197–202, 1985.
66. Marshall LF, et al: Deterioration after spinal cord injury: a multicenter study. *J Neurosurg* 66:400–404, 1987.
67. Rivlin A, Tator CH: Effect of duration of acute spinal cord compression in new acute spinal cord injury model in the rat, *Surg Neurol* 10:39–43, 1978.
68. Gertzbein SD, et al: The neurological outcome following surgery for spinal fractures, *Spine* 13:641–644, 1988.
69. Hardcastle P, Bedbrook G, Curtis K: Long term results of conservative and operative management in complete paraplegics with spinal cord injuries between T10 and L2 with respect to function, *Clin Orthop* 224:88–96, 1987.
70. Rimoldi RL, et al: The effect of surgical intervention on rehabilitation time in patients with thoracolumbar and lumbar spinal cord injuries, *Spine* 17:1443–1449, 1992.
71. Suyama T, et al: Spinal flexibility activities of daily living for the thoracic and lumbar spinal cord injured—comparison of a non-operated group with an internal spinal fused group, *Nippon Seikeigeka Gakkai Zasshi* 64:1155–64, 1990.
72. Anderson PA, Bohlmann HH: Anterior decompression and arthrodesis of the cervical spine: long-term motor improvement: II. Improvement in complete traumatic quadriplegia, *J Bone Joint Surg* 74A:671–682, 1992.
73. Anderson PA, Bohlmann HH: Later anterior decompression of thoracolumbar spine fractures, *Semi Spinal Surg* 2:54–62, 1990.
74. Benzel EC, Larson SJ: Functional recovery after decompressive operation for thoracic and lumbar spine fractures, *Neurosurgery* 19:772–778, 1986.
75. Bohlman HH, Anderson PA: Anterior decompression and arthrodesis of the cervical spine. Long-term motor improvement: I. Improvement in incomplete traumatic quadraparesis, *J Bone Joint Surg* 74A:659–670, 1992.
76. Clohisy JC, et al: Neurologic recovery associated with anterior decompression of spine fractures at the thoracolumbar junction (T12-L1), *Spine* 17:S325–S330, 1992.
77. Delamarter RB, et al: Experimental lumbar spinal stenosis: Analysis of cortical evoked potentials, microvasculature, and histopathology, *J Bone Joint Surg* 72A:110–120, 1990.
78. Delamarter RB, Sherman JE, Carr JB: Spinal cord injury: the pathophysiology of spinal cord damage and subsequent recovery following immediate or delayed decompression. Paper presented at 21st annual meeting of the Cervical Spine Research Society, New York, December, 1993.
79. Donal EJ, Tator CH, Endrenyi L: The value of decompression for acute experimental spinal cord compression injury, *J Neurosurg* 53:749–755, 1980.
80. Esses S, Botsford D, Kostuik J: Evaluation of surgical treatment for burst fractures, *Spine* 15:667–675, 1990.
81. Sutton DC, et al: Thoracolumbar burst fractures treated with anterior decompression and posterior compression instrumentation, *Orthop Trans* 17:137, 1993.
82. Cammisa FP, Eismont FJ, Green AB: Dural laceration occurring with burst fractures and associated laminar fractures, *J Bone Joint Surg* 71A:1044–1052, 1989.

13

LUMBAR FRACTURES OF THE SPINE

Jeffrey Wang
Rick B. Delamarter

Fractures in the lower lumbar spine levels L3 through L5 account for less than 4% of all spinal fractures.[1,2] There is a great deal of literature on the treatment of thoracolumbar fractures; however, there is very little written about low lumbar spine fractures. The unique anatomy of the lower lumbar spine accounts for the increased stability inherent in this region. There is normally approximately 30° to 60° of lordosis in the lumbar spine. The facet joints in the lumbar spine are oriented vertically and laterally inclined. As a result, rotation in this area is minimal, whereas flexion and extension is maximal. The amount of sacral inclination varies among individuals and accounts for the different amount of spinal curvatures seen in the lumbar area.[3]

Fractures seen in the lumbar spine often take on familiar patterns because of the inherent curvature and coupled motions in the bony architecture. In addition, neural compromise in this area may differ markedly from injuries sustained at other levels. The actual spinal cord usually ends around the L1 level with the cauda equina extending below. Encroachment into the area available for the dural sac impinges on the cauda equina rather than the spinal cord itself. The cauda equina is more resistant to trauma than the actual spinal cord, and there is more space available for the neural elements compared to other levels.[1] Low lumbar injuries usually present as a lower motor neuron lesion because the nerve roots have branched off at higher levels.

Treatment of deformities in the lumbar spine must be structurally directed at preserving the normal anatomy of the region. The normal lordotic curvature of the lumbar spine contributes to the kinematics of normal spinal movement and coupled motions. Any disruption of the standard interactions of the bony and soft tissue interactions may result in complications such as pain, degenerative change, and abnormal body mechanics. Patients with "flat-back" syndrome, with loss of the normal lordotic lumbar curvature, may develop severe low back pain that may impair their everyday activities. Any conservative or surgical management of lumbar spine fractures must attempt to preserve the normal anatomy.

DIAGNOSIS

The diagnosis of low lumbar spine fractures must start with a high index of suspicion. Victims of high-energy trauma must be treated as if the spine is unstable until injury is ruled out. Patients must be protected during transport, log rolled only, and kept on a backboard until they can be fully evaluated. Although low spine fractures may occur with various types of trauma, certain mechanisms of injury are more likely to be associated with low lumbar spine fractures. Falls from heights in which the spine is loaded axially can be associated with thoracolumbar spine fractures as well as lower lumbar spine fractures. Fractures of the calcaneus may indicate that a lumbar spine fracture is also present.

In addition, fractures in other areas of the spine also may be associated with low lumbar spine fractures. Calenoff has reported several patterns of noncontiguous spine fractures in which low lumbar spine fractures are associated with certain spinal column fractures.[4] Noncontiguous multilevel injuries were found in 4.5% of the cases with 50% of these being missed initially. The delay in the diagnosis averaged 52 days. Other studies have demonstrated similar findings.[5] Thus, if a fracture of the spine has occurred in one area, the entire spine must be carefully evaluated.

Seatbelts that cross the lower abdomen can provide a fulcrum point at which flexion or flexion-distraction injuries can typically occur in the lumbar spine. Other factors that can raise the index of suspicion include external signs of trauma such as a lumbar or abdominal hematoma, lacerations, and localized pain or deformity.

A history of previous compression fractures, especially in elderly patients, may indicate severe osteoporosis and a propensity for low lumbar compression fractures. Severe osteopenia noted on skeletal radiographs may also aid in making the diagnosis of osteoporosis. These osteoporotic compression fractures are usually markedly different from fractures resulting from high-energy trauma.

Full spinal radiographs should be taken for any patient with suspected spinal trauma, Magnetic resonance imaging (MRI) may help if the patient is neurologically compromised without evidence of injury on plain radiographs. Computed tomography (CT) scans may help fully define the fracture if one is identified on plain radiographs. Canal compromise and fracture stability can be fully assessed.

PRINCIPLES OF TREATMENT

The general principles of treatment depend on the type of fracture, and each patient represents an individual case. The overall patient treatment plan in low lumbar fractures, therefore varies according to the neurologic status and fracture type.

NEUROLOGIC STATUS

The neurologic status plays a key role in the determination of a treatment plan. If a patient is neurologically intact, one may assume that the neural elements are also intact and the treatment may not be emergent. The physician has time for complete radiographic studies and addressing other concurrent injuries. The patient may have a full medical work-up while the neurologic status is being monitored for any deterioration.

If the patient is partially neurologically compromised, the work-up must proceed expeditiously. The administration of methylpnednisolone may aid in neurologic recovery if started within 8 hours of the time of injury.[6] The cause of the neurologic injury must be discovered and treatment implemented. The decision for operative versus nonoperative treatment is made after adequate studies are done.

If the patient is fully neurologically compromised, again, it is necessary to determine quickly the cause of the neural injury. A careful examination must be performed to assess any amount of distal sparing no matter how minimal it may seem. If the patient is still in spinal shock, this determination cannot be made until the return of the bulbocavernosus reflex. This is the lowest cord-mediated reflex and is, therefore, the first to return, usually within 48 hours in 99% of the cases.[7] If there is continued neural compression, the treatment plan may necessitate alleviating the compression by surgical or nonsurgical methods.

FRACTURE PATTERN

The radiographic studies reveal the fracture pattern, which can suggest the mechanism of injury. Compression of the anterior structures denotes some type of flexion injury has occurred. Distraction of posterior structures indicates a flexion-distraction mechanism (Fig. 13-1). Severe comminution of the vertebral body with disruption of the middle column structures may denote an axial component. From the deforming forces, one can predict which structures may still be intact and which forces must be applied to the spinal column to reduce the fracture and maintain stability. This is especially important when considering surgical treatment. In general, the deforming forces should be reversed to realign the spine and remove any residual neural compression.

The decision for operative versus nonoperative treatment depends on many factors, which are discussed in more detail later. In general, the decision is made on the overall stability of the fracture and the neurologic status.

Late complications do occur after low lumbar fractures and must be taken into account when formulating a treatment plan. The normal lordotic contour of the low lumbar spine must be restored to preserve normal mechanics and prevent the "flatback" syndrome from occurring. This can result in continued pain and dysfunction and may require surgical correction. Low back pain can occur in many patients years after their initial lumbar fracture. Degenerative disease and late spinal stenosis also may occur as complications after lumbar fractures. Initial treatment aimed at restoring the normal anatomic alignment of the spinal column can minimize these late problems.

OSTEOPOROTIC FRACTURES

Patients with severe osteoporosis caused by a variety of factors can sustain compression fractures from minimal traumatic episodes. This is a major problem in our society today as large numbers of elderly patients have not built up their bone mass early in their lives and continue to lose the integrity of their bony skeleton. Patients with hormone and dietary deficiencies and those on certain chronic medications may experience this problem.[8]

Osteoporotic fractures should be evaluated initially as other types of fractures. In addition to generalized treatment principles, the medical management of the osteoporosis must also be addressed. Calcitonin can be administered in the acute phase to inhibit further resorption of bone and to help replenish stores of bone.[8,9] It is FDA approved for use in metabolic bone disease and can help with the acute pain of the fracture. Calcium and vitamin D supplementation can help decrease bone resorption; however, the cause of the metabolic bone disease must be discovered and treated in the appropriate manner. (For further information, see Chapter 6, Spinal Cord Injuries from Minor Trauma.)

A B

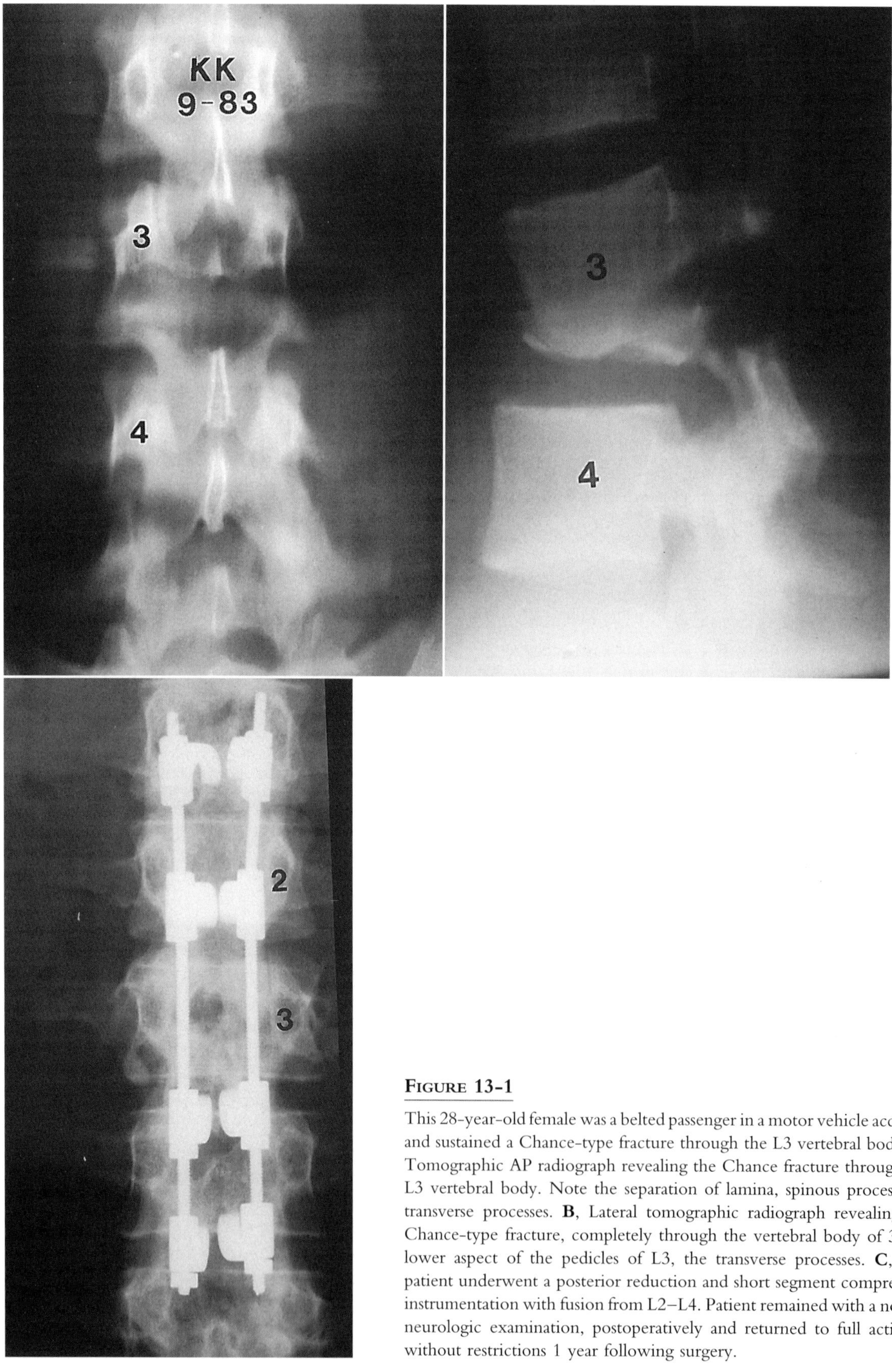

C

FIGURE 13-1

This 28-year-old female was a belted passenger in a motor vehicle accident and sustained a Chance-type fracture through the L3 vertebral body. **A**, Tomographic AP radiograph revealing the Chance fracture through the L3 vertebral body. Note the separation of lamina, spinous process and transverse processes. **B**, Lateral tomographic radiograph revealing the Chance-type fracture, completely through the vertebral body of 3, the lower aspect of the pedicles of L3, the transverse processes. **C**, The patient underwent a posterior reduction and short segment compression instrumentation with fusion from L2–L4. Patient remained with a normal neurologic examination, postoperatively and returned to full activities without restrictions 1 year following surgery.

FRACTURE CLASSIFICATION

There are many classification systems for lumbar spine fractures. The benefit of a complete classification system is that it allows for one physician to easily communicate the fracture to another physician. Some classification systems are arranged by the mechanisms of injury. Patterns associated with injury to different stabilizing elements direct the reduction, treatment, and the forces necessary to stabilize the segments.

The fracture pattern allows the physician to determine the stability of the spine and, thus, guides the need for bracing, reduction, decompression, and the type of stabilization. This plays a key role in determining whether operative or nonoperative treatment is initiated. As the technology of imaging spinal fractures increases, understanding the injury pattern becomes more complete.

Denis Three-Column Theory of Spinal Stability. Holdsworth and Whitesides and Shah popularized the idea of the spine having two main columns for stability.[10,11] Denis introduced and defined the concept of the three-column stability of the spine.[12] The anterior column is comprised of the anterior vertebral body, anterior annulus fibrosis, and anterior longitudinal ligament. The middle column consists of the posterior longitudinal ligament, posterior annulus fibrosis, and posterior wall of the vertebral body. The posterior facet joints and facet capsules, the ligamentum flavum, the interspinous ligaments, and the posterior aspect of the neural arch make up the posterior column. Major injuries to the spine are classified into four different categories defined by the degree of involvement of the three columns. Biomechanical studies have confirmed the validity of the three-column theory of spinal stability and have placed particular value on the status of the middle column as the key to restoring spinal stability.

Compression fractures have failure of the anterior column under compression. The middle column is intact and acts as the fulcrum for partial failure of the posterior column in very severe compression fractures. The preserved middle column is of extreme importance, because it prevents subluxation and does not fragment and retropulse into the neural elements. Patients with compression fractures are usually neurologically intact.

Burst fractures are failures of both the anterior and middle columns of one or both endplates of the vertebral body. These usually result from an axial load and may involve part of the posterior column. There are five types of burst fractures.

Type I—Both endplates of the vertebra are fractured.
Type II—The superior endplate of the vertebra is fractured (most common).
Type III—The inferior endplate of the vertebra is fractured.
Type IV—A burst fracture with rotation is present.
Type V—A burst fracture with lateral flexion is present.

Seat–belt injuries are the third type of fracture in the Denis classification and represent a failure of the posterior and middle columns usually under a tension force with the anterior column as the fulcrum point. The anterior column may or may not fail under compression. The middle and posterior columns may either fail through the bone or through ligamentous disruption (see Fig. 13-1). There is usually no subluxation, which would then classify this as a dislocation.

Fracture-dislocations of the spine represent the final category of spinal injury. This is the most unstable situation with failure of all three columns under any type of mechanism or force (tension, compression, shear, rotation). Subtypes of this fracture include flexion-rotation fracture-dislocation, shear type of fracture-dislocation, and flexion-distraction fracture-dislocation. Fracture-dislocations are rare in the lower lumbar spine.

McAfee and associates classified spinal injury in terms of mechanisms of injury to the middle column.[13] They devised six main categories of fractures.

1. Wedge compression fractures results from failure of only the anterior column in compression. There is no posterior or middle column injury; therefore, the injury is usually stable. Usually no treatment is required except when the degree of compression exceeds 50%.
2. A stable burst fracture results in failure of the anterior and middle columns, usually secondary to an axial load. There is no injury to the posterior column; therefore, this injury is usually stable. There is minimal retropulsion of the bony fragments, and the resulting deformity is usually mild. Nonoperative management usually suffices.
3. An unstable burst fracture results from axial load and has failure of the anterior, middle, and posterior columns (Fig. 13-2). The posterior column may fail under tension or compression. Surgical treatment is normally needed to restore stability and for decompression of neural elements.
4. The fourth type of fracture is the Chance-type fracture and results in disruption of the posterior and middle columns. The failure may occur through bone or soft tissue and normally is a result of a seatbelt injury. Treatment depends on the individual case (see Fig. 13-1).
5. A flexion-distraction injury results in disruption of the posterior elements and failure of the anterior column in compression. The fulcrum may be located in the middle column.
6. The last type of fracture is the translational injury.

A B C

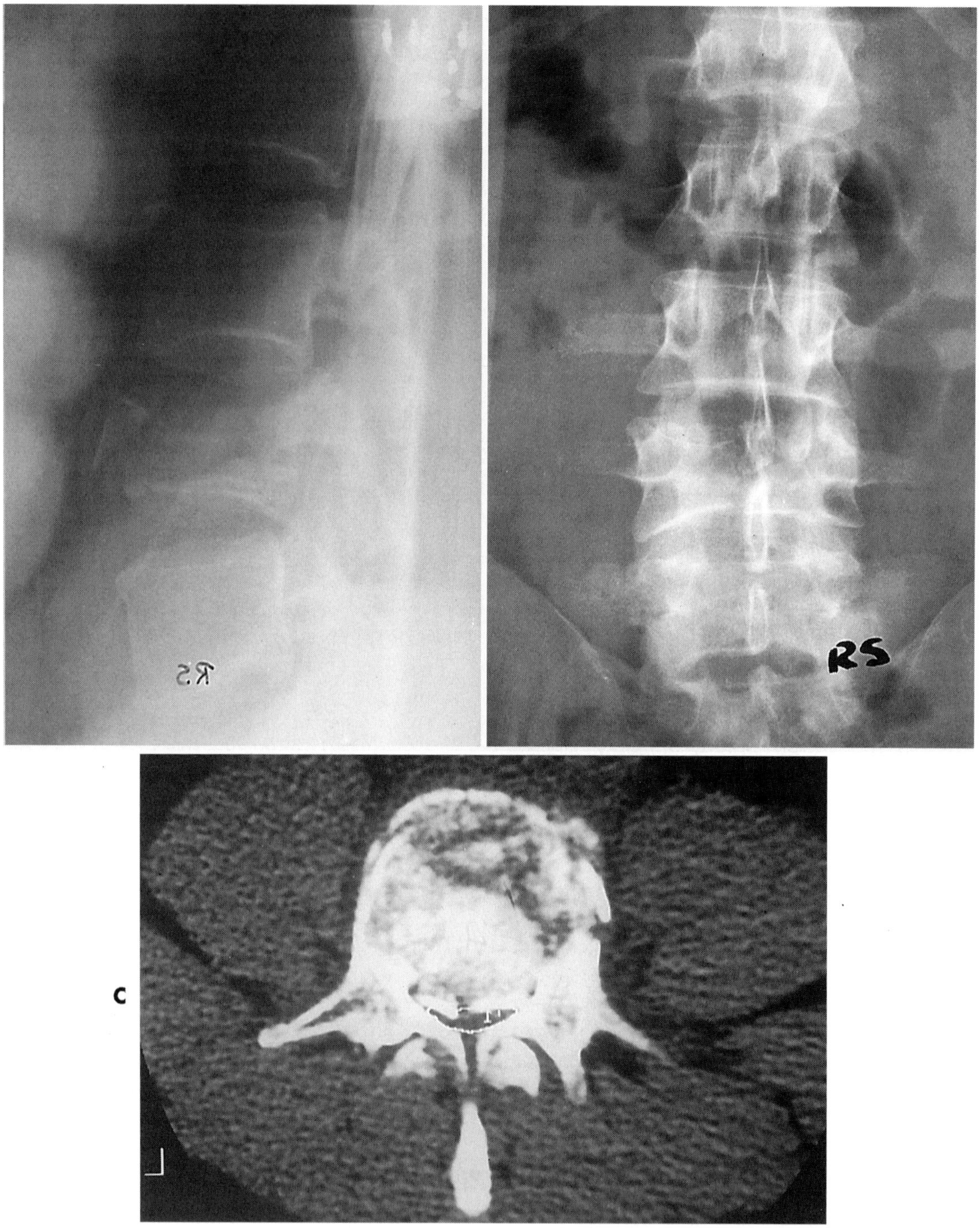

FIGURE 13-2

This 42-year-old male fell off a roof three stories high, landing on his buttocks and was brought to the emergency room an L4 paraplegic. **A**, Lateral radiograph revealing severe compression burst fracture of L4 vertebral body. **B**, Plain anterioposterior radiograph revealing widening of the L4 pedicles and decreased vertebral body height of the L4 vertebra. **C**, A computed tomography (CT) scan through the L4 vertebral body revealing severe canal stenosis from burst fragments. The residual spinal canal measured approximately 2 mm.

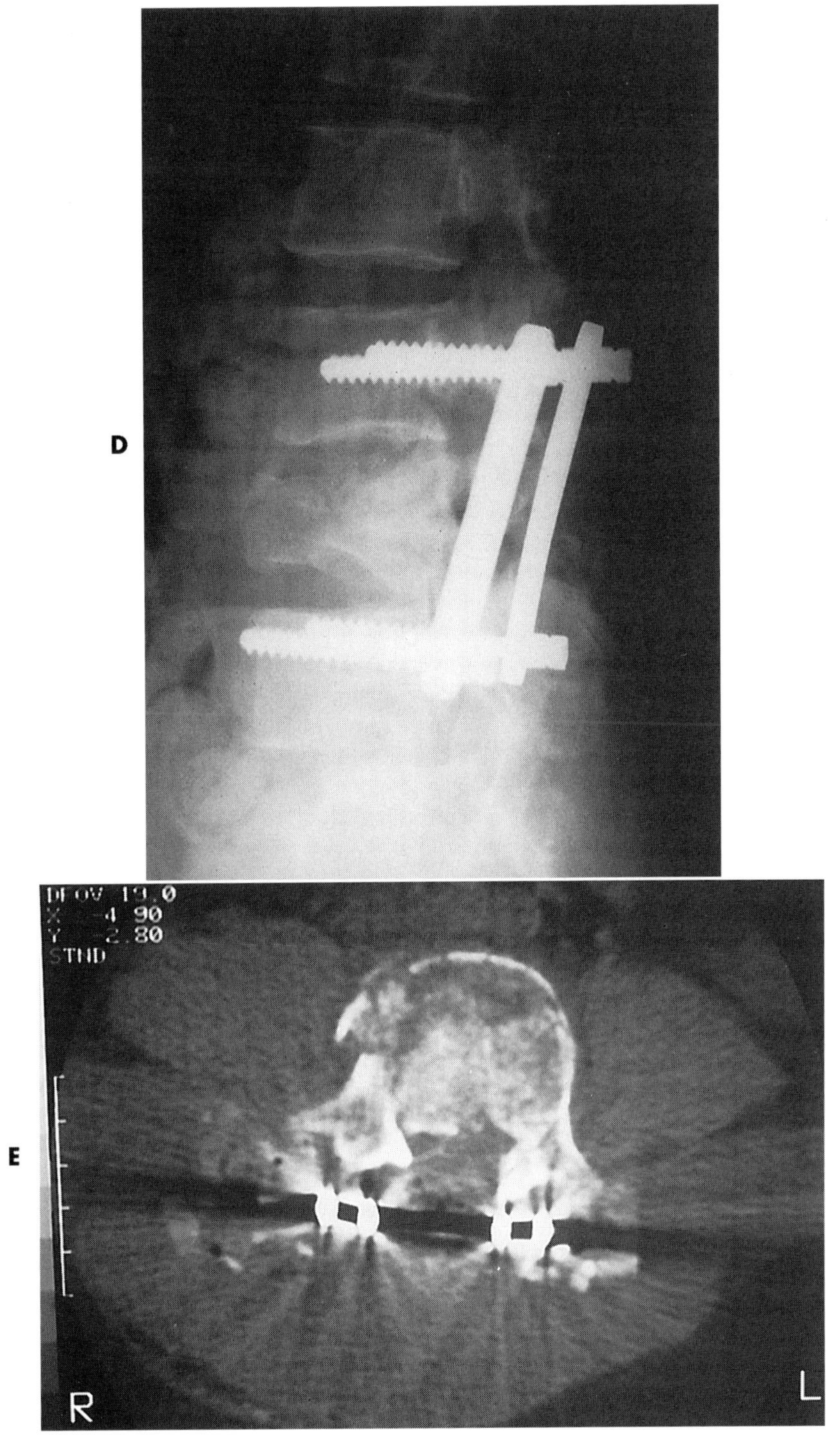

FIGURE 13-2

D, Patient underwent an emergent L4 laminectomy, direct burst fragment decompression and posterior fusion with pedicle screw instrumentation. This figure reveals a 1-year lateral radiograph showing excellent maintenance of vertebral body alignment. **E**, A postoperative CT scan revealing spinal canal decompression and burst fragment excision. Two years postoperatively, this patient recovered the ability to ambulate with a single leg AFO and returned to normal bowel, bladder, and sexual function.

All three columns are injured, and the alignment of the neural canal is disrupted. This is a highly unstable situation and may be caused by a variety of forces. Surgery is usually indicated in this type of fracture.

There are several other classification systems in the literature. Gertzbein has a complete classification system based on mechanisms of injury, which is modified from the AO classification.[14] Categories are based on compression, distraction, and multidirectional force with translation. In a review of 1,445 consecutive thoracolumbar injuries, a comprehensive classification of thoracic and lumbar fractures has recently been proposed. This system is based on mechanism of injury, pathomorphologic uniformity, and on the prognostic and healing potential.[15]

Load-Sharing Classification System. The concept of a load-sharing classification system is important for fully defining the fracture and assessing its stability and capacity to heal without further deformity. This concept was introduced by McCormack and takes into account the amount of displacement and apposition of the fracture fragments and assesses their ability to transfer load.[16] Three factors are independently graded from 1 to 3 depending on severity of the fracture: the amount of comminution, the apposition of the fragments, and the amount of deformity that is to be corrected. Points are assigned for each of three quantities and the final score indicates ability of the fracture to share the load. The lowest score is 3 and the highest score is 9.

In a study of short-segment pedicle screw instrumentation, no screw breakage was noted in patients with scores of 6 or less.[16] Patients with scores of more than 6 need some type of anterior support, because the ability of the anterior structures to share the load transmitted across the injured vertebra is compromised. This classification system does not assess amount of soft tissue and ligamentous injury, which plays a key role in assessing overall stability of the spine and therefore, is not useful to base the decision for operative or nonoperative treatment. It does, however, help direct the proper approach and surgical instrumentation of those fractures that are taken to surgery.

OPERATIVE VERSUS NONOPERATIVE TREATMENT

Making the decision to treat a lumbar spine fracture operatively or nonoperatively depends on several factors. The overall status and health of the patient must be fully and completely assessed before an appropriate decision can be made. All necessary studies should be completed, and a full history and physical examination must be documented. The goal of any treatment is to restore the normal anatomy and function of the spine and to prevent any late deformities or functional compromise that may occur. There are many factors to consider.

NEUROLOGIC FACTORS

Neurologically Intact Patients. Patients who are fully awake and neurologically intact without evidence of neural injury do not need emergency surgical decompression. More time can be taken to further assess and observe the patient, and any necessary tests can be obtained. The decision for operative or nonoperative treatment is primarily dictated by the overall stability of the fracture and the resulting deformity. Complete tests should be done to assess the three columns of the spine and, depending on the fracture pattern, the amount of canal encroachment. Although neurologically intact, there may be a relatively large amount of canal encroachment and some neural compression.

The fracture pattern is the determining factor for operative management in neurologically intact patients. Anterior column compromise only does not destabilize the spine. If the middle column is also compromised, the fracture is considered unstable and surgical stabilization may be indicated. Recent biomechanical fracture studies have validated the three-column approach for assessing spinal stability.[17] Each of the three columns must be evaluated independently for stability of both bone and soft-tissue elements. Recent biomechanical studies have shown that the posterior column may be the key for spinal stability, and treatment should focus on the preservation and restoration of the posterior structures.[18] A complete evaluation of fracture stability, therefore, should be performed. The highly unstable three-column fractures should be considered for more aggressive operative treatment, whereas the more stable fractures should be considered for nonoperative treatment. Orthotic devices may posturally reduce and stabilize the spine while the fracture heals. These orthotics are used successfully for treatment of lumbar fractures.[2,19] They do not always provide complete fracture reduction but are definitely an option for nonoperative treatment.

Kyphosis over the injured segment also is a factor in making the decision for operative treatment. The amount of kyphosis over the entire injured segment is added for injuries that involve more than one vertebra. The normal amount of lordosis must be taken into account when analyzing the amount of deformity present. Although there is no magical number or percentage of collapse or kyphosis that mandates operative treatment, the goal is to preserve the normal lordosis and alignment of the lumbar spine. Residual kyphosis in the normally lordotic lumbar spine that cannot be reduced with nonoperative measures often requires operative treatment. Loss of lordosis may cause problems with back pain and fatigue from a "flat-back deformity."[1,19,20] Normal biomechanics of the lumbar spine are disrupted, which alone can result in late problems and deformity. Severe kyphosis may progress leading to late complications.

Comminution of fracture fragments plays a key role in the decision for operative treatment. As stated earlier, the load-sharing classification of spinal fractures must be considered when determining spinal stability. By examining the number of columns involved and the amount of comminution and separation of the fragments, the ability of the injured segment to transmit and bear axial load may be estimated. Fractures with minimal comminution may have the ability to share considerable load. These fractures are amenable to nonoperative treatment without the worry of late deformity; however, severely comminuted fractures are highly unstable and may worsen with continued axial load. These fractures may be treated operatively to restore stability and prevent late collapse. Comminution has implications for the type of surgical approach and instrumentation and is discussed later in this chapter.

Although the patient may be neurologically intact, there still may be significant canal encroachment and neural compression. Patients with disruption of the middle columns may have retropulsion of bone into the neural canal. In unstable fractures, progression of deformity or movement of the unstable segment may result in further neural compression and neurologic damage. Some studies recommend allowing less than 50% canal encroachment for conservative treatment in these neurologically intact patients. Others suggest if there is significant neural compression despite the absence of neurologic damage, surgical decompression should be performed. Long-term, follow-up studies demonstrate that fragments in the canal usually resorb over time.[20] Stenosis as a result of the fracture fragments, however, can develop and cause great disability. In addition, degenerative changes may be accelerated at the injured levels resulting in late spinal and foraminal stenosis, which can be accentuated by the canal space already compromised by fractured fragments.

The soft tissue structures that constitute the columns of the spine must be carefully evaluated. Extent of soft tissue injuries are not assessed by normal radiographs and must be diagnosed by the displacement of the bony structures and the subluxation seen in dynamic studies. Fractures of bony structures may heal and the stability may then be restored. The soft tissue structures may not heal appropriately to restore stability to the injured spine.

Patients With Partial Neurologic Injury. Making the decision for operative treatment in patients with partial neurologic injury also should be based on several important factors. Here, the decision is based upon the fracture pattern and the restoration of the normal neurologic function.

Evidence of spinal injury is not always present in radiographic studies. This usually occurs in children after motor vehicle accidents.[21] Patients who do not have any abnormalities on plain radiographs should have an MRI scan. Hemorrhage or edema of the neural elements and ligamentous injury may be diagnosed by changes seen on MRI scans.

If neural compression is identified, steps should be taken to relieve the neural compression for the best chance at neurologic recovery. Postural reduction has been reported to be an option and may grossly align the spine when there is obvious malalignment; however, this may be insufficient when small bony fragments are retropulsed into the canal. Kyphosis may be corrected by extending the spine into lordosis; however, distraction is difficult to apply nonoperatively to the lumbar spine. Manipulation of the spine in a neurologically compromised patient with an unstable spine is not recommended.

Surgical decompression is the treatment of choice in patients with neural deficits and neural compression. Operative treatment allows direct removal of the offending fracture fragments and full decompression of the neural structures. Better anatomic reduction also may be accomplished.[1,18] The offending fragment causing the compression must be fully defined before surgical treatment can be properly planned. Computed tomography scans with or without myelography are helpful in assessing the amount of canal encroachment and the number and location of fracture fragments. Magnetic resonance imaging scans can help identify soft tissue and neural injury and assess the stabilizing structures that are important for a proper reduction. From these studies, the proper approach to provide the optimal decompression can be ascertained. An anterior or posterior approach can be planned to allow access to the fragments for complete decompression. Anterior or posterior stabilizing procedures may then be considered to recreate the normal lordosis of the spine and stabilize the injured segments.

A direct or indirect decompression may be used. If the posterior longitudinal ligament is intact and the normal height of the injured segment is decreased, applied distraction may indirectly reduce the fracture fragments from the canal. Contouring rods appropriately preserve the normal anatomic lordosis of the lumbar spine. Conversely, an anterior approach allows complete access to the anterior fragments causing the compression. This may be the only option for decompression if the treatment comes several days after the injury, because fragments may not move on attempted indirect reduction.[22]

Timing of surgical decompression is controversial. Patients with progressive neurologic deficit should be taken for operative decompression and spinal alignment on an emergent basis. Patients with neural compromise with some neurologic sparing and a grossly dislocated spine should also be taken to surgery on an urgent basis for realignment and decompression. Patients with a stable neurological status and evidence of compression on radiologic studies, however, may either be taken to the operating room immediately or after a short waiting period.

Proponents of waiting for a period of a few days before taking patients with stable neurologic status feel that edema and swelling has time to subside, facilitating surgery and decreasing the chance of neural injury.[20] Studies have shown that waiting a few days before undertaking surgery results in a decrease in the intraoperative blood loss.[10] Other reasons include the ability to fully mobilize a well-trained operative team with the appropriate instrumentation. Waiting also allows the diagnosis and work-up of all injuries including those that were not initially detected. Full studies of the spine may be obtained and a complete operative plan may be implemented.

The authors advocate early operative intervention in those patients who are partially neurologically compromised even if their examination does not indicate deterioration. We feel the best chance of neurological recovery is with early decompression. Delamarter et al. performed an animal study examining the timing of decompression of the spinal cord at the lumbar level.[23] Compression of 50% of the diameter of the spinal cord resulting in paraplegia was performed with decompression at certain time intervals. All of the subjects treated with decompression in 1-hour recovered the ability to walk. When the time of compression exceeded 6 hours, no neurologic recovery was seen and there was progressive necrosis of the spinal cord. The percentage of recovery of evoked potentials was related to the total time of compression. We recommend early decompression of these patients with partial neurological injury as soon as they are systemically and medically stable to maximize their neurologic recovery. Other advantages of early surgery include the ability to mobilize the patient earlier to avoid complications associated with prolonged bedrest. Waiting too long may make the fracture more difficult to reduce or decompress. Psychologically, early stabilization and decompression allows early progression and can hold some psychological advantages for both patient and family.

Patients With Complete Neurologic Injury. Patients with complete absence of neurologic function are treated according to the same basic principles although this is not frequently seen with only a lumbar fracture. One must be sure that the patient has had resolution of spinal shock before the injury can be graded complete. In addition, a careful neurologic examination must be performed to assure that there is no sparing and no spine lesion above the lumbar area. Sometimes the presence of minimal perianal sensation is enough to discount that the lesion is complete.

We recommend early decompression of any injury with obvious neural compression based on the underlying principles that maximize neural recovery. The principles of surgical stabilization of these fractures is similar to the treatment of patients with partial neurologic injury. The spine should be aligned by nonoperative or operative means in a timely manner. The evaluation and work-up of these patients also is similar. Decisions regarding operative or nonoperative treatment follow the same basic guidelines. The prognosis for recovery is grim if the lesion remains complete after the resolution of spinal shock. Aggressive stabilization of complete lesions aids in the overall mobilization of these patients and should be instituted when appropriate.

OTHER CONSIDERATIONS FOR OPERATIVE TREATMENT

In any decision regarding the treatment of a lumbar fracture, the major symptoms of the patient must be taken into consideration. Patients who are neurologically intact yet severely impaired by pain, discomfort, and immobility may benefit from early rigid surgical fixation to allow early mobilization. Bracing may allow patients with minimal pain the ability to ambulate early with little discomfort. There are many other factors that influence the decision for operative or nonoperative treatment. The overall health of the patient must be taken into account. If the patient has multiple severe medical problems that would preclude an extensive spinal operation, conservative management should be used. The surgical risk may be the determining factor in fractures that could be properly treated either with or without surgery.

The older, not very active patient may do well with nonoperative treatment when the fracture is minimal. Late complications may not be of great concern with such a patient. If the patient is not able to tolerate prolonged bedrest or orthotic treatment without a multitude of potential complications, however, he or she may be a candidate for surgical treatment for earlier mobilization.

Young patients wishing to remain active are good candidates for operative treatment. Care should be taken to properly restore the normal anatomic alignment and stability of the lumbar spine to prevent late pain, deformity, and degenerative changes from causing significant disability in their later years. If nonoperative management is feasible, however, avoidance of a lumbar fusion in this population would be ideal.

Many patients have several associated injuries along with a lumbar spine fracture. These must be taken into account in the treatment plan. If the patient is too ill from other injuries for a surgical procedure, conservative management should be used. If the patient has other injuries and needs early mobilization, surgical treatment may allow early ambulation and avoidance of a long recumbency period.

Nonoperative Treatment

Nonoperative treatment of lumbar spine fractures involves several modalities. For certain fractures, this is the preferred method of treatment and should be used when the fracture is amenable.

Indications for Nonoperative Treatment. General health issues may preclude surgical treatment because the patient is not an acceptable risk for surgery. If the patient is neurologically intact, there is not an absolute need for surgical treatment of lumbar spine fractures. When deformity caused by the fracture is minimal, the patient will most likely do well with nonsurgical treatment. Ideally the kyphosis is minimal or reduced in extension so that relative lordosis of the lumbar spine is preserved. Stable injuries without disruption of more than two of the three columns are amenable to nonoperative management. Progression of deformity is rare.

Many authors have set guidelines in the literature for surgical or nonoperative treatment of lumbar fractures. Bohlman and Brown both recommend surgical treatment for fractures with loss of 40% of body height and more than 1 cm of retropulsion of fracture fragments.[24,25] Willen recommends operative treatment for fractures with 50% compression and 50% canal compromise.[26] Dunn operates using canal compromise of 50% as the criteria.[27] Jacobs recommends operative treatment for any fracture that may result in permanent neurological deficit.[28] He also includes loss of 40% vertebral body height and loss of posterior ligamentous stability. Denis suggests operative treatment for fractures involving the middle column with severe obstruction of the spinal canal.[29] Similarly, Ferguson reserves surgical treatment for those fractures that he calls "tension blowout," which is a severe middle-column failure fracture.[30] Kostuik recommends surgery for any fracture with significant retropulsion, while Krompinger recommends surgery for fractures with neurological compromise, rotational fracture-dislocations, or translational injuries with more than 50% canal compromise and more than 30° of total kyphosis.[31,32] Stauffer classifies unstable fractures as those with more than 25° of kyphosis, canal compromise of more than 50%, or a combination of greater than 50% loss of vertebral height and kyphosis of more than 15°.[20] He recommends operative treatment for three-column injuries that are unstable. Dewald operates on all burst fractures and uses a combination of anterior surgery for those with canal diameters less than 10 mm.[33] Garfin recommends surgery for those with more than 50% of vertebral body compression.[34] Weitzman uses surgical treatment for those fractures with 50% wedging of the vertebral body and fractures with posterior interspinous ligament, lamina, or pedicle injuries.[35] Roy-Camille recommends surgery for fractures with any neurologic deficit or with any fragments producing dural compression greater than one third body collapse.[36]

We recommend surgical treatment for any fracture with neurologic compromise. Any unstable fracture with significant loss of vertebral body height, canal compromise, or significant kyphotic deformity should also be considered for operative treatment. We reserve nonsurgical treatment for those patients with no neurologic compromise, minimal deformity, minimal canal compromise, and little chance of progressive deformity.

PROBLEMS WITH SURGICAL TREATMENT

Progressive spinal stenosis and kyphotic collapse or deformity have been treated nonoperatively in the past. There has been a recent progression toward operative management of lumbar fractures; however, recent studies have shown that neurologically intact patients with selected fractures can be managed successfully with nonoperative measures.[31,37,38,39]

Nicoll in 1949 recognized many problems in dealing with lumbar spine fractures using an operative approach.[40] These problems have resurfaced in several recent studies.[1,41,42] Problems with using spinal instrumentation in this area are well documented. In addition, severe long-term back pain and disability in a high percentage of patients is seen with immobilization and fusion of the important low lumbar segments. Application of posterior distraction with instrumentation can result in a kyphotic deforming force that results in a loss of the normal anatomic lordosis and the possible development of a flatback syndrome.[1,43] In the area of the low lumbar spine, there is a high pseudoarthrosis rate and a high incidence of instrumentation failure especially with fusions to the sacrum.[1] Surgical treatment in this area usually requires a spinal fusion, which must extend one or two levels above and below the injured segment. In the low lumbar spine, the preservation of these important motion segments is critical. Conservative care usually preserves these segments and is without the risk of surgical complications. In addition, surgical treatment introduces the risk of iatrogenic complications such as bleeding, infection, inadequate decompression, late degenerative changes above and below the fusion mass, and neurologic damage.

Forms of Nonoperative Treatment

Advocates of nonoperative treatment cite studies that support its use. Research has shown that there is no correlation between the amount of canal encroachment and the initial neurologic examination.[13,44,45] In addition, there is no correlation between residual deformity and neural recovery rate.[46] Posttraumatic spinal stenosis, although a concern of nonoperative management, has been shown in many studies to be of little concern with a low incidence of occurrence.[46] In fact, the fragments retropulsed into the canal usually resorb and the amount of encroachment usually decreases over time.[46]

Postural reduction and prolonged bedrest is the classic method of nonoperative treatment. Patients are kept recumbent for long periods of time, and a bump or towel may be placed at the point of maximal deformity to reduce the kyphosis by extending the spine. After the fracture is reduced by posture alone, the patient may be placed in a brace that provides stability until the fracture is healed. The customary brace is a plastic thoracolumbar-sacral orthosis (TLSO). The duration of bed rest and the timing of bracing varies, and there are no hardfast rules. This treatment has been less practical in the new era of health care.

Weitzman advocates early ambulation and feels that prolonged bed rest would be detrimental to the overall status of the patient.[35] The average length of recumbency was 8 days for the fractures he chose to treat nonoperatively. Bedbrook recommended a total of 6 to 8 weeks of bed rest followed by ambulation without a brace.[47] Some have recommended 4 to 6 weeks of bed rest followed by bracing, while still others recommend 8 to 12 weeks of bed rest followed by bracing depending on the severity of the injury.[10,32] The more unstable the injury, the longer the usual amount of time both at bed rest and in the brace.

A recent study by Mumford examined the clinical efficacy and outcome of nonoperative management of lumbar fractures.[46] The amount of time at bed rest averaged about 4 weeks. The amount of time then spent in the brace averaged 12 weeks. The shortest period of time was 1 week, while the longest time spent at bed rest was 10 weeks. The amount of bed rest depended on the severity of the fracture and the amount of instability present. Patients with injuries at the low lumbar levels generally need more time at bed rest before they may ambulate without fear of progressive deformity. By these guidelines, Mumford found a very small complication rate with no patients requiring surgery for a progressive deformity, instability, or stenosis. Only one patient managed by these guidelines had neurologic deterioration and required surgical decompression. There was little change in the amount of lordosis present at final follow-up. In addition, the amount of canal compromise decreased over time with partial resorption of the fragments in the canal. A high percentage of the patients were able to return to work, and overall they did very well.

In a similar study by Cantor and Eismont in which patients specifically had preservation of the posterior column, patients were treated with early mobilization in a brace as soon as their medical condition allowed.[48] No attempt was made to reduce the fracture, and the patients were treated with the specific goal of early mobilization and reduction of the time allotted for bed rest. The results seen in this study were excellent for preservation of the neurological function with minimal progression of deformity. Ninety-five percent of the patients in this study were able to return to their previous level of activity with minimal restrictions and pain.

In a separate biomechanical study by James et al., this concept was validated.[18] A burst fracture model was used to determine the stability of the spine when the anterior and middle column are compromised but with the posterior column intact. Biomechanical testing of these burst fractures confirmed that the status of the posterior column is a better indicator of fracture stability. Fractures with preservation of the posterior column usually have enough inherent stability to warrant nonsurgical treatment.

Patients with fractures amenable to nonoperative treatment must first be stabilized and fully evaluated. The patient is initially kept at bed rest. The patient is moved by "logrolling" only 30° side to side for daily care and the prevention of decubitus ulcers. This small amount of movement performed in the proper manner should not compromise the unstable spine. The patient must be carefully monitored for any signs of neurologic change. Serial radiographs should be taken if there is any suggestion of movement of the spine or progression of deformity.

Injuries to the anterior column only, such as compression fractures, are quite stable provided there is no posterior column injury. These patients may be ambulated early in an extension orthosis, such as a Jewett hyperextension brace. Studies have shown that this brace may limit motion in the sagittal plane by as much as 50%.[49] This brace should be worn for approximately 4 to 6 weeks although the discomfort from the fracture pain usually subsides well before then, and many patients discontinue the brace when the pain has disappeared. Patients should refrain from heavy lifting and work for approximately 12 weeks. Rehabilitation programs that include isometric strengthening may begin at the 2-week period and become more aggressive at approximately 6 weeks. Radiographs should be taken when the patient first ambulates with the brace and at intervals to assure that the fracture remains stable.

Fractures involving the anterior and middle columns with preservation of the posterior column have more inherent stability than three-column fractures. If there is mild deformity, mild canal compromise, and minimal loss of vertebral height, these patients may ambulate after a short period of bed rest when their medical condition permits. Bed rest may range from 1 to 6 weeks depending on the severity of the fracture.[2] These fractures are unstable in more than one plane as confirmed by biomechanical studies.[50] A Jewett hyperextension brace provides stability in only the sagittal plane; therefore, a body cast or TLSO should be used to control more motion of the upper body in several planes and more efficiently immobilize the injured segments. To immobilize the lumbosacral junction we favor a TLSO with a unilateral pantaloon extension for 8 to 12 weeks until stability of the spine has been restored.

Fractures involving all three columns are highly unstable and require an average of 4 weeks of bed rest if nonoperative treatment is chosen. During this time, the patient must be carefully monitored for progression of neurologic deficits or increased deformity. The patient should have a body cast or TLSO with a unilateral pantaloon extension for about 12 to 16 weeks. Radiographs should be taken with the patient in the brace to assure that the alignment of the spine is preserved and there is no progressive deformity.

TREATMENT OF OSTEOPOROSIS FRACTURES

With the increased prevalence of osteoporosis in our society the number of osteoporotic lumbar fractures also is increasing. Although these occur more commonly at the thoracolumbar junction, these fractures can occur in the low lumbar spine and result in great disability for these usually older individuals.

Most osteoporotic fractures resulting from low-energy trauma are anterior column compression fractures and do not involve the middle or posterior columns. These are usually stable fractures and can be treated with an extension brace such as a Jewett extension brace. Conservative care usually suffices, and the incidence of neurologic damage is very small. Operative treatment is rarely used in these types of fractures differentiating these fractures from the high-energy trauma victims. In addition to the brace for structural support, the mainstay of treatment lies in identifying the underlying cause of the osteoporosis and instituting medical treatment aimed at increasing bone stock. As discussed earlier in this chapter, calcitonin helps with fracture pain while the fracture heals.

Patients who are immunosuppressed such as those who have received organ transplants may have metabolic bone disease as a result of the various immunosuppression medications and can sustain compression fractures. Again, there are many health issues in these patients and the treatment must be individualized.

COMPLICATIONS OF NONOPERATIVE TREATMENT

There are potential problems with the use of nonoperative management for the treatment of low lumbar fractures of the spine. Neurologic deterioration can occur and can progress to complete paraplegia.[46] This is obviously one of the most devastating complications and may immediately require surgical intervention. Neurologic damage can occur during postural reduction or during the course of conservative management. In a study by Davies, 6% of the patients experienced neural deterioration during the postural reduction; however, this was only a temporary condition.[51] Another study reported an approximate 1% incidence of neurologic deterioration during the course of conservative management.[52] Denis reported that 21% of his patients developed neurologic complications as a result of conservative management.[29] One study reported a 1% to 2% incidence of decubitus ulcers and a 12% to 20% incidence of deep venous thrombosis.[51] This may happen despite taking the necessary precautions. Frequent turning with examination of the pressure points when the patient is in bed may detect the formation of these ulcers; however, once formed, they prove to be formidable challenges. Any patient who requires prolonged bed rest is at increased risk for deep venous thrombosis. This can be minimized by early mobilization (if the fracture allows), anticoagulants, and pressurized stockings.

In one series of nonsurgical fracture management, there was an overall 32% complication rate, which included spinal cord infarction, neural deterioration, pulmonary embolism, and an increased deformity.[53] Operative treatment may be required at a later time for problems such as instability or stenosis. Willen reported that 11% of his conservatively treated patients required decompression with or without fusion 3 to 16 months after injury.[54] In a separate study by Weinstein looking at the long-term treatment of lumbar fractures, 7% of the patients required late operations for instability or stenosis.[55] Frankel had only a 1 % reoperation rate for late instability.[52]

A certain amount of residual pain is expected with nonoperative management. The incidence of some residual pain as a result of the lumbar fracture is very high. The incidence of pain is reported to be as high as 90%.[46] The majority of those reporting pain, however, consider it minor, and the degree of pain is very low. Studies in the literature do not feel that this is a significant problem. For the most part, a large percentage of people do return to their previous level of work or some form of modified work. Only 10% to 15% of the patients are unable to return to work.[46] Overall, nonoperative management of lumbar spine fractures is successful in selected fractures. Proper evaluation and recognition of the fracture pattern allow for the institution of conservative care and avoid the complications associated with surgery. Improper selection of fractures, however, may lead to grave complications associated with nonoperative management.

OPERATIVE TREATMENT

INDICATIONS FOR OPERATIVE TREATMENT

The operative treatment of low lumbar spine fractures has been associated with many long-term complications, which led several early studies to conclude that nonoperative treatment should be used whenever possible.[41,42] Operative treatment with older instrumentation systems was fraught with complications, and several of these studies recommended decompression and fusion without the use of spinal instrumentation.[1] The risk of pseudoarthrosis in the low lumbar levels, the need for fusing important low lumbar levels, and the loss of lumbar lordosis with older surgical instrumentation techniques were all of major concern.

With the advent of newer sophisticated pedicle screw systems and anterior instrumentation, there are several more recent studies demonstrating excellent results with operative instrumentation and fusion for low lumbar spine fractures.[1,2] Operative treatment is an excellent way to correct fracture deformity and stabilize the spine. Patients may be spared prolonged bedrest and be mobilized more quickly thereby avoiding the complications of conservative treatment. Early stabilization provides the best chance of preventing further deformity or neurologic deficit. We feel that any patient with evidence of canal compromise and neurologic compromise should be taken for surgical treatment through either direct or indirect decompression. In addition, any patient with significant canal encroachment, significant loss of vertebral height, or loss of the normal anatomic lumbar lordosis should be considered for operative intervention regardless of the neurologic status.

The guidelines for the amount of canal encroachment, loss of vertebral height, and kyphotic deformity that would mandate operative treatment as determined by several authors were presented earlier in the chapter. Because of the potential risks of flat-back deformity, late kyphosis and instability, and neurologic deterioration, we recommend operative treatment for those patients with loss of anatomic lordosis, canal encroachment causing neurologic compromise, or significant loss of vertebral body height.

ANTERIOR VERSUS POSTERIOR SURGERY

The goals of spinal instrumentation for low lumbar fractures are anatomic reduction, adequate decompression, and spinal stabilization. These can be achieved with operative treatment using either an anterior or posterior approach. One of the primary goals of surgery is to fully decompress the neural structures. In unstable burst fractures, retropulsion commonly results in anterior neural compression. An anterior approach allows direct visualization of the offending fragments and direct decompression of the neural structures. Posterior surgery relies mainly on ligamentotaxis and an intact posterior longitudinal ligament to indirectly decompress the neural structures when distraction is applied.

Posterior Surgery. Low lumbar spine fractures treated operatively are most commonly undergo posterior decompression and fusion. Several early studies looking at the treatment of these fractures with hooks and rods concluded that the use of instrumentation was fraught with complications at this level and should not be used.[40,41,42] These studies concluded that treatment should consist of either bed rest with subsequent bracing or surgical decompression and fusion without instrumentation.

POSTERIOR INSTRUMENTATION. The early use of instrumentation in the spine consisted of Harrington rods or rod-sleeve constructs. These had been used with great success in the thoracolumbar spine for stabilization of fractures. These often required fusion of several levels above and below the injured segment to form a stable construct that could adequately resist the forces placed upon the spine. The motion segments in the lumbar spine are vital for the normal kinematics of the spine and extended fusions at this level requires fusion to the sacrum. This results in a high rate of pseudoarthrosis and implant failure.[1,40,41,42]

In addition, these implants relied on distraction placed posteriorly on the spine to restore the vertebral body height and for the indirect reduction of fracture fragments. Distraction placed posteriorly on the spine produces a kyphotic deforming force and can result in a loss of lordosis and the development of a flat-back deformity. The combination of a loss of lordosis and loss of motion segments in the low lumbar spine can lead to back pain and long-term disability.

With the advent of pedicle screw technology, more recent studies have demonstrated success with short segmental instrumentation in the low lumbar spine. An et al. published a study comparing conservative care to instrumentation using either Harrington and Luque rods and a pedicle screw construct for the treatment of low lumbar burst fractures.[1] The patients treated with the distraction rod systems had much less lumbar lordosis when compared to the pedicle screw system. Furthermore, the maintenance of lordosis produced a good result. The rod constructs required fusion of more levels than pedicle screw systems, which allowed the fusion to extend only one level above and below the injured segment. Complaints of persistent back pain were noted in the group with longer fusion levels and rod systems. Pedicle screw system cases had superior results with no cases of pseudoarthrosis or implant failure.

Levine and Edwards published their results of the treatment of low lumbar burst fractures with the rod distraction systems and pedicle screw instrumentation.[2] The patients treated with distraction rod systems experienced the same complications of loss of lumbar lordosis and residual kyphosis, longer fusion lengths, and increased incidence of pseudoarthrosis and instrumentation failure. Patients treated with pedicle screws did very well with preservation of lordosis, shorter fusion lengths, no instrumentation failures, and high fusion rates.

A distinct advantage of the pedicle screw systems is

the ability to allow for flexibility in contouring the rods and positioning the pedicle screws. This allows for the independent application of a lordotic and distraction force to the spine and provide more correction. A biomechanical study compared the ability of instrumentation systems with indirectly reduce retropulsed fracture fragments and recreate the normal anatomy of the lumbar spine.[56] Instrumentation systems that allowed for the independent application and correction of distraction best restored anatomic lordosis, vertebral body height, and provided for the most canal clearance through indirect reduction of fracture fragments (Fig. 3-3).

Pedicle screw instrumentation systems are the treatment method of choice for operative treatment of low lumbar spine fractures. They provide for a stable, rigid construct that has the ability to withstand the loads place upon the lumbar spine. They allow for optimal restoration of the normal vertebral anatomy and allow canal decompression through indirect or direct decompression, and they allow for the shortest possible fusion length and preservation of the critical lumbar motion segments.

Low lumbar fractures characteristically have fracture comminution of the upper one third of the vertebral body and usually allow for placement of pedicle screws into the injured segment, which increases the stability of the construct.[52] Most pedicle screw systems allow for the variable positioning of the screws to gain purchase in the structurally sound portion of the vertebral body.

AUTHORS' METHOD OF POSTERIOR SURGERY. We routinely treat low lumbar spine fractures with posterior pedicle screw instrumentation for indirect canal decompression and posterior-lateral fusion with iliac crest bone grafting. Pedicle screws are placed one level above and one level below the injured segment. A screw also is placed into the injured vertebra if the fracture is accommodating for added stability.

Rods connecting the pedicle screws are contoured to recreate the normal anatomic lordosis of the lumbar spine. Screws allow for the positioning of the vertebral bodies in lordosis (extension) and for the recreation of vertebral body height and indirect canal decompression via distraction. Studies have shown that distraction is the main force that governs indirect reduction of fracture fragments by tensioning the posterior longitudinal ligament.[57] Since placing a lordotic force on the vertebral body may decrease slack in the posterior longitudinal ligament, we recommend applying the distraction force before the lordotic force to obtain the optimal amount of canal clearance. This principle has been confirmed by biomechanical studies.[18]

Fragments encroaching on the spinal canal must be examined carefully. If the fragment appears rotated, patency of the posterior longitudinal ligament may be compromised and the fragment does not reduce by ligamentotaxis. If the fracture has been present for more than 4 to 6 days, the fracture may have already consolidated to the point where indirect reduction may not suffice. Intraoperative ultrasound helps evaluate the amount of canal decompression, but a partial laminotomy to allow the probe to be placed on the dura must be performed. If the fragments cannot be reduced by an indirect method, a direct posterior decompression may then be performed by a laminectomy or transpedicle decompression.[58] Vertebral body fragments may be impacted by placing an impacter underneath the dura directly on the posterior bony fragments. Adequate reduction of the bony fragments may be assessed by palpating the fragments underneath the dura. We have found this to be an excellent method of reducing anterior fragments impinging on the neural elements.

TECHNIQUE. The patient is brought to the operating room using all the principles of spinal precautions. The patient is positioned by log-rolling and moving the spine as one unit. The patient is placed on bolsters to allow the abdomen to hang free to prevent venous congestion, and the spine is placed in the neutral position. We recommend using a radiolucent table to allow for plain radiographs and fluroscopy if needed. This will allow for assessment of reduction, restoration of normal alignment, and direct visualization of the pedicles.

A standard posterior approach is used to expose the injured segment as well as one level above and one level below. A lateral radiograph is taken to confirm that the appropriate level has been reached. Careful examination of the injury radiographs should concentrate on fracture or disruption of posterior lamina and bony structures. Exposure of fractured lamina requires careful dissection without any downward pressure to avoid injury to the dura. Normal levels with intact posterior elements to be included in the fusion should be exposed first to establish some normal anatomic relationships, which facilitate exposure of the fractured elements. It is important not to disturb facet joints of the levels that are not to be fused to prevent late instability or degenerative changes in these important motion segments.

Pedicles are identified using the anatomic landmarks available. The proper orientation for angling the screw superior or inferior can be determined by looking at the angle of the pedicle in a cross table, lateral radiograph that was used for localizing the appropriate level. The screw must also be angled medially approximately 5° to 10° to assure it follows the pedicle into the vertebral body. In the fractured segment, the screw may be angled to assure that the screw has the best bone purchase.

Once the posterior entry point has been defined for the pedicle, we use a burr to decorticate the posterior cortex. A pedicle finder is carefully used to find the pathway for the screw, and a small wire is placed into the path. These wires can then be visualized by plain radiograph or under fluoroscopy to assure they are in

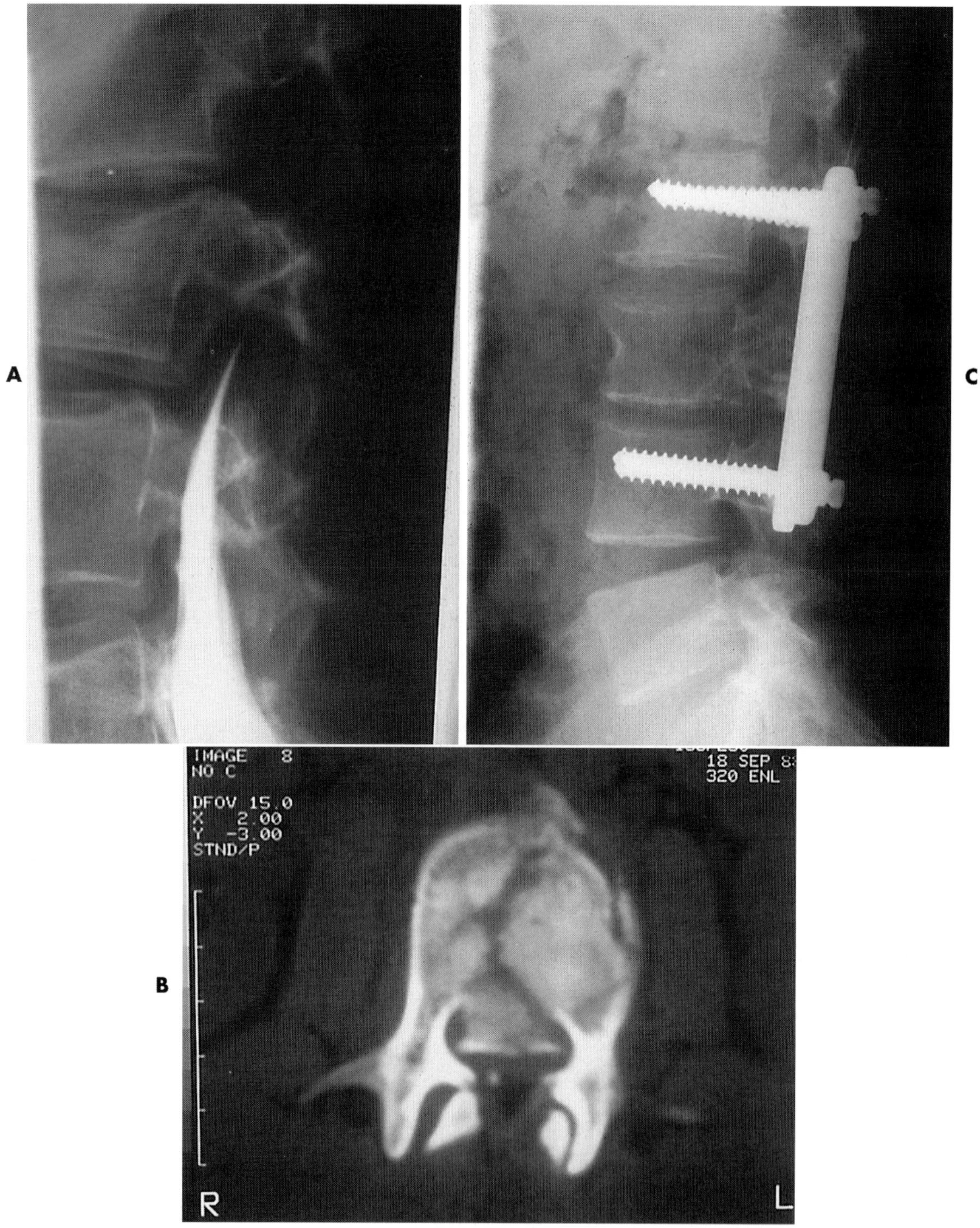

FIGURE 13-3

Twenty-six-year-old male was involved in a motorcycle accident and rendered paraplegic. He was transferred to our hospital 4 days after the injury with no motor function of the lower extremities but with slight perineal and rectal sensation. **A**, Lateral anteroposterior myelogram reveals the burst fracture of the L3 vertebral body and complete blockage of the myelographic dye. **B**, computed tomography scan reveals the large burst fragment occluding approximately 80% of the spinal canal with complete blockage of the myelographic dye. **C**, Patient was taken to the operating room and underwent indirect reduction of the burst fragment with distraction and a small hemilaminotomy site for ultrasound confirmation of burst fragment reduction. Additionally, a posterolateral fusion with pedicle screw instrumentation was performed. This figure reveals an 18-month follow-up radiograph with excellent lateral alignment and restoration of vertebral body heighth. The patient did return to ambulate with a single cane and bilateral AFOs but did not have the return of bowel and bladder function.

the pedicles. This pedicle may then be tapped, and a pedicle "feeler" may be used to feel the grooves for the threads of the screw along the circumference of the pedicle pathway. An appropriate screw length is then inserted into the anterior portion of the vertebral body being careful not to penetrate the anterior cortex.

Indirect reduction is then performed by distracting the spine along rods contoured for the normal amount of anatomic lordosis in the lumbar spine. Extension or lordosis of the screws may then be added if the system allows for the independent positioning of the screws in relationship to the contoured rods. For low lumbar spine fractures, which usually do not have a large amount of loss of vertebral body height or kyphotic deformity, indirect reduction using ligamentotaxis performed within 48 hours usually suffices for reduction of canal encroachment (see Figs. 13-2 and 13-3).[1,2,46,56] In cases where indirect decompression is inadequate, a laminectomy with direct removal of the encroaching fragments is necessary.

A laminectomy may be performed, and the anterior fragments may be impacted forward as described earlier in this chapter. Care must be taken in those patients with lamina fractures because they may have dural tears. In some of our cases with lamina fractures, the dura is torn and the nerve roots are protruding through the lamina fracture. The neural elements must not be injured during the exposure of the fracture, and the dural tears must be carefully repaired.

The area involved in the fusion must be properly decorticated to form a proper bed for the bone graft. Iliac crest bone graft is then taken and placed posterolaterally for an intertransverse process fusion. We prefer to use a morselized bone graft, which is harvested from the iliac crest using a small acetabular reamer. This bone paste has been shown to provide for a faster and more reliable fusion.[59]

Postoperatively, the patient is placed into a custom-molded TLSO. The patient is allowed to ambulate in the brace as soon as possible. Radiographs are checked when the patient first ambulates to assure that the position of the construct has not changed. Serial radiographs are taken, and the fusion is usually solid in 3 to 6 months.

Excellent results have been shown with this technique.[1,2,60] Fractures with minimal deformity are appropriately managed with conservative measures. However, when surgical treatment is necessary, the treatment of choice is short segmental pedicle screw instrumentation using a posterior approach. Occasionally, an anterior decompression is needed to supplement posterior surgery.

Anterior Surgery. Anterior surgery requires more expertise and is less commonly used for fractures of the low lumbar spine. In the more common thoracolumbar spine fractures, anterior decompression and instrumentation provides an optimal environment for neural decompression and recovery.[61] Its use is extremely limited in the less common low lumbar spine fractures, however, and there are no long-term studies to support its general use over posterior instrumentation in low lumbar fractures.

ADVANTAGES OF ANTERIOR SURGERY. The primary benefit of an anterior approach is the ability for direct decompression of the spinal canal. Several studies have indicated that indirect posterior reduction alone may not provide sufficient neural decompression, and either a direct transpedicle posterior decompression or a second stage anterior decompression may be necessary (Fig. 13-4).[13,27,61,62] In a biomechanical fracture model, anterior surgery with instrumentation provided more canal decompression when compared to posterior indirect decompression.[61] This decompression combined with an anterior strut graft and instrumentation provide for immediate stability. In unstable burst fractures, the anterior and middle columns are compromised. By reconstructing the anterior and middle columns via an anterior approach, spinal stability can be restored.

Another theoretic advantage of anterior instrumentation is the load sharing aspect of an anterior reconstruction. When the lumbar fracture is severely comminuted and the fragments are widely separated, the ability of the anterior vertebral body to transmit load is markedly compromised. When these fractures are treated with posterior instrumentation alone, the load is transmitted posteriorly through the posterior construct and the anterior vertebral body has little resistance to axial compression resulting in more motion at the injured segment. The ability of posterior instrumentation systems to control motion at the anterior spine when there is minimal load sharing capabilities of the vertebral body is poor.[63] This situation may occur when a decompression results in a partial corpectomy or in severely comminuted, collapsed fractures. The posterior fixation may fail and a kyphotic deformity may ensue.

The load sharing classification system described earlier in this chapter can help recognize which fractures are poorly controlled with posterior fixation and which require some type of anterior support. Using this system, the authors who described the classification were able to predict failure of posterior instrumentation.[16] Biomechanical studies have shown that stability can be restored in these fractures by using anterior strut grafting combined with posterior fixation.[63]

Another distinct advantage of anterior instrumentation is the stability it affords when used in place of posterior constructs. In a biomechanical study on unstable burst fractures, anterior reconstruction with grafting and instrumentation was found to be more stable than posterior devices.[61] The constructs were tested in axial compression, rotation, and flexion-

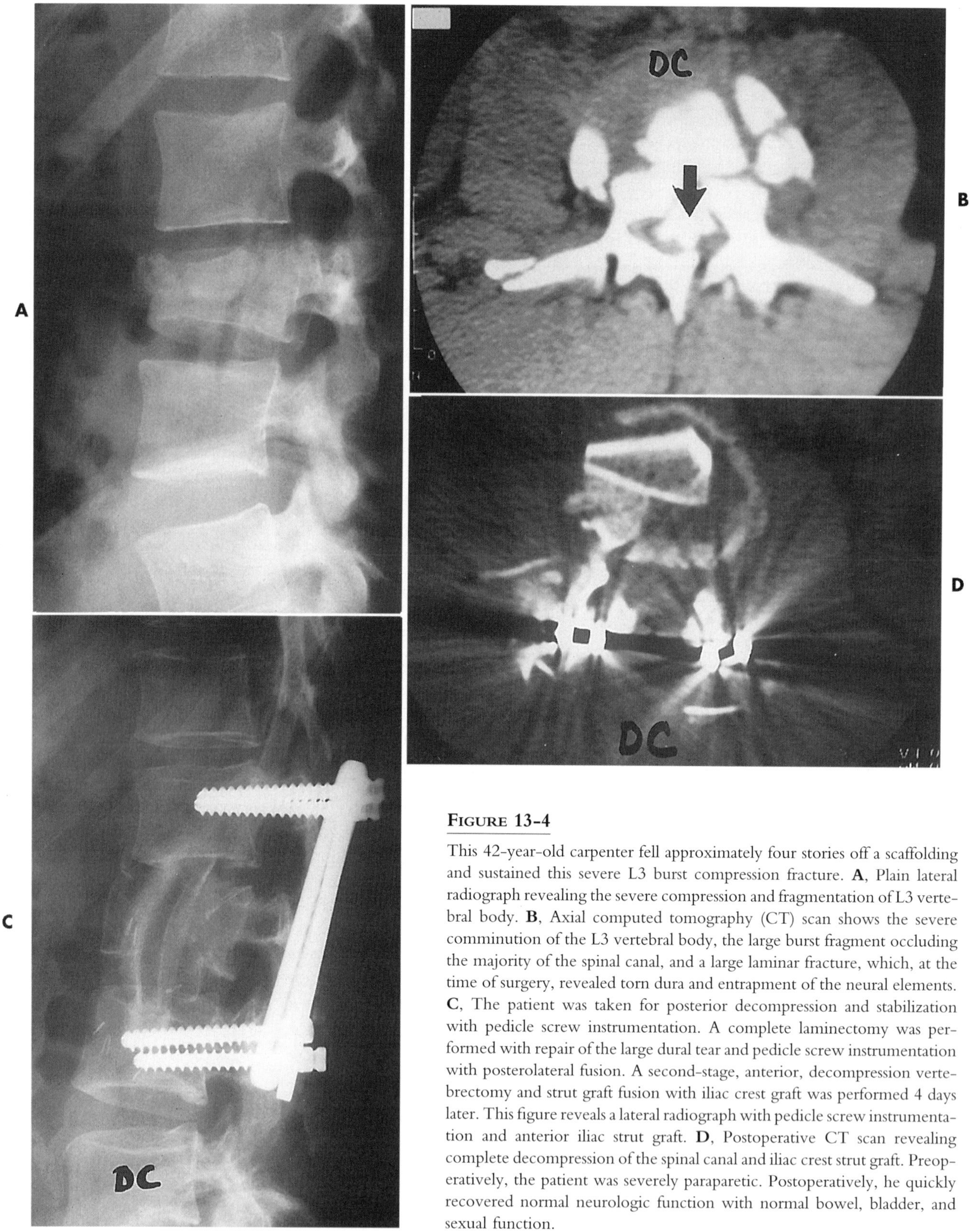

FIGURE 13-4

This 42-year-old carpenter fell approximately four stories off a scaffolding and sustained this severe L3 burst compression fracture. **A**, Plain lateral radiograph revealing the severe compression and fragmentation of L3 vertebral body. **B**, Axial computed tomography (CT) scan shows the severe comminution of the L3 vertebral body, the large burst fragment occluding the majority of the spinal canal, and a large laminar fracture, which, at the time of surgery, revealed torn dura and entrapment of the neural elements. **C**, The patient was taken for posterior decompression and stabilization with pedicle screw instrumentation. A complete laminectomy was performed with repair of the large dural tear and pedicle screw instrumentation with posterolateral fusion. A second-stage, anterior, decompression vertebrectomy and strut graft fusion with iliac crest graft was performed 4 days later. This figure reveals a lateral radiograph with pedicle screw instrumentation and anterior iliac strut graft. **D**, Postoperative CT scan revealing complete decompression of the spinal canal and iliac crest strut graft. Preoperatively, the patient was severely paraparetic. Postoperatively, he quickly recovered normal neurologic function with normal bowel, bladder, and sexual function.

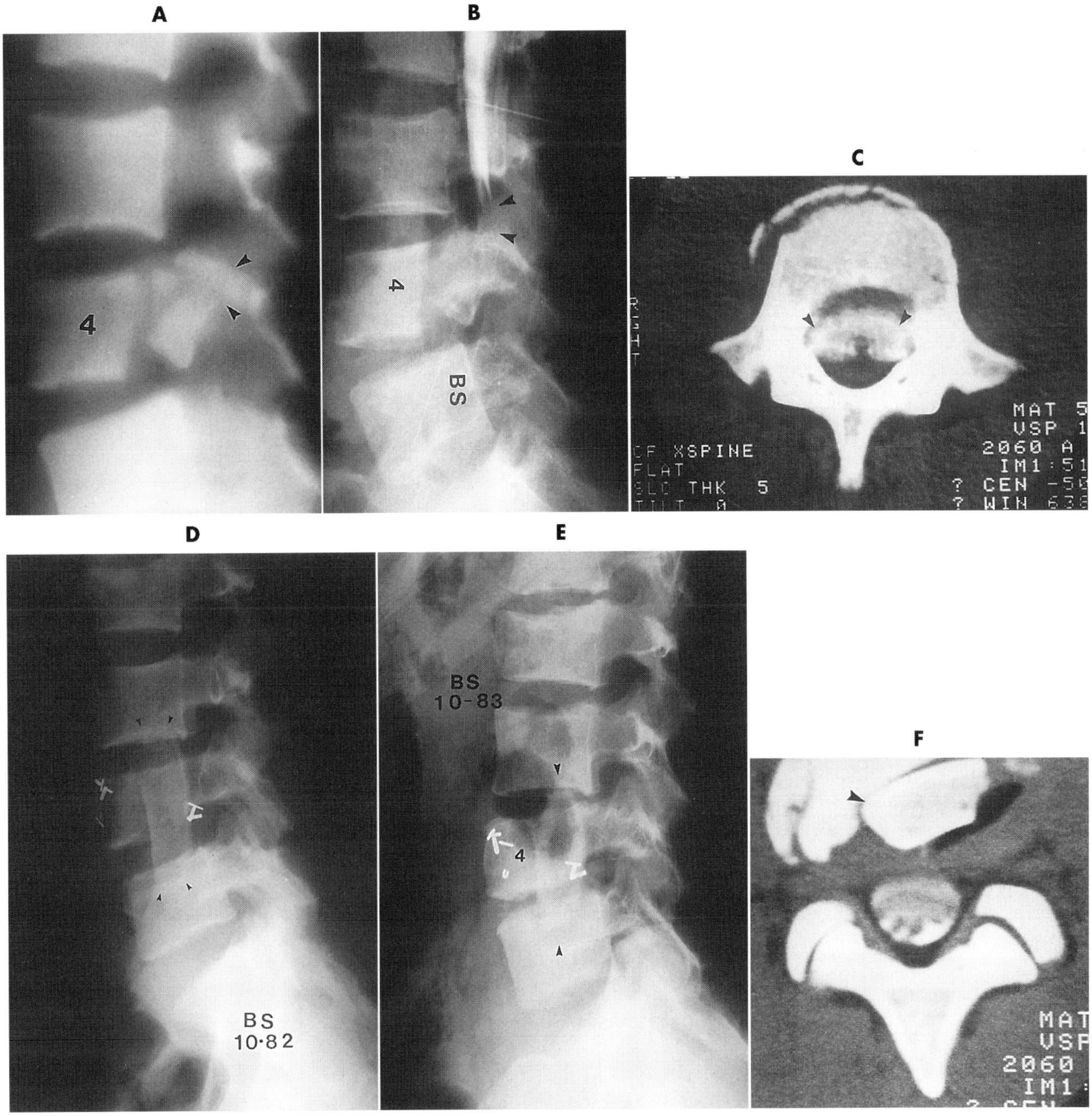

Figure 13-5

This 33-year-old officer in the United States Army was involved in a motor vehicle accident and sustained a severe L4 vertebral body fracture. **A**, Lateral tomogram revealing the burst fragments of L4 vertebral body protruding significantly into spinal canal. **B**, This lateral myelographic view shows complete block of the myelographic dye beginning at the top of L4 burst fragments. **C**, Axial computed tomography (CT) scan shows the large burst fragment occluding approximately 75% of the spinal canal. **D**, The patient was taken for anterior decompression, vertebrectomy, and fusion with iliac crest bone graft. This figure is an immediate postoperative radiograph showing excellent alignment of the lateral lumbar spine and maintenance of normal vertebral body height. **E**, A 1-year postoperative radiograph shows continued maintenance of vertebral body height and normal sagittal alignment. This patient had complete return of neurologic function. **F**, Postoperative CT scan reveals the complete spinal canal decompression and the arrow notes the iliac crest strut graft.

extension, and, in all cases, the anterior instrumentation surpassed the posterior devices. This makes sense when one remembers that unstable burst fractures disable the anterior and middle columns, which can be directly reconstructed by anterior strut grafting and solid instrumentation.

The use of older posterior instrumentation, such as Harrington rods, required the fusion of several levels above and below the fractured vertebra. Anterior instrumentation allows for reconstruction of the fractured segment and fusion of only one level above and below the fracture. This allows for the preservation of motion segments in the low lumbar spine where each segment is valuable. With the advent of pedicle screw instrumentation, however, which also allows for fusion of the minimal number of levels, this advantage of anterior instrumentation is no longer absolute.

INDICATIONS FOR ANTERIOR SURGERY. In certain low lumbar fractures, anterior grafting or decompression along with posterior instrumentation may be needed. We recommend the use of anterior decompression only in the rare instance when posterior indirect reduction of the fracture fragments is inadequate. We also recommend anterior supplemental grafting in fractures that have required a significant amount of anterior bone removal for the decompression or grossly unstable fractures that are not sufficiently stabilized by posterior instrumentation alone.

TECHNIQUE. Anterior surgery should be performed by experienced surgeons. The retroperitoneal approach is commonly used and has been shown to provide excellent access to the low lumbar levels.[62] In many institutions, general surgeons collaborate with the orthopedic surgeon for the approach. Decompression is performed under direct visualization and strut grafting is commonly used (Fig. 13-5).

The grafting that is used must reconstruct the anterior and middle columns and withstand the axial loads place on the spine to achieve immediate stability. Commonly, iliac crest bone graft or fibular graft is used. Allograft with iliac crest bone graft placed inside the allograft ring may also be used. These grafting techniques provide for load sharing of the anterior portion of the lumbar spine. Metal cages with bone graft placed inside also are sometimes used. If anterior instrumentation is necessary, many forms of anterior plating systems are available. Instrumentation placed in the anterior portion of the low lumbar spine approximates several important structures such as the aorta or iliac veins. The complications of anterior instrumentation could prove disastrous if the hardware is prominent and erodes into these vital structures. We currently do not recommend the use of anterior instrumentation devices below the L3 or L4 vertebrae. This recommendation is supported by other authors.[64] Posterior instrumentation with distraction and lordosis usually provide adequate decompression. If further decompression is necessary, a second stage anterior decompression with bone grafting for support can be used.

Many surgeons do not recommend the use of an anterior approach to the lumbar spine for fractures at the level of L4 and L5 because of the problems with anterior fixation at these levels.[60] They also believe that decompression at these levels, especially of root lesions, are better treated by posterior decompression. Other authors have cited the fact that dural tears associated with neurologic deficits occur most commonly on the posterior surface and are more properly addressed by a posterior approach.[65]

REFERENCES

1. An HS, et al: Low lumbar burst fractures: comparison among body cast Harrington rod, Luque rod, and Steffee plate, *Spine* 16(8 suppl.):S440–S444, 1991.
2. Levine AM, Edwards CC: Low lumbar burst fractures: reduction and stabilization using the modular spine fixation system, *Orthopedics* 11(10):1420–1432, 1988.
3. Benson DR, Mintz LJ. Spondylolysis and spondylolisthesis: congenital and isthmic. In Kasser JR, editor: *Orthopedic knowledge*, Update 5, Park Ridge, Illinois, 1996, American Academy of Orthopedic Surgeons.
4. Calenoff L, et al: Multiple level spinal injuries: importance of early recognition, *Am J Roentgenol* 130:665–669, 1978.
5. Keenen TL, Antony J, Benson DR: Non-contiguous spinal fractures, *J Trauma* 30(4):489–491, 1990.
6. Bracken MB, et al: A randomized, controlled trial of methylprednisolone or naloxone in the treatment of acute spinal-cord injury: results of the Second National Acute Spinal Cord Injury Study, *N Engl J Med* 322:1405–1411, 1990.
7. Spivak JM, Vaccaro AR, Cotler JM: Thoracolumbar spine trauma: evaluation and classification, *J Am Acad Orthop Surg* 3:345–352, 1995.
8. Lane JM, Riley EH, Wirganowicz PZ: Osteoporosis: diagnosis and treatment, *J Bone Joint Surg* 78A:618–632, 1996.
9. Einhorn TA, Bone metabolism and metabolic bone disease, In Kasser JR, editor: *Orthopedic knowledge*, update 5, Park Ridge, Illinois, 1996, American Academy of Orthopedic Surgeons.
10. Holdsworth F, Fractures, dislocations and fracture-dislocations of the spine, *J Bone Joint Surg* 52A:1534–1551, 1970.
11. Whitesides TE Jr, Shah SGA: On the management of unstable fractures of the thoracolumbar spine: rationale

for use of anterior decompression and fusion and posterior stabilization, *Spine* 1:99–107, 1976.
12. Denis F: Spinal instability as defined by the three-column spine concept in acute spinal trauma, *Clin Orthop* 65–76, 1984, 189.
13. McAfee PC, et al: The value of computed tomography in thoracolumbar fractures, *J Bone Joint Surg* 65A:461–473, 1983.
14. Classification of thoracic and lumbar fractures. In Gertzbein SD: *Fractures of the thoracic and lumbar spine*, Baltimore, 1992, Williams & Wilkins.
15. Magerly F, et al: A comprehensive classification of thoracic and lumbar injuries, *Eur Spine J* 3(4):184–201, 1994.
16. McCormack T, Karaikovic E, Gaines R: The load sharing classification of spine fractures, *Spine* 19:1741–1744, 1994.
17. Panjabi MM, et al: Validity of the three-column theory thoracolumbar fractures: a biomechanical investigation, *Spine* 20(10):1122–1127, 1995.
18. James KS, et al: Biomechanical evaluation of the stability of thoracolumbar burst fractures, *Spine* 19(15):1731–1740, 1994.
19. Frederickson BE, Yuan HA, Miller H: Burst fractures of the fifth lumbar vertebrae, *J Bone Joint Surg* 64A:1088–1094, 1982.
20. Thoracolumbar spine fractures without neurologic deficit. In Stauffer ES: *American Academy of Orthopaedic Surgeons Monograph Series*. Rosemont, 1993, AAOS.
21. O'Brien J, Betz R, Berman A: A comparison of children with spinal cord injury with and without radiographic abnormality. Presented at the annual meeting of the American Orthopaedic Association, Pittsburgh, March 29–April 1, 1995.
22. Kinoshita H, et al: Conservative treatment of burst fractures of the thoracolumbar and lumbar spine, *Paraplegia* 31(1):58–67, 1993.
23. Delamarter RB, Sherman J, Carr JB: Pathophysiology of spinal cord injury, *J Bone Joint Surg* 77A:1042–1049, 1995.
24. Bohlman HH: Current concepts review: treatment of fractures and dislocations of the thoracic and lumbar spine, *J Bone Joint Surg* 67A:165–169, 1985.
25. Brown GA: Bone resorption in the canal following a thoracolumbar fracture with a displaced diaphyseal fragment, *Iowa Orthop J* 9:69–71, 1989.
26. Willen J, Lindahl S, Nordwall A: Unstable thoracolumbar fractures: a comparative clinical study of conservative treatment and Harrington instrumentation, *Spine* 10:111–122, 1985.
27. Dunn HK: Anterior spine stabilization and decompression for thoracolumbar injuries, *Orthop Clin North Am* 17:113–119, 1986.
28. Jacobs RR, Casey MP: Surgical management of thoracolumbar spina injuries, *Clin Orthop Rel Res* 189:22–35, 1984.
29. Denis F, et al: Acute thoracolumbar burst fractures in the absence of neurologic deficit: a comparison between operative and nonoperative treatment, *Clin Ortho Rel Res* 189:142–149, 1984.
30. Ferguson RL, Allen BL: An algorithm for the treatment of unstable thoracolumbar fractures, *Orthop Clin North Am* 17:105–112, 1986.
31. Kostuik JP: Anterior fixation for fractues of the thoracic and lumbar spine with or without neurologic involvement, *Clin Orthop* 189:142, 1984.
32. Kropinger WJ, et al: Conservative treatment of fractures of the thoracic and lumbar spine, *Orthop Clin North Am* 17:161–170, 1986.
33. Dewald RL: Burst fractures of the thoracic and lumbar spine, *Clin Ortho Rel Res* 189:150–161, 1984.
34. Garfin SR: Thoracolumbar spine trauma. In Poss R, editor: *Orthopedic knowledge*, update 3, Park Ridge, Illinois, 1990, American Academy of Orthopedic Surgeons.
35. Weitzman G: Treatment of stable thoracolumbar spine compression fractures by early ambulation, *Clin Ortho Rel Res* 76:116–122, 1971.
36. Roy-Camille R, Saillant G, Mazel C: Plating of thoracic, thoracolumbar and lumbar injuries with pedicle screw plates, Clin Orthop North Am 17:147–154, 1986.
37. Johnsson R, et al: Spinal canal remodeling after thoracolumbar fractures with intraspinal bone fragments, *Act Orthop Scand* 62(2):125–127, 1991.
38. Ried D, et al: The nonoperative treatment of burst fractures of the thoracolumbar junction, *J Trauma* 28:1188, 1988.
39. Shulman WP, et al: Thoracolumbar burst fractures: CT dimensions of the spinal canal relative to postsurgical improvement, *AJNR* (6)337–342, 1985.
40. Nicoll EA: Fractures of the dorso-lumbar spine, *J Bone Joint Surg* 31A:376–394, 1949.
41. Court-Brown CW, Gertzbein SD: The management of burst fractures of the fifth lumbar vertebrae, *Spine* 12:308–312, 1987.
42. Frederickson BE, Yuan HA, Miller H: Burst fractures of the fifth lumbar vertebrae, *J Bone Joint Surg* 64A:1088–1094, 1982.
43. Lagrone MO, et al: Treatment of symptomatic flatback after spinal fusion, *J Bone Joint Surg* 70A:569–580, 1988.
44. Gertzbein SD, MacMichael D, Tile M: Harrington instrumentation as a method of fixation in fractures of the spine, *J Bone Joint Surg* 64B:526–529, 1982.
45. Keene JS, et al: Diagnosis of vertebral fractures, *J Bone Joint Surg* 64A:586–595, 1982.
46. Mumford J, et al: Thoracolumbar burst fractures: the clinical efficacy and outcome of nonoperative management, *Spine* 18(8)955–970, 1993.
47. Bedbrook GM: Treatment of thoracolumbar dislocation and fractures with paraplegia, *Clin Ortho Rel Res* 112:27–43, 1975.

48. Cantor JB, et al: Nonoperative management of stable thoracolumbar burst fractures with early ambulation and bracing, *Spine* 18(8)971–976, 1993.
49. Patwardhan AG, et al: Orthotic stabilization of thoracolumbar injuries: a biomechanical analysis of the Jewett hyperextension orthosis, *Spine* 15:654–661, 1990.
50. Panjabi MM, et al: Thoracolumbar burst fracture: a biomechanical investigation of its multidirectional flexibility, *Spine* 19(5)578–585, 1994.
51. Bedbrook GM: A balanced viewpoint in the early management of patients with spinal injuries who have neurological damage, *Paraplegia* 23:8–15, 1985.
52. Frankel HC, et al: The value of postural reduction in the initial management of closed injuries of the spine with paraplegia and tetraplegia, *Paraplegia* 7:179–192, 1969.
53. Davies WE, Morris JH, Hill V: An analysis of conservative (nonsurgical) management of throacolumbar fractures and fracture dislocations with neural damage, *J Bone Joint Surg* 62A:1324–1328, 1980.
54. Willen J, Anderson J, Toomoka K, Singer K: The natural history of burst fractures at the thoracolumbar junction *J Spinal Disord* 3:39–46, 1990.
55. Weinstein JN, Collalto P, Lehman TR: Thoracolumbar "burst" fractures treated conservatively: a long-term follow-up, *Spine* 13:33–38, 1988.
56. Zou K, et al: Mechanics of anatomic reduction of thoracolumbar burst fractures: comparison of distraction versus destraction plus lordosis, in the anatomic reduction of the thoracolumbar burst fracture, *Spine* 18(2):195–203, 1993.
57. Harrington RM, et al: Biomechanics of indirect reduction of bone retropulsed into the spinal canal in vertebral body fracture, *Spine* 18(6):692–699, 1993.
58. Hardaker WT Jr, et al: Bilateral transpedicular decompression and Harrington rod stabilization in the management of severe throacolumbar burst fractures, *Spine* 18:692–699, 1992.
59. Kushwaha VT, Minchew JT, Delamarter RB: Rapid lumbar fusion using an alternative graft harvesting technique. Presented at the annual meeting of the American Academy of Orthopaedic Surgeons, Orlando, Florida, Feb. 20, 1995.
60. Levine AM: Surgical techniques for thoracic and lumbar trauma. In Rothman RH, Simeone FA, editors: *The spine*, ed 3, Philadelphia, 1992, WB Saunders.
61. Shono Y, McAfee PC, Cunningham BW: Experimental study of thoracolumbar burst fractures: a radiographic and biomechanical analysis of anterior and posterior instrumentation systems, *Spine* 19(15)1711–1722, 1994.
62. McAfee PC, Bohlman HH, Yuan HA: Anterior decompression of traumatic thoracolumbar fractures with incomplete neurological deficit using a retroperitoneal approach, *J Bone Joint Surg* 67A:89–104, 1985.
63. Maiman DJ, et al: Effects of anterior vertebral grafting on the traumatized lumbar spine after pedicle screw-plate fixation, *Spine* 18(15)2423–2430, 1993.
64. Shonnard NH, Anderson PA: Low lumbar (L3–L5) spinal fractures, *Semin Spine Surg*, 7(2):116–127, 1995.
65. Cammisa FP, Eismont FJ, Green AB: Dural laceration occurring with burst fractures and associated laminar fractures, *J Bone Joint Surg* 71A:1044–1052, 1989.

14

FRACTURES OF THE SACRUM AND COCCYX

Steven Nagelberg
Hillel Sperling

Given the complexity associated with treatment of fractures of the sacrum and coccyx, relatively little has been written on this subject, especially compared with the recent research concerning fractures of the lumbar and cervical spine. Significant information on sacrum and coccyx fractures is infrequently published. With the publication of the Denis' classification of sacral fractures, however, there is some increased interest.[1] This may be related to the fact that this landmark classification system links the zone of injury with a likely neurologic prognosis.

To understand and treat sacral fractures, one must have an excellent understanding of the morphology of the sacrum and its neurological relationships. With increased incidence of injury to the spine because of vehicular accidents, the incidence of sacral fractures has increased. While high-impact trauma is the most common cause of sacral fractures, Newhouse et al. have presented a series of 17 occult sacral fractures, in osteopenic patients.[2] These fractures were present without significant associated trauma. Technology has enabled us to better appreciate and diagnose sacral fractures when previously we depended on plain radiographs alone.

We attempt in this chapter to review the current state of both diagnosis and treatment of sacral fractures, after presenting the normal anatomy and morphology of the sacrum and coccyx.

ANATOMY OF THE SACRUM AND COCCYX

The sacrum is a composite bone consisting of five fused vertebra. Its shape is shield-like or triangular with an anterior concave surface and a posterior convex surface. In the coronal plane, it is widest superiorly and tapers inferiorly towards its apex. The anterior surface of the sacrum forms the posterior wall of the pelvis, and its lateral portions, the pars lateralis, opposite the first three sacral segments, articulate with the iliac bones forming the sacroiliac joints. These joints are stabilized by the very thick posterior sacroiliac ligaments and the anterior sacroiliac ligaments. Additional stabilizers of the sacrum, found more caudally, are the sacrospinous and sacrotuberous ligaments. The cranial surface of the sacrum contains the endplate for the lumbosacral disk and superior articular processes, which articulate with the inferior articular processes of the last lumbar vertebra. In the erect position, the upper aspect of the first sacral vertebra is tilted forward at an angle of approximately 30° to 40°.[3]

The anterior surface of the sacrum contains the promontory, which is the superior margin of the first sacral vertebra projecting forward in a sharp lip. At its inferior surface, the sacrum articulates with the superior surface of the coccyx by a fibrocartilaginous disk. The ventral surface contains ridges at the sites of the remnants of the anterior vertebral disks.[4] These ridges point laterally toward neural foramina and lateral masses of the fused vertebra. The lateral masses of the first sacral segment expand to form the sacral alae, which have the appearance of wings. The neural foramina are formed by the resultant anterior and posterior lateral mass fusion and fusion of the vertebral bodies. Through the anterior sacral foramina emerge the sacral ventral rami and their vessels. The rami later converge to form the sacral plexus. The size of the ventral neural foramina decreases successively in a cephalad to caudad direction. The ridges of bone that separate the anterior sacral foraminal are very prominent and form the origin of the piriformis muscle.[5]

The posterior convex surface of the sacrum exhibits a series of longitudinal ridges. The middle ridge is known as the middle sacral crest and is formed by the fusion of spinous tubercles, which are a continuation of the spinous processes of the lumbar vertebra. A sacral groove on either side of the middle sacral crest separates it from the medial sacral articular crest, which represents the fused articular processes. The most cephalad portion of these crests forms the superior articular processes of the first sacral vertebra and contributes to the formation of the lumbosacral articulation. The roof of the sacral spinal canal is a continuous one, formed by the fusion of the neural arches of the first four sacral segments. The fifth sacral segment is devoid of a complete neural arch and contains a rudimentary articular process and pedicle on each side. It is these prominences of the fifth sacral segment that form the cornua of the sacrum. The sacral hiatus is the opening of the spinal canal on the posterior surface, and it is bounded by the sacral cornua and the caudal edge of the neural arch of the fourth sacral segment. The fifth sacral vertebral body is flattened on its caudal surface to facilitate articulation with the coccyx.[5,6]

On the dorsal surface there are additional paired neural foramina formed by fusion of the posterior elements of the sacrum. It is through these posterior foraminae that sacral dorsal rami exit from the spinal canal. On the lateral aspects of the posterior foramina, lateral crests and sacral tuberosities serve as attachments for dorsal sacroiliac ligaments. These ligaments and the sacrum are anterior to the posterior iliac spines, creating a space that contains the origin of the inferior portion of spinal extensor muscles. Multifidus muscles lie in grooves between the median spinal crest and the articular crests. Origins of the iliocostal and iliolumbar muscles are dorsal and lateral to the origins of the multifidus muscles.[5,7]

Soft tissue structures are in intimate proximity to the sacrum and can be injured as a result of sacral fracture. The spinal canal, which is curved and triangular in cross section, contains the dural sac, which usually ends at S2. Beyond this point, the filum terminale extends and continues to insert into the coccyx. On the anterior surface of the sacrum, the ventral rami exit through the foramina and continue on to form the lumbosacral plexus. Other structures nearby are the ureters and internal iliac vessels and their branches, which also may be injured.[8,9]

IMAGING OF SACRAL FRACTURES

If the practitioner suspects that injury and fracture of the sacrum has occurred, various imaging techniques can be used to assess the type and extent of the injury. High-energy trauma should always raise suspicion.

Radiography. Because of the shape and orientation of the sacrum, exact detail of the sacrum cannot be completely visualized on an anteroposterior (AP) radiograph of the pelvis. Because of its curvature, an AP film of the pelvis reveals the upper half in end on fashion and shows more detail of the lower half. An AP view taken with the beam projected cephalad 30° permits a better assessment of the upper portion of the sacrum with its neural foramina.[1] Transverse fractures of the sacrum are difficult to detect on a radiograph, especially on AP views. They may be seen on lateral views of the sacrum and, most likely, only if they are displaced in the AP plane. Findings on an AP radiograph may include disruption or blurring of the trabecular pattern of the lateral sacral mass, asymmetry of the sacral notch, and irregularity or discontinuity of the arcuate lines (roofs of the sacral foramina).[10] Sacral fractures should also be suspected when other associated findings such as fracture of the transverse process of the lowest lumbar vertebra are seen on the AP radiograph. When viewing an AP view of the pelvis, if there is presence of a significant fracture of the anterior portion of pelvis but no posterior pelvic lesions, a sacral fracture should be suspected.[9] Plain radiographs, however, still miss 20% to 30% of traumatic fractures of the sacrum; therefore, detection requires other imaging studies.[11]

Tomography. Anteroposterior and lateral tomograms can be helpful in visualizing sacral fractures. Anteroposterior tomograms are helpful in outlining zone I and zone II injuries, and lateral tomograms are helpful in delineating zone III injuries. Lateral tomograms are especially useful in visualizing transverse fractures of the sacrum.[1]

Computed Tomography Imaging. Computed tomography (CT) scanning with multiplanar reformatted images is a valuable tool in the assessment of sacral fractures. Bone windows and soft tissue sections taken in 5-mm intervals can demonstrate the orientation and type of fracture, and its relationship to the neurologic structures.[9] Zone I fractures, especially displaced ones, which can damage the obturator nerve and lumbosacral trunk, can be adequately visualized with CT scanning. Fractures in zone II, which involve the neural foramina with potential damage to the sacral nerve roots, and zone III fractures, which involve the spinal canal, can be assessed with great detail, especially when adding multiplanar reformations. These are helpful in assessing the degree of comminution and direction of fragment displacement.[12]

In addition, CT scanning can simultaneously identify presacral hematoma and other associated lesions such as sacroiliac dislocations and fractures of the pelvis. Computed tomographic scanning also is useful in diagnosing sacral insufficiency fractures, which occur usually in older patients, predominately women.[13] These fractures can occur by themselves or can be associated with fractures around the pubic symphysis. These usually occur in patients with osteoporosis and rheumatoid arthritis, and in those who have received radiotherapy. Plain radiographs show these fractures in approximately 30% of cases, and CT scanning and radionuclide scanning are helpful in detecting these types of fractures.[2,14]

Magnetic Resonance Imaging. Sagittal magnetic resonance imaging (MRI) sections are most useful in identifying and demonstrating transverse fractures of the sacrum. To date, the exact place for MRI scanning in the evaluation of sacral fractures is not known, because vast experience with MRI imaging is lacking. It may become a useful tool in the evaluation of damage to soft tissue structures in the vicinity of the sacrum.

Myelography. Denis, Davis, and Comfort state that myelography is of limited use in sacral fractures, and its limitation is usually due to poor visualization of the roots within the foramina.[1] Traumatic avulsion of the lumbosacral nerve roots may lead to posttraumatic pseudomeningoceles. Myelography can detect these pseudocysts and may exhibit vanishing of the sacral nerve roots in the foramina or absence of lumbosacral trunk at the lumbosacral fossa.[11] Myelography can be supplemented with postmyelography CT scanning. Myelography may only be useful in high injuries of the sacrum, because the dural sac ends at S2.[9]

Neurologic Evaluation

Sacral fractures may be associated with neurologic injury, from single nerve root injuries with dermatomal sensory loss only to a more serious involvement, accompanied by loss of bowel, bladder, and sexual function. Careful neurologic evaluation is essential and helps determine both the site of injury and prognosis. For higher nerve root injuries, such as L5 and S1, patients may present with dermatomal sensory loss, motor deficit, reflex changes, or all three.

Lower neurologic injury may present with dermatomal sensory loss, bowel, bladder, or sexual dysfunction. It is essential that a very careful and thorough neurologic evaluation be performed including dermatomal evaluation and rectal examination, which assesses bulbocavernous reflex and anal sphincter tone. In patients with relatively minor injuries, these evaluations are simple and straightforward. In the multiinjured patient, however, this type of evaluation often can be overlooked in the face of more serious life threatening problems.

Neurological Injuries

Unfortunately at times, neurologic injury is discovered later on in the patient's treatment course as the patient improves, when the patient cannot void following removal of the urinary catheter or has loss of volitional bowel function.

The L5 nerve root dysfunction presents with weakness of great toe extension (EHL) and weakness of gluteus medius function, that is, hip abduction. There is associated diminished sensation along the lateral leg and dorsum of the foot. The S1 nerve root dysfunction presents with weakness of foot eversion, secondary to weakness of the peroneus longus and brevis and weakness of hip extension and gluteus maximus. There can be a loss of the Achilles tendon reflex with diminished sensation along the lateral malleolus and lateral and plantar side of the foot. The S2, S3, and S4 nerves are the principal nerve supply to the bladder. Obviously, bladder muscles cannot be separately tested on manual examination; however, these nerve roots also supply the intrinsic muscles of the foot, and abnormalities in this area should be looked for. There are no specific reflex changes associated with this injury. Dermatomal sensory loss however, is more easily tested for dermatomes associated with the S2, S3, and S4-S5 nerve roots are concentrically arranged around the anus. In addition, the superficial anal reflex should be checked. To perform this, the skin around the anus is simply lightly touched and the sphincter should contract in response.

Although neurodiagnostic testing, that is, electromyography and nerve conduction studies, may have an important place in evaluation of injuries to the lumbar and cervical spine, it is much less useful in the evaluation of sacral injuries. In addition, these tests are of little use until at least 3 weeks following the traumatic event. They may, however, have some usefulness in attempting to separate injuries of distal lumbar and sacral nerve roots from peripheral nerve injuries.

Because of the difficulties in evaluating the multiinjured patient and the occasional lack of easily tested results, we, along with many other authors, recommend the use of cystometrograms in the early phase of evaluation in patients who have sustained sacral fractures involving the sacral canal.

Given the difficulties sometimes associated with the diagnosis of sacral fractures from a radiographic standpoint, careful neurologic evaluation is essential. This evaluation can lead one to suspect injury when it is not obvious on plain radiographs. Unfortunately, as has already been noted, neurologic evaluation in this area and the associated findings are frequently overlooked.

Classification of Sacral Injuries

A number of authors have presented classification systems of sacral fractures. The first system was presented by Bonnin in 1945.[15] That system, however, had several deficiencies. It was not until the system presented by Denis et al. in 1987 that a simple system was proposed, which related location of fracture to a likelihood of neurologic injury (Fig. 14-1). The importance of this system is that it helped the clinician relate the prognosis of the injury to the fracture itself. The usefulness of this system was confirmed by Gibbons in 1990 in a retrospective analysis of 253 patients with pelvic or sacral fractures.[16]

We would like to suggest a fourth category of fracture: occult sacral fractures in osteopenic patients, as these injuries occur without significant trauma.

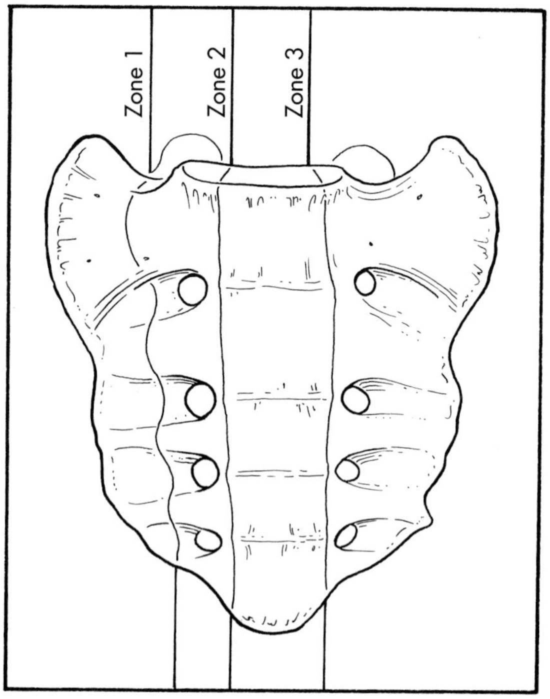

FIGURE 14-1

The three zones of injury as suggested by Denis.[1]

Zone I. Zone I injuries involve a fracture of the sacrum lateral to the lateral most aspect of the foraminal line. Fractures in this category may be of two types: minimally displaced fractures and severely displaced fractures, such as seen in vertical sheer fractures. As noted by Denis, neurologic deficit is relatively uncommon in this category, occurring no more that 6% of patients. These injuries would include either injury to the L5 nerve root or the sciatic nerve.

Zone II. Zone II fractures involve one or more foramina. The incidence of neurologic injury associated with the fractures in Denis' study is 28%. Suggested by this classification, this can involve one or more neural foramen. Bowel and bladder involvement, although uncommon, can be present as well.

Zone III. In zone III injuries, the fracture involves primarily the central sacral canal. One can see multizonal injuries; however, these fractures are still classified in zone III. As one might predict, the likelihood of neurologic injury is far higher in this category, with Denis' study suggesting frequency of neurologic injury greater than 56%. Bowel and bladder dysfunction also were quite common. In one study, it was greater than 76%.[1]

Occult Sacral Insufficiency Fractures (Suggested Zone IV). Newhouse et al. presented a separate category of sacral fractures in 1992.[2] These fractures are somewhat unique in they are frequently seen in elderly women, and they usually occur without trauma. Associated medical conditions were common in this group, including a history of malignancy of the pelvis with and without radiation treatment. Symptoms universally resolved as long as other conditions were not present.

TREATMENT

The treatment of sacral fractures may be accomplished by nonsurgically or surgically. The method of treatment depends on the type and extent of injury and should address skeletal instability and neurologic injury.[9] The classification of Denis et al. is helpful in delineating treatment.[1,17,18]

ZONE I FRACTURES

Fractures of the sacral ala are usually stable and not displaced and usually cause no neurologic injury. These may be treated symptomatically with an initial period of bed rest and subsequent early mobilization. Mobilization should consist of nonweight-bearing or partial weight-bearing with a walker or crutches, as the patient's symptoms dictate.

Sacral fractures can occur in conjunction with fractures of the pelvis. The pubic rami may be fractured in addition to the sacral fracture; however, this situation may remain stable. Lateral compressive injuries to the pelvis also are stable as long as the posterior sacroiliac ligaments remain intact. When the pain diminishes, mobilization may be begun early to allow weight-bearing on the uninjured side.

In the presence of unstable sacral ala fractures and anterior pelvic instability, anterior pubic rami fractures are treated with application of an external fixator. If symphyseal disruption is present, however, this should be treated with open reduction and internal fixation plating. If there is no vertical shear component to the sacral fracture, then early mobilization is possible with nonweight-bearing or partial weight-bearing.

Vertically unstable alar fractures may produce a traumatic "far-out" syndrome, by crushing the L5 nerve root in between the superiorly migrated alae fragment and the transverse process of L5. Initial treatment consists of traction to allow for decompression and reduction of tension on the L5 nerve root. When the patient has stabilized, surgical treatment can consist of open reduction and internal fixation of the sacral fracture and the anterior pelvic fracture. An alternate approach is open reduction, internal fixation of the sacral fracture, and an external fixation device anteriorly. In patients with vertical shear injuries it is recommended that even after open reduction, internal fixation can be maintained with bed rest for 3 to 4 weeks.

ZONE II FRACTURES

The anterior pelvic rings are stable in these types of fractures, and the sacral fractures are usually nondisplaced or minimally displaced. Patients with these types of fractures usually do not have sciatica and can be treated with early mobilization with nonweight-bearing of the extremity on the side of foraminal involvement. Those patients who have sciatica should be treated with bed rest until the sciatica has adequately improved, and nonweight-bearing or partial weight-bearing on the side of the foraminal fracture may be started at that time. If the patient has persistent sciatic symptoms after 6 to 8 weeks of rest and CT evidence reveals that the S1 or S2 foramina are narrowed by at least 50%, then sacral foraminotomy is indicated. Motor deficit is also an indication for surgical decompression.

Unstable zone II fractures may be seen in conjunction with lateral compression or "open book-type" injuries and with vertical shear injuries. The vertical shear sacral-type fractures also can cause the traumatic "far-out" syndrome involving the L5 nerve root. These also are treated with closed reduction by using traction, keeping the fracture reduced, and removing pressure from the L5 nerve root. When the patient's condition stabilizes, treatment consists of open reduction, internal fixation posteriorly and anteriorly, or open reduction with internal fixation posteriorly and external fixation anteriorly. Zone II sacral fractures, in conjunction with lateral compression and "open book pelvic-type" injuries are treated similar to the zone I sacral fractures that have these similar associated pelvic injuries.

ZONE III FRACTURES

Zone III injuries without neurologic deficits are treated by stabilization. In those patients with neurologic injury, surgery is planned by obtaining an accurate diagnosis of the pathoanatomy from CT scanning. This imaging study allows detailed visualization of foraminal encroachment and neural involvement in the central sacral spinal canal.

Denis et al. have described the sacral burst fracture in which the sacral vertebral body has retropulsed into the central spinal canal without concomitant fracture of the sacral lamina.[1] Early surgical decompression is indicated, as delayed surgery appears to yield poor results.

Low transverse fractures usually occur through S4 and are usually treated symptomatically. High transverse fractures require decompression of the sacral spinal canal. If displacement is severe, with intractable pain, reduction may be required. Threaded pins inserted into the particular portion of the sacrum can assist in providing purchase for fractures that cannot be manually reduced. On occasion, obtaining and maintaining reduction of a sacropelvic injury can allow decompression of neural structures so that no further surgery may be required.

Surgical methods for open reduction and internal fixation of fractures of the sacrum are usually achieved with a posterior incision.[14,19] An additional vertical incision is made on the opposite side so that both iliac crests can be spanned if the posterior tension band approach is to be used. Types of fixation devices available for this are threaded, metal rod assemblies and large, double cobra plates. Another method of fixation is by internal fixation with cannulated lag screws, transfixing the fracture from the iliac wing to the body of the sacrum.[20] This should be performed with the assistance of an image intensifier. Pohlemann et al. also have described a stabilization technique of local osteosynthesis using adapted standard AO/ASIF small fragment implants.[21]

COCCYX

ANATOMY

The coccyx has no supportive functional role in the spine. It is one of the points of origin of the gluteus maximus muscle posteriorly and of the muscles of the pelvic diaphragm anteriorly.[5] The coccyx, like the sacrum, is a composite of three to five fused rudimentary vertebral bodies. The first coccygeal vertebra has vestigial transverse processes and cornua that can become large enough to articulate with the sacral cornua.[3,8] The coccygeal cornua are vestigial superior articulating processes. The first coccygeal vertebra articulates with the apex of the sacrum.

The vertebral canal does not continue into the coccygeal vertebra; however, the sacral hiatus provides egress for the S5 and coccygeal nerves. These nerves are the sensory innervation of the coccyx. The coccygeal nerves and the dorsal rami of S4 and S5 join to innervate the skin of the gluteal cleft over the coccyx.[6,9]

DIAGNOSIS OF COCCYDYNIA

A careful history and thorough physical examination are essential to the diagnosis of coccydynia. Coccydynia is usually associated with falls, especially falls directly onto the buttocks. Patients typically describe intense pain with sitting and with straining, which is relieved by lying down. Symptoms can be persistent and partially disabling.

Other potential causes of perceived coccygeal pain need to be investigated. These would include gynecologic problems, neoplasms, and more proximal intraspinal causes. Physical examination should include observation of the skin and surrounding tissues, rectal examination, and in a female patient, a pelvic examination. The one constant in evaluation of patients with coccydynia is pain associated with motion of the coccyx. In true coccydynia, patients almost always have pain associated with motion of the coccyx. When other causes are present, such as a referred pain to the coccyx, motion of the coccyx is not typically painful.

TREATMENT

The treatment of chronic coccygeal pain, or coccydynia, involves the treatment of the symptoms. Treatment may include the use of a rubber donut, a firm narrow board, and/or antiinflammatory medications. Use of other invasive treatments, such as local anesthetic and/or steroid injections into the area may result in reduced symptoms. There are those that believe coccygeal manipulation has a place in the management of coccydynia, although the literature does not necessarily confirm this. Frequency of sitting may be reduced by severity of symptoms.

Given the chronicity of symptoms in many patients, alternative types of treatments such as acupuncture and biofeedback training have been recommended by some. The use of antidepressants may have a place in patients who develop chronic incapacitating pain.

We believe it is rarely, if ever, indicated to consider coccygectomy in the management of these symptoms. We urge clinicians who are considering this procedure to have their patients evaluated by a psychiatrist or psychologist before this, given the significant incidence of functional overlay in this particular group of patients.

SUMMARY

Fractures of the sacrum and coccyx can be overlooked, but with multiple trauma, evaluation of the area is critical. Special radiographic views and CT imaging may be required to diagnose and classify the injury. The Denis classification provides sufficient information to guide treatment and predict outcome. Nontraumatic related conditions can contribute to fracture in this region and must be considered.

REFERENCES

1. Denis F, Davis S, Comfort T: Sacral fractures: an important problem. Retrospective analysis of 236 cases, *Clin Orthop* 227:67–81, 1988.
2. Newhouse KE, El-Koury EY, Buckwalter JA: Occult spinal fractures in osteopenic patients, *J Bone Joint Surg (Am)* 74(10):1472–1477, 1992.
3. White AH, Schofferman JA: *Spine care,* St. Louis, 1995, Mosby–Year Book.
4. Rockwood CA Jr, Green DP: *Fractures in adults,* Philadelphia, 1984, JB Lippincott.
5. Rothman RH, Simeone FA: *The spine,* ed 2, Philadelphia, 1982, WB Saunders.
6. Crafts RC: *A textbook of human anatomy,* New York, 1966, Ronald Press.
7. Rothman SLG, and Glenn WV Jr: *Multiplanar CT of the spine,* Baltimore, 1985, University Park Press.
8. Grant JCB: *Grant's atlas of anatomy,* ed 6, Baltimore, 1972, Williams & Wilkins.
9. Frymoyer JW: *The adult spine. Principles and practice,* New York, 1991, Raven Press.
10. Farrah M, et al: Radiographic evaluation of the acutely traumatized thoracolumbar spine and sacrum. *Spine: State of the Art Reviews,* 3(2):299–311, 1989.
11. Manelfe C: *Imaging of the spine and spinal cord,* New York, 1992, Raven Press.
12. Fishman EK, et al: Fractures of the sacrum and sacroiliac joint: evaluations by computerized tomography with multiplanar reconstruction. *South Med J* 81(2):171–177, 1988.
13. Peh WCG, et al: Imaging of pelvic insufficiency fractures, *Radiographics* 16:335–348, 1996.
14. American Academy of Orthopaedic Surgeons: *Orthopaedic Knowledge,* update 2, Park Ridge, Illinois, 1987, AAOS.
15. Bonnin JG: Sacral fractures and injuries of the cauda equina, *J Bone Joint Surg* 27:113, 1945.
16. Gibbons KJ, Soloniuk DS, Razack N: Neurology injury and patterns of sacral fractures. Department of Neurology, State University of New York, Buffalo, *J Neurosurg* 72(6):889–903, 1990.
17. Samberg CL, Kurz LT, Herkowitz HN: Lumbar spine injuries, *Spine: State of the Art Reviews,* 3(2):269–277, 1989.
18. Crenshaw AH: *Campbell's operative orthopaedics,* ed 8, St. Louis, 1992, Mosby–Year Book.
19. American Academy of Orthopaedic Surgeons: *Orthopaedic Knowledge,* update 3, Park Ridge, Illinois, AAOS, 1990.
20. American Academy of Orthopaedic Surgeons: *Orthopaedic knowledge,* update 4, Rosemont, Illinois, 1993.
21. Pohlemann T, et al: Fixation of transforaminal sacrum fraction a biomechanical study, *J Orthop Trauma* 7(2):107–117, 1993.

15

PEDIATRIC INJURIES OF THE SPINE: DIAGNOSIS AND MANAGEMENT

Christian H. Dee
Sean E. Nork
Serena S. Hu

INCIDENCE AND DEMOGRAPHY

Injuries to the spine in children and adolescents are relatively rare, accounting for between 2% to 7% of all injuries to the spine.[1–7] In one retrospective review of 57 children with spinal injuries, vehicular trauma accidents were the cause in 46% of cases. This percentage decreased to 29% in children under the legal driving age of 16. Spinal cord injury without radiographic abnormality (SCIWORA) occurred in 38% of children under 13 compared with 12% of children over 13.[8] Reviewing spinal injuries in children under 16 years of age, 70% involved the cervical spine.[9] The most common injury in children age 13 or older was flexion-distraction injury of the lumbar spine often associated with abdominal trauma similar to injury patterns in adults.

Another review from the Mayo Clinic of 143 patients between 2 months and 15 years of age showed similar demographics.[10] Children less than 11 years of age suffered an increased proportion of upper cervical spine injuries most commonly from a fall from a height. These injuries resulted in a high proportion of neurologic injuries with higher mortality rates. Injuries in children between 11 and 15 years of age were more commonly caused by sports and other recreational activities and were predominantly located in the lower cervical spine. Adults had a similar injury pattern. Similarly, Birney and coworkers in their review of 84 consecutive children with traumatic cervical spine injuries found that 38% were results of a fall from a height, 17% were from road traffic accidents, and the remainder were from various sports and recreational activities. Upper cervical spine injuries were more common in younger children, who had a 21% incidence of SCIWORA.[11]

Hamilton and coworkers reviewed 174 pediatric patients with spinal column injuries of which 42% involved the cervical spine. Overall, 52% were injured as a result of motor vehicle accidents in their series. Patients up to 9 years of age were more likely to be pedestrians struck by a car or to have fallen from a height (79%). Patients 15 years of age or older were more likely to be drivers or passengers in motor vehicle accidents (63%). Children accounted for only 5.3% of all patients admitted for spinal column injuries, with a disproportionately high percentage of spinal cord injuries (45% overall) particularly in the group up to aged 9 and older (74%) when compared with adults. Injuries between the occiput and C2 represented 67% of cervical spine injuries in the up to 9 age group compared with 6% in the 10- to 14-year-old age group and 7% in children between ages 15 to 17. In the 0- to 9-year old age group, 50% of children with SCIWORA had complete deficits compared with 11% in the 15- to 17-year old age group.[12]

The developing spine has numerous physes that fuse at predictable times during a child's development. Any physician involved in the treatment of spinal injuries should be aware of normal development and its variations in order to accurately diagnose the abnormal. Spinal cord injury may occur before vertebral column failure in the young child and frequently requires techniques such as magnetic resonance imaging (MRI) to document the injury.

When a child's spine requires surgical stabilization, it must be remembered that the child's smaller size makes the use of internal fixation less feasible. When used, it is often limited to wiring techniques supplemented by external fixation devices such as Minerva casts or halo vests. Expert help from other specialists such as those in rehabilitation medicine, urology, psychiatry, anesthesiology, pediatrics, and physical and occupational therapy is preferred as an integral part of the SCI health care team.

DEVELOPMENT OF THE SPINE

Embryology

The development of the spine is a complex series of programmed events that begin very early during the first 8 weeks after conception. By the third week of development, three germ layers develop by gastrulation to form three structures: the primitive streak, the notochord, and the neural tube. The primitive streak is a midline thickening of the epiblast from which forms the mesoderm, which then forms the nucleus pulposus and induces formation of the neural plate and serial segmentation of the centra. The ectoderm in the midbody region forms a precursor to the spinal cord called the neural tube formed from the neural plate. The paraxial mesoderm forms paired segments along the neural tube called somites, which develop into the paraspinal musculature (myotomes), connective tissues of the skin (dermatomes), and the vertebral column (sclerotomes).

The embryonic period follows (fourth to eighth week of development). During this period, the embryo is most vulnerable to teratogenic insults with potential formation of neural tube defects (spinal dysraphisms), and congenital spinal anomalies. The somites grow dorsolaterally with some trailing cells surrounding the notochord. The sclerotomes dorsally form the vertebral arch and ventrally form the vertebral column as segmental condensations of cells, which are loosely arranged at their cephalic ends. The intervertebral disks are formed from densely packed cells of the sclerotomes, which migrate to the center of their respective myotomes. The residual densely packed cells at each sclerotome combine with the loosely grouped cells of the caudal adjacent sclerotome to form the centrum. The caudal half of each sclerotome fuses with the cephalic half of the sclerotome below to form the mesenchymal vertebral body. Each centrum forms two cartilaginous centers by the sixth week, which then fuse to form a single cartilaginous centrum. Cartilaginous centers appear on each side of the arch and fuse with one another.

By the end of gestation each cartilaginous vertebra contains three primary ossification centers: one for each vertebral body and two for each neural arch.

Ossification

By birth, ossification of the vertebral centrum and developing arches is well under way. The ossific center of each vertebral centrum is separated from the neural arch by a broad cartilaginous neurocentral junction, which fuses usually between 3 and 6 years of age. Occasionally bipartite centers (anterior and posteriorly) associated with anomalous vessel arrangements may be encountered. Such normal variants result in coronally clefted vertebrae, which usually fuse by 4 years of age. The ossification center is ovoid on a lateral radiograph and approximately the same height as the disk space. The ossification centers of the vertebral arches usually fuse between 2 and 4 years of age.

As growth continues, the bodies appear more rectangular with visible indentations on the anterior surface of the vertebral body because of vascular channels that persist until the end of growth. Superior and inferior steplike recesses appear on the anterior edge of the vertebral bodies at 5 years of age. Small calcific foci begin to form in these cartilaginous regions between 6 and 8 years of age in girls and 7 and 9 years of age in boys. These foci fuse and form the bony vertebral ring apophysis at 12 years of age.

The spinous processes are formed by an amalgamation of the neural arches. This begins in the lumbar area soon after birth and spreads to the cervical area by 2 years of age. Union may occur in the atlas as late as 6 years of age and in the sacrum at 10 years of age. The neurocentral synchondroses ossify in the cervical region by 3, continuing caudally to reach the sacrum by 6 or 7 years of age.

The Atlas

The atlas is formed from three ossification centers, one in the body and one in each neural arch (Fig. 15-1). The ossification centers appear in utero in the seventh week. The body of the atlas is not visible radiographically until the second year of life. The synchondrosis of the posterior spinous process usually has fused by 3 years of age. The synchondroses located at each side of the body have usually fused by 7 years of age. Failure of fusion of the ossification centers may be mistaken for a fracture.

The Axis

There are four main ossification centers that form the axis: the odontoid, the body, and two halves of the neural arch (Fig. 15-2). The odontoid originates from two ossification centers that fuse in the midline in the seventh fetal month. A secondary ossification center appears at the tip of the dens between 3 and 6 years of age and fuses with the odontoid by 12 years of age. The synchondrosis between the body and odontoid fuse by 3 to 6 years of age but may still be visible until 11 years of age. This synchondrosis is a common source of confusion during interpretation of posttrauma cervical spine radiographs. The arches fuse posteriorly by 2 to 3 years of age.

C3 to C7 and Thoracic and Lumbar Spine

The vertebral body arises from a single ossification center that appears by the fifth fetal month (Fig. 15-3). The neural arches appear by the eighth fetal week and fuse posteriorly by the third year of life. The synchondroses between the body and arches fuse by

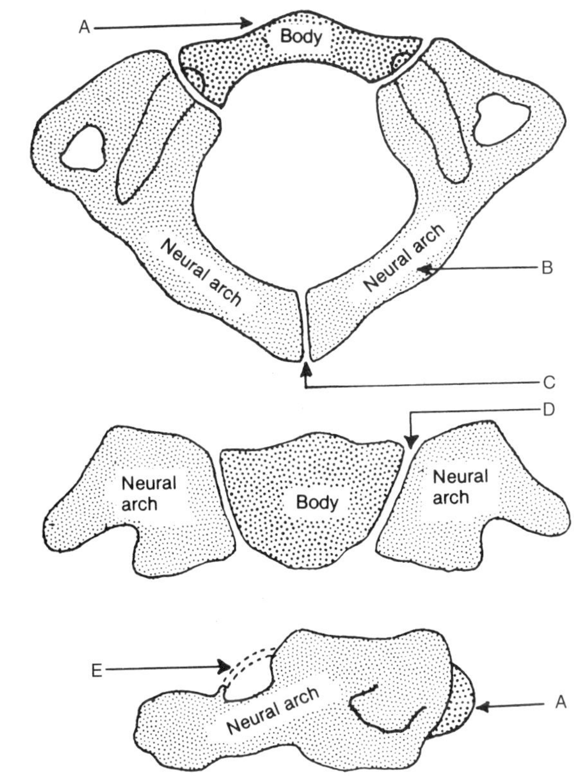

FIGURE 15-1

Diagram of the first cervical vertebra (atlas). **A** Body. The body is not ossified at birth; the center (occasionally two centers) appears during the first year of life. The body may fail to develop resulting in forward extension of the neural arches. **B** Neural arches. These appear bilaterally at about the seventh fetal week. The most anterior portion of the superior articulating surface is usually formed by the body. **C** Synchondrosis of the spinous processes. Union may rarely be preceded by the appearance of a secondary center within the synchondrosis. **D** Neurocentral synchondrosis. This fuses by approximately 7 years of age. **E** Ligament surrounding the superior vertebral notch. This may ossify, especially later in life. (From Bailey DK: Normal cervical spine in infants and children, *Radiology* 59: 712–719, 1952.)

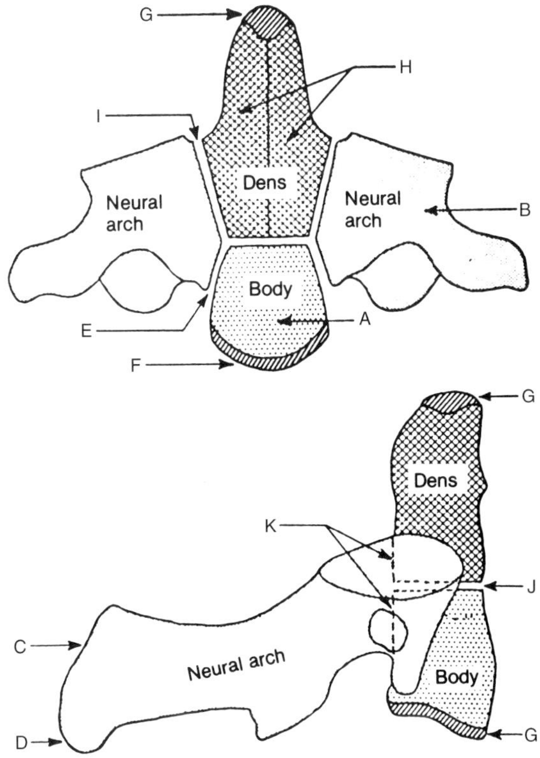

FIGURE 15-2

Diagram of the second cervical vertebra or axis. **A** Body. One center (occasionally two) appears by the fifth fetal month) **B** Neural arches. These appear bilaterally by the seventh fetal month. **C** Neural arches. These fuse posteriorly by the second or third year. **D** Bifid tip of the spinous process (occasionally a secondary center is present in each tip). **E** Neurocentral synchondrosis. This fuses at 3 to 6 years of age. **F** Inferior epiphyseal ring. This appears at puberty and fuses at about 25 years of age. **G** "Summit" ossification center for the odontoid. This appears at 3 to 6 years of age and fuses with the odontoid by 12 years of age. **H** Odontoid (dens). Two separate centers appear by the fifth fetal month and fuse with each other by the seventh fetal month. **I** Synchondroses between the odontoid and neural arch. This fuses at approximately 3 to 6 years of age. **J** Synchondrosis between the odontoid and the body. This fuses at 3 to 6 years of age. **K** Posterior surface of the body and odontoid. (From Bailey DK: Normal cervical spine in infants and children, *Radiology* 59:712–719, 1952.)

the third to sixth year of life. Secondary ossification centers in the superior and inferior epiphyseal rings appear by puberty. These are subject to avulsion fractures in the thoracolumbar spine in flexion distraction injuries. There are three additional secondary ossification centers that appear around the same time of the bifid spinous process tips and each transverse process. In the lumbar spine, the mamillary processes also develop from secondary ossification centers. All secondary ossification centers have fused by 25 years of age.[13,14]

PATHOANATOMY

There are some important anatomical considerations that are unique to the pediatric patient. The orientation of the facet joints changes during the child's development. For example the angle of the C1-C2 facet is 55° from the horizontal in the newborn and increases to 70° at maturity. In the lower cervical spine, the angles of the facet joints are 30° at birth and increase to 70° at maturity. The more horizontal inclination of the facet joints and increased ligamentous laxity explain the increased motion seen in dynamic cervical spine radiographs in the child.

The higher proportion of C1-C2 injuries in the under 8-year-old age group appears to the result of the wedge-shaped vertebral bodies in the developing spine and the more cephalad fulcrum of neck motion. The disproportionately large head predisposes small children to flexion injuries in the upper cervical region.

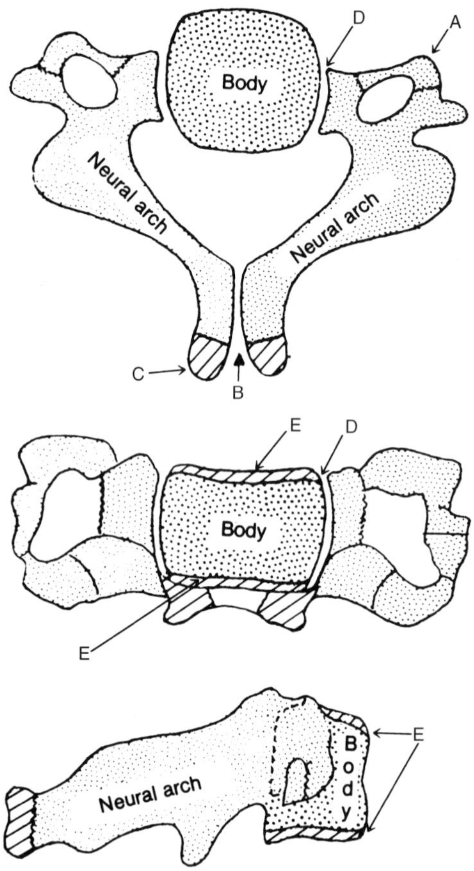

Figure 15-3

Diagram of the typical cervical vertebra, C3–C7. The body appears by the fifth fetal month. **A** Anterior portion of the transverse process. This may develop from a separate center, which appears by the sixth fetal month and joins the arch by the sixth year. The neural arches appear by the seventh to ninth fetal week. **B** Synchondrosis between the spinous processes. This is usually united by the second or third year. **C** Secondary centers for bifid spine. These appear by puberty and unite with the spinous process by 25 years of age. **D** Neurocentral synchondrosis. This fuses at 3 to 6 years of age. **E** Superior and inferior epiphyseal rings. These appear at puberty and unite with the body at approximately 25 years of age. The seventh differs slightly because of a long powerful nonbifid spinous process. (From Bailey DK: Normal cervical spine in infants and children, *Radiology* 59:712–719, 1952.)

Maturation of the spinal cord vascular supply also is an important variable. Indeed the tenuous blood supply of the immature spine may help to explain the increased proportion of SCIWORAs in children who sustain injuries in this region. The anterior two-thirds of the spinal cord is supplied by a solitary anterior median spinal artery and posterior third by two posterolateral spinal arteries with very little anterior-posterior anastomosis. These arteries anastomose with a variable number of medullary feeder arteries, which are themselves supplied by segmental arteries that terminate at the intervertebral foramen at every level. A medullary feeder as low as L4 or L5 may be on occasion the sole source of blood for the conus medullaris. The surgically important artery of Adamkiewicz is on the left side of the lower thoracic spine in 80% of patients.

The immature spine has an increased physiologic mobility compared with the adult spine. This is attributed to an increased ligamentous laxity and more horizontally inclined facet joints discussed above. During injury the osteocartilaginous vertebral column may lengthen as much as 2 inches before failure. The spinal cord can only tolerate 0.25 inches of stretching before disruption occurs.[15,16] This finding is one factor that may help explain the SCIWORA phenomenon seen in children under 8 years of age.

In the cervical spine, the vertebral artery is contained within the foramen transversarium from C6 to C2. At C1, the vessel passes through the foramen and courses over the superior surface of the atlas to enter the foramen magnum posteriorly approximately 1.5 cm from the midline in the adult. This distance is less in the child. At C7 the artery runs anterior to the transverse process. The spinous process of C7 is not bifid, is easily palpable, and is a useful anatomic landmark during planning of surgical incisions in this region.

The conus medullaris in the infant is at the level of L4. It ascends to the adult level of L1 by 2 months of age, because the vertebral column grows faster than the spinal cord.[17]

IMMOBILIZATION AND TRANSPORT

Adequate immobilization of any patient with a cervical spine injury is critical in preventing further injury. The pediatric patient, when placed on a flat spine board, has his or her cervical spine forced into kyphosis because of the disproportionately large head (Figure 15-4).[18]

Herzenberg demonstrated an increase in deformity and kyphosis in a clinical series of 10 children with cervical spine injuries when the patients were placed on an adult spine board. This displacement of upper cervical spine fractures was reduced when the thorax of the patients were elevated by folded towels or mattress under the thorax. This resulted in a more neutral alignment of the spine and reduction of fracture.[19] Head circumference increases logarithmically from birth, whereas chest circumference increases linearly. A child usually has reached 50% of his or her adult head circumference by 18 months of age but does not reach 50% of adult chest circumference until 8 years of age.[20] This explains the disproportionate size between the head and the chest. In children under the age of 10, a pediatric spine board with cut-out area for the occiput should be used routinely to maintain neutral alignment of the spine. If this is not available, an adult board may be used with a double mattress pad or folded towels to raise the chest. The amount of padding required to safely maintain neutral alignment is not known. Each case should be monitored with a lateral radiograph

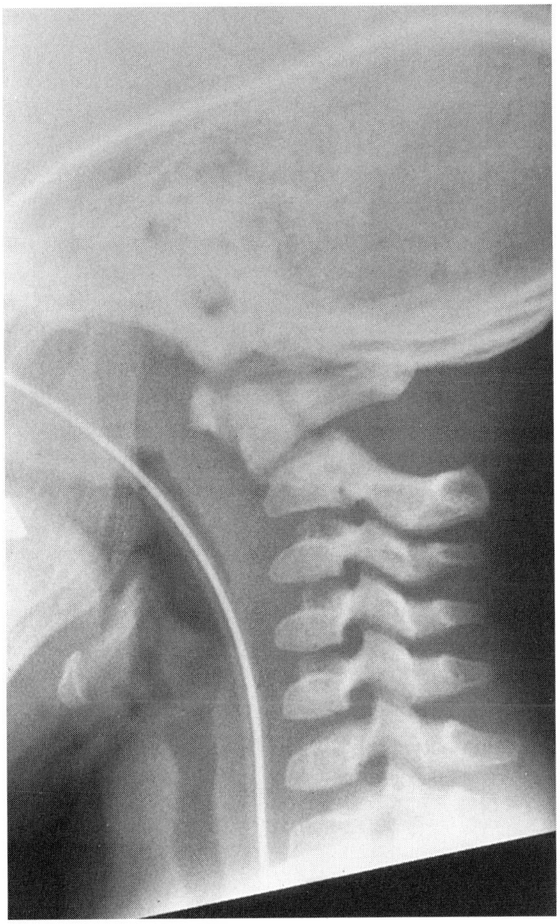

FIGURE 15-4

Lateral cervical spine radiograph of a 2 1/2-year-old female after a fall. The disproportionately large head produces flexion of the neck. In this case, forward displacement of C1 on C2 has occurred. (Courtesy of Children's Hospital, Oakland.)

to check the alignment of the spine. This has been confirmed by Nypaver and Treloar who were unable to show a linear relationship between the patient's age and amount of padding required under the thorax to obtain neutral alignment of the spine.[21] By approximately age 10 the adult backboard may be used; however, surveillance lateral radiographs should be obtained to confirm that the spine is in neutral alignment.

Curran and coworkers performed a prospective study of 118 children who were immobilized for suspected cervical spine injuries. Only 11% of the children presented with their spines in a neutral alignment. Sixty-one percent of the children transported had C-spine radiographs with more than 5° of kyphosis or lordosis. Most of these patients were in excessive flexion. The degree of cervical kyphosis did not correlate with the patient's age. A variety of acceptable immobilization techniques were used. These included 1) hard collar and board with towels under the thorax; 2) collar, board, and blocks under the thorax; and 3) collar, board, and other padding under the thorax. No single immobilization technique was shown to be superior. Children up to 12 years of age in their series had significant flexion of the spine despite precautions being taken to avoid this. They emphasized the importance of obtaining surveillance lateral C-spine radiographs even in children with an adult body habitus.[22] Huerta and coworkers have suggested that all children suspected of cervical injuries should have their heads immobilized with a correctly fitting rigid cervical collar with supplemental sandbag and tape.[23]

EVALUATION OF THE INJURED PEDIATRIC SPINE

In the emergency room, all trauma patients should be evaluated in a sequential and coordinated fashion. The cervical spine should be immobilized with a Philadelphia collar and the head stabilized with sandbags during transportation. The patient's airway, breathing, and circulation are evaluated and appropriately addressed in that order. Orotracheal airways in patients with basilar skull fractures or nasotracheal intubation in patients with compromised airways should be instituted, thus protecting the cervical spine by avoiding extension. The use of gentle in-line manual traction to maintain bony alignment is recommended during intubation. The entire spine is immobilized until cleared radiographically. All patients should be carefully examined for any stepoffs or tenderness over the spine region. Searching for ecchymoses from seat belts or direct blows to the spine may provide useful clues to an underlying spinal injury. Associated periorbital ecchymosis or head injury requires careful evaluation for an associated cervical spine injury.

Initial radiographic evaluation of the cervical spine is performed after the patient is resuscitated. The patient is examined, and a history is carefully taken. A detailed neurologic examination of all extremities should be performed, including motor, sensory, reflexes, and rectal examination. These findings should be carefully documented in the medical record and changes investigated. The entire spine is immobilized as described above to prevent potentially adverse motions of unidentified injured regions of the spine. The initial radiographic series is taken when the patient is still, on the backboard, and generally consists of a lateral and open-mouth odontoid view.

RADIOLOGY OF THE PEDIATRIC SPINE

Adequate cervical screening includes a lateral cervical spine radiograph, odontoid view, and, if needed, to view down to the C7-T1 interspace, a swimmer's view or computed tomographic (CT) scan.

Familiarity with the normal growth centers of the pediatric spine, particularly when evaluating patients less than 8 years of age, is essential to identify injuries of the spine. Normal physiologic wedging because of normal incomplete ossification of the superior or inferior endplates should not be confused with fracture (Fig. 15-5). The presence of similar wedging in adjacent vertebrae help differentiate normal ossification from compression fractures. Normal variations in curvature and displacement can make interpretation difficult. Synchondroses and ossification centers have smooth margins. A common variant is the os odontoideum. The dens is usually fused to the body of C2 by 6 years of age, but if delayed, this synchondrosis may be mistaken for a fracture. Fractures tend to have irregular margins. An os odontoideum, which is thought to be caused by an infantile traumatic event, usually reduces with cervical flexion while an odontoid fracture usually reduces with cervical extension.

An open-mouth view of the odontoid may on occasion show an apparent fracture or radiolucency at the base of the odontoid. This line, known as Mach's band, is due to the appearance of dark and light lines appearing at the border of structures of different densities. The use of tomography or sagittal CT scan and MRI scans help differentiate this artifact from pathologic conditions in such cases. The entire spine should be assessed radiographically to exclude other spinal injuries.

Flexion-extension views are useful studies, which help to assess ligamentous instability. They should never be obtained in the comatose patient and should be physician-supervised only in a cooperative patient (Fig. 15-6). They are often not useful in the acute phase of injury because muscle spasm can mask any underlying instability. The atlanto-dens interval (ADI) is normally less than 4 mm in children (3 to 15 years of age) compared with 2.5 mm in patients 15 years of age or older. At C1, one-third of the spinal canal is occupied by the spinal cord, one-third by the odontoid, and one-third is free space. Both the Powers ratio (defined as the ratio of the distances between basion and posterior arch of the atlas and the distance between the anterior arch of the atlas and the opisthion) as well as the dens-basion distance should be measured to determine ligamentous injuries between the occiput and atlas (Fig. 15-7). A Powers ratio greater than 1 suggests an anterior dislocation and less than 1 suggests a posterior dislocation. Traction should be applied gradually starting well below 5 lb to prevent over distraction. Traction is applied to reduce and maintain spinal alignment. Overdistraction should be avoided in the pediatric population. Three-dimensional CT reconstruction has been used in some centers to identify areas of instability instead of dynamic studies in the acute phase.

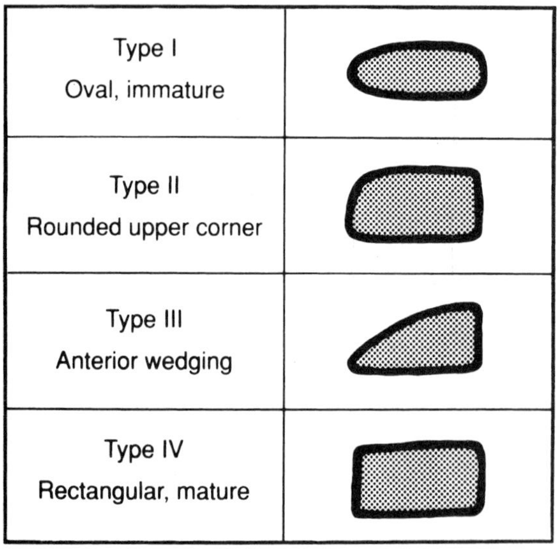

FIGURE 15-5

Cervical wedging is a normal radiographic appearance due to the sequence of ossification of the vertebral bodies. Ossification of the superior body occurs last and explains this appearance, which can be mistaken for a compression fracture. Adjacent vertebrae usually have a similar appearance in the normal developing spine. CT scanning may be helpful in equivocal cases. (Swischuk LE, Swischuk PN, John SD: Wedging of C-3 in infants and children: usually a normal finding and not a fracture, *Radiology* 188: 523–526, 1993.)

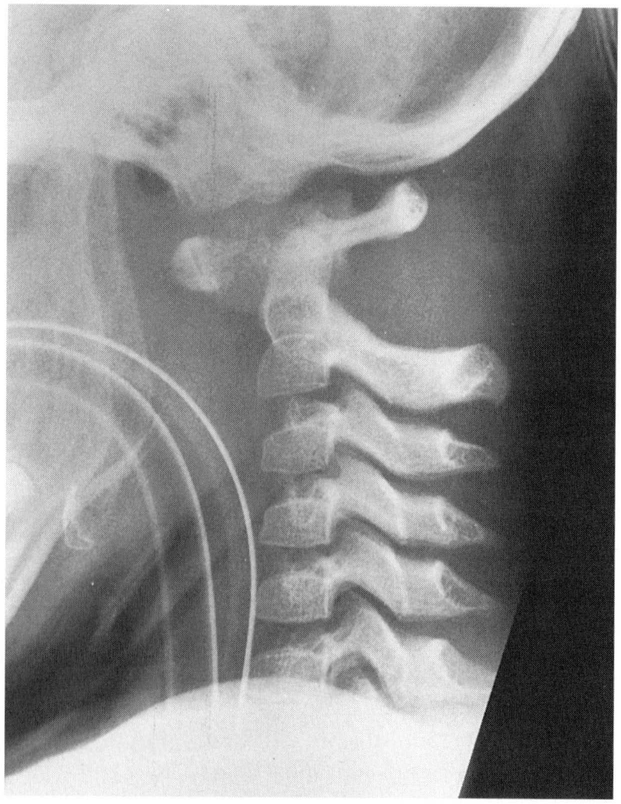

FIGURE 15-6

Lateral flexion radiograph obtained in a 3 1/2-year-old female who was found comatose after a motor vehicle accident. Note C1 on C2 ligamentous injury with increased ADI and C1-C2 subluxation. (Courtesy of Children's Hospital, Oakland.)

Use of the line drawing method described by Swischuk, which is described in the next section is useful in discriminating pseudosubluxation of C2-C3 from pathologic injury. A C2-C3 pseudosubluxation of 3 mm or more is found in 20% of children under 9 years of age.

Increase in the retropharyngeal soft tissue may be the only indication of an underlying spine injury. The reliability of this measurement is variable. The soft tissue swelling can be increased in the crying child. It is measured from the anteroinferior aspect of the second vertebral body to the posterior wall of the pharynx on a lateral cervical spine radiograph. A value greater than 7 mm in both children and adults is pathologic. The retrotracheal space is measured from the anteroinferior aspect of the body of C6 to the posterior aspect of the trachea. It ranges from 5 to 14 mm (average 7.9 mm) in children under 15 years of age. Measurements of this space greater than 14 mm in children and 22 mm in adults warrant further investigation.

PSEUDOSUBLUXATION

Because of the increased ligamentous laxity, more obliquely aligned facets, higher axis of rotation in the sagittal plane to flexion, and immaturity of the joints of Luschka, the pediatric spine undergoes more physiologic motion than the adult spine (Fig. 15-8). To differentiate pathologic from physiologic motion, Swischuk has described a line that can be drawn to assess the alignment of the spinous processes of C1, C2, and C3 on a lateral radiograph. In their review of 26 sets of radiographs, they found that a straight line could be drawn along points made on the anterior surface of the posterior arches of C1 through C3 (Fig. 15-9). Occasionally the line would miss the anterior laminar line of C2 by 1 mm but never more than this in the normal subject. If a fracture or ligamentous instability were present at C2 the line drawn along these points was never straight. It is important that a true lateral be obtained or else erroneous interpretation may result. Flexion-extension of the spine is not required for the use of Swischuk's line; however, occasionally if muscle spasm is present, this causes angulation of C2 may reduce the physiologic offset between C2 and C3 giving a false positive result.[3,24–26] Up to 14% of normal children under the age of 16 may show a loss of cervical lordosis, therefore, this cannot be used as an indicator of muscle spasm or underlying cervical spine injury.[24]

ATLANTOOCCIPITAL INJURIES

The atlantooccipital joint is stabilized primarily by the ligaments that insert into the atlas and axis. The tectorial membrane, the cruciate ligament, the paired alar ligaments, and the apical ligament insert into the axis (Fig. 15-10). The two articular capsules and atlantooccipital membranes insert into the atlas. Flexion-extension is

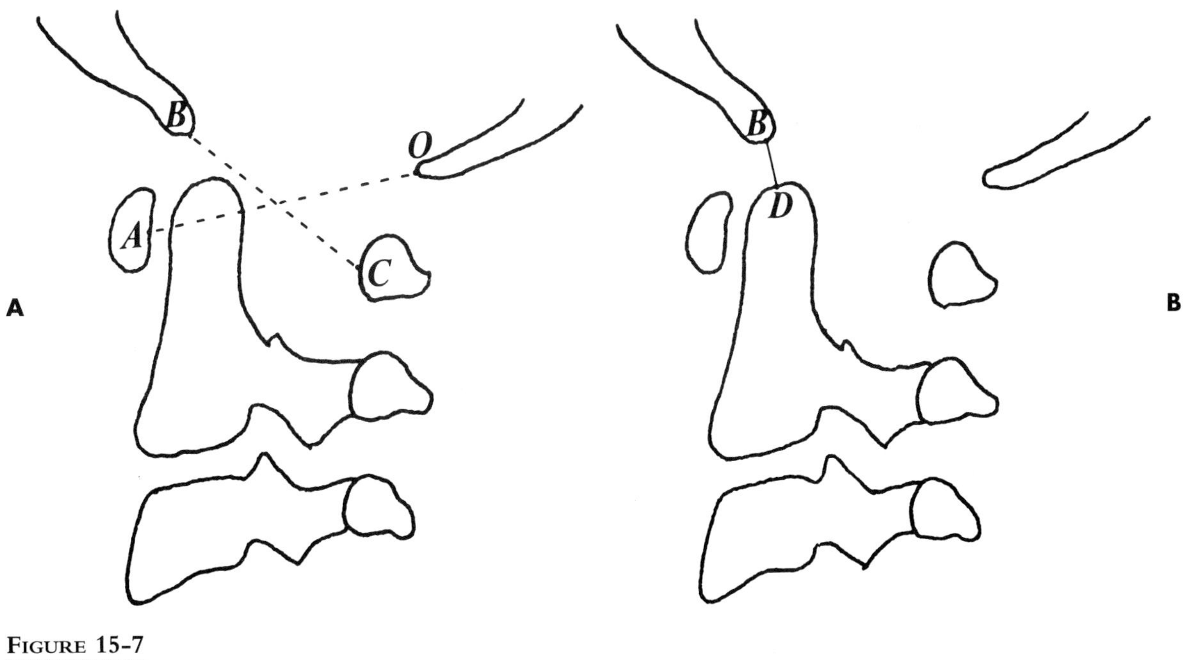

FIGURE 15-7

A, Diagram illustrating the Power's Ratio. (*A*) Anterior arch of C1. (*C*) posterior arch of C1. (*B*) Basion of the skull. (*O*) Opisthion of the skull. A ratio of BC/OA of greater than 1.0 is considered pathologic. **B**, Diagram illustrating the dens-basion distance (DB). D = dens, B = basion of the skull. Normal values determined by Bulas et al. are 8.3 mm ± 4.2 mm. (From Bulas DI, et al: *Radiology* 188:155–158, 1993.)

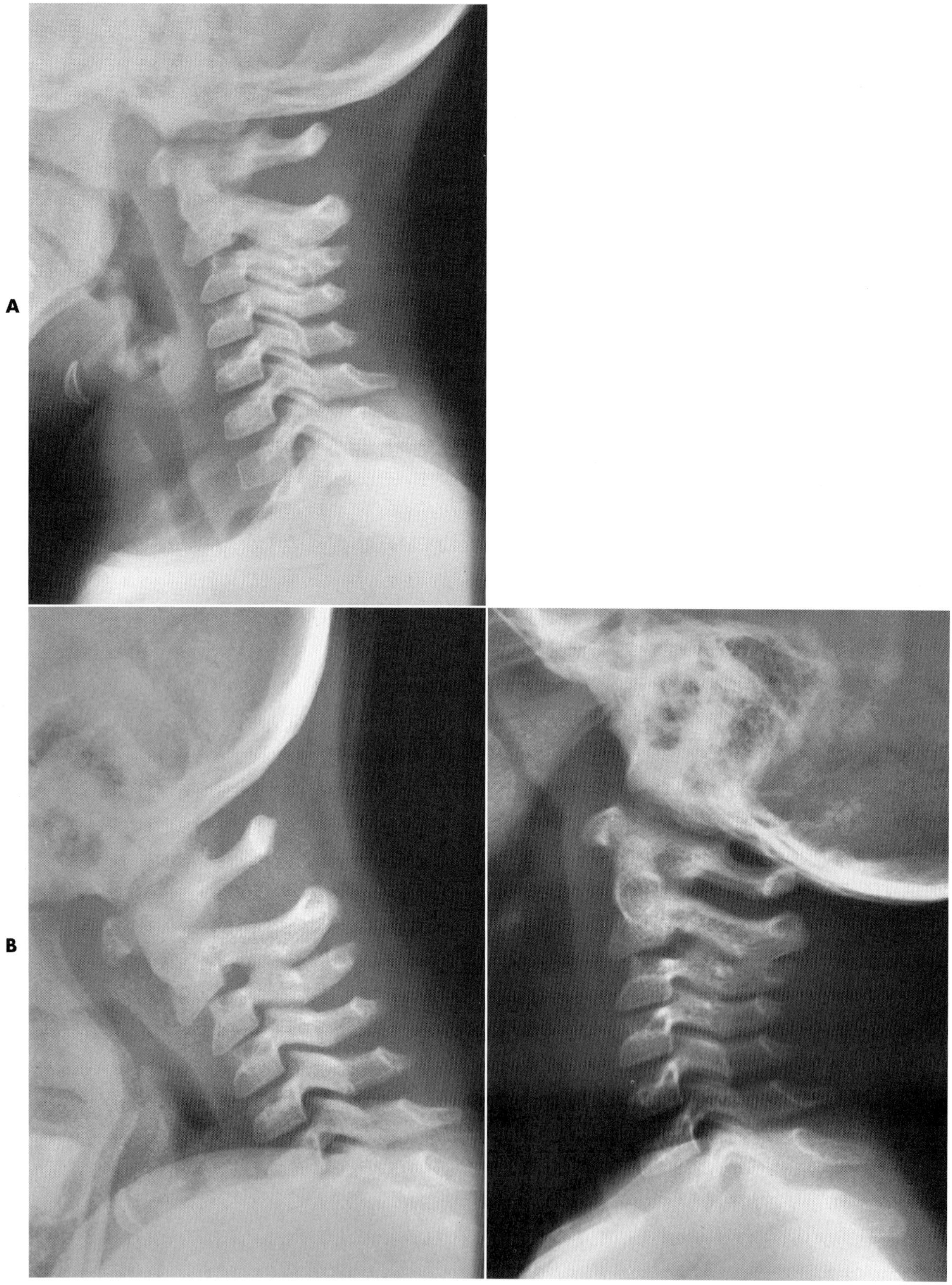

FIGURE 15-8

Pseudosubluxation of the cervical spine. **A**, A 3-year-old girl fell off a fence and complained of neck pain. C2 on C3 subluxation was noted on lateral radiograph. Flexion **B** and extension **C** views were obtained. Despite obvious motion at C2-C3, the spinolaminar line was normal. (Courtesy of Children's Hospital, Oakland.)

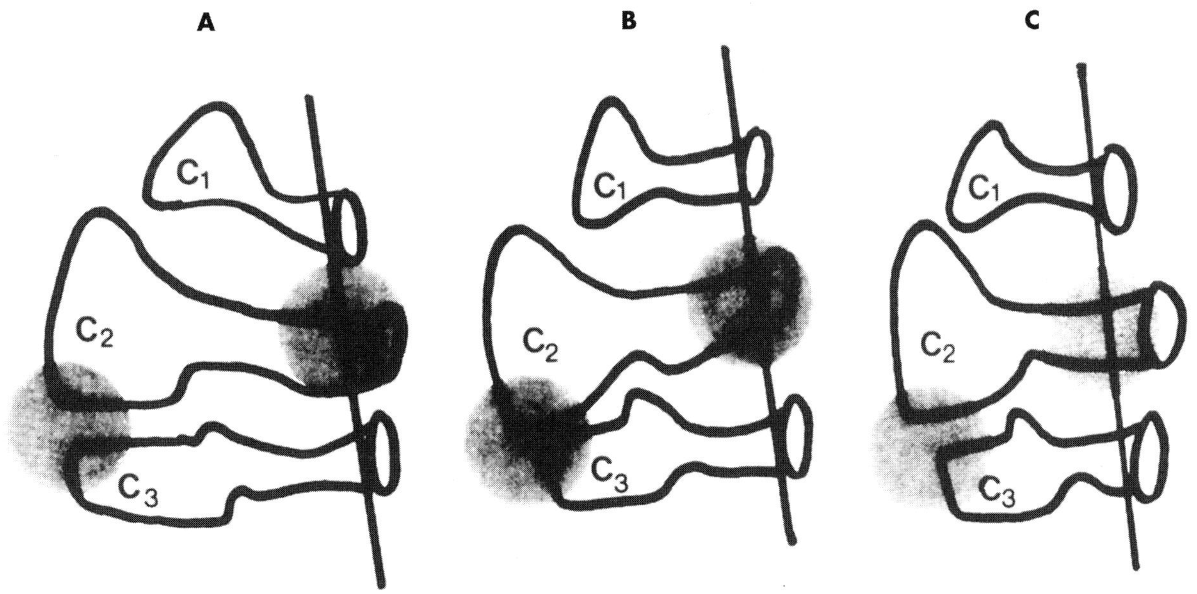

FIGURE 15-9

B, **C** The posterior cervical line (*PCL*) is drawn by connecting the anterior aspect of the spinous processes of C1 and C3. This line is only reliable for determining pathologic motion of the upper cervical junction in radiographs in which C2 is displaced anteriorly on C3. **A**, There is no subluxation of C2 on C3, and, consequently, the PCL can not be reliably used. **B**, Pseudosubluxation is present and the anterior aspect of the spinous process of C2 lies on the PCL (*NORMAL*). **C** Subluxation is present and the anterior aspect of spinous process of C2 misses the PCL by × 2 mm. This finding is suggestive of a Hangman's fracture of C2 (*ABNORMAL*). (From Fesmire FM, Luten RC: *J Emerg Med* 7:139, 1989.)

the main plane of motion at this joint, and the joint is disrupted by hyperextension and traction.

Severing of both the tectorial membrane and the paired alar ligaments is required to produce atlantooccipital dislocation. Children are particularly vulnerable to this injury because of a disproportionately large head and lax ligaments (Fig. 15-11). The outcome is usually fatal.[27]

Hamilton and coworkers performed autopsies in 31 pediatric deaths from multiple trauma including cervical spine trauma. Mortality rate from spinal injury was 2.5 times more likely than their adult counterparts. Of their series, 40% had atlantooccipital dislocation.[28] The most common cause is motor vehicle accident. In one series of 11 children with this injury, seven were pedestrians struck by motor vehicles, and four were passengers. Presentation varies from no neurologic involvement to frank cardiopulmonary failure. Cranial nerve palsies can occur, particularly of the sixth, seventh, and twelfth nerves, and upper cervical root injury.[29] Prognosis is related to the degree of neurologic injury at presentation. Death from cardiopulmonary failure can be secondary to subarachnoid hemorrhage, cerebral edema, intraventricular hemorrhage, and associated skull fractures.

Maves and coworkers reviewed 10 cases of atlantooccipital disruption and reported motor vehicle accidents as the sole cause usually with a pedestrian being struck by a car.[30] They stressed the importance of screening all children radiographically with this history of injury. Soft tissue swelling anterior to the arch of C1 of greater than 7 mm was pathologic in 90% of cases. The atlantooccipital distance described by Kaufman of greater than 5 mm was pathologic in all cases.[31] These authors described the usefulness of the dens-clivus line in determining whether dislocation was anterior, posterior, or longitudinal. Normally this line bisects the tip of the dens on a lateral radiograph.

Accurate radiographic diagnosis is crucial if diagnosis is to be made and appropriate treatment is to be instituted. Clinical diagnosis is unreliable in diagnosing this condition. Bucholz's review of 112 postmortem examinations of multiple trauma victims found atlantooccipital disruption in nine patients.[32] Death had been instantaneous in all victims. In their series, the incidence of injury to the atlantooccipital joint was 15% for children and 6% for adults. Appropriate transportation from the accident scene on pediatric spinal boards with careful immobilization of the head may allow the patient who survives the initial injury to reach a facility with the expertise necessary to diagnose and treat such injuries. Atlantooccipital injuries are rarely isolated and frequently associated with head injuries. Radiographic diagnosis can occasionally be

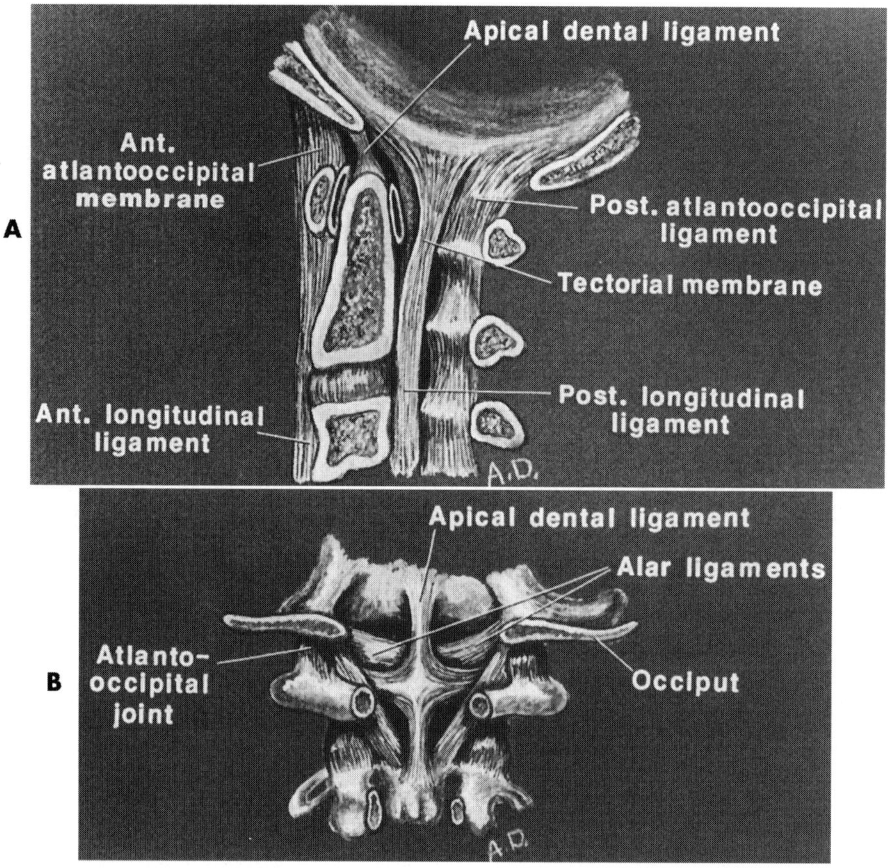

FIGURE 15-10

The stabilizing ligaments of the craniocervical junction are depicted in the sagittal and coronal planes. (From Georgopoulos G, et al: *J Bone Joint Surg* 69A:432, 1987.)

made from the Powers ratio; however, this ratio is unreliable in the young child, reported as being positive in only 6 of 11 patients with this condition in one series.[33] The distance from the tip of the dens to the basion has been used with a distance of more than 12.5 mm considered pathologic. Measurement of the retropharyngeal space may be useful in identifying an upper cervical spine injury but is nonspecific and can be normal as in 2 of the 11 patients with this injury reported by Bulas and coworkers.[34]

An incidence of this injury of 0.7% was found in 1,600 children who had a cross table lateral radiograph following trauma. The normal dens-basion (DB) distance in this series was 8.3 mm ± 4.2 mm. All 11 children with atlantooccipital dislocation had a DB distance greater than 14 mm with a mean of 17 mm.

Treatment usually requires immobilization in a halo vest with minimal traction. Associated respiratory support measures such as ventilation or tracheostomy may be necessary. Posterior cervical fusion with internal fixation is warranted if reduction cannot be maintained. Georgopoulos and coworkers reported their results of five cases treated operatively (including two with congenital abnormalities). They recommend surgical stabilization in all patients by posterior spinal fusion.[29]

FRACTURES OF THE PEDIATRIC SPINE

C1: JEFFERSON FRACTURE

The mechanism of injury of a Jefferson fracture is axial loading by a direct blow to the head such as from a fall or motor vehicle accident. In a recent review of 143 children with cervical spine injuries, only eight had an isolated Jefferson fracture and two had this injury in combination with injury at a different level.[10] Pain along the course of the greater occipital nerve with muscle spasm may be the only presenting complaint. Occasionally, the patient may present with a torticollis.[35] This fracture rarely presents with neurologic symptoms due to the large canal in this region of the spine and the fact that the fracture results in an

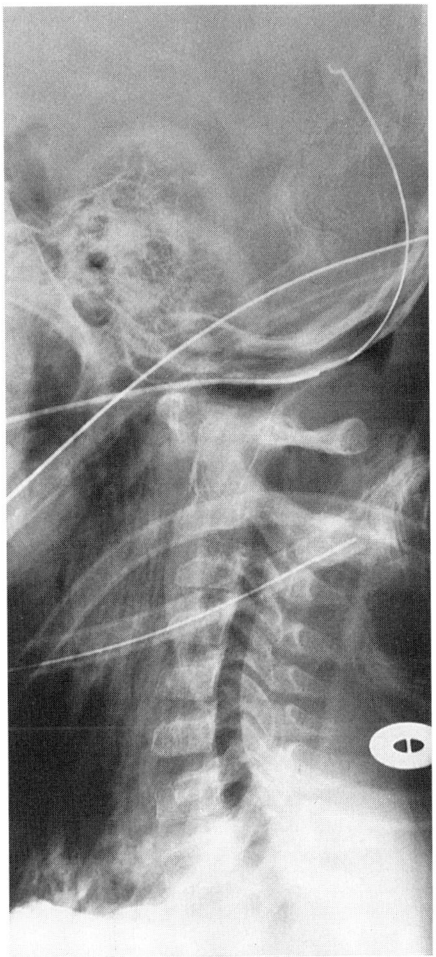

Figure 15-11

Atlanto-occipital dissociation. A 5-year-old male pedestrian, struck by a motor vehicle, was found to be unresponsive at the time of evaluation. A single radiograph was obtained. The patient expired shortly thereafter. (Courtesy of Children's Hospital, Oakland.)

enlargement of the canal. Radiographs are frequently normal, and thin-slice axial CT scanning is often helpful in confirming the diagnosis (Fig. 15-12).

The ring of C1 is made up of three ossification centers, one for the anterior arch and one for each lateral mass. The synchondrosis of the posterior arch ossifies by 4 years of age and the two synchondroses between the anterior and posterior arch ossify by 8 years of age. These synchondroses can fail as a result of trauma, and fractures through the synchondrosis do occur. Differentiating synchondrosis from congenital anomalies, such as anomalous posterior ossicles from true fractures, is facilitated by the use of thin-slice axial CT.[36] Occasionally, the anomalous posterior ossicle of C1 can be differentiated from a fracture by tomography because of its smooth margin and absence of instability on flexion extension views.[37] Patients can usually be successfully treated with a cervicothoracic brace for 3 months.[38] Gehweiler and coworkers in their review of 36 patients with malformations of the atlas and 10 patients with a fracture of the atlas, noted lateral mass offsets of less than 2 mm on either or both sides in normal patients. This so-called pseudospread of the atlas may be confused with a fracture. Offsets greater than 3 mm, however, were pathologic in all cases.[39]

Suss and coworkers described gradual increase of pseudospread during early childhood; infants developed 1 mm offset of C1 compared with C2, increasing to 2 mm in the second year of life, and 3 mm each in the third year. After this point, the offset decreased and returned to zero (although they did have two normal patients older than this with 8 mm of total spread). They also devised an "atlas spread index," which looked at the distances between the upper outer and lower outer corners of the opposite lateral masses and the distance between the medial tubercles of the lateral masses of C1. From these indices, a number of normal ratios were determined to differentiate normal from abnormal spread.[40]

Treatment of C1 fractures is universally nonoperative and is managed with immobilization in a halo cast or brace or Minerva jacket for up to 3 months. Other bony or ligamentous injuries of the spine may be present. Late instability can be treated by limited posterior spinal fusion from C1 to C2, although fusion to the occiput may be required to maintain stability.

FRACTURES OF THE ODONTOID

Fractures of the odontoid process are the most common type cervical injury seen in the under-8-year-old age group, comprising up to 60% of fractures in some series. Most can be managed nonoperatively in a halo vest or cervicothoracic orthosis. The fracture occurs through the weak synchondrosis at the base of the dens in most cases, usually as a result of hyperextension or flexion with rotation (Fig. 15-13). This zone fuses by 7 years of age but may be delayed to as late as 12 years of age. The use of sagittal CT was recently shown by Vining and coworkers to be effective in identifying this fracture, and it confirmed that the injury could occur as a synchondrotic slip in young patients.[41] This injury can even occur in children less than 1 year of age; it was a result of birth trauma in one case.[42,43]

Sherk and coworkers reported 11 patients less than 7 years of age with fractures of the odontoid process.[14] All fractures occurred through the cartilaginous plate between the odontoid process and the body of C2. Diagnosis was made by radiography in all cases. Six patients were treated in a Minerva jacket, four in a halo vest, and one infant in a soft collar. All fractures healed without evidence of growth disturbance as late as 13 years after fracture, unlike the results in adult odontoid process fractures.

A

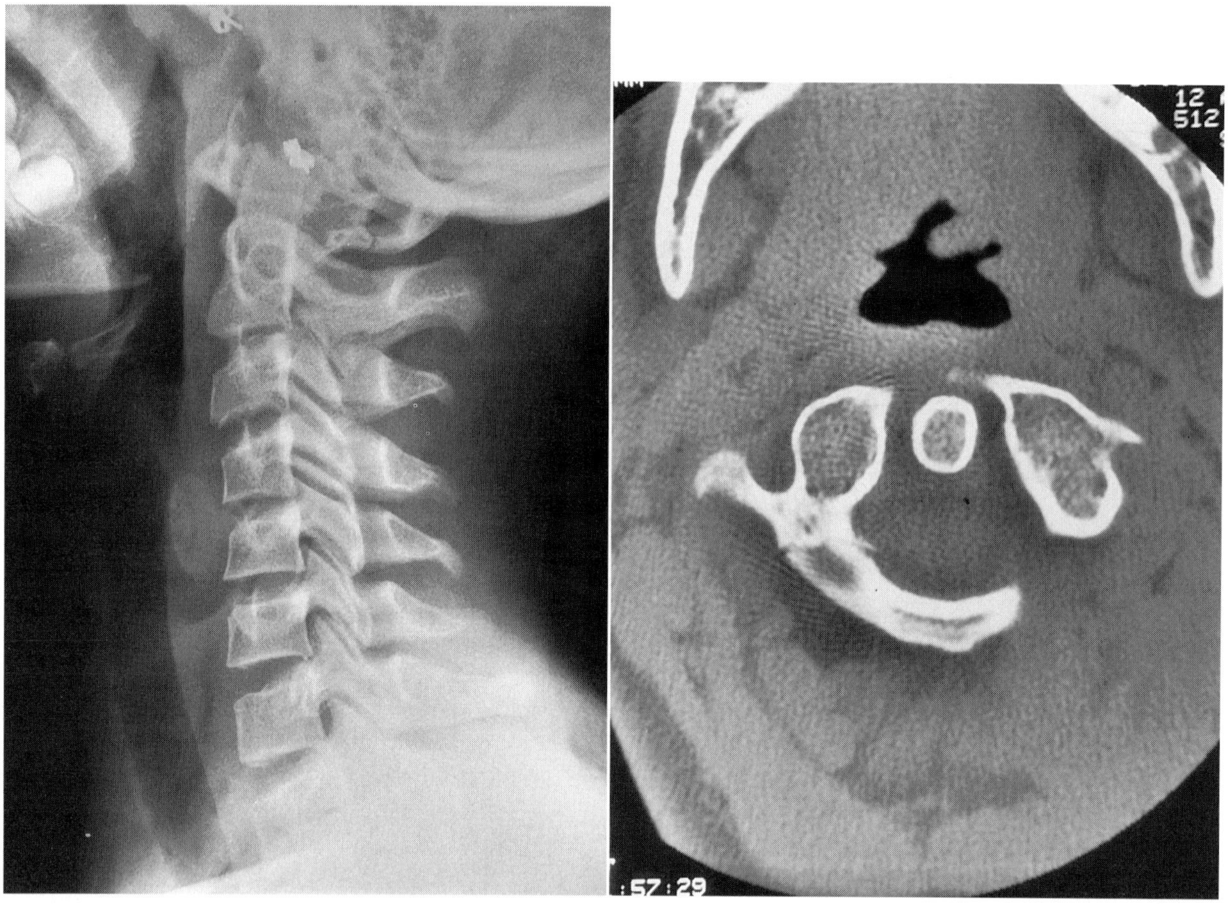

B

FIGURE 15-12

Jefferson fracture. A 12-year-old male who suffered an injury after a diving accident with axial loading to the cervical spine. **A**, lateral radiographs demonstrate a fracture of the posterior arch of C1. **B**, Thin-cut CT scanning is often necessary to clearly demonstrate this injury. (Courtesy of Children's Hospital, Oakland.)

SPONDYLOSIS OF C2 (HANGMAN'S FRACTURE)

The so called "Hangman's fracture" is a traumatic spondylolisthesis caused by bilateral fractures through the pedicles of C2. Fracture lines can extend through the pars interarticularis or foramen transversalis. Hyperextension with axial loading creates the injury. It is relatively uncommon in children.[44] In a review of 143 children with cervical spine injuries, only one patient in the 11- to 15-year-old age group presented with this fracture.[10] Evans and coworkers reported only one of these injuries in 24 consecutive cervical spine trauma cases.[45] Another review by Birney reported eight children with this injury out of 84 children with cervical spine injuries.[11] Ruff and coworkers reported a case of a Hangman's fracture in an 18-month-old infant. Diagnosis was delayed as the infant's torticollis was initially attributed to tonsillitis. Radiographs taken in flexion confirmed the diagnosis.[46] Most cases can be successfully diagnosed on plain radiographs; however, the use of thin-slice CT is particularly sensitive (Fig. 15-14). Measurement of the posterior laminar line of Swischiuk as described earlier demonstrates an abnormal posterior displacement of the arch of C2 in most cases. Equivocal cases may require axial thin-slice CT scans for diagnosis.

Young patients may be successfully treated in a well-padded Minerva cast for 2 months. Older children may be managed in a halo vest or Minerva jacket. Posterior fusion of C1 to C3 may be indicated for persistent instability or nonunion. Atlantoaxial instability as a result of trauma in children is thought to be caused by increased strain as a result of more horizontally aligned facet joints placed on the relatively more elastic ligaments. McGrory reported nine cases of atlantoaxial instability in 143 children treated for cervical spine injuries.[10] When isolated ruptures of the transverse ligament occur, they are treated nonoperatively with generally good results.[47] Surgery is reserved for late onset of instability and consists of posterior C1-C2

A B

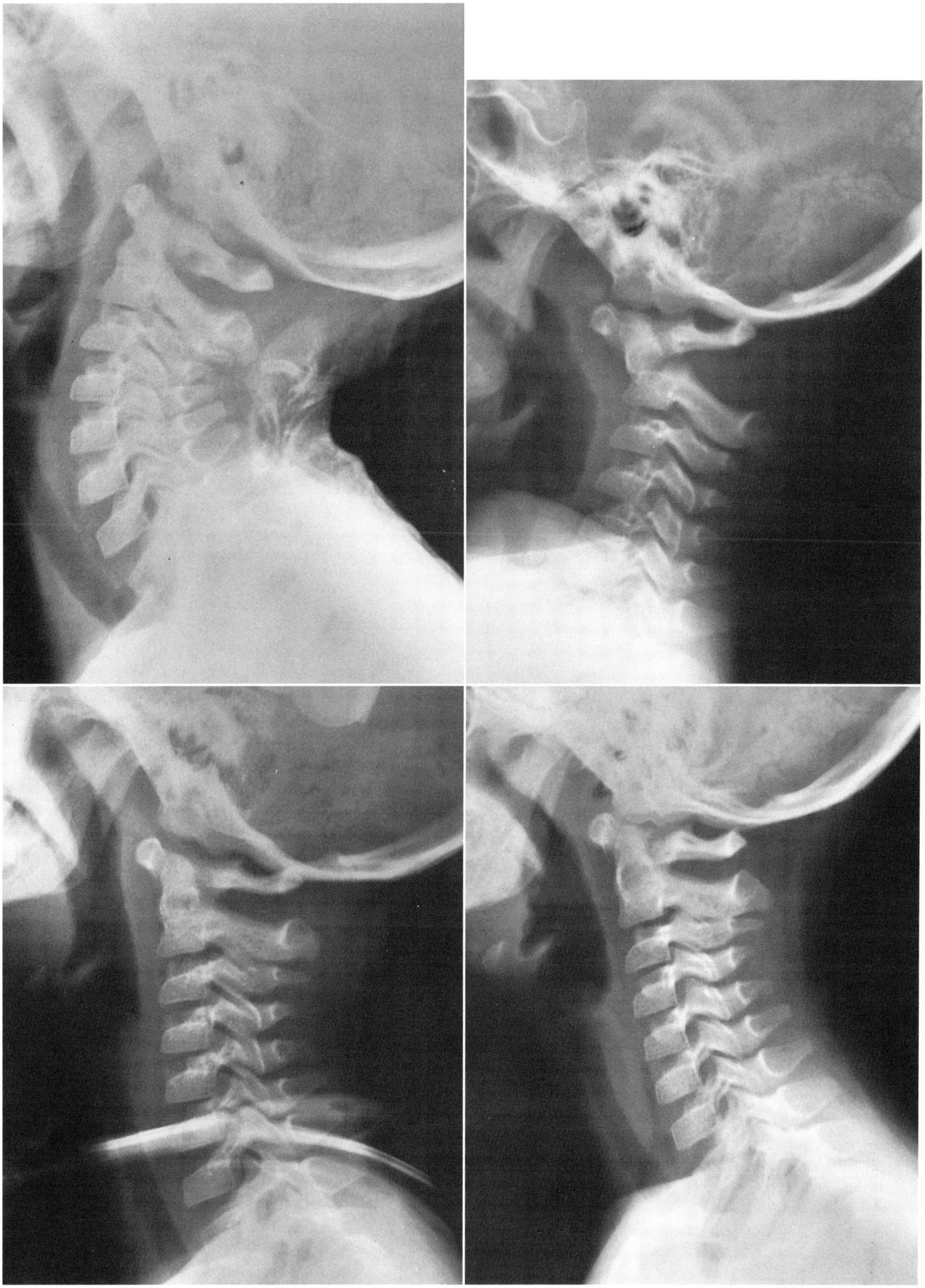

C D

FIGURE 15-13

Odontoid fracture (synchondrotic slip). A 3 1/2-year-old female complained of neck pain after a fall. **A**, Initial radiographs read as normal. **B**, Flexion radiographs demonstrate obvious C2 fracture at the base of the dens (synchondrotic slip). **C**, Alignment in halo. **D**, Healed at 16 weeks. (Courtesy of Children's Hospital, Oakland.)

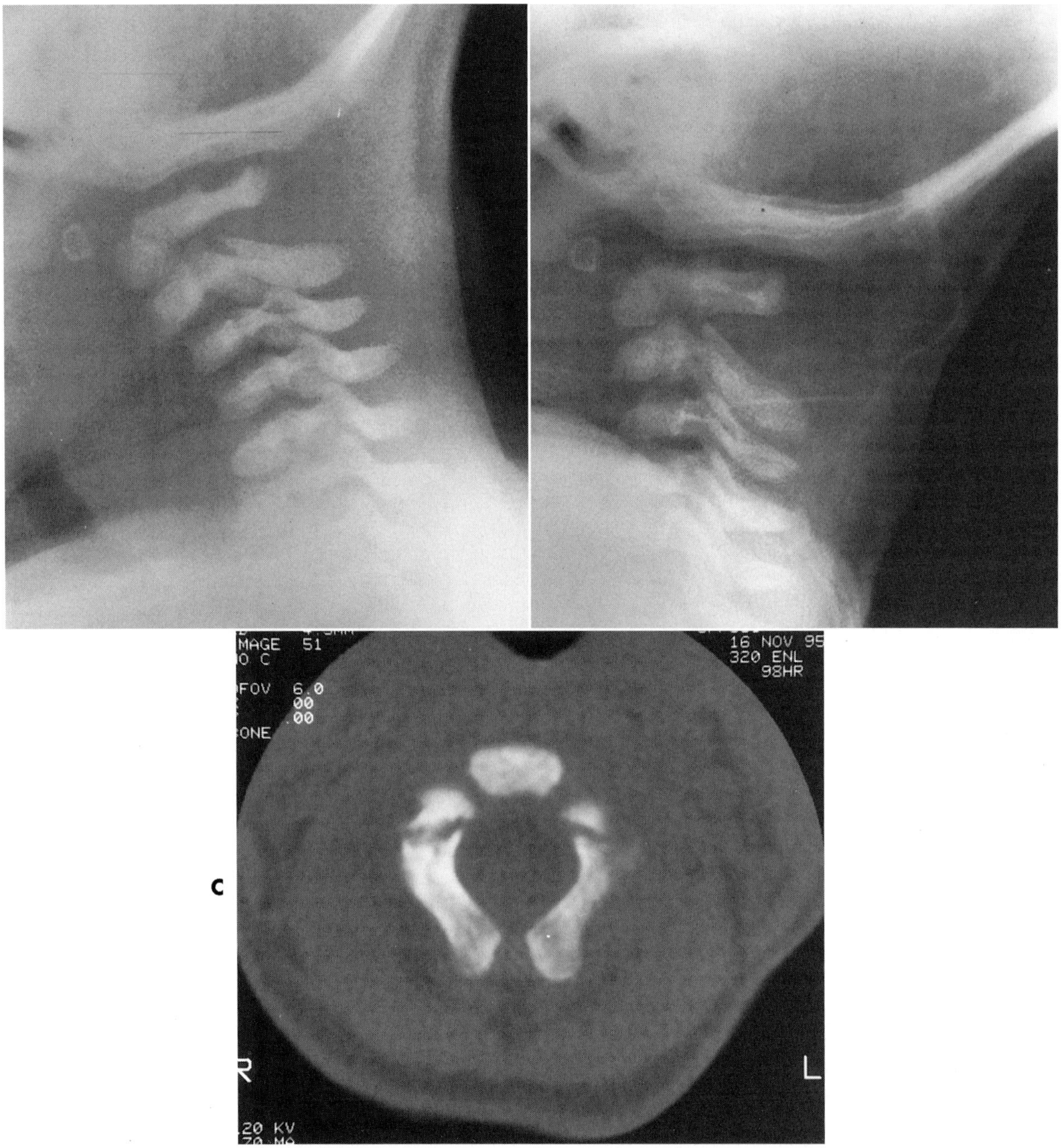

FIGURE 15-14

Hangman's fracture (C2 pars fractures). A 14-month-old boy, victim of child abuse, was found to have bilateral C2 pars interarticularis fractures and other cervical injuries. **A**, Injury radiographs. **B**, Flexion view. **C**, Axial CT scan. The patient was treated in a soft collar. (Courtesy of Children's Hospital, Oakland.)

fusion and halo or Minerva cast immobilization until fused.

VERTEBRAL ANOMALIES AND TRAUMA

There are a number of common vertebral anomalies that deserve separate discussion. These are classically divided into failure of segmentation and failure of formation.[48]

Greenberg is credited with first classifying cervical anomalies in the atlantoaxial region (Fig. 15-15). Five subtypes are described. In type 1, the normal dens does not fuse to the C2 body. Known as os odontoideum, this congenital anomaly is thought to be caused by a traumatic event interfering with normal development of the dens. Occasionally, it can be mistaken for an acute fracture. An increase in ADI may gradually develop or may be exacerbated by trauma. An ADI of greater than 1 cm or neurologic findings warrant a

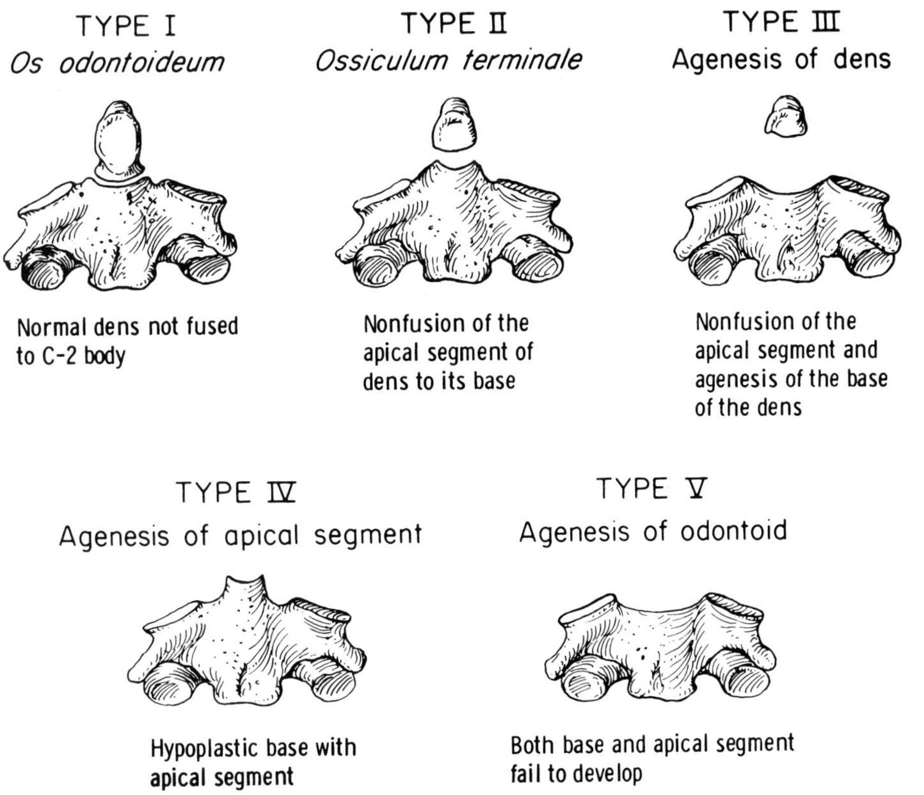

FIGURE 15-15

Greenberg's classification of congenital anomalies of the atlantoaxial junction. These anomalies may be symptomatic or may present with frank quadriplegia. Patients' symptoms may be exacerbated by a minor fall and require careful evaluation to exclude pathologic instability. (From Dawson EG, Smith L: *J Bone Joint Surg* 61A:583, 1979.)

posterior C1-C2 fusion. Acute injuries with less displacement or with no associated cord compression can be managed in a halo for 2 months and monitored for instability. Type 2 anomalies, or ossiculum terminale, are caused by nonfusion of the apical segment of the dens to its base, the so called ossiculum terminale. This is the most common atlantoaxial anomaly, seen in 80% of cases in one series by Dawson and coworkers.[48] Other anomalies are more uncommon. Type 3 is nonfusion of the apical segment of the dens and agenesis of the base of the dens. Type 4 is a hypoplastic odontoid base with a separate apical segment. Type 5 is complete agenesis of the odontoid.

Klippel-Feil syndrome has been extensively described. The syndrome may include congenital fusion of two or more cervical vertebra, congenital scoliosis, Sprengel's deformity, deafness, short neck, and low posterior hairline. The clinician should be aware that this group of patients is more susceptible to injury in the cervical spine region because of the longer lever arm adjacent to the levels of congenital fusion. There have been a number of reported cases of sudden death or quadriplegia after minor falls due to cervical instability in these patients. A high index of suspicion should be maintained in the diagnosis and treatment of this at-risk patient population.[49]

Patients with Down syndrome should be screened for chronic atlantoaxial instability. Generalized ligamentous laxity secondary to a defect in collagen synthesis predisposes these patients to atlantoaxial instability. A decreased tensile strength of the growth plate additionally predisposes this group to avulsion fractures of the odontoid process. Such patients involved in any kind of trauma from a minor fall to a motor vehicle accident require careful evaluation and treatment.[50] Normal ADI in children with Down syndrome has been defined by Martel and coworkers to be 5 mm and 4 mm in the skeletally immature child.[51,52] Values over this are pathologic until proved otherwise, particularly in the presence of neurologic symptoms. Additional osseous anomalies are very commonly seen in Down syndrome, such as ossiculum terminale or congenital fusion of C1 to the skull. Surgical intervention has been recommended in patients with neurologic findings or symptoms or an ADI greater than 1 cm. High complication rates, however, such as pseudoarthrosis with surgical intervention for atlantoaxial instability in Down syndrome have been reported in the literature.[50,53-55] Treatment is individualized and may be influenced by the patient's activity level, space available for the cord, (occiput C, instability) and presence of symptoms such as torticollis pain or myelopathy.

Participation in sports is allowed if ADI is 4 to 8 mm and the patient has no symptoms. Magnetic resonance imaging is helpful in assessing space available for the cord. Most authors advocate either a C1-C2 posterior fusion or occiput to C2 fusion and halo-vest immobilization, in patients with symptoms and ADI less than 8 mm.

SPINAL CORD INJURY WITHOUT RADIOGRAPHIC ABNORMALITY

Increased incidence of cervical spine injuries without associated radiographic findings in the under 8-year-old age range has been well established in the literature.[2,13,56–60] As described earlier, the immature spinal cord has a unique pathoanatomy and physiology that predisposes it to injury. In one review of 926 patients with SCI, 9.6% were under 16 years of age. Of these 35%, 31 patients, showed no radiographic evidence of fracture or subluxation. Of the group with SCIWORA, 71% were under 8 years of age, and 95% of these had the most severe cord injuries. Ten were neonates who sustained cord injury as a result of birth injuries during breech extraction. Ten patients, all under 8 years of age, sustained their injury from falls from a height. Neurologic syndromes included complete cord injury in 40%, partial cord injury in 35%, and central cord syndrome in 20%.[56]

The injuries are usually in the cervical spine with the upper cervical spine being particularly susceptible in the under-3-year-old age group. The spinal column is more elastic in the child and, when deformed by injury, causes compromising strain within the spinal cord without associated ligamentous or bony failure. The disproportionately larger head of the child under 2 years of age with weaker supporting musculature and higher fulcrum of flexion also predisposes to cord injury.

Hyperextension is thought to be the main mechanism of injury. An inward bulging of the ligamentum flavum can result in up to 50% reduction in the anteroposterior (AP) diameter of the spinal canal. Vascular spasm of the vertebral arteries may also occur causing ischemia and infarction in some cases.

A SCIWORA can present hours and occasionally days after injury. The clinician may overlook the injury on initial examination in some cases. Neurologic findings may be subtle and missed in the early phase of presentation. Many such patients may recall transient neurologic symptoms at the time of injury, such as paresthesias, numbness, or paresis.[57,58] Two theories exist to explain this delay in onset of neurologic symptoms following injury. One implies a single insult to the cord as proposed by Ahman and coworkers, with resulting vessel spasm and infarction of the cord.[61] The other theory proposed by Pang and coworkers, for a small group of patients with SCIWORA suggests the development of instability not detectable on dynamic films following injury. Multiple microtraumas to the cord may result in the final neurologic syndrome with delayed or recurrent SCIWORA.[57]

Diagnosis requires careful physical examination and confirmation with MRI. Surgically treatable lesions such as herniated disks or extradural hematomas are rarely found. The use of high-dose steroids has been recommended but is not proved in this age group with SCIWORA. Spinal angiography rarely demonstrates vessel occlusion. CT myelography may occasionally show extravasation of contrast extradurally into the chest and is a poor prognostic indicator in such patients.

Pollack and coworkers described this entity in 42 children and described a treatment algorithm based on their results. Initial management consisted of hard collar immobilization for 2 months and restriction of contact sports. In their series, eight experienced recurrent cord injury during the 2-month period of immobilization because of poor compliance. The reinjury was associated with a minor hyperextension occurring during sports and was associated with a recurrence or worsening of neurologic symptoms. Flexion-extension radiographs failed to demonstrate any instability probably because such dynamic studies are ineffective in detecting the small amount of instability that explains the SCIWORA. Somatosensory evoked potential (SSEP) data was found to be useful in the evaluation of these children, differentiating cranial from cord injury in those with combined head and spine trauma. Due to the significant rate of recurrent SCIWORA, Pollack and coworkers recommended admission to hospital, bed rest with a hard collar for a few days until muscle spasm subsided, and flexion-extension studies. All patients were immobilized in a Guilford brace for 3 months. All sports activities were disallowed during this time period. They monitored SSEPs at presentation and at 6 weeks. The SSEPs appeared to match the clinical course. Patients were returned to full activities only if flexion-extension radiographs did not demonstrate instability.[59]

All patients should have the spine immobilized with a Philadelphia collar, with custom collars fashioned, if needed, for infants. Immobilization is maintained for 3 months at which time flexion-extension radiographs are taken to exclude instability. Aggressive respiratory care including early tracheostomy and ventilatory support should be provided if needed. Meticulous skin care with rotorest beds were indicated and sequential compression stockings for deep vein thrombosis (DVT) prophylaxis is recommended. A multidisciplinary approach at centers that specialize in the care of patients with SCI is advisable.

Prognosis is universally poor for neurologic return in patients under 8 years of age with SCIWORA. This age group comprises 95% of the most severe cord injuries in the pediatric spine. Surgery has little or no place in the early management of these patients. Most can be managed in a collar for up to 3 months. Flexion extension views at that time identify the small number of children who require a posterior cervical fusion.

ATLANTOAXIAL ROTATORY SUBLUXATION

Rotatory atlantoaxial subluxation (RAAS) is an unusual condition that is often misdiagnosed. The cause is poorly understood but results in abnormal relationships in the axis of rotation of the C1-C2 joint. Fifty percent of cervical rotation occurs at this joint with the transverse ligament being the main stabilizing ligament. The affected child typically has a torticollis and restricted range of motion of the neck. Associated factors may include upper respiratory tract infections, minor trauma, oral surgery, or rheumatoid arthritis, although in most cases no cause is found.

Other considerations include congenital abnormalities of the spine, tumors of the central nervous system (particularly of the posterior fossa and cervical spine), syringomyelia, Arnold-Chiari malformation, infection, or bony or soft tissue tumors, and certain ophthalmologic conditions.

Diagnosis can be made with plain radiographs, although this may be difficult. The normal motion of the C1-C2 joint resulting from the inclination of the C1-C2 facet joint causes the distance between the dens and the lateral masses to decrease on the right when the subject is looking to the left. The opposite occurs when looking to the right. In RAAS, these distances do not change with rotation of the head. If the transverse ligament also is ruptured, an increase in the ADI occurs. An ADI of less than 4 mm is considered unstable and may warrant fusion in such cases. Dynamic CT, described below, is probably the gold standard for diagnosis (Fig. 15-16).

Fielding and Hawkins in their classic review of 17 cases noted an average delay of 11.6 months before diagnosis. Of their 17 patients, 13 were treated with some form of upper cervical fusion following halter or halo traction (Figs. 15-17 and 15-18). They classified the condition into four subtypes:

Type 1—rotatory fixation with no anterior displacement of the atlas

Type 2—rotatory fixation with 3 to 5 mm of anterior displacement

Type 3—rotatory fixation with anterior displacement of more than 5 mm

Type 4—rotatory fixation with posterior displacement.[62]

More recently Philips and Hensinger reported treatment results for 23 children with this condition. The patient group had a mean age of 7.5. Eight children had type 1 RAAS and 14 had type 2. Dynamic axial CT using 3-mm cuts was used for diagnosis. This method requires axial cuts parallel to C1 from occiput to below C2. Scanning is done in neutral and left and right rotation. Positive scans demonstrated no motion

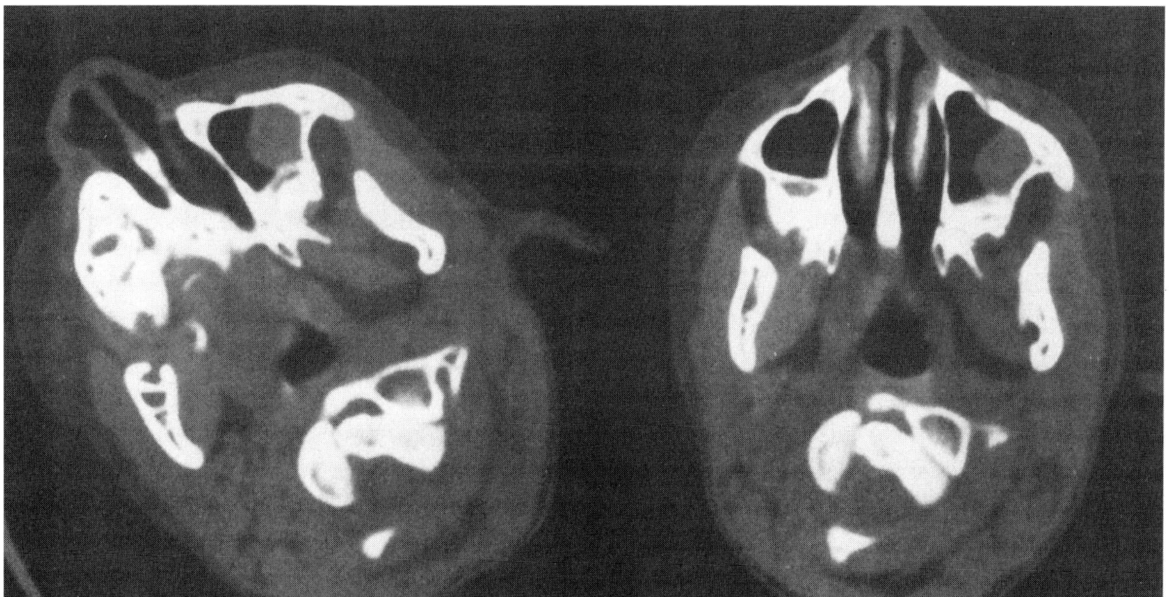

FIGURE 15-16

Dynamic CT scans of C1-C2 in a patient with rotatory atlantoaxial subluxation. *Left.* The head is rotated to the left 45°. *Right.* When looking to the right the patient is unable to achieve full rotation and the relationship between the lateral masses and the dens remain unchanged *(ABNORMAL).* (From Philips W, Hensinger RN: *J Bone Joint Surg* 71A:664–668, 1989.)

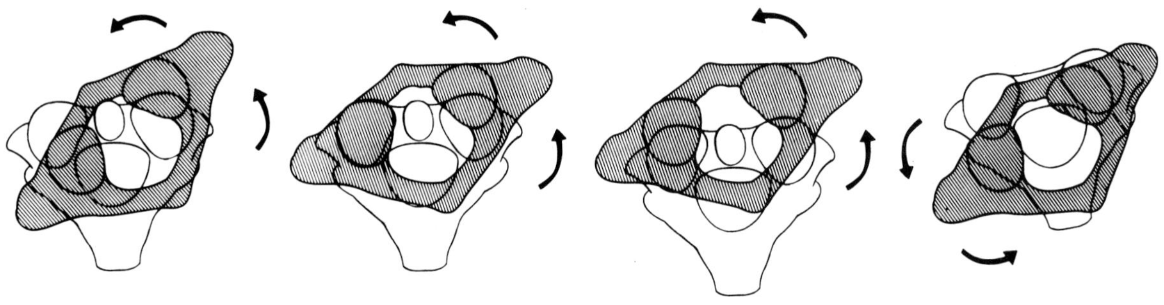

Figure 15-17

Classification of rotatory subluxation of C1-C2 is depicted above. **A** Type 1 rotatory fixation with no anterior displacement and the odontoid acting as the pivot. **B** Type 2 rotatory fixation with anterior displacement of 3 to 5 mm, one lateral articular process acting as the pivot. **C** Type 3 rotatory fixation with anterior displacement of more than 5 mm. **D** Type 4 rotatory fixation with posterior displacement. (From Fielding JW, Hawkins RJ: *J Bone Joint Surg* 59A:37–44, 1977.)

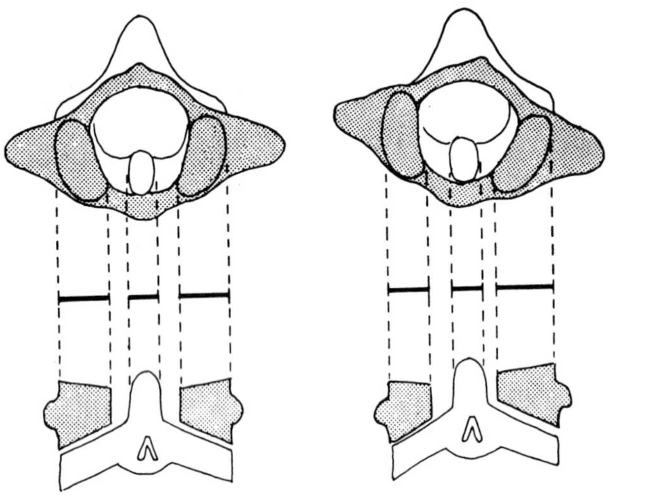

Figure 15-18

Diagram of the atlantoaxial joint viewed from above and anteriorly. The normal relationships of the lateral masses to the dens are shown. In this case the patient is depicted looking to the left. (From Wortzman G, and Dewar FP: Rotary fixation of the atlantoaxial joint: Rotational atlantoaxial subluxation, *Radiology* 90: 479, 1968.)

or asymmetrical motion at C1-C2. Only three children in their series required surgical stabilization and fusion due to late presentation and diagnosis. No attempt at reduction was made in these cases.[63] The remainder were successfully treated with halo or chin halter traction for less than a week followed by a Philadelphia collar until full motion had been regained and dynamic studies were normal.

Recently Crockard reported two cases of traumatic atlantoaxial rotatory dislocation, which were reduced using an extreme lateral approach and fusion with good results.[64] Schwarz and coworkers described two cases in which diagnosis was delayed 3 months. A 2-year-old patient was successfully treated with closed reduction; however, resubluxation requiring surgical stabilization occurred in a 13-year-old patient.[65]

Treatment is usually dictated by the duration of the torticollis prior to treatment. A soft collar or Philadelphia collar can be used in minor reducible RAAS; however, if diagnosis is delayed for more than 1 week, a period of halter traction is warranted followed by some form of occipital-cervicothoracic immobilization. The period of immobilization ranges between 4 to 6 weeks. If diagnosis is delayed more than 1 month, traction is attempted for up to 3 weeks. Open reduction with arthrodesis is indicated if reduction cannot be achieved in this time frame.[63]

LOWER CERVICAL SPINE INJURIES

When evaluating any child with an upper cervical spine injury, evaluating the entire cervical spine radiographically is mandatory. Frequently, additional injuries are found at the cervicothoracic junction. The incidence is lower than in adult populations because of the altered pathoanatomy of the skeletally immature child. Treatment is maintenance of reduction in a halo vest until healing is achieved, usually 3 months. Late instability can be stabilized by posterior cervical fusion if needed. Patients with neurologic symptoms should be evaluated by MRI. All patients should be evaluated with CT to better delineate the fracture pattern and determine the canal size (Fig. 15-19).

SPINAL INJURIES IN BATTERED CHILDREN

First described by Caffey in 1946, spinal injuries in battered children are still overlooked by the clinician.[66,67] He reported six cases of fractures of the limbs associated with chronic subdural hematomas.[68] In 1974, Caffey identified a number of cases of the "whiplash

A

B

C

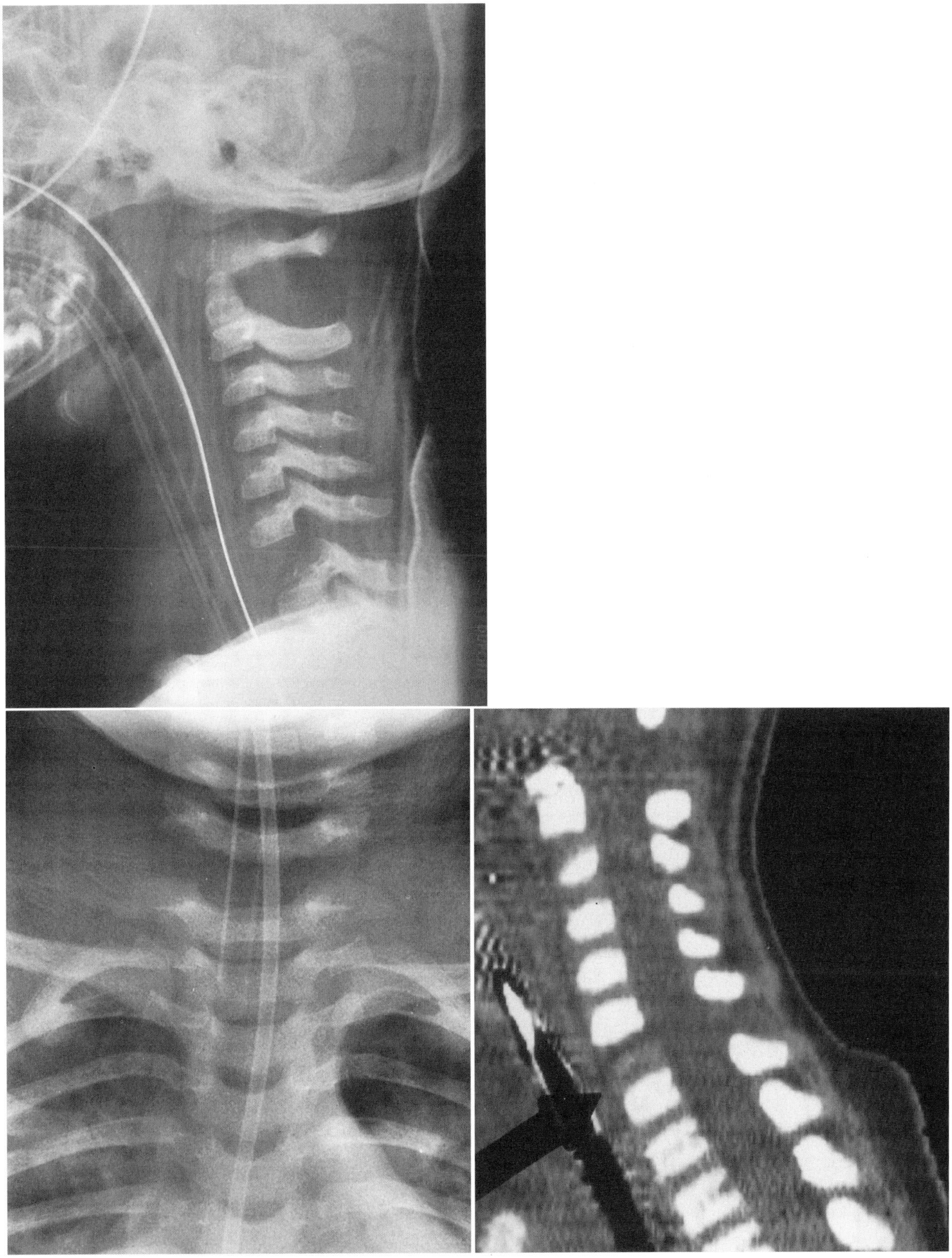

Figure 15-19

C6-C7 dislocation. 11-month-old female involved in a high-speed motor vehicle accident. Patient was found to have a C6-C7 dislocation on anteroposterior **A** and lateral **B** radiographs. **C, D, E** Sagittal and three-dimensional CT scan images confirm the diagnosis. **F** MRI demonstrates C1-C7 cord edema and infarction. The patient expired. (Courtesy of Children's Hospital, Oakland.)

D

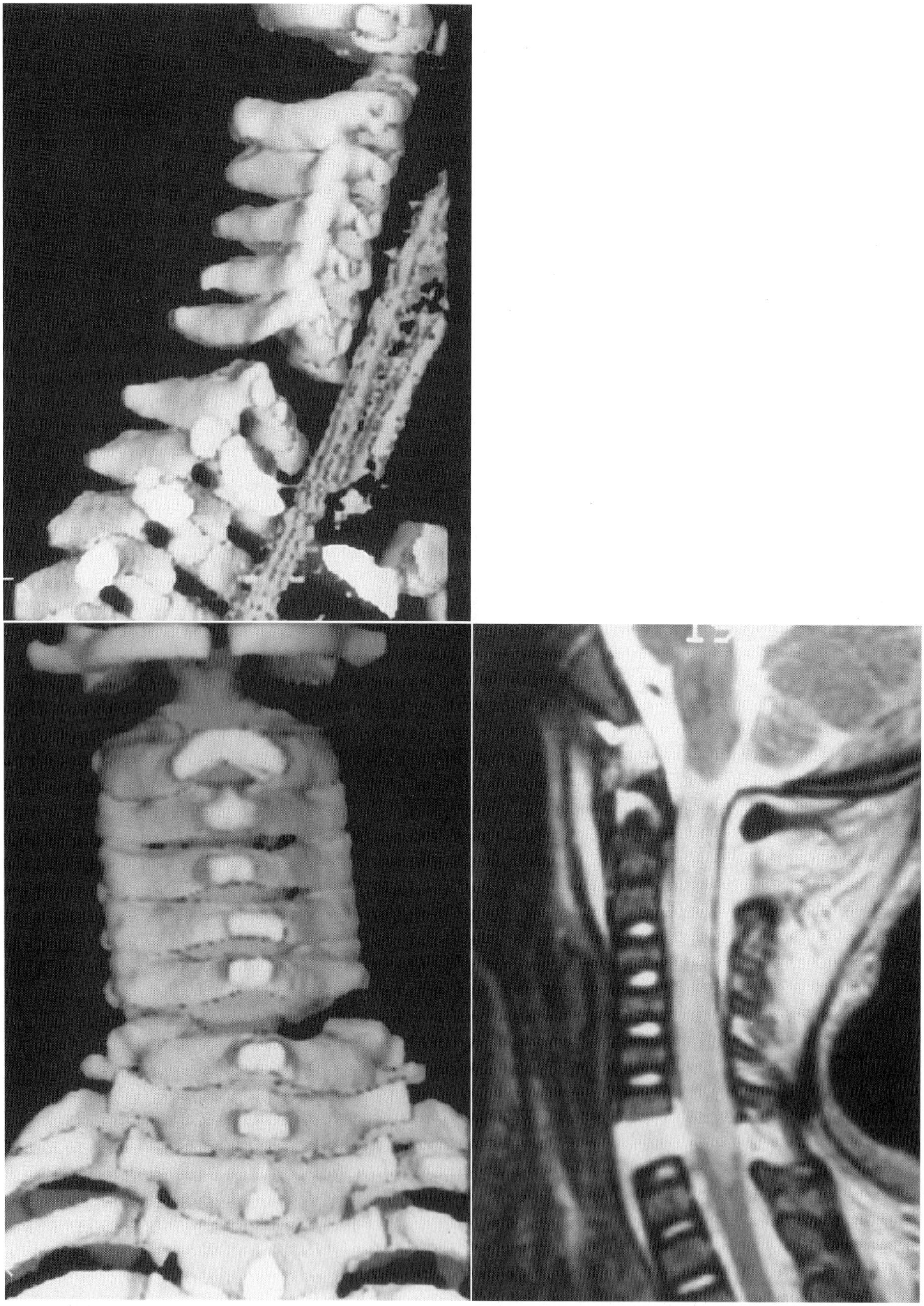

E F

Figure 15-19 *Continued*

shaken baby syndrome."[69] This leads to subdural hematomas and intraocular bleeding, which frequently go undetected. Usually history is lacking from the parents and family. Associated vomiting or hyperirritability may be attributed to a host of unrelated common complaints. The disproportionately large head and lack of head control predisposes infants to upper cervical spine injury.

Cullen and associates reported the cases of five young children with radiographic evidence of spine injuries as a result of physical abuse. All were under the age of 2. None of the children had neurologic injury. All children had associated injuries of either the skull or long bones.[70]

Diamond reported a 12-month-old child who sustained a thoracolumbar spine fracture dislocation with cord compression, which was initially interpreted as a congenital spondylolisthesis. Other soft tissue injuries were present; however, a skeletal survey was negative.[71] Child abuse is usually associated with spiral fractures of the long bones. Typically the femur and humerus are affected. Involvement of the spine is rare, and, consequently, such injuries are often missed by the clinician. Anteroposterior and lateral routine views of the spine should be taken in all cases of suspected child abuse.[71] If radiographic evidence is absent but there are neurologic findings, an MRI should be obtained.

HALO FIXATION IN CHILDREN

Use of halo fixation in a child carries a much higher risk of dislodgment, loosening, and pin protrusion than in the adult. Letts and coworkers had a 40% incidence of pain, loosening, and pin migration in children under 10 years of age when treated for over 4 weeks.[72] A bone window CT scan of the skull should be obtained before pin insertion in the young child or infant. Skull thickness can be as low as 2 mm in the very young child, and, consequently, pin site planning aided by the scan before pin insertion is recommended. The frontal sinus may be a variable distance from the midline in the developing child. Usually there is sufficient room anterolaterally to place one pin; however, the remaining pins should be placed in the parietal and occipital regions. Skull thickness begins to increase 1 mm per year by 10 years of age reaching adult mean thickness of 7 mm by 16 years of age. Congenital skull abnormalities with wide variations in skull thickness are found on CT. Six to eight pins should be used to improve fixation and reduce the chance of pin penetration in children under 10 years of age. An MRI compatible halo and pins are suggested as the study provides superior imaging of osteocartilaginous and neural structures of the spine.

Garfin and coworkers performed a CT study of 18 pediatric skulls. From this data they determined the optimal sites for placement of the halo pins were posterolaterally and anterolaterally, where the bones were the thickest. Insertion of pins in the temporal fossa was determined to be dangerous due to the thin cortex and cranial suture being located in this region of the skull. Even if pin penetration were not a significant risk, pressure at the temporalis muscle would interfere with the process of mastication. From their study, halo usage in children under 2 years of age was not recommended. The use of other external immobilization devices such as cervicothoracic cast braces with helmet extensions can be considered. Between 2 and 5 years of age, a halo may be used with six pins at 4 to 6 inches per pound of torque. The accuracy of torque screwdrivers varies widely. Friction between the screw and halo thread is one major source of error as are changes in friction due to autoclaving, antiseptic solutions, and damaged threads.[72] New pins are recommended. Once skull thickness approaches that of the adult then four pins at 8 inch-lb of torque may be used. Absolute contraindications to halo use include associated skull fracture, poor patient compliance, or cardiopulmonary complications.[73,74]

SURGICAL TREATMENT

Most cervical spine injuries in children can be managed nonoperatively. External immobilization such as casts, cast braces, or halo vests may be used up to 12 weeks in up to 80% of cases.[75] Surgery is reserved for late instability following closed treatment, loss of reduction, failure to reduce with closed treatment, or spinal cord compression with incomplete neurologic deficits.[33,75]

As discussed, the most common site of injury is in the upper cervical spine of children younger than 8 years of age.[75] Posterior figure of eight interspinous wiring is recommended for persistent instability following closed treatment or for failure to maintain acceptable spinal alignment with external immobilization techniques. Bilateral facet dislocations and irreducible unilateral facet dislocations require stabilization with posterior interspinous wiring and fusion due to the high incidence of late instability. There was a 14% incidence of kyphosis in one series of 24 cervical spine fractures of all types.[45] Sublaminar wiring at C1 and interspinous wiring at C2 and below is generally used (Fig. 15-20). The smaller spinal canal in the child poses a theoretic increased risk of neurologic injury.

Surgery is performed with the patient in a prone position with reduction maintained by Gardner Wells tongs or halo traction. Particularly in the skeletally immature child, surgical exposure should be limited to the region to be fused to prevent unwanted extension of the fusion beyond the injured region. Needle localization of levels can be confirmed radiographically

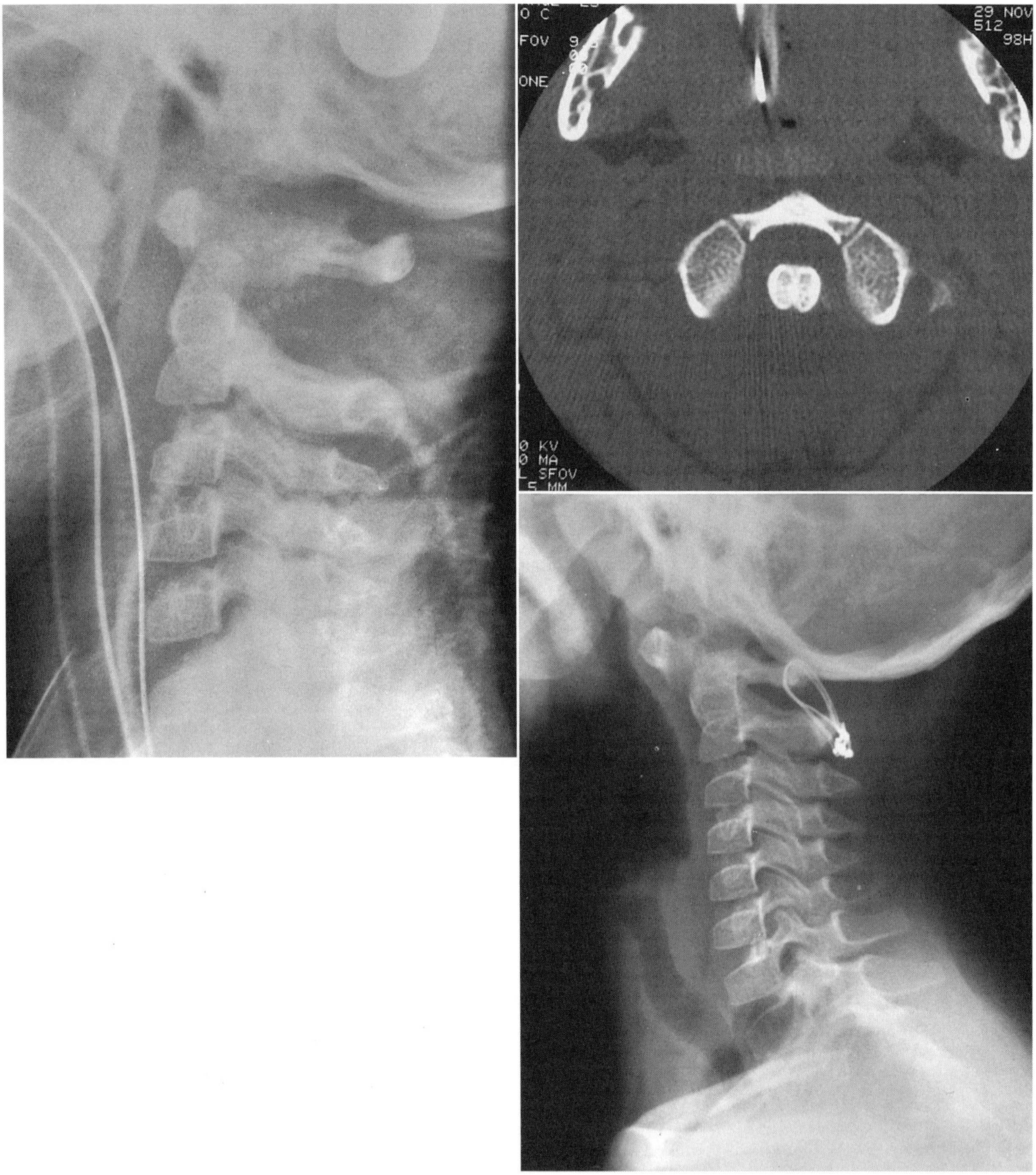

A

B

C

FIGURE 15-20

A, B Posterior wiring for C1-C2 subluxation in a 3-year-old female, hit by an automobile. C1-C2 subluxation noted on lateral radiograph and CT scan. Note wide separation of odontoid process and anterior arch of C1 on axial CT image. **C** The patient was treated with posterior wiring. (Courtesy of Children's Hospital, Oakland.)

prior to incision. The loop end of 18-gauge double-stringed wire or MRI-compatible titanium braided wire is then passed inferiorly underneath the posterior arch of C1, and the free end of the wire is passed through the loop to secure the arch of C1. The wire is then passed inferiorly to the spinous process of C2 or through a hole in the base of the spinous process if it is large enough. Bone graft is placed after decortication. Children are placed in a skull occiput mandibular immobilization (SOMI) brace for 8 to 12 weeks until fusion is achieved. Halo immobilization may be used if fixation or bone quality is deemed tenuous at the time of surgery if skull thickness is adequate. Fusion is confirmed by radiographs or tomography or flexion extension views if appropriate.

Cell saver is routinely used if significant blood loss (greater than 1 liter in larger children) is anticipated. A "wake-up test" should be performed in all cases if practical. SSEP monitoring can be used, but SSEP does not monitor motor pathways as does the wakeup-test; its false negative rate, however, is low in experienced hands. Anesthetic agents that lower the cortical wave amplitude such as nitrous oxide are avoided if SSEPs are used. The use of anticoagulants for DVT in any patients undergoing spine surgery is not routinely recommended. The incidence of DVT in the pediatric population is almost unheard of, and the complications from such routine anticoagulation are serious after spine surgery.

For patients with significant spinal canal encroachment and an incomplete neurologic deficit, anterior decompression and fusion may be indicated. Shaked and coworkers reported on six children with lower cervical spine fractures with significant vertebral collapse and canal encroachment or major kyphotic deformity treated by an anterior approach, decompression, and fusion. One child was 3 years of age while the remainder were between 6 and 14 years of age. All children experienced marked neurologic improvement following decompression while no patient experienced late instability. They attributed this success to meticulous sizing and shaping of the tricortical graft. The graft should be at least 4 mm larger than the space left from the corpectomy to prevent graft dislodgment. Most patients were managed in a Philadelphia collar until fusion was solid. All patients were followed for at least 4 years with no evidence of deformity.[76]

In contrast, Stauffer reported a series of 16 young patients treated for similar indications with an interbody dowel fusion technique. All had postoperative instability with angular deformity after surgery.[77]

INJURIES TO THE THORACOLUMBAR SPINE IN CHILDREN

Injuries of the thoracic and lumbar spine are relatively uncommon in the pediatric population. Elasticity of the ligaments, wedge-shaped vertebra, horizontally oriented facets, a flexible intervertebral disk, and the presence of cartilagenous endplates may all be protective in children. Mechanisms of injury include motor vehicle accidents, falls from height, sports injuries, and child abuse.

FLEXION-DISTRACTION INJURIES

Seat belts are effective in decreasing the overall morbidity and mortality of motor vehicle accidents in both children and adults.[78–82] The use of lap belts, however, is associated with both flexion-distraction injuries of the spine and injury to the intraabdominal hollow viscus, aorta, and pancreas.[80,83–98] Despite increasing use of a shoulder harness to augment the lap belt, injury still occurs and may be associated with the restraining device itself or with improper use of the seat belt.[83,87,99–101] The high incidence of this injury in children can largely be attributed to the use of lap belts only, a higher center of gravity, an underdeveloped pelvis, and a poorly fitting seat belt.

In 1948 G.Q. Chance first described the horizontal split of the spine and neural arch, which occurred after a flexion force.[102] Smith and Kaufer are credited with first detailing the biomechanics of lumbar spine injuries associated with lap belts. In a deceleration injury, the combined forces of hyperflexion and rotation, both centered anterior to the vertebral bodies, produce failure of both the anterior and posterior structures in distraction. As a result, there is longitudinal disruption of the posterior elements (ligamentous, osseus, or both) combined with minimal loss of anterior vertebral body height.[95] (Fig. 15-21). In the pediatric population, the lap belt is often worn above the level of the pelvis and may produce a flexion moment at the compressed abdominal surface in a rapid deceleration injury.

Several studies have looked specifically at the incidence of intraabdominal injury associated with flexion distraction injuries with seat belt use.[80,84,86,88,90,92–94,103] The overall incidence of intraabdominal injury associated with seat belt–related flexion distraction has been as high as 50% to 84%.[84,86,88,103] In a study by Anderson and coworkers, 90% of skeletally immature patients with flexion-distraction spine injuries had an associated abdominal injury.[84] Similarly, Reid and coworkers reported concomitant abdominal injury in 50% of patients with spine injuries. Additionally, over 80% of patients wearing a seat belt restraint had evidence of the "seat belt sign," a bandlike ecchymosis over the anterior abdomen.[93] This bruising across the pelvis and abdomen has been found to have an extremely high association with both intraabdominal injury and spine injury.[84,92–95,98] Given these results, the clinician must have a high index of suspicion for major intraabdominal pathology in any patient who presents with a flexion distraction injury of the spine. Diagnostic peritoneal lavage or contrast CT should be considered in most if not all patients with a flexion distraction injury of the spine. Similarly, a careful examination of the spine should be performed in any child with belt-like abdominal and pelvic ecchymosis or intraabdominal injury. This should include lateral spine radiographs, palpation of each spinous process, and CT as needed. In a study by Sivit and coworkers, 21% of 61 children evaluated with a CT scan for intraabdominal injury were found to have a lumbar spine fracture not previously apparent on plain radiographs.[94] Similarly, if

A B

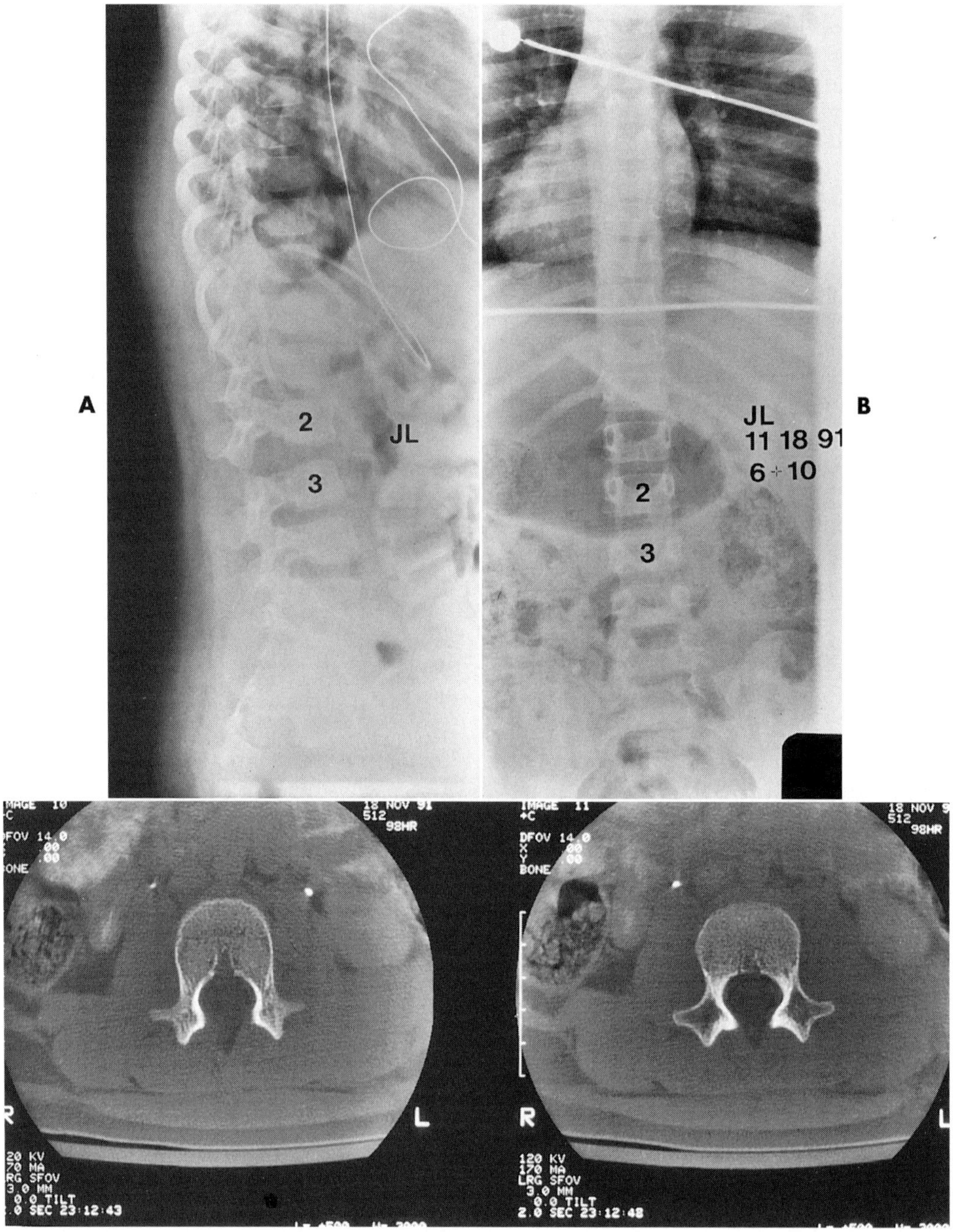

C

Figure 15-21

A, B Ligamentous flexion-distraction injury. Six-year-old male, wearing lap belt only, involved in rapid deceleration injury in a moto vehicle. Anteroposterior and lateral T-L spine films show L2-L3 flexion-distraction injury. **C** CT scan shows minimal involvement o the vertebral bodies and may actually miss the injury.

D

E

F

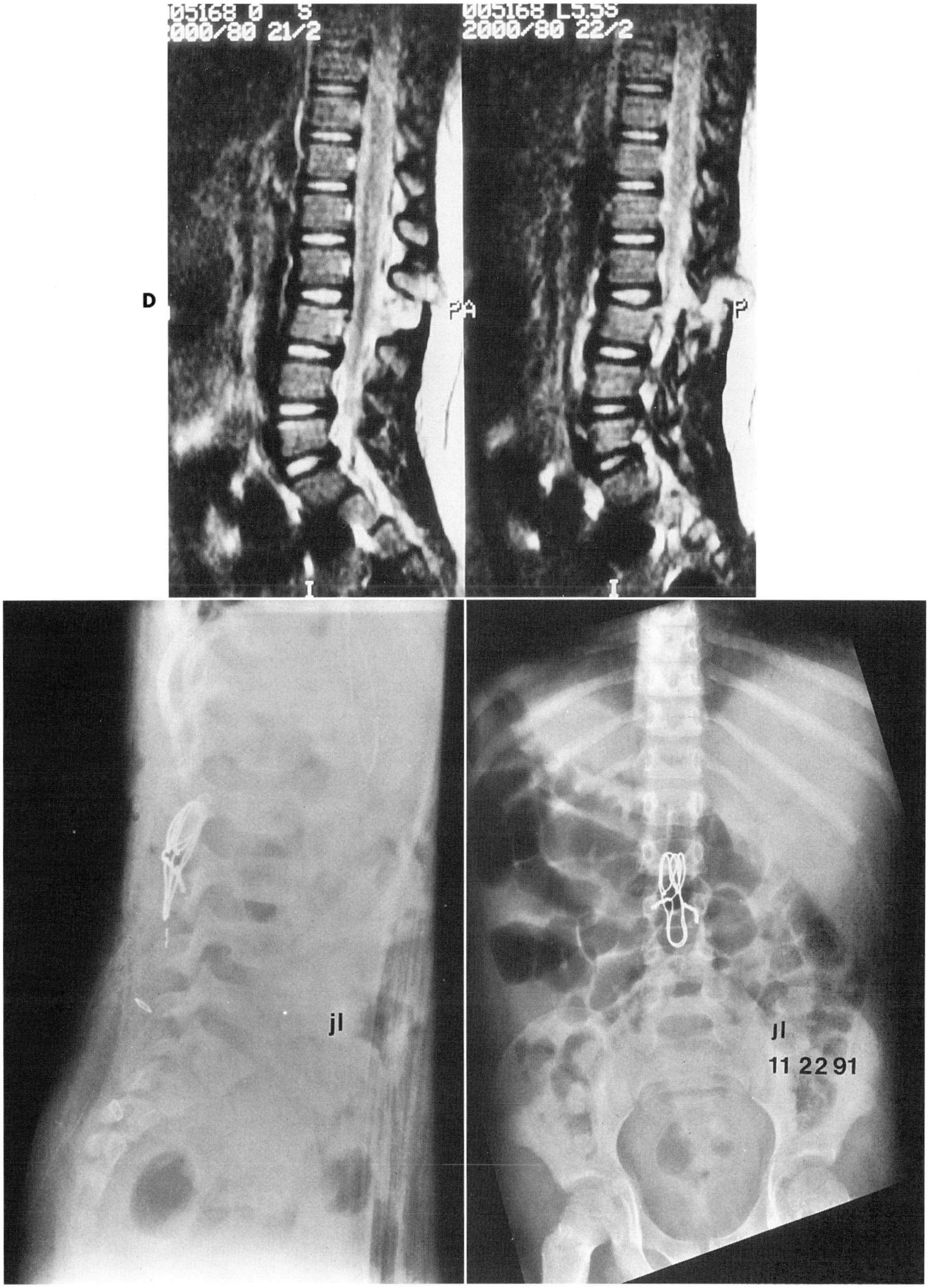

FIGURE 15-21 *Continued*

D, MRI shows soft tissue injury to posterior ligaments with swelling and separation at L2-L3. **E, F** Patient was treated with posterior wiring in compression.

children with this injury mechanism have undergone a CT scan that is negative, lateral radiographs should be taken to increase the overall yield.[104]

Glass and coworkers reviewed 35 children with injuries to the lumbar spine who had axial CT scans with 1-cm cuts performed in this region to rule out intraabdominal pathology.[105] They found that spine abnormalities could not be demonstrated in 57% of the cases. The lateral lumbar spine radiograph identified the injury in all cases. These authors recommend a cross table lateral scout view to screen for lumbar spine injuries in patients undergoing an abdominal CT scan. If identified, thinner slice CT (3 mm) in the region of injury can then be performed to reduce radiation exposure and save time in the scanner. The CT scan is particularly useful in assessing canal encroachment, visualizing endplate avulsion fractures, visualizing laminar fractures, and assessing the overall fracture configuration.[105]

Although several authors have proposed classification systems for the flexion-distraction injuries of the lumbar spine, no universal system is widely accepted.[89,106] Injury may involve disruption through the ligaments and soft tissues, through the osseus elements, or a combination of the two. The level of injury is usually in the lumbar spine or at the thoracolumbar junction.[83,84,89,90,93,103]

Treatment of these injuries is usually based on the perceived stability of the injury. Purely bony injuries (Chance fractures) have been successfully treated nonoperatively with extension casting.[84,90,93,95,103,107,108] Operative treatment is usually advisable for ligamentous flexion-distraction injuries, significant kyphosis (>15°), or polytrauma or severe intraabdominal injury.[84,103]

Where indicated, in children, thoracolumbar injuries can be stabilized posteriorly with interspinous wiring techniques. Wiring can be combined with hyperextension casting if fixation or stability of the construct is a concern. Sublaminar wiring is not recommended in this region. Pedicle screw fixation should be reserved for the almost skeletally mature individual because small pedicle size often precludes the use of this mode of instrumentation in skeletally immature patients. In general, larger children over 13 years of age may be treated with similar techniques used for adults with such injuries, with hooks and/or screws used according to the anatomic level of the fracture, the size of the patient, and surgeon preference. Careful preoperative planning is mandatory to ensure implants are suitable for the smaller skeleton.

FRACTURE DISLOCATIONS

Fracture dislocations of the thoracic and lumbar spine are rare in children. As with adults, these are often associated with neurologic deficits. In a recent review by Kewalramani and Tori, 97 children admitted to a rehabilitation unit were studied.[109] Of these, only four dislocations and eight subluxations in the thoracic and lumbar spine were noted. Hubbard reported on six cases of a fracture dislocation in the thoracic and lumbar spine in 42 children under the age of 18.[1] All six patients were treated with operative stabilization, and two underwent decompression for neurologic loss. Fifty percent of these patients had significant neurologic injury at initial presentation. In a review of long-term follow-up on 48 patients with thoracic and lumbar fractures, Horal and coworkers noted no fracture dislocations.[110] Although this injury is uncommon, it demands prompt attention and often requires surgical stabilization of the fracture dislocation (Fig. 15-22).

COMPRESSION FRACTURES

The combination of increased elasticity of the intervertebral disks, endplates, and ligaments, and the presence of the ribcage, protects the thoracic spine in traumatic injuries. As a result, fractures of the thoracic and lumbar spine are relatively uncommon in children.[1,111,112] Additionally, they are rarely associated with significant morbidity even with long-term follow-up.[1,110,111] The location of compression fractures in children is more often in the thoracic spine and at the thoracolumbar junction.[1,109,110] (Fig. 15-23) The relative increase in the incidence of traumatic compression fractures of the thoracic spine in children when compared with adults has been attributed to the increased mobility of the thoracic spine in children when compared with the mature, adult spine.[110]

Horal and coworkers, in a review of 48 children under the age of 17 (average age of 6) with thoracic and lumbar fractures, found a preponderence of compression-type fractures (71%) with only 5% to 7% of the fractures classified as compression with vertebral body fragmentation. At minimum 13-year follow-up, 38% of the patients complained of some pain at the site of previous fracture. This was believed to be similar to the overall incidence of back pain in the general population and, therefore, considered benign.[110] Similarly, Hubbard reported a benign overall clinical course in 42 children with traumatic injuries of the spine. Sixty-seven percent of these patients sustained a stable, usually vertebral body, fracture of the spine. Of these patients, none had evidence of neurologic injury, and all were treated nonoperatively. Hubbard emphasized, however, some abnormalities may result in rapid progression of deformity and may require surgical treatment.[1] These injuries tended to be either unstable injuries with abnormal alignment initially or injuries associated with paralysis or neurologic loss.

The actual biomechanic and pathologic changes of the spine associated with compression were best described in a classic study by Roaf in 1960. He found

A C B

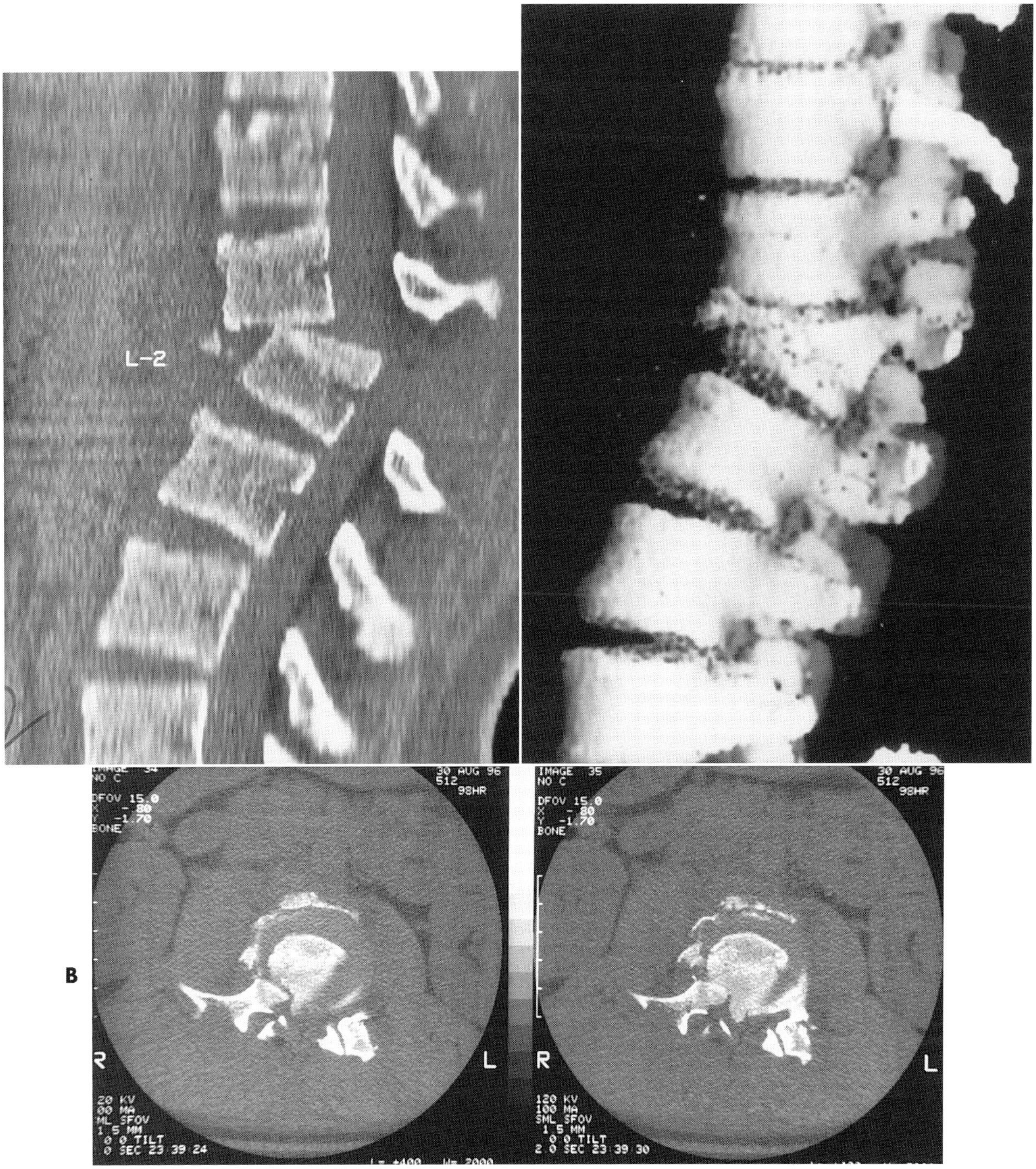

FIGURE 15-22

Fracture dislocation of the lumbar spine. An 11-year-old girl had inadequate routine radiographs after a high-speed motor vehicle accident. **A, B, C, D** CT scan images demonstrate L2 burst fracture with injury to the pedicles, facets, and ligamentous complex. Partial dislocation is noted. **E, F** The patient was neurologically intact. Treatment consisted of posterior stabilization and partial reduction only. (Courtesy of Peter Slabaugh, MD, Children's Hospital, Oakland.)

D

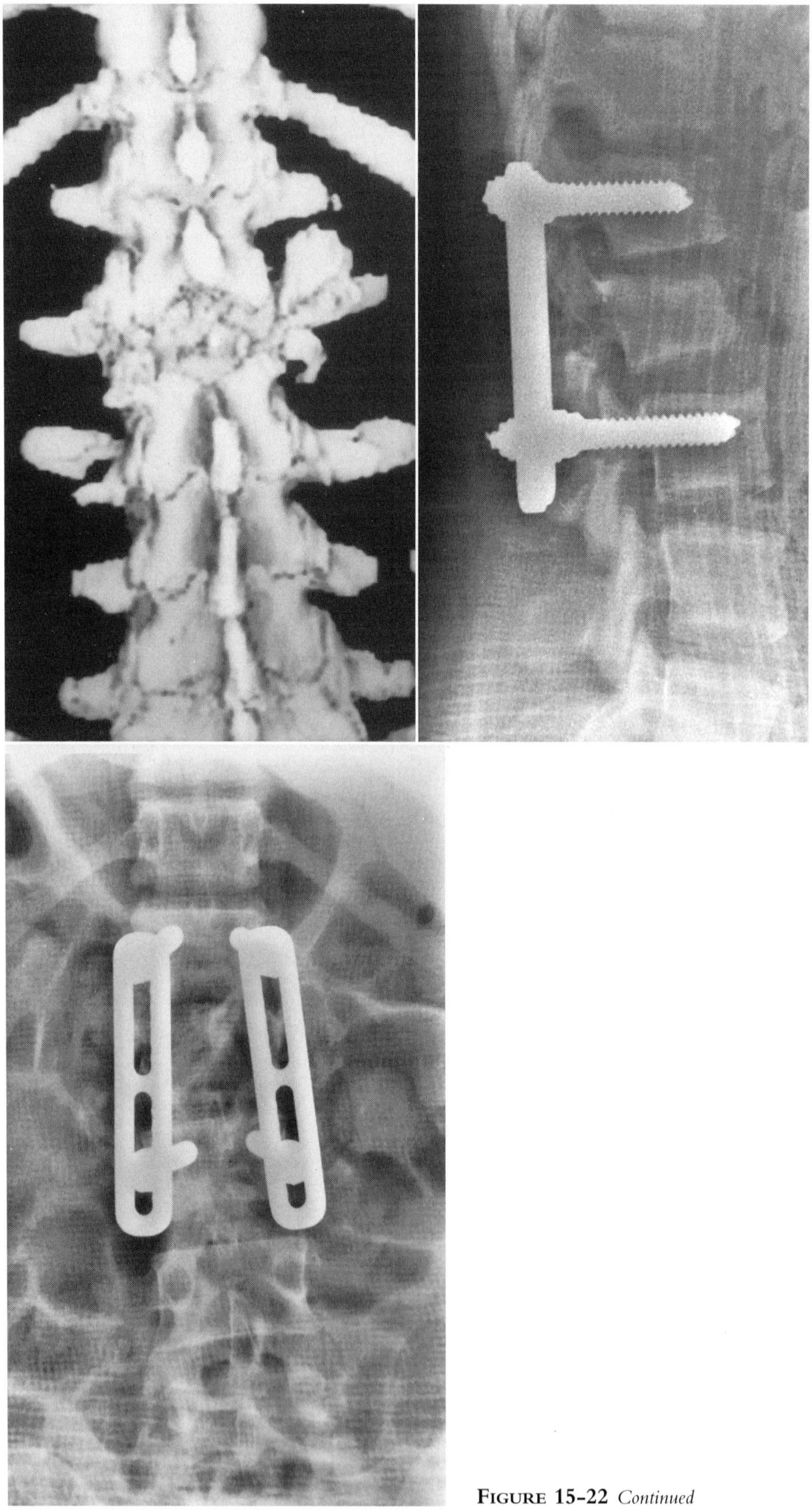

E

F

FIGURE 15-22 *Continued*

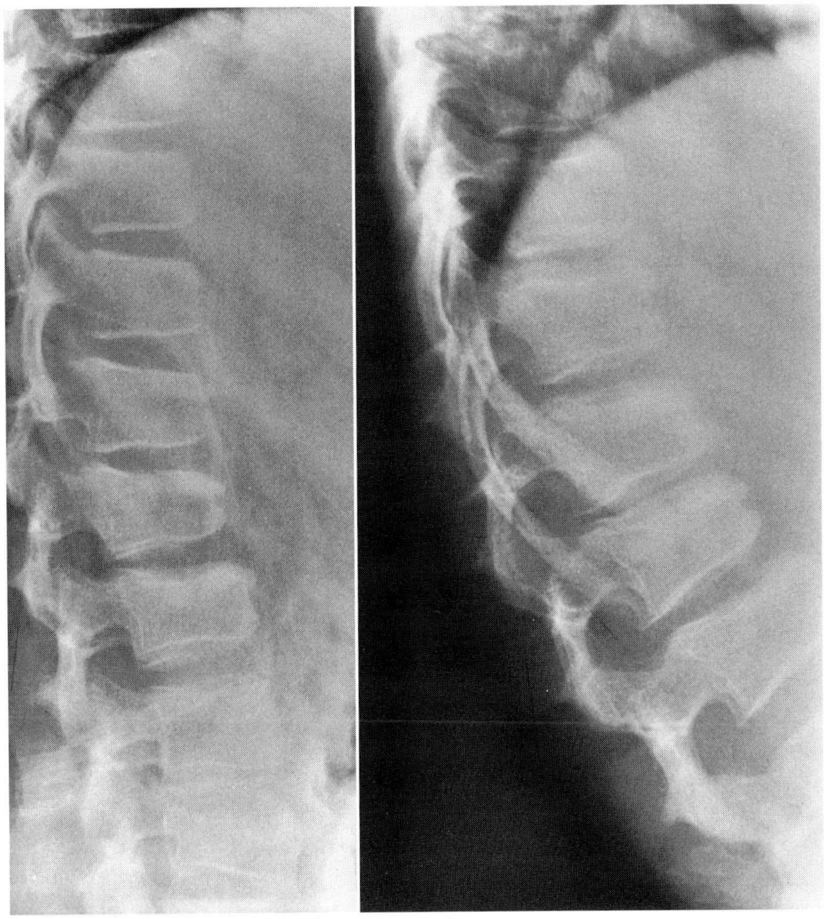

FIGURE 15-23

Multiple compression fractures of the thoracic spine. **A** Supine and **B** sitting radiographs demonstrate increased kyphosis and loss of anterior height in this 13-year-old male who suffered a fall. (Courtesy of Children's Hospital, Oakland.)

that with axial loading of an uninjured human, cadaveric spine (mostly children and adolescents), the major deformation occurred at the vertebral endplate and not at the nucleus pulposus. As a result of loading in compression, blood is squeezed from the vertebral bodies. Extrusion of blood from cancellous bone is a major indication of energy absorption. Endplate failure occurs with increasing pressure and, it is at this time that the annulus undergoes significant bulging and deformation. In compression, the intact disk is more resistant to axial loading than the vertebral endplates. This provides an understanding of compression injuries in the child and young adult. The combination of an intact intervertebral disk with a fluid nucleus pulposus probably contributes to the low incidence of these injuries in children.[112]

SLIPPED VERTEBRAL APOPHYSIS

Rupture of the cartilagenous portion of the vertebral body is uncommon and has been previously reported only in numerous case reports and small series.[113–117] This entity is typically associated with either repetitive trauma or a single, severe episode, although spontaneous fracture of the lumbar vertebral ring apophysis may occur.[113,117]

The ring apophysis normally appears at the age of 6 and fuses with the vertebral body at approximately 18 years of age.[113] Typically, injury to the ring apophysis occurs in males between 13 and 16 years of age, and usually involves the inferior, posterior rim of the apophysis.[113–116] In up to 80% of previously reported cases, the level of injury is L4, with the remainder at the L3 and L5 levels.[113–117]

Endplate fractures are most often associated with disk herniations at the same level.[113–116] Radiographic evaluation with plain films have demonstrated the pathology in only 50% of cases.[113] CT or MRI, therefore, should be obtained in any patient in this age group with onset of lower extremity neurologic signs and symptoms, especially if associated with weight lifting, trauma, or sports injury. Treatment for lesions with

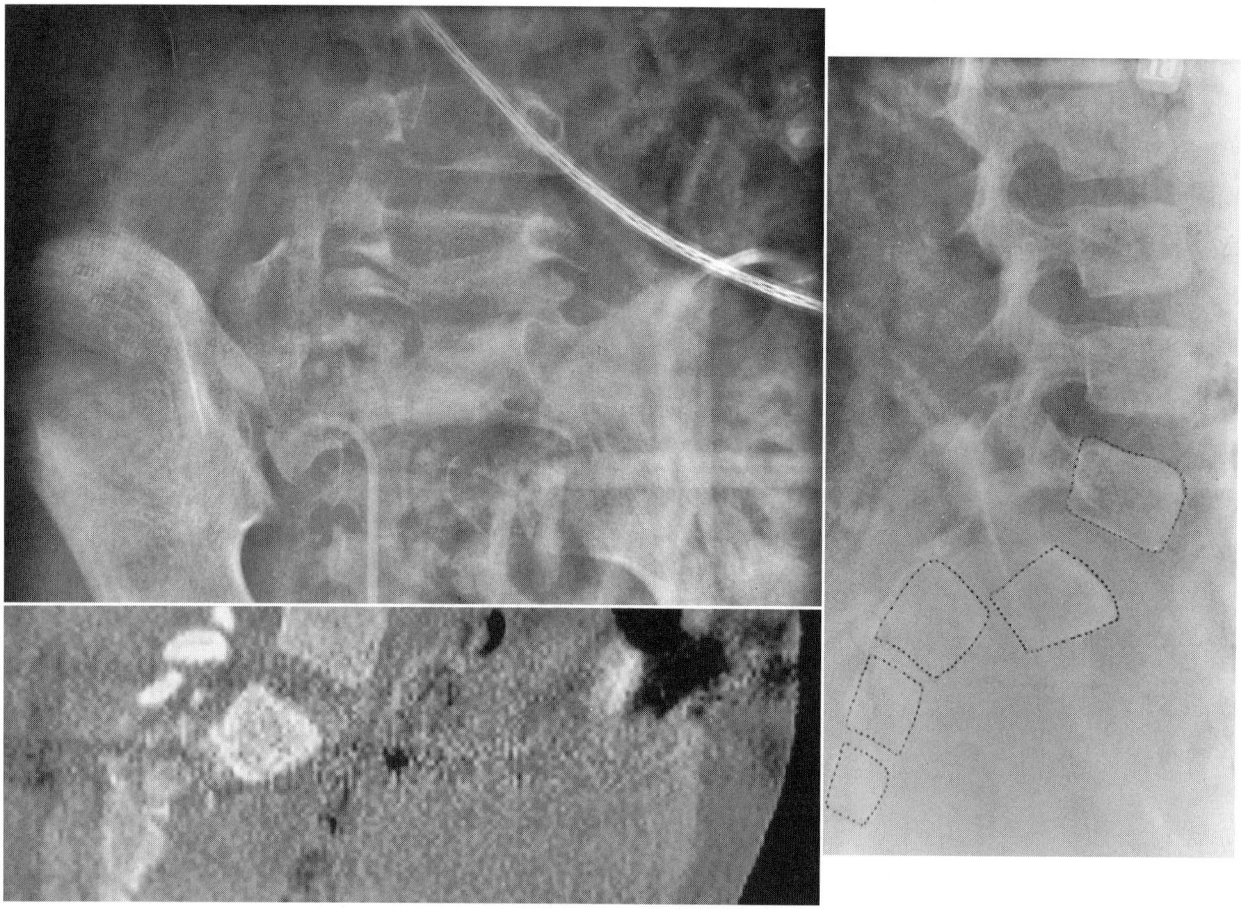

Figure 15-24

A and **B**, Eight-year-old female, thought to be an unrestrained rear-seat passenger in a severe motor vehicle accident. Anteroposterior and lateral radiographs demonstrate pelvic fracture and S1-S2 traumatic spondylolisthesis. **C**, CT reconstruction shows comminution and angulation of the fracture. **D** and **E**, Patient underwent posterior spinal fusion from L5-sacrum. The fracture was reduced and iliosacral screws connected by a rod were used to reduce the S1-iliac joints holding the fracture reduced. The patient was immobilized with a double-pantaloon spica. Lateral radiograph shows antibiotic beads, which were placed at a later operation when a deep infection developed. **F** and **G**, The patient eventually underwent hardware removal after consolidation of fusion. She is doing well at most recent follow-up. (Case courtesy of William R. Steven, MD, William Beaumont Army Medical Center, El Paso, Texas.)

neurologic symptoms consists of posterior laminotomy with decompression of the neural elements.

Traumatic Spondylolysis

Defects of the pars interarticularis, although often developmental, can be secondary to acute trauma.[118–123] Although most cases of fracture of the pars interarticularis are the result of cyclic loading in flexion and extension with subsequent fatigue of the bone, sudden lumbar extension loading may produce acute disruption.[120,121,124–128] Activities most often associated with fracture of the pars interarticularis include weight lifting, gymnastics, diving, and hockey; though these injuries likely represent fatigue fractures.[120,121,126,127] Acute spondylolysis is often the result of high-energy trauma such as motor vehicle accidents, pedestrian–motor vehicle injuries, and falls from height. Because of compromised ligamentous restraints, these injuries may be quite unstable (Fig. 15-24).[121]

Although risk of progression in patients with isthmic lumbar spondylolysis with spondylolisthesis in young patients is quite low (0.6% per year), the risk of progression after an acute spondylolysis appears to be far greater.[124] In a report by Hilibrand and coworkers of three patients under 16 years of age with acute fractures of the pars interarticularis with spondylolisthesis, progression of the slip occurred in two patients 14 and 15 years of age) with one cauda equina syndrome as a complication. The single patient without progression of the spondylolisthesis (5 years of age) was effectively treated with extension casting. The authors concluded that children may be managed with cast immobilization whereas adolescents may require operative stabilization and fusion to prevent progression of the deformity.[121]

D

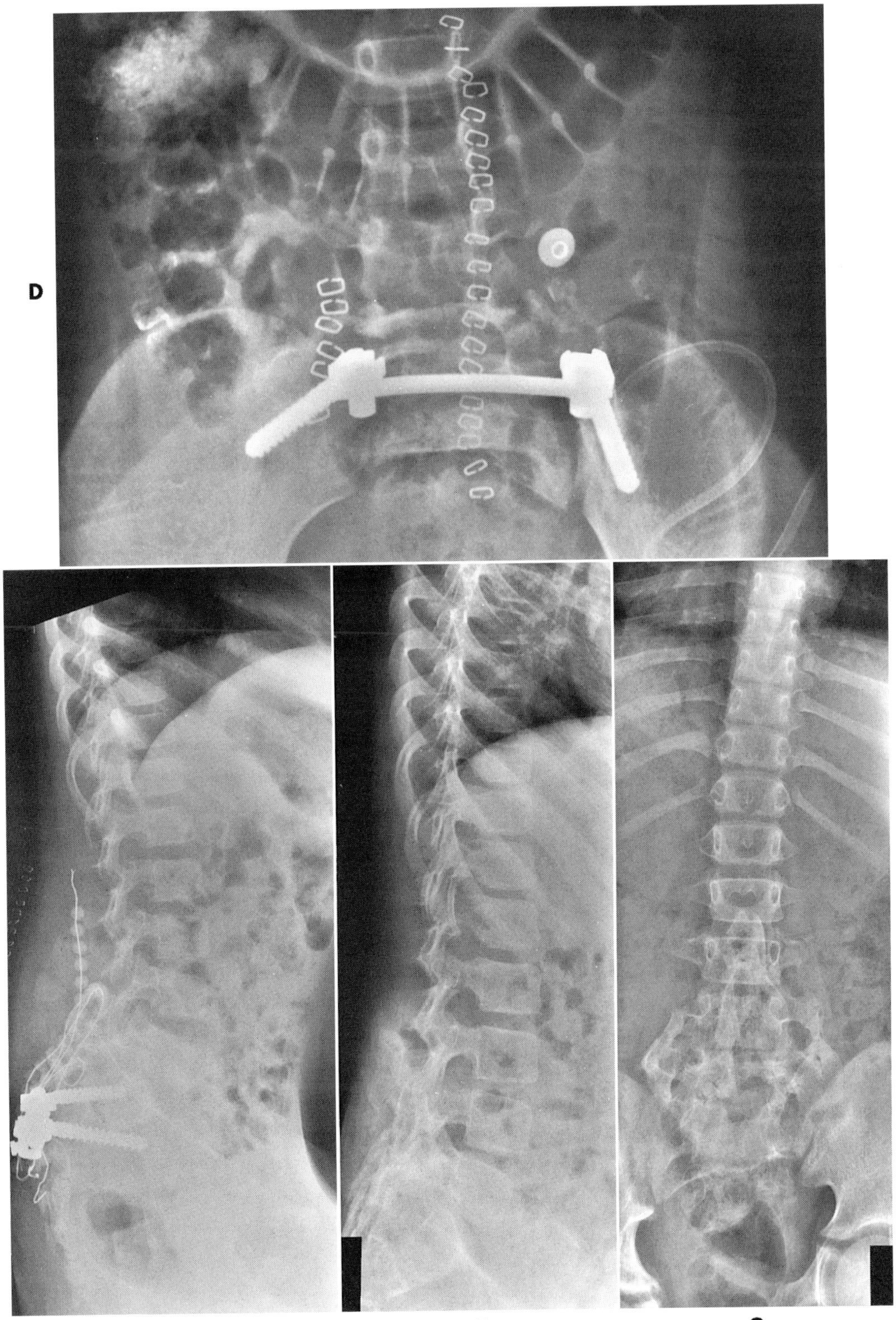

E F G

Figure 15-24 *Continued*

LONG-TERM SEQUELAE IN CHILDREN WITH SPINAL CORD INJURY

Following SCI, the paralyzed child may develop a multitude of problems because of loss of function below the level of injury similar to problems in adult cord injury. These include pressure sores over insensate areas, particularly over bony prominences such as the greater trochanter and ischial tuberosity, respiratory difficulties because of recumbency, joint contractures, recurrent urinary tract infections caused by multiple self-catheterizations, and development of spinal deformity. Many of these can be prevented with thorough patient and family education and a team approach to SCI rehabilitation. Good nursing care and physical therapy are important in the prevention of skin breakdown and joint contractures. Occupational therapy and the judicious use of orthotics also are important in the prevention of these deformities.

Spinal deformity following SCI is seen in some patients. Loss of sitting balance and pelvic obliquity often result in skin breakdown over the ischial tuberosity. The magnitude of the curve is related to the age of onset of SCI and the presence of spasticity. In one study by Lancourt and coworkers, 90% of children less than 10 years of age with an SCI developed scoliosis. Children older than 10 years of age were less likely to develop a significant deformity. The presence of spasticity can lead to the development of a postparalytic deformity. Bracing is poorly tolerated over insensate skin, particularly in the presence of spasticity, and does not appear very effective in controlling these curves. Once curves reach 40° or when sitting balance or skin integrity becomes compromised, posterior spinal fusion from T2 to the sacrum using the Galveston technique is indicated.[129,130]

Fusion ideally should be performed after 10 years of age to prevent the crankshaft phenomenon. Posterior procedures usually are adequate. Severe, stiff curves, particularly with fixed pelvic obliquity may require combined or staged anterior and posterior fusion.

Development of posttraumatic syringomyelia has been reported in 1% to 2% of patients with posttraumatic spinal deformities. Neurologic deterioration above the level of previous cord injury is typical. MRI diagnostic and neurosurgical consultation is indicated.[131]

ACKNOWLEDGMENTS

A special thank-you to Ellen Bair, R.N. and James Betts, M.D. from Childrens Hospital, Oakland, California for providing the numerous excellent illustrative cases. Thanks to Elizabeth Jameson and Susan Averbach for preparation of the manuscript.

REFERENCES

1. Hubbard D: Injuries of the spine in children and adolescents, *Clin Orthop* 100:56–65, 1974.
2. Ruge JR, et al: Pediatric spinal injury: the very young, *J Neurosurg* 68:25–30, 1988.
3. Sherk HH, Schut L, Lane JM: Fractures and dislocations of the cervical spine in children, *Orthop Clin North Am* 7:593–604, 1976.
4. Stauffer ES, Mazur JM: Cervical spine injuries in children, *Pediatr Ann* 11:502–508, 510–511, 1982.
5. Steele AG, Aks SE: Infant involved in a motor vehicle accident, *Ann Emerg Med* 26:508–514, 1995.
6. Agran PF, Dunkle DE, Winn DG: Motor vehicle accident trauma and restraint usage patterns in children less than 4 years of age, *Pediatrics* 76:382–386, 1985.
7. Buckley SL, et al: The relationships of skeletal injuries with trauma score, injury severity score, length of hospital stay, hospital charges, and mortality in children admitted to a regional pediatric trauma center, *J Pediatr Orthop* 14:449–53, 1994.
8. Mann DC, Dodds JA: Spinal injuries in 57 patients 17 years or younger, *Orthopedics* 16:159–164, 1993.
9. Meyer PR, Jr: Posterior stabilization of thoracic, lumbar, and sacral injuries, *Instr Course Lect* 35:401–419, 1986.
10. McGrory BJ, et al: Acute fractures and dislocations of the cervical spine in children and adolescents, *J Bone Joint Surg* 75:988–995, 1993.
11. Birney TJ, Hanley EN, Jr: Traumatic cervical spine injuries in childhood and adolescence, *Spine* 14:1277–1282, 1989.
12. Hamilton MG, Myles ST: Pediatric spinal injury: review of 174 hospital admissions, *J Neurosurg* 77:700–704, 1992.
13. Fesmire FM, Luten RC: The pediatric cervical spine: developmental anatomy and clinical aspects, *J Emerg Med* 7:133–142, 1989.
14. Sherk HH, Nicholson JT, Chung SM: Fractures of the odontoid process in young children, *J Bone Joint Surg* 60:921–924, 1978.
15. Levanthal H: Birth injuries of the spinal cord, *J Pediatr* 56:557–563, 1960.
16. Weinstein SL, editor: *The pediatric spine: principles and practice,* New York, 1984.
17. Wilson DA et al: MRImaging determination of the location of the normal canvus medullaris throughout childhood. *AJR* 152(5):1029–1032, 1989.
18. Schriger DL, et al: Spinal immobilization on a flat backboard: does it result in neutral position of the cervical spine? *Ann Emerg Med* 20:878–881, 1991.
19. Herzenberg JE et al: Emergency transport and positioning of young children who have an injury of the cervical spine. The standard backboard may be hazardous. *J Bone Joint Surg* 71A:15–22, 1989.
20. Snyder R, Schneider LW, Owings CL: *Anthropometry of infants, children, and youths to age 18 for product safety*

design SP-40, Warrendale, 1977, Society of Automotive Engineers.

21. Nypaver M, Treloar D: Neutral cervical spine positioning in children, *Ann Emerg Med* 23:208–211, 1994.
22. Curran C, et al: Pediatric cervical-spine immobilization: achieving neutral position? *J Trauma* 39:729–732, 1995.
23. Huerta C, Griffith R, Joyce SM: Cervical spine stabilization in pediatric patients: evaluation of current techniques (see comments), *Ann Emerg Med* 16:1121–1126, 1987.
24. Cattell H, Filtzer, DL: Pseudosubluxation and other normal variations in the cervical spine in children, *J Bone Joint Surg* 47A:1295–1309, 1965.
25. Swischuk LE: Anterior displacement of C2 in children: physiologic or pathologic, *Radiology* 122:759–763, 1977.
26. Swischuk LE, Swischuk PN, John SD: Wedging of C-3 in infants and children: usually a normal finding and not a fracture, *Radiology* 188:523–526, 1993.
27. Levine AM, Edwards CC: Traumatic lesions of the occipitoatlantoaxial complex, *Clin Orthop* 293:53–68, 1989.
28. Hamilton MG, Myles ST: Pediatric spinal injury: review of 61 deaths, *J Neurosurg* 77:705–708, 1992.
29. Georgopoulos G, Pizzutillo PD, Lee MS: Occipito-atlantal instability in children. A report of five cases and review of the literature, *J Bone Joint Surg* 69A:429–436, 1987.
30. Maves CK, et al: Traumatic atlanto-occipital disruption in children, *Pediatr Radiol* 21:504–507, 1991.
31. Kaufman RA, et al: Traumatic longitudinal atlanto-occipital distraction injuries in children, *AJNR* 3:415–419, 1982.
32. Bucholz RW, Burkhead WZ: The pathological anatomy of fatal atlanto-occipital dislocations, *J Bone Joint Surg* 61A: 248–250, 1979.
33. Bohlman HH: Acute fractures and dislocations of the cervical spine. An analysis of three hundred hospitalized patients and review of the literature, *J Bone Joint Surg* 61A:1119–1142, 1979.
34. Bulas DI, Fitz CR, Johnson DL: Traumatic atlanto-occipital dislocation in children, *Radiology* 188:155–158, 1993.
35. Routt ML, Jr, Green NE: Jefferson fracture in a 2-year-old child, *J Trauma* 29:1710–1712, 1989.
36. Wirth RL, Zatz LM, Parker BR: CT detection of a Jefferson fracture in a child, *AJR* 149:1001–1002, 1987.
37. Georgopoulos CE, Jones DG, Davies DM: Injury to the upper cervical spine: fracture versus congenital anomaly, *Am J Emerg Med* 4:235–237, 1986.
38. Mikawa Y, et al: Fracture through a synchondrosis of the anterior arch of the atlas, *J Bone Joint Surg* 69B:483, 1987.
39. Gehweiler JA, Jr, Daffner RH, Roberts L, Jr: Malformations of the atlas vertebra simulating the Jefferson fracture, *AJR* 140:1083–1086, 1983.
40. Suss RA, Zimmerman RD, Leeds NE: Pseudospread of the atlas: false sign of Jefferson fracture in young children, *AJR* 140:1079–1082, 1983.
41. Vining DJ, Benzel EC, Orrison W: Childhood odontoid fractures evaluated with computerized tomography. Case report, *J Neurosurg* 77:795–798, 1992.
42. Clasper JC, Pailthorpe CA: Delayed diagnosis of an odontoid process fracture in an infant, *Injury* 26:281–282, 1995.
43. Savader SJ, Martinez C, Murtagh FR: Odontoid fracture in a nine-month-old infant, *Surg Neurol* 24:529–532, 1985.
44. Francis WR: Traumatic spondylolisthesis of the axis, *J Bone Joint Surg* 63B:313–318, 1981.
45. Evans DL, Bethem D: Cervical spine injuries in children, *J Pediatr Orthop* 9:563–568, 1989.
46. Ruff SJ, Taylor TK: Hangman's fracture in an infant, *J Bone Joint Surg* 68B:702–703, 1986.
47. de Beer JD, Hoffman EB, Kieck CF: Traumatic atlantoaxial subluxation in children, *J Pediatr Orthop* 10:397–400, 1990.
48. Dawson EG, Smith L: Atlanto-axial subluxation in children due to vertebral anomalies, *J Bone Joint Surg* 61A:582–587, 1979.
49. Elster AD: Quadriplegia after minor trauma in the Klippel-Feil syndrome. A case report and review of the literature, *J Bone Joint Surg* 66A:1473–1474, 1984.
50. Davidson RG: Atlantoaxial instability in individuals with Down syndrome: a fresh look at the evidence, *Pediatrics* 81:857–865, 1988.
51. Martel W: Observations on the spine in mongoloidism, *AJR* 97:630–638, 1966.
52. Burke SW, et al: Chronic atlanto-axial instability in Down syndrome, *J Bone Joint Surg* 67A:1356–1360, 1985.
53. Goldberg MJ: Spine instability and the special olympics, *Clin Sports Med* 12:507–515, 1993.
54. Rizzolo S, Lemos MJ, Mason DE: Posterior spinal arthrodesis for atlantoaxial instability in Down syndrome, *J Pediatr Orthop* 15:543–548, 1995.
55. Tredwell SJ, Newman DE, Lockitch G: Instability of the upper cervical spine in Down syndrome, *J Pediatr Orthop* 10:602–606, 1990.
56. Osenbach RK, Menezes AH: Spinal cord injury without radiographic abnormality in children, *Pediatr Neurosci* 15:168–175, 1989.
57. Pang D, Wilberger JE, Jr.: Spinal cord injury without radiographic abnormalities in children, *J Neurosurg* 57:114–129, 1982.
58. Pang D, Pollack IF: Spinal cord injury without radiographic abnormality in children—the SCIWORA syndrome, *J Trauma* 29:654–664, 1989.
59. Pollack IF, Pang D, Sclabassi R: Recurrent spinal cord injury without radiographic abnormalities in children, *J Neurosurg* 69:177–182, 1988.

60. Yngve DA, et al: Spinal cord injury without osseous spine fracture, *J Pediatr Orthop* 8:153–159, 1988.
61. Ahmann PA, et al: Spinal cord infarction due to minor trauma in children, *Neurology* 25:301–307, 1975.
62. Fielding JW, Hawkins RJ: Atlanto-axial rotatory fixation. (Fixed rotatory subluxation of the atlanto-axial joint), *J Bone Joint Surg* 59:37–44, 1977.
63. Phillips WA, Hensinger RN: The management of rotatory atlanto-axial subluxation in children, *J Bone Joint Surg* 71A:664–668 1989.
64. Crockard HA, Rogers MA: Open reduction of traumatic atlanto-axial rotatory dislocation with use of the extreme lateral approach. A report of two cases, *J Bone Joint Surg* 78A:431–436 1996.
65. Schwartz N: Fixed atlanto-axial rotational dislocation—a rare cause of torticollis. *Unfallchirug*, 98:532–534 1995.
66. McGrory BE, Fenichel GM: Hangman's fracture subsequent to shaking in an infant, *Ann Neurol* 2:82, 1977.
67. Dickson RA, Leatherman KD: Spinal injuries in child abuse: case report, *J Trauma* 18:811–812, 1978.
68. Caffey J: Multiple fractures in the lone bones of infants suffering from subdural hematoma, *AJR* 56:163, 1946.
69. Caffey J: The whiplash shaken infant syndrome: manual shaking by the extremities with whiplash-induced intracranial and intraocular bleedings, linked with residual permanent brain damage and mental retardation, *Pediatrics*, 54:396–403, 1974.
70. Cullen JC: Spinal lesions in battered babies, *J Bone Joint Surg* 57B:364–366, 1975.
71. Diamond P, Hansen CM, Christofersen MR: Child abuse presenting as a thoracolumbar spinal fracture dislocation: a case report, *Pediatr Emerg Care* 10:83–86, 1994.
72. Letts M, Kaylor D, Gouw G: A biomechanical analysis of halo fixation in children, *J Bone Joint Surg* 70B:277–279, 1988.
73. Garfin SR, et al: Complications in the use of the halo fixation device, *J Bone Joint Surg* 68A:320–325, 1986.
74. Garfin SR, et al: Skull osteology as it affects halo pin placement in children, *J Pediatr Orthop* 6:434–436, 1986.
75. Crawford AH: Operative treatment of spine fractures in children, *Orthop Clin North Am* 21:325–339, 1990.
76. Shacked I, Ram Z, Hadani M: The anterior cervical approach for traumatic injuries to the cervical spine in children, *Clin Orthop* 292:144–150, 1993.
77. Stauffer ES, Kelly EG: Fracture-dislocations of the cervical spine. Instability and recurrent deformity following treatment by anterior interbody fusion, *J Bone Joint Surg* 59A:45–48, 1977.
78. Campbell BJ: Safety belt injury reduction related to crash severity and front seated position, *J Trauma* 27:733–739, 1987.
79. Evans L: Fatality risk reduction from safety belt use, *J Trauma* 27:746–749, 1987.
80. Hoffman MA, et al: The pediatric passenger: trends in seat belt use and injury patterns, *J Trauma* 27:974–976, 1987.
81. Huelke DF, Sherman HW: Seat belt effectiveness: case examples from real-world crash investigations, *J Trauma* 27:750–753, 1987.
82. Newman RJ: A prospective evaluation of the protective effect of car seatbelts, *J Trauma* 26:561–564, 1986.
83. Agran PF, Dunkle DE, Winn DG: Injuries to a sample of seatbelted children evaluated and treated in a hospital emergency room, *J Trauma* 27:58–64, 1987.
84. Anderson PA, et al: Flexion distraction and chance injuries to the thoracolumbar spine, *J Orthop Trauma* 5:153–160, 1991.
85. Arajarvi E, Santavirta S, Tolonen J: Aortic ruptures in seat belt wearers, *J Thorac Cardiovasc Surg* 98:355–361, 1989.
86. Denis R, Allard M, Atlas H, Farkouh E: Changing trends with abdominal injury in seatbelt wearers, *J Trauma* 23:1007–1008, 1983.
87. Freeman CP: Isolated pancreatic damage following seat belt injury, *Injury* 16:478–480, 1985.
88. Green DA, et al: Flexion-distraction injuries to the lumbar spine associated with abdominal injuries, *J Spinal Disord* 4:312–318, 1991.
89. Gertzbein SD, Court-Brown CM: Flexion-distraction injuries of the lumbar spine. Mechanisms of injury and classification, *Clin Orthop* 227:52–60, 1988.
90. Greenwald TA, Mann DC: Pediatric seatbelt injuries: diagnosis and treatment of lumbar flexion-distraction injuries, *Paraplegia* 32:743–751, 1994.
91. Miller JA, Smith TH: Seatbelt induced chance fracture in an infant. Case report and literature review, *Pediatr Radiol* 21:575–577, 1991.
92. Newman KD, et al: The lap belt complex: intestinal and lumbar spine injury in children, *J Trauma* 30:1133–1138, 1990.
93. Reid AB, Letts RM, Black GB: Pediatric Chance fractures: association with intraabdominal injuries and seatbelt use, *J Trauma* 30:384–391, 1990.
94. Sivit CJ, et al: Safety-belt injuries in children with lap-belt ecchymosis: CT findings in 61 patients, *AJR* 157:111–114, 1991.
95. Smith W, Kaufer, H: Patterns and mechanism of lumbar injuries associated with lap seat belts, *J Bone Joint Surg* 51A:239–254, 1969.
96. Woelfel GF, et al: Severe thoracic and abdominal injuries associated with lap-harness seatbelts, *J Trauma* 24:166–167, 1984.
97. Hudson I, Kavanagh TG: Duodenal transection and vertebral injury occurring in combination in a patient wearing a seatbelt, *Injury* 15:6–9, 1983.
98. Johnson DL, Falci S: The diagnosis and treatment of pediatric lumbar spine injuries caused by rear seat lap belts, *Neurosurgery* 26:434–441, 1990.
99. Muwanga CL, et al: Cardiac contusion in patients wearing seat belts, *Injury* 17:37–39, 1986.

100. States JD, et al: Fatal injuries caused by underarm use of shoulder belts, *J Trauma* 27:740–745, 1987.
101. Sato TB: Effects of seat belts and injuries resulting from improper use, *J Trauma* 27:754–758, 1987.
102. Chance G: Note on a type of flexion fracture of the spine, *Br J Radiol* 21:452–453, 1948.
103. LeGay DA, Petrie DP, Alexander DI: Flexion-distraction injuries of the lumbar spine and associated abdominal trauma, *J Trauma* 30:436–444, 1990.
104. Taylor GA, Eggli KD: Lap-belt injuries of the lumbar spine in children: a pitfall in CT diagnosis (published erratum appears in *AJR* 151(3):preceding 641, 1988), *AJR* 150:1355–1358, 1988.
105. Glass RB, et al: Lumbar spine injury in a pediatric population: difficulties with computed tomographic diagnosis, *J Trauma* 37:815–819, 1994.
106. Gumley G, Taylor TK, Ryan MD: Distraction fractures of the lumbar spine, *J Bone Joint Surg* 64B:520–525, 1982.
107. Gallagher DJ, Heinrich SD: Pediatric chance fracture, *J Orthop Trauma* 4:183–187, 1990.
108. McGuire RA, Freeland AE: Flexion-distraction injury of the thoracolumbar spine, *Orthopedics* 15:379–381, 1992.
109. Kewalramani LS, Tori JA: Spinal cord trauma in children. Neurologic patterns, radiologic features, and pathomechanics of injury, *Spine* 5:11–18, 1980.
110. Horal J, Nachemson, A, Scheller, S: Clinical and radiological long term follow-up of vertebral fractures in children, *Acta Orthop Scand* 43:491–503, 1972.
111. Hadley MN, et al: Pediatric spinal trauma. Review of 122 cases of spinal cord and vertebral column injuries, *J Neurosurg* 68:18–24, 1988.
112. Roaf R: A study of the mechanics of spinal injuries, *J Bone Joint Surg* 42B:810–823, 1960.
113. Handel SF, et al: Posterior lumbar apophyseal fractures, *Radiology* 130:629–633, 1979.
114. Lippitt AB: Fracture of a vertebral body end plate and disk protrusion causing subarachnoid block in an adolescent, *Clin Orthop* 116:112–115, 1976.
115. Keller R: Traumatic displacement of the cartilagenous vertebral rim: a sign of intervertebral disc prolapse, *Radiology* 110:21–24, 1974.
116. Lowrey J: Dislocated lumbar vertebral epiphysis in adolescent children: report of three cases, *J Neurosurg* 38:232–234, 1973.
117. Techakapuch S: Rupture of the lumbar cartilage plate into the spinal canal in an adolescent. A case report, *J Bone Joint Surg* 63A:481–482, 1981.
118. Chapman P: Traumatic spondylolysis—a case report, *J R Army Med Corps* 133:96–97, 1987.
119. Cope R: Acute traumatic spondylolysis. Report of a case and review of the literature, *Clin Orthop* 162–165, 1988.
120. Hensinger RN: Spondylolysis and spondylolisthesis in children and adolescents, *J Bone Joint Surg* 71A:1098–1107, 1989.
121. Hilibrand AS, Acute spondylolytic spondylolisthesis. Risk of progression and neurological complications, *J Bone Joint Surg* 77A:190–196, 1995.
122. Kleinberg S, Burman, MS: Spondylolisthesis. Report of three cases in adults with forward displacement of the vertebra below the level of the laminar defect, *J Bone Joint Surg* 24:899–906, 1942.
123. Klinghoffer L, Murdock MG: Spondylolysis following trauma. A case report and review of the literature, *Clin Orthop* 72–74, 1982.
124. Danielson BI, Frennered AK, Irstam LK: Radiologic progression of isthmic lumbar spondylolisthesis in young patients, *Spine* 16:422–425, 1991.
125. Letts M, et al: Fracture of the pars interarticularis in adolescent athletes: a clinical-biomechanical analysis, *J Pediatr Orthop* 6:40–46, 1986.
126. Morita T, et al: Lumbar spondylolysis in children and adolescents, *J Bone Joint Surg* 77B:620–625, 1995.
127. Stinson JT: Spondylolysis and spondylolisthesis in the athlete, *Clin Sports Med* 12:517–528, 1993.
128. Wiltse LL, Widell EH, Jr, Jackson DW: Fatigue fracture: the basic lesion is inthmic spondylolisthesis, *J Bone Joint Surg* 57A:17–22, 1975.
129. Lancourt JE, Dickson JH, Carter RE: Paralytic spinal deformity following traumatic spinal-cord injury in children and adolescents, *J Bone Joint Surg* 63A:47–53, 1981.
130. Mayfield JK, Erkkila JC, Winter RB: Spine deformity subsequent to acquired childhood spinal cord injury, *J Bone Joint Surg* 63A:1401–1411, 1981.
131. Griffiths ER, McCormick CC: Post-traumatic syringomyelia (cystic myelopathy), *Paraplegia* 19:81–88, 1981.

16

RECOGNITION AND AVOIDANCE OF COMPLICATIONS IN SURGERY FOR SPINE TRAUMA

Daniel A. Capen

To achieve optimal outcomes in care and treatment of spinal trauma, avoidance of complications remains an important goal for the treating surgeon. Surgical and nonsurgical management, in the best of hands, has complications. At present, the health care environment necessitates minimizing all complications for the patient, the physician, and the health care agency subsidizing the treatment. Benefit to the patient remains the primary concern in the attempt to avoid complications. Increased time of treatment of the complications and delay in recovery are undesirable. For the physician the complications of care create significant stresses, especially with the present-day litigation epidemic. Patient well-being remains a heartfelt commitment for the practitioner. Medical-legal issues and, in an era of capitation, time and effort expenditure are considerations for the treating doctor. Lastly, expense of complications always increases the cost of treatment for the carrier. For all these reasons and many more this chapter focuses on many avoidable and reducible complications in the treatment of spine trauma.

GENERAL PREPARATION

Preparation by the surgeon in reviewing the anatomy of the spine is important in formulating an effective care plan. A complete understanding of the biomechanics of the spine also is valuable.

The Allen classification of instability, if understood, can eliminate inappropriate or ineffective use of the halo. It also can assist in selecting the optimum surgical stabilization technique. In a large series review at Rancho, the problems of anterior surgery in primarily posterior instability have been documented by Capen.[1] Both Nelson[2] and Garfin[3] have documented complications of halo immobilization. In the best of circumstances, there is a 20% complication rate with pin problems and loosening and failure to heal after 3 months in the halo for compressive and distraction-flexion injuries. The halo vest has success in upper cervical injuries, for lateral flexion and distraction-extension trauma, and in vertical compression injuries. The correct application of the device and the appropriate fitting of the vest are essential.

Before undertaking treatment there also must be a working knowledge of the equipment and the postoperative care requirements. Assembly of a well-trained trauma team is essential. Lastly, there must be facility capability to deal with all patient needs before and after surgery to facilitate recovery. If all of these factors are addressed, there still will be complications but many problems can be avoided. In the past 15 years, there has been a plethora of specialty trained fellows with specific interest in the spine for all practitioners to consult.

COMPLICATIONS

Cervical Complications

Complications in the treatment of cervical trauma occur primarily for five reasons.

1. Severity of systemic effects of spinal cord injury
2. Errors in understanding or fully appreciating cervical instability.
3. Inappropriate decisions regarding the timing of surgery
4. Technical errors with the halo or surgical fixation
5. Failure to recognize multilevel injury and extent of instability.

Obviously, the severity of complications are far reaching in terms of the potential for loss of root or cord function. Attention to detail is critical. At Rancho Los Amigos Medical Center (RLAM), cases have often been previously treated in the early stages of the injury at facilities where the injury may be only partially diagnosed, without full understanding of instability and cord injury. This may be a factor in some complication. The redo surgery rate at RLAM for cervical trauma is 30% to 35% of all patients undergoing care for cervical spine trauma. Most revisions result from failed stabilization or partial stabilization.

The pansystemic effects of injury to the cervical spinal cord renders the patient very susceptible to pulmonary, renal, intestinal, and vascular disasters early in the course of recovery.[4] Quadriplegia or quadriparesis together with the multisystem effects of missile trauma and high-speed vehicular injury, create a very delicate environment for the patient and the spinal surgeon. Life-saving, emergency, nonspinal surgery further compromises the patient in the early stages of recovery and increases medical complications from spinal surgery. Post–spinal surgery, deep vein thrombosis, pulmonary embolism, and infection rates are increased.[5]

The postsurgery cord recovery is adversely impacted by hemodynamic instability and cord edema. Many complications are avoidable by appropriate surgical timing and presurgical treatment. Appropriate fluid management and presurgery bowel and bladder and respiratory care are essential. If all of these ancillary supports are not present, transfer to a secondary or tertiary center after emergency care would serve the patient better than emergency surgery without the ability to deal with or avert postsurgical problems, unless clear neurologic deterioration precludes transfer. In the event that emergency surgery is required, early transfer to a cord injury center after the operation may be preferable to reduce potential complications. The skilled care at a spine center may prevent some of the disasters that can occur.

Very little evidence exists documenting the need or benefit of emergency spinal surgery. Except for the rare case of injury followed by clear progression of neural deficit with documented canal compromise, the trauma to the cord at the time of injury determines outcome.[6] The use of corticosteroids, the realignment of the spine, and the stabilization by halo or tongs remain primary emergency treatment goals.[7] Exact diagnosis is essential to permit surgical planning. The reflex operation for "decompression" either by destabilizing laminectomy or anterior decompression not only invites disaster but has no foundation for use based on outcome data.[8] The issue of spinal shock must be addressed by the surgeon before any operation can be considered. The potential for recovery based on surgery is not clear if the patient remains in spinal shock. Postlaminectomy kyphosis requires posterior or sometimes anterior fixation. The fact that anterior bone decompression is not possible often necessitates a second decompression anteriorly. Outcome studies of nonsurgerically treated patients provide sufficient information to dispel the myth that emergency surgery for all paralysis is required.

In this text, the authors of the cervical and lumbar chapters clearly state situations in which to operate emergently and to wait for clarification of neurologic diagnosis. From the information presented, it seems very clear that until the patient emerges from spinal shock, no one can make an accurate neurologic diagnosis. From long-term studies presented in chapters by Waters, Cotler, and Ragnarsson, prognosis or outcome is directly linked to initial diagnosis.

The research done by Delamarter clearly shows the benefits of emergency decompression in animals within 6 hours of injury. The evidence would seem to indicate that except for the few patients injured close enough to an equipped center to allow emergency care, diagnosis, and surgery within 6 hours of injury, the best course to eliminate complications would be to establish a diagnosis, stabilize the patient, and operate under optimal circumstances.

Decompression surgery can improve function and enhance recovery, but the timing of the surgery can permit adequate work-up and stabilization of medical conditions. Also, because of the technical requirements, assembling a rested team that is familiar with tools and procedures is vastly superior to an ill-advised, hastily convened spinal team that inefficiently performs the decompression.

Many cases of partial decompression and poor stabilization are the product of surgery that did not need to be done as an "emergency." The disservice to the patient, which must be subjected to additional corrective procedures, far exceeds the benefit of the initial procedure. All recent experimental animal studies show that a definite time window for recovery exists, but it is quite a broad window. The surgeon must avoid self or patient-family pressure to rush to a surgical solution, hoping that neurologic recovery depends on emergency surgery. This most often is a prelude to a complication. The very focus, that is, neural recovery of this ill-advised effort is often imperiled by the complication itself, especially if the surgery is not successful at complete decompression. At smaller hospitals and larger facilities, the night and weekend staff is often a mix of people familiar with spine procedures and those who are not. The ill-timed operation with inadequate team support often results in a complication of incomplete surgical decompression and fusion. The need to reoperate occurs at RLAM in 30% to 40% of cases in which surgery was performed at the time of injury. Many of these situations would be avoided by appropriate planning.

The window of surgical opportunity is open for 48 to 72 hours after injury, then closes for 7 to 10 days, followed by indefinite opening. Surgical manipulation of the spinal cord during the closed window presents a very high risk of neurologic failure.[9] It is the time when ascending deficit is seen because of cord edema, and it also is the period of ascending hematomyelia. Even nondecompressive manipulation is risky. The RLAM experience with posterior arthrodesis either with cord monitoring or with awake anesthesia is that neurologic injury is substantially increased during the period of risk.[10] Caution here can prevent neurologic compromise by surgical judgment rather than technique.

Errors in technique obviously create complications, but prevention depends on special understanding of cord injury and spine trauma. Full knowledge of instability and complete familiarity with fixation devices are required. The postfixation effects also must be understood. Reoperation at RLAM and other tertiary centers is frequently done to permit maximum function. Excessive levels included in the fusion mass and inadequate or excessive instrumentation are problems. A cervically complete patient relies upon and significantly stresses the cervical spine. With better life expectancy for quadriplegics and normal life expectancy for neurologically normal patients, cervical function is an important long-term consideration. Initial surgery must minimize segments fused to permit maximum function of the upper spine.

In trauma surgery, the anatomy of the vertebral artery location and the neural foramen location is an important consideration. Application of anterior plates depends on placing the plates in the anterior midline. Posterior lateral mass plates placement require knowledge of the specific anatomy of the pedicle and the cephalad orientation. Finkelstein and Anderson in Chapter 10 discuss the correct lateral and cephalad angulation required to achieve secure and complication free fixation. Although there is information that vertebral artery injury may be tolerated in some instances, avoiding the injury is best.[12]

Although rare, the spinal surgeon must be aware of the potential development of mediastinitis. It may inadvertently invade the esophagus, and it can occur after anterior surgery or from plate erosion. High mortality rates have been associated with this complication even when anterior cervical edema or gas is recognized and antibiotics and drainage are initiated.[12]

Completeness of decompression can vary according to surgeon experience. Maintaining midline dissection is critical. Preoperative scaling of a malleable instrument (paperclip) on the computed tomography (CT) scanner can serve as a medial lateral guide because it can be sterilized for in vivo use. Proximity of the vertebral artery must counterbalance the surgeons vigor to "widely" decompress. Anterior decompression can be more difficult for spondylotic myelopathy because of increased tortuosity of vertebral arterial anatomy.[14]

Whitecloud[15] has described the many potential complications of anterior surgery on the cervical spine. Carotid artery injury, vocal cord paresis, and esophageal injury should be reduced by meticulous attention to anatomy and dissection. Hoerner's syndrome dysphagia and dysphonia are retraction and exposure related and may not be completely avoidable.

THORACIC COMPLICATIONS

Thoracic spinal trauma complications are, in general, uncommon for several reasons. The area is more forgiving because of the added stabilization of chest wall structures. Capen and coworkers showed the effects of nonsurgical successful arthrodesis in the upper thoracic region.[16] It is clear that these fractures will heal. Certainly if no neurologic deficit exists, there is no reason to perform surgical fixation of added levels because it has less impact on spine function in this region.

Decompression in the upper thoracic region may present some unique challenges. Intraoperative identification of the exact level can prove difficult whether counting ribs or radiographing the spine. The importance of being in the correct location can not be overstated. The area of true spinal cord is manipulation sensitive whether posterior or anterior decompression is performed. Delicate technique together with cord monitoring, preferably by motor evoked potential, is required. The role of spinal cord monitoring in spine surgery is discussed in Chapter 8.

Spine fixation creates potential for complication, especially when nonoperative treatment can be successful. The lower thoracic region fixation often involves the upper lumbar segments but in general can accommodate longer fusion without serious impact on long-term outcome. The major concern in fixation of these fractures is sagittal balance preservation especially in ambulatory cases. Creating a flat-back can result in late difficulty for this group.[17]

Spinal fixation must be planned and performed to enhance rehabilitation in neurologically complete patients.[18] Whether the patient is neurologically intact or not, the surgery goal must be specific, keeping in mind that one cannot improve on an intact patient. The benefit of root improvement for any case from T2 to T12 is negligible, so outcome, especially in this era of cost containment and insurance profit, must be considered. If these factors are kept in mind, complications will be reduced. Injuries with overdistraction can be reduced by fixation systems, but technique and familiarity remain important. The postsurgical management with orthosis when appropriate can reduce the incidence of rod cut-out. Anterior plates for the thoracic spine are emerging as an adjunct to surgical decompression, but, to date, they do not permit brace-free postsurgical management.

Diagnosis of injury is difficult in the thoracic spine, often requiring imaging in addition to plain radiographs. Burst-type injuries are the most difficult to completely diagnose as appearance is often confused with simple compression fracture. Ballock[19] has noted only 54% accuracy with plain radiograph analysis.

Although causation of fracture from high-energy trauma is clear, thoracic fracture from low-energy trauma may have an alternative cause. The practitioner should maintain an index of suspicion for possible infection, tumor, or bone disease. Gilbert and coworkers[20] discuss incidence and treatment. Early diagnosis is important for these problems. Age groups in which primary carcinoma may occur and patient groups with medical conditions predisposing them to infection are clearly at greatest risk.

LUMBAR SPINE SURGERY COMPLICATIONS

Although somewhat more forgiving in terms of neurologic injury, lumbar surgical complications remain a problem for the practitioner. Much has been published about the importance of pedicle anatomy, fixation failure, neurologic injury, infection, and inadequate decompression. All require extensive extra treatment as pedicle screw fixation has become the standard fixation in lumbar trauma. Because it may lead to distraction, compression, and preservation of lordosis, insertion of screws is prone to complication from insecure fixation or inadvertent nerve injury from medial or inferior placement of the screw.[21,22,23] Anterior penetration is rare.[24] Anatomic considerations are paramount in the angulation and orientation of the screws. Preoperative CT, intraoperative radiograph, and endoscopic visualization are the preferred methods of ensuring accurate and safe placement of the screws. Regardless of insertion method, the "missed pedicle" rates are between 3% and 10%. Experience can reduce the missed pedicle rate.

To minimize operative time and minimize intraoperative encumbrances, direct visualization by endoscopic technique provides the best hope for accurate screw placement. I prefer this visual examination technique to multiple radiographs or C arm because all four quadrants plus depth can be visually inspected in the obviously desirable effort to avoid canal penetration. Electrical stimulation and evoked potentials also have been described.[25,26] None of these methods have been scientifically proved.

Probably the single most frequently seen complication in spine trauma surgery for the lumbar spine is infection. The lumbar spine musculature is thicker. Blood loss tends to be greater. Dissection to expose the pedicles either by the Wiltse paraspinous approach or the midline approach results in postsurgical blood loss, edema, and a high percentage of patients with residual hematoma and seroma problems.[27] The hematoma can often become infected.

Kayvanfar[28] showed in elective lumbar surgery that there are some risk factors for infection including smoking, obesity, and persistent drainage. Obviously, with trauma, control of smoking and obesity is not possible; however, drainage of seroma and making sure of adequate hemostasis are important. Kayvanfar shows that drains should be left in place if 8-hour drainage totals exceed 30 ml. Surgical technique and postsurgical continuous cold therapy may be helpful.

In the case of persistent seroma, open irrigation and reclosure is my preferred method to avoid repeated aspirations and to prevent infection. Once infection is suspected, the immediate open irrigation and wound care along with appropriate antibiotics are essential. Severe problems obviously occur if the infection becomes deep and necessitates instrumentation removal. Delayed closure when granulation tissue is present, along with 6 weeks of antibiotics, is often successful at preventing deep infection. Preservation of instrumentation is the goal in posttrauma surgery infection, and it is best achieved by early recognition of the complication and immediate treatment.

Decompression in the lumbar area can be performed anteriorly or posteriorly with equal efficacy as shown by Hu.[29] Complications of inadequate decompression may be less severe but are best avoided by accurate imaging and appropriate surgical technique. There continues to be some controversy in the literature regarding the recovery with stabilization alone, which theoretically permits fragment resorption and restoration of canal area.[30,31] Certainly, the authors highly recommend this course of treatment for the neurologically normal patient with some canal compromise. The so-called prophylactic decompression has yet to be scientifically presented as beneficial.

Loss of sagittal balance has now been clearly defined as a complication for ambulators.[17] Whether the spinal surgery is for scoliosis, degeneration, or trauma, preservation of lordosis is important. Selection of an instrument system that permits this is imperative. Distraction alone can produce the flat-back syndrome. The use of rods alone present this problem, which is at least partially solved by Levine blockers in the rods and further prevented by screw-hook component systems.

Certain obvious advantages of the modern surgical tables and frames are undeniable and have scored to make spinal easier for the practitioner; however, loss of lumbar lordosis remains a risk. The surgeon must be aware of this in the preparation for surgery as well as the actual performance of the corrective operation.

GRAFT COMPLICATIONS

All areas of the spine are arthrodesed with bone graft. Autologous graft remains the gold standard in terms of rapidity of healing. Newer scientifically investigated components such as bone morphogenic protein, collograft, and coral provide some hope for a better, less complicated arthrodesis but are not yet proved.

Complications of graft harvest can present the practitioner with a challenge. Graft donor site traditionally is the pelvis. Early information on the complication of use of the tibia and fibula have led us away from use of these important skeletal structures. There remain several undesirable problems with harvesting graft from the iliac crest including clinical nerve injury, pelvic penetration, and sciatic nerve or lateral femoral cutaneous nerve injury.[32] Pelvic fracture, especially the anterior superior crest region is a problem that can result from too anterior a harvest.

Banwart and coworkers[33] nicely review and categorize major and minor complications of harvest. The series of 261 cases of graft by a single, experienced surgeon had no major complications of superior gluteal artery injury or sciatic nerve injury. Even with the experienced surgeon, however, 39% of the patients had minor complications. Clearly, it remains impossible to harvest fusion autologous bone graft without morbidity.

Careful attention to surgical detail during harvest of graft is important. Minimal soft tissue dissection can help avoid cluneal nerve injury. Complete layered closure must be performed to prevent hernia. Avoidance of complications requires that this part of the spinal procedure be performed with complete attention of the surgical team. The zones of safety for harvest of posterior iliac crest are outlined by Xu and coworkers.[34] They note a safe area free of potential injury to cluneal nerves or the superior gluteal artery and vein.

In the harvest of block corticocancellous plugs, the surgeon must be aware of the actual harvest process. In the author's experience, the use of osteotomes produces graft fracture which can lead to graft collapse. It is the author's preference to use the oscillating saw to harvest the graft instead of an osteotome to prevent graft fracture. Other spine surgeons have related similar experiences to the author.

Extension and flexion of the hip creates significant vector forces that can fracture the spine. Caution when harvesting for anterior surgery is required to avoid meralgia paresthetica and iliac fracture. A bolster under the side of harvest helps to permit more lateral iliac access.

Chronic donor site pain and, more often in women, cosmetic problems also are described with donor procedures.[35] Although not completely preventable, all of these problems can be reduced.

DURAL INJURY

In recognizing and repairing of dural injury, the surgeon must minimize complications. In anterior decompressive procedures repair of inadvertent durotomy ranges from difficult to impossible. Dural sealant and drainage with prolonged bedrest may be the only option. Prevention of meningocele, fistula, and infection are the main objectives once the tear has occurred.

Posterior surgery affords the opportunity for repair more frequently. Water-tight repair is the objective to avoid need for reexploration. Drainage remains an option in this approach. Early decompressive surgery, missile fragment removal surgery, and redo surgery provide the practitioner with greatest risk for durotomy. Chapters 13 and 19 in this book contain further reference. Kaar[36] and Camissa[37] in separate articles address appropriate techniques for recognition and repair.

In some surgical cases, one of the more dangerous complications is an unrecognized dural tear. Postsurgical precautions would not be instituted. Delay in recognition creates increased risk of infection. The presence of headache and clear drainage must always alert the practitioner. Cerebrospinal fluid flow studies and G<inf>2</inf> transferrin assay may be required for diagnosis.[38] Reexploration is the treatment of choice especially with meningocele. Cerebrospinal drainage also is an option. Untreated meningitis and fistula can result.

AVOIDANCE OF COMPLICATIONS

Major spinal reconstructive surgical efforts can result in deep venous thrombosis. Various authors site incidence ranging from 10% to 70%, however, little has been determined in terms of the actual benefit of compression stocking, compression boot, or anticoagulation. All of these have had some support in the literature to suggest a reduction in the incidence; however, recent elective spinal surgical information from Rokito and coworkers[39] suggests that mechanical prophylaxis by graduated compression stocking and medicompression boots are preferable to anticoagulation. My preference surgery for trauma victims is to avoid stomach anticoagulants unless there is a history of previous deep venous thrombosis and pulmonary embolism. I also prefer mechanical compression.

QUALITY OF DIAGNOSIS

The practitioner must keep in mind that spinal fractures from seemingly low-energy or minor trauma can be a simple result of a fractured osteopenic vertebrae. Ruling out the presence of possible spinal vertebral infection or spinal metastatic infiltration is critical, especially in patients with a previous history of neoplasm or immune system compromise. It is important to ensure that the fracture does not contain infected or neoplastic tissue. Using CI, MRI, and bone scanning may be required in the work-up of some of these patients. This would avoid a potential complication of worsening of the spinal condition by missing the diagnosis. Appropriate overall patient care also would be compromised if the osteoblastic or osteoclastic processes are not identified. Severe osteoporosis, multiple myeloma, and neoplastic disease may be the primary cause of this lesion. Pain prior to the trauma would be a critical piece of information, as this is frequently the most prominent feature of spinal metastatic disease. At presentation, neurologic involvement is rare. Later, development of neurologic defect is a risk in metastatic disease or infection, especially if minor trauma is the diagnosis and recognition of the underlying process is delayed.

The overlooked spine trauma associated with lumbar transverse process fracture also is a potential problem. At U.C. San Diego, there were 3 of 28 patients with significant spine trauma that was missed on plain radiographs but was diagnosed by CT scan. The study of seemingly benign transverse process fractures by CT scan to avoid overlooking serious injury is recommended.[40]

PENETRATING TRAUMA

Experience with missile trauma is unparalleled at Rancho Los Amigos and other urban cord injury centers. Low-velocity trauma to the spine is discussed in Chapter 19. Avoidance of complications in this group depends on the knowledge of which cases potentially benefit from surgery. The decompression of missile fragments must be confined to cervical and lumbar injured patients. Instability is rare. Complications arising from unessential stabilization surgery and from inappropriate destabilizing decompression surgery are completely preventable.

CONCLUSION

Elimination of treatment complications may be impossible but should remain a goal in spine care. Elimination of spinal surgery that is not based on sound decision-making certainly reduces the number of complications. Awareness of the potential complications for all spine treatment should assist in early recognition and appropriate treatment of any complication as it occurs. Reducing complications of treatment and early treatment when a complication develops provides the best environment for successful outcomes in spine care. In spine trauma, nonsurgical treatment also can result in some complications. The checklist format is recommended to assure quality of care and optimal outcome.

SUMMARY

Avoidance of complications in surgery for problems caused by trauma to the spine is difficult; however, some basic considerations may be helpful for the practitioner and the patient. The surgeon must ask the following questions:

1. Do I understand the spinal injury, anatomy, and surgical techniques required for treatment?
2. Is the surgery I am contemplating required at this time for optimal outcome, and can the team and I accomplish the task safely and completely?
3. Am I aware of all surgical and postsurgical requirements, and can the facility provide all of the patient needs?
4. Do I understand the entire patient condition, and am I prepared to recognize and treat all potential complications?

If there questions can be answered with four affirmative responses, then complications will be kept to a minimum and outcomes will be successful in the vast majority of case.

REFERENCES

1. Capen DA, Garland DE, Waters RL: Stabilization of the cervical spine: a comparison of anterior and posterior cervical fusion, *Clin Orthop* 196:229–237, 1985.
2. Nelson R, et al: Halovest stabilization of cervical spine fractures and dislocations. A series review and long-term followup. Presented at the American Academy of Orthopaedic Surgeons Annual Meeting, Atlanta, 1984.
3. Garfin SR, et al: Complications in the use of the halo fixation device, *J Bone Joint Surg* 68A:320–325, 1986.
4. Belleman JF, et al: Complications of trauma; care and risk analysis of pneumonia in 10,000 adult trauma patients, *Am Surg* 62(3):207–211, 1996.
5. Ragnarsson KT, et al: Management of pulmonary, cardiovascular, and metabolic conditions after spinal cord injury. In SL Stover, JA DeLisa, GG Whiteneck, editors: *Spinal cord injury: clinical outcomes from the model systems*, Gaithersburg, 1995, Chapter 5, pps. 79–99.
6. Waters RL, et al: *Recovery following spinal cord injury. A clinician's handbook*, Downey, 1995, Los Amigos Research and Educational Institute.
7. Bracken MB, et al: A randomized, controlled trial of methylprednisolone or naloxone in the treatment of acute spinal-cord injury: results of the Second National Acute Spinal Cord Injury Study, *N Engl J Med* 322:1405–1411, 1990.
8. Capen DA: Decompressive laminectomy in cervical spine trauma orthopedic transactions, *J Bone Joint Surg* 9(3):465, 1985.
9. Capen DA, Zigler JE, Garland DE: Surgical stabilization in cervical spine trauma, *Contemp Orthop* 14(2):25–32, 1987.

10. Capen DA et al: Posterior cervical fusion with local anesthesia, the awake patient as the ultimate spinal cord monitor *Spine* 12(3):206–208, 1987.
11. Stover SL, DeLisa JA, Whiteneck GG, editors: *Spinal cord injury: clinical outcomes from the model systems,* Gaithersburg, 1995, Aspen.
12. Ebraheim NA, Xu R, Yeasting RA: The location of the vertebral artery foramen and relation to posterior alteral mass screw fixation, *Spine* 21:11, 1291–1295, 1996.
13. McDonnel MF, et al: Perioperative complications of anterior procedures on the spine, *J Bone Joint Surg* 78(A)839–847, 1996.
14. Oga M, et al: Tortuosity of the vertebral artery in patients with cervical myelopathy: risk factor for the vertebral artery injury during anterior cervical decompression, *Spine* 21:9, 1085–89, 1996.
15. Whitecloud TS: Complications of anterior cervical fusions. In *American Academy of Orthopedic Surgeons Instructional Course Lectures*, St. Louis, 1978, St. Louis Press.
16. Capen DA, et al: Non-operative management of upper thoracic spine fractures, *Orthop Rev* 23(10):818–821, 1994.
17. Lagrone MO, et al: Treatment of symptomatic flatback after spinal fusion, *J Bone Joint Surg* 70A:569–580, 1988.
18. Rimoldi RL, et al: The effect of surgical intervention on rehabilitation time in patients with thoracolumbar and lumbar spinal cord injuries, *Spine* 17(12):1443–1449, 1992.
19. Ballock RT, et al: Can burst fractures be predicted from plain radiographs? *J Bone Joint Surg* 74B:147–150, 1992.
20. Gilbert RW, Kim JW, Posner JD: Epidural spinal cord compression from metastatic tumors. Diagnosis and treatment, *Ann Neurol* 3:40–51, 1978.
21. Louis R: Fusion of the lumbar and sacral spine by internal fixation with screw plates, *Clin Orthop* 203:18–33, 1986.
22. Roy-Camille R, Saillant G, Berteaux D: Early management of spinal injuries. In McKibben B, editor: *Recent advances in orthopedics*, New York, 1979, Churchill Livingstone.
23. West J, Bradford D, Ogilvie J: Results of spinal arthrodesis with pedicle screw plate fixation, *J Bone Joint Surg* 73A:1179–1184, 1991.
24. Castron HM, et al: Accuracy of pedicle screw placement in lumbar vertebrae, *Spine* 21(11):1320–1324, 1996.
25. Darden BV II, Wook KE, Hatley MK: Evaluation of pedicle screw insertion monitored by intraoperative evoked electromyography. Presented at the 8th Annual North American Spine Society Meeting, San Diego, October 14–16, 1993.
26. Wingo DH: Electrical stimulation to guide pedicle fixation. Proceedings of 27th annual Scoliosis Research Society Meeting, Kansas City, Sept 24–26, 1992.
27. Wiltse LL: Paraspinal approach to the lumbar spine, *Clin Orthop* 91:48–57, 1973.
28. Kayvanfar JF, et al: Wound infections after instrumented posterolateral adult lumbar spine fusions. Presented at the North American Spine Society, Annual Meeting, San Diego, Oct, 1995.
29. Hu S, et al: The effect of surgical decompression on neurologic outcome after lumbar fractures, *Clin Orthop* 288:166–173, 1993.
30. Willen J, et al: The natural history of burst fractures at the thoracolumbar junction, *J Spin Disord* 3:39–46, 1990.
31. Weinstein JN, Collalto P, Lehman TR: Thoracolumbar "burst" fractures treated conservatively: a long-term follow-up, *Spine* 13:33–38, 1988.
32. Kurtz LT, Garfin SR, Booth RE: Harvesting autogenous iliac bone grafts: a review of complications and techniques, *Spine* 14(12):1324–1331, 1989.
33. Banwart JC, Asher MA, Hassanein RS: Iliac crest bone graft harvest donor site morbidity. A statistical evaluation, *Spine* 20(9):1055–1060, 1995.
34. Xu R, et al: Anatomic considerations for posterior iliac bone harvesting, *Spine* 21(9):1017–1020, 1996.
35. Fernyhough JC, et al: Chronic donor site pain complicating bone fraft harvesting from posterior iliac crest for spinal fusion, *Spine* 17(12):1474–1480, 1992.
36. Kaar GF, Briggs M, Bashir SH: Thecal repair inpost-surgical menigocel, *Br J Neurosurg* 8:703–708, 1994.
37. Cammisa FP, Eismont FJ, Green AB: Dural laceration occurring with burst fractures and associated laminar fractures, *J Bone Joint Surg* 71A:1044–1052, 1989.
38. Ryall RG, Peacock MK, Simpson DA: Usefulness of G<inf>2</inf> transferrin assay in detection of cerebrospinal fluid leaks, *J Neurosurg* 77:737–739, 1992.
39. Rokito SE, Schwartz MC, Neuwrith MG: Deep vein thrombosis after major reconstructive spinal surgery, *Spine* 21(7):853–859, 1996.
40. Krueger MA, et al: Overlooked spine injuries associated with lumbar transverse process fractures, *Clin Orthop* 327:191–195, 1996.

17

OSSEOUS HEALING IN SPINAL INJURIES

Robert T. Greenfield III

Fracture healing involves a complex series of cellular, biomechanical, biochemical, and bioelectric interactions, which result in the restoration of the functional and anatomic properties of the skeleton. Although most spinal fractures heal in spite of position, reduction and stabilization of spinal fractures may be critical in preventing ongoing or impending neurologic damage. Reduction and stabilization may be achieved by internal or external means supplemented with an arthrodesis. Healing of fractures and arthrodeses follow the same three sequential phases.[1] It is important to understand the process of fracture healing and the factors that effect fracture healing to properly manage these injuries operatively and nonoperatively.

At the site of the fracture, osteoblasts do not exist in sufficient numbers to restore the tissues to their preexistant state.[2,3] A local tissue response, however, initiates the inflammatory, reparative, and remodelling phases of fracture healing. Local and systemic mediators magnify and expand the response, promote cell proliferation and differentiation, expedite removal of tissue debris, and reestablish vascular supply and the production of new skeletal matrices.[4] Failure of this response results in nonunion or pseudarthrosis.

The inflammatory phase is the shortest phase lasting 5 to 7 days.[4,5,6] The inflammatory phase is important because the degree of inflamation in early callus correlates with the quantity of cartilage in the callus and subsequent osteogenesis.[7] A fracture damages the soft tissue envelope rupturing vascular channels and leading to hematoma formation. The hematoma accumulates within the medullary cavity between fracture end and under the periosteum. Vasogenic angiogenic pyrogens and kallekriens are released from vascular tissues and initiate vasodilatation. The relative hypocalcemia created by the hematoma results in release of parathyroid hormone, which also has vasodilatory effects.[4]

Polymorphonuclear cells, macrophages, and lymphocytes migrate to the fracture site to resorb necrotic tissue and cellular debris.[5,8] This mass of inflammatory tissue becomes a self-sustaining organ composed of primative mesenchymal cells, fibroblasts, macrophages, and lymphocytes among others. Each cell type elicits mediators, which through autocrine or paracrine mechanisms, promote cell differentiation and proliferation. Lymphocytes and macrophages produce interleukin I (IL-I), which may increase the rate of mitoses of cells within the fracture matrix.[2,3] Platelets release platelet-derived growth factor (PDGF), epidermal growth factor (EGF), and transforming growth factor beta (TGF-B). These mediators help initiate a rapid acceleratory process that enhances chondrogenesis and osteogenesis.[4,9] Angiogenic factors encourage development of endothelial cells and new vessels.[2,3] Guenther and coworkers have shown that endothelial cells produce endothelial cell–derived growth factor (ECDGF), which results in the proliferation of bone cells.[10] In addition to degrading necrotic bone and other devitalized tissue, the fracture exudate, through its high hyaluronic acid content, promotes migration and proliferation of mesenchymal and endothelial cells, which, in turn, produce other mediators, which stimulate osteogenic and chondrogenic precursors.[2,3,7] At the conclusion of the inflammatory phase, an osteogenic organ has created an environment suitable for cartilage and bone production (Fig. 17-1).

The reparative phase or "callus phase" lasts between 1 and 4 months, overlapping both the inflammatory and the remodelling phases.[6] As early as the fourth day, nests of cartilage cells and osteoid tissue from endothelial cells are seen.[8] Chondroblasts and osteoblasts in the granulation tissue synthesize extracellular organic matrix. The matrix consists of glycosaminoglycans, proteoglycans, and types I and II collagen, among others. Neutral proteinases and alkaline phosphatase remove these substances, dissolve proteoglycans, and hydrolyze adenosine triphosphate (ATP) into phosphate to produce hydroxyapatite. Osteoblasts deposit calcium filled matrix vesicles into "hole zones" of type I collagen resulting in formation of fracture callus.[5,6,8] Increased callus formation reduces interfragmentary motion thus decreasing strain and promoting tissue differentiation to fibrocartilage and then bone.[11]

McKibbon[12] has described a model of callus formation from two different origins. Determined osteoprogenitor cells (DOPC) present in the periosteum and marrow produce membraneous bone. Induceable osteoprogenitor cells (IOPC) form pleuripotential cells with chondrogenic potential and synthesize external callus. Within 1 to 3 weeks, osteoid is mineralized and endochondral ossification occurs along blood vessels established by capillaries. This resembles a model of the preexistant trabecular pattern. Endochodral ossification in the reparative phase leads to restabilization and continuity between the fractured parts.[2,3]

Remodelling is the process by which early callus is removed and remodelled into lamellar bone resulting in formation of new cortical osteons and restoration of the marrow cavity.[5] The remodelling phase is the longest phase of bone healing and may last as long as 7 years.[6] The duration is dependent on the location, severity, and treatment of the fracture.

The cornerstone of the modelling phase is the basic multicellular unit (BMU). The basic multicellular unit

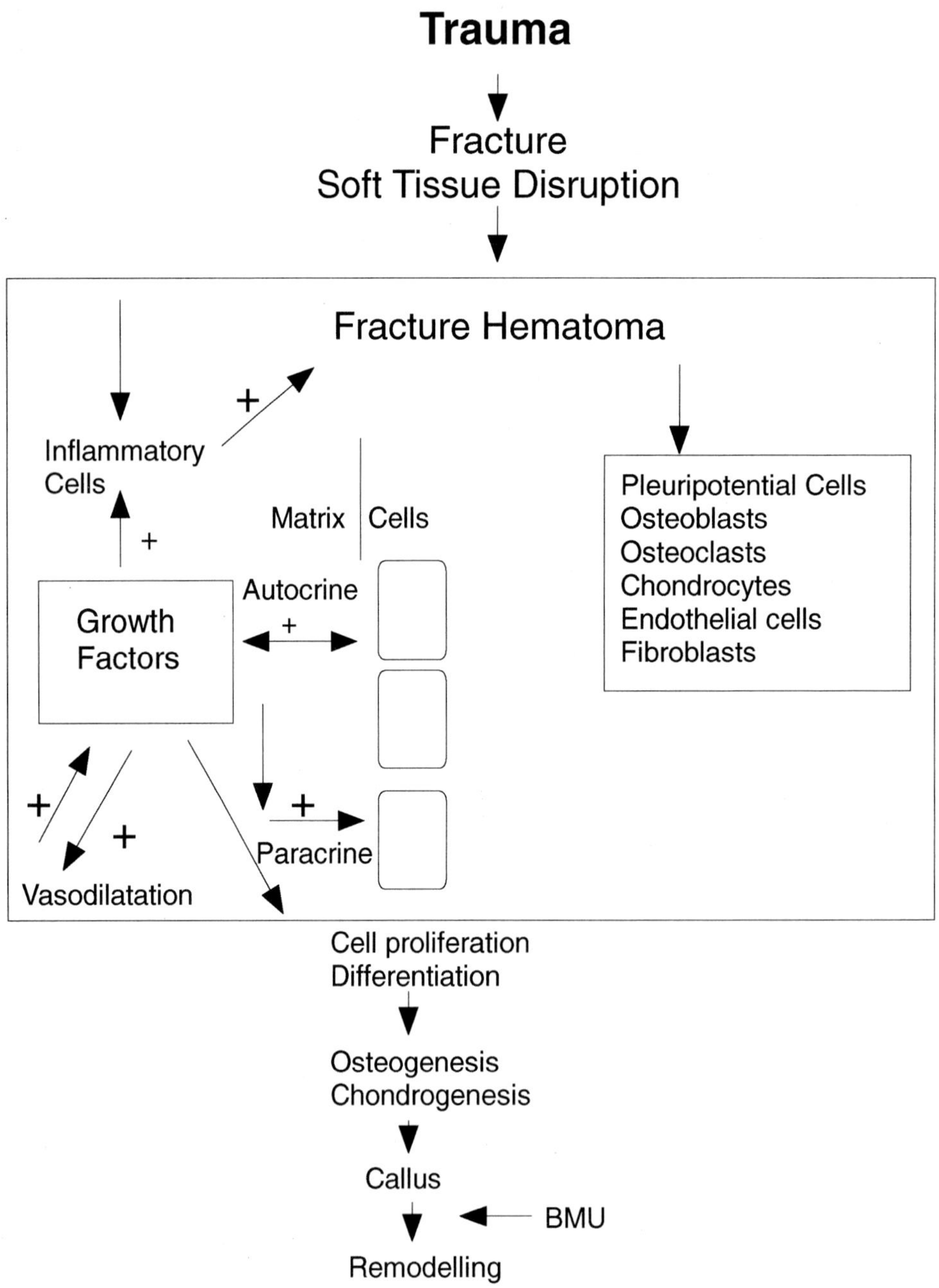

FIGURE 17-1

Schematic representation of fracture healing and interaction of growth factors. (Modified from Subburaman M, Baylink DJ: Bone growth factors, *Clin Orthop* 263:3–43, 1991.)

consists of a front of osteoclasts, which resorb bone from old necrotic trabeculae followed by osteoblasts, which produce bone in an activation resorption formation.[6] A population of strain-sensitive cells restore the biomechanical properties of the tissue along new lines of force. Remodelling of the cortical and trabecular architecture reestablishes an optimal strain environment, which restores the biomechanical substance of bone (Fig. 17-2).[8]

MEDIATORS

As stated previously, when a fracture occurs, local tissues do not contain enough osteogenic potential to heal the fracture.[6] The process is catalyzed by a complex interaction between mediators and cells that have synthesized them (autocrine) and other cells present in the matrix (paracrine). These effects elicit a rapid acceleration process (RAP) by activating previous dormant local precursor cells to produce new cell populations.[6] Most of these factors are produced by bone and stored within the bone matrix.[13] The mediators may exert more control over osteogenic sequences than systemic agents. Their dysfunction may be responsible for nonunion and pseudarthrosis, and their effectiveness may reflect the importance of blood supply in a vascularized graft (Table 17-1).[6] Research on oseoinductive and osteoconductive growth factors has intensified because the problem with nonunion has not been completely eliminated through use of internal fixation.[14]

Bone morphogenetic protein (BMP) is a glycoprotein that has osteoinductive properties by stimulating recruitment, activation, and differentiation of local progenitor cells into chondrocytes or osteoblasts.[15] First isolated from bovine bone by Urist, BMP is a member of a large group of the TGF-β superfamily, which has been proved to induce endochondral bone formation in ectopic bone studies.[16] Sampath and Reddi isolated BMP from demineralized bone matrix and have identified-bone inducing activity.[5] In studies using BMP with coral or demineralized bone matrix as carriers, Boden et al.[17] have seen migration and differentiation of mesenchymal cells from surrounding soft tissue into chondrogenic and osteogenic cells. Recombinant human BMP mixed with demineralized bone matrix has

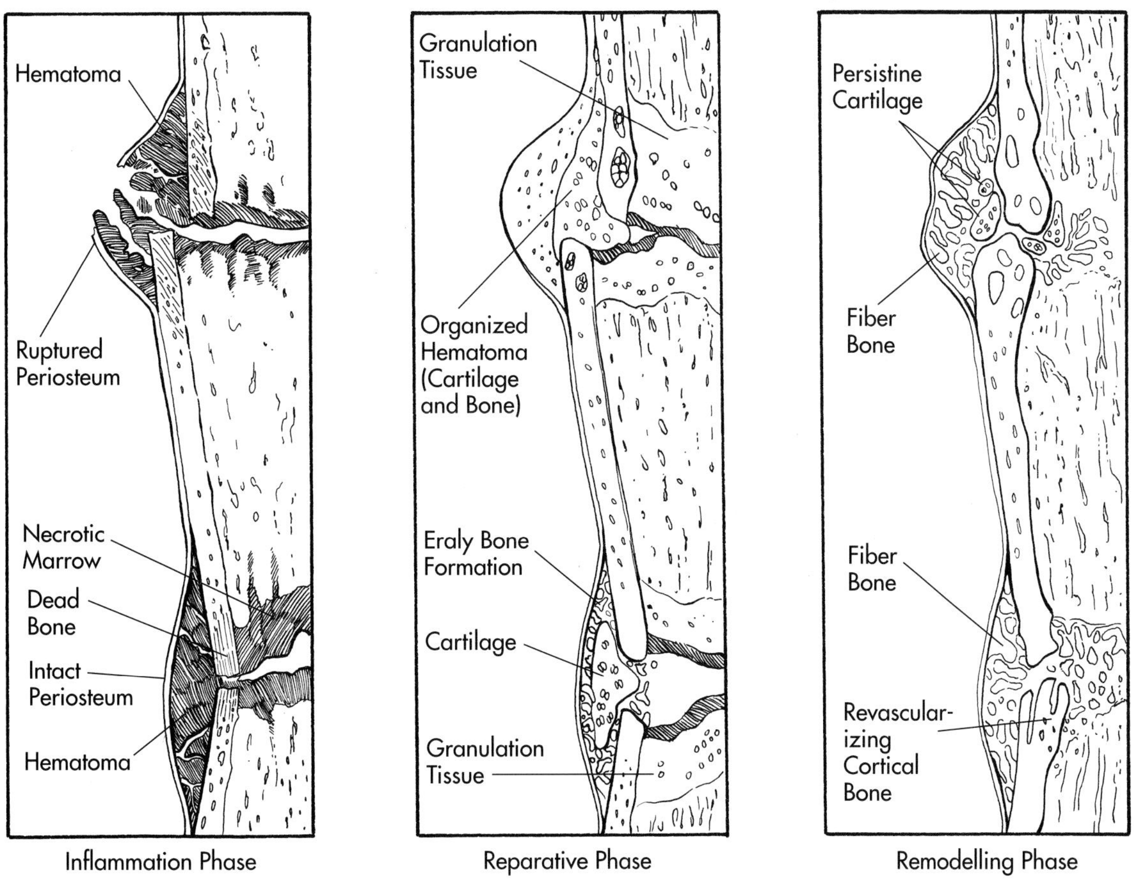

FIGURE 17-2

Phases of osseous healing. **A**, The inflammatory phase. **B**, The reparative phase. **C**, The remodeling phase.

Table 17-1. Bone Growth Factors

	Relative Abundance		Actions on Osteoblasts	
Factor	Bone	Bone Cell CM	Proliferation	Differentiation
IGF-I	+	+	+	+
TGF-B	+++	++	+/−	+
FGF	+	?	+	?
PDGF	+	=/−	+	+
BMP	+	?	?	?
IL-I	?	+	?	+

Modified from Subburaman M, Baylink DJ: Bone growth factors, *Clin Orthop* 263:30–43, 1991.

been effective in healing 2.5 cm long midiaphyseal plate-stabilized segmental defects in adult sheep femora.[18]

The TGF-β is a member of a family of proteins related by amino acid sequence homology, and it is produced by osteoblasts and stored in bone matrix. It induces chondrogenesis in muscle-derived cells, stimulates prostaglandin-mediated bone resorption, and inhibits formation of multinucleated osteoblast-like cells in human marrow culture.[13] Among other functions, fibroblast growth factor (FGF), insulin growth factor (IGF), ECDGF, and PDGF are present in the matrix and stimulate types I and II collagen production, chondrocyte and osteoblast proliferation, and, in some cases (PDGF, TGF-B), bone resorption.[13] In addition, platelets release PDGF, which is mitogenic for fibroblasts, EGF and TGF-β.[2,9] Chondroblasts produce the mitogens collagen growth factors (CGF) I and II, which are required for type II collagen synthesis, and hyaluronic acid thus providing an optimal environment for osteogenesis.[19]

Osteonectin regulates mineralization by binding to calcium salts, crystals, and type I collagen.[15] Osteocalcin regulates ossification through inhibition of mineral formation.[3]

ELECTRICAL STIMULATION

Bioelectric phenomena play an important role in fracture healing. In addition to generating the release of mediators and growth factors, mechanical stresses in bone produce electrical potentials, a process called *piezoelectricity*.[3,8] Yasuda reported that concave portions of hydrated long bone were negatively polarized and convex portions were positively polarized. Electrical currents can influence cell activation and bone growth by the proliferation of cellular components of callus.[8]

The discovery of endogenous potentials and the generation of these potentials by electromechanical means has led to an effort to determine if exogenous electrical stimulation of bone stimulates growth and healing. Osteogenesis occurs around the cathode, between electrodes, and around the anode. Direct current is more effective than alternating current or pulsed current. Consumption of dissolved oxygen and an increase in the local pH at the stainless steel cathode produce a low oxygen tension and a high pH, which are favorable to osteogenesis.[20]

Current may be generated by inductive or capacitive coupling. Inductive coupling is an invasive method in which time-varying magnetic fields (PEMF) are produced by electric coils resulting in the generation of electric current. Capacitive coupling is a noninvasive method in which an electric field is produced through placement of capacitor plates on the skin. Invasive and noninvasive methods have shown the same healing rates.[20–23]

Early clinical applications with electrical stimulation included treatment of congenital pseudarthrosis of the tibia and the treatment of tibia nonunions with 70% to 85% and 65% success rates respectively.[24,25] These clinical applications have been extended to the treatment of spine fusions. Tejano et al.[25] have shown that direct current stimulation in multilevel lumbar fusion is equal to instrumented fusion. In a study of canine spinal fusions, Kahanovitz[26] reported an increased incidence of facet fusion with direct current stimulation. Kane[27] reported a statistically significant higher incidence of lumbar spine fusions treated with electrical stimulation. Despite these studies, further information is required before definitive conclusions and recommendations can be made regarding the use of electrical stimulation for the treatment of spinal fusions.[20]

INTERNAL FIXATION

Fractures rigidly stabilized with internal fixation heal by primary bone healing. Lamellar bone forms across the fracture site with extension of osteons across the fracture.[5] Rigid fixation enhances healing in spinal fusions as well.[28] Although motion between the fracture fragments stimulates the release of prostaglandin E, (PGE_2) and other mediators, internal fixation promotes a low oxygen tension, which stimulates chondrogenesis and endochrondral ossification by decreasing compressive forces.[29,30]

BONE GRAFTS AND SPINAL FUSIONS

Osseous healing in spinal fusions does not differ markedly from osseous healing in fractures. Osteogenesis occurs by influx of polymorphonuclear cells, lymphocytes, macrophages, fibroblasts, and mesenchymal cells followed by revascularization and callus formation and remodelling.[31] In an analysis of posterolateral intertransverse process arthrodesis in New Zealand rabbits, Boden et al.[1] identified inflammatory, reparative, and remodelling phases. These phases occurred in sequence but in delayed fashion in the central zone as compared with the outer transverse process zone. Membraneous bone formation is identified in the transverse process zone as the predominant mechanism of healing. In the reparative phase (weeks 4 to 5) solidification of the fusion with remodelling of cancellous bone occurred near the transverse processes. Differentiation of osteoblasts and chondroblasts with resorption of the cortical portion of the iliac grafts occurred in the central zone. Chondrogenesis in the central zone may be secondary to the limited blood supply in this zone contrasted with that in the transverse process zone (Fig. 17-3). In the remodelling phase (weeks 6 to 10), the ratio of cortical to cancellous bone drops and a peripheral cortical rim forms extending to the center zone. Adequate decortication of the transverse processes prior to arthrodesis is an important technique in minimizing the incidence of nonunion.[1]

Bone graft plays a critical role in the stabilization and healing of spinal fractures. Graft may be osteoinductive and/or osteoconductive. Osteoinduction is the process by which tissue is influenced to form osteogenic elements. Mesenchymal cells and stem cells differentiate into osteoblasts and chondroblasts when stimulated by mediators supplied locally and by the graft.[31] Osteoconduction is the process of capillary ingrowth and deposition of osteoprogenitor cells and osteoid from the recipient into the trabecular scaffold. Many of the graft cells survive and synthesize bone.

Cancellous grafts differ from cortical grafts in the rate of revascularization.[2] Cancellous are completely revascularized, but cortical grafts remain an admixture of viable and necrotic bone. The rate of revascularization for cortical grafts is approximately one half that of cancellous grafts. Osteoclastic resorption of the grafts is followed by vascular penetration of Volkman's and the haversian canals. After resorption is initiated by osteoclasts, osteoblasts fill these spaces with osteoid, which is then converted to woven and then lamellar bone.

Autogenous bone is the "gold standard" for bone grafting, because it is osteoinductive in that it provides growth factors and viable osteoblasts, and because it is osteoconductive providing the strongest structural support. However, morbidity associated with harvesting autogenous bone and the inflammatory response and brittleness associated with allografts have led to the use of "bone substitutes," which when combined with growth factors also have osteoconductive and osteoinductive properties (Table 17-2).

Ceramics are composed of tricalsium phosphate, hydroxyapatite, or combinations of the two. They are brittle and, therefore, do not provide adequate struc-

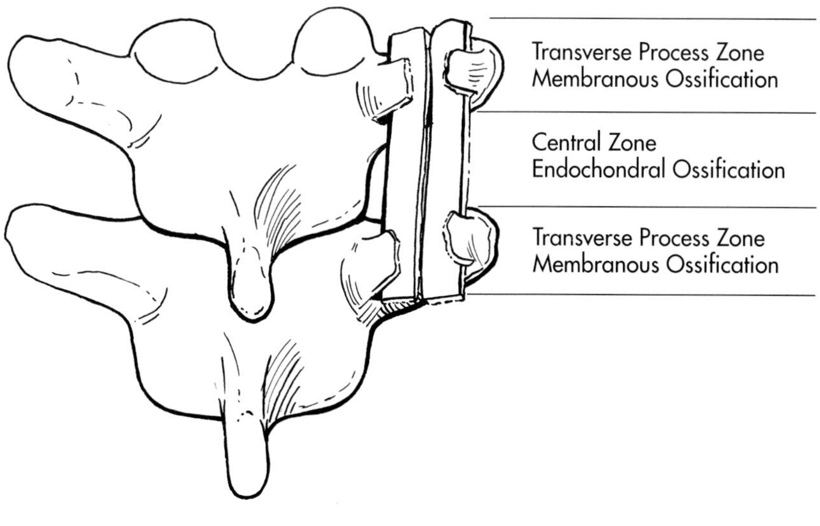

Figure 17-3

Osseous healing in posterolateral arthrodesis.

Table 17-2. Properties of Bone Graft Alternatives

Material	Osteoconduction	Osteoinduction
Cancellous autograft	++++	++
Cortical autograft	+	+/−
Freeze-dried allograft	+	+/−
Frozen allograft	+	+/−
Ceramics	+	−
Demineralized bone matrix	+	++
Bone marrow	−	+/−
Ceramic with bone marrow	++	+/−

Modified from Gazdag AR, et al: Alternatives to autogenous bone graft: efficacy and indications, *J Am Acad Orthop Surg* 3:1–8, 1995.

tural support. They may be used as fillers in bony defects. When used in spinal fusions, they create a dense radiographic appearance, which makes evaluation of fusion healing quite difficult.

Demineralized bone matrix (DBM) is formed by acid extration of bone, which leaves the noncollagenous proteins, bone growth factors, and collagen as a composite Grafton. It is available as a powder, granules, or in an injectable form, which may be spread across the graft bed. Although DBM provides no structural support, it does have osteoinductive and osteoconductive properties, and we employ it as a supplement to autogenous bone graft.

Composite grafts are defined as any combination of materials that have both an osteoconductive matrix and an osteoinductive material. Collagraft (Zimmer, Warsaw, Inc., Collagen Corporation, Palo Alto, California) is such a composite consisting of deantigenated bovine fibrillar collagen and porous calcium phosphate ceramic. When combined with autogenous bone and marrow, Collagraft is both osteoinductive and osteoconductive, but it does not provide structural support. We have noticed a tendency for it to flow and break when not handled delicately in a dry environment. In a study of posterolateral arthrodesis in New Zealand rabbits, composites consisting of BMP and either coral, DBM, autograft were compared. Bone protein fusions (using coral or DBM) were more homogenous and biomechanically stronger than those using autograft.[17,32] If similar results occur in human beings, this may represent a solution to the problem of nonunion and pseudarthrosis in management of spinal fractures.

COMPLICATIONS

Causes of delayed union and nonunion include infection, comminuted fractures, poor blood supply, pathologic fractures and soft-tissue interposition among others. Excluding type II odontoid fractures, vertebral fractures have a very low incidence of nonunion. Much of the vertebral fractures involve cancellous, which usually unites quite rapidly.[5] Failed fracture healing is caused by biologic and technical failures. Technical failures include infection, poor reduction-distraction, repeated motion, and loss of the local blood supply.[6] Evidence suggests that most biologic failures stem from problems caused by mitogens, differentiating and priming agents, growth factors, and other labile biochemical messengers and signals in the region of the fracture itself. Failures that are not biologic are technical failures and are secondary to fracture instability.[6]

Other systemic factors may retard bone healing. Corticosteroids compromise fracture healing by inhibiting differentiation of osteoblasts from mesenchymal cells and by decreasing the synthesis of bone organic matrix components necessary for repair.[5] Steroid administration also may decrease bone density and predisposes one to vertebral fractures. Diabetics have reduced osteoblastic and osteoclastic activity, cell proliferation, ground substance production, vascular ingrowth, and remodelling.[33] Open spinal fractures secondary to penetrating injuries have not shown a predisposition to nonunion as long as appropriate measures, including antibiotics and debridement, have been taken to prevent infection.[34] Restoration of fragment apposition and stabilization through external and or internal means supplemented with arthrodesis minimizes the incidence of nonunion.[5,30,35]

SUMMARY

1. Osseous healing of spinal fractures and spinal arthrodeses is comprised of inflammatory, reparative, and remodeling phases.
2. The success of fracture healing is dependent on the production of mediators from cells present in the

matrix. Through paracrine and autocrine effects, the mediators magnify the response and increase the rate of fracture repair.

3. The basic multicellular unit consisting of a blood supply, osteoclasts, and osteoblasts is the cornerstone of fracture remodelling.
4. Direct current electrical stimulation of bone results in low oxygen tension and high pH, which is a favorable environment for chondrogenesis and osteogenesis.
5. Bone grafts play a critical role in the stabilization and healing of spinal fractures. Autogenous grafts are osteoinductive and osteoconductive.
6. Alternatives to autogenous bone are available and have osteoinductive and/or osteoconductive properties.

REFERENCES

1. Boden SD, et al: The use of osteoinductive growth factor for lumbar spinal fusion, *Spine* 20:2626–2632, 1995.
2. Huluth A: Fracture healing—more biology than mechanics, *Clin Orthop* 156:259, 1981.
3. Huluth A: Current concepts of fracture healing, *Clin Orthop* 249:265, 1989.
4. Simmons DJ: Fracture healing perspectives, *Clin Orthop* 200:100, 1985.
5. Buckwalter JA, et al: Bone biology. II: Formation, form. Modelling, remodelling and regulation of cell function, *Instr Course Lect* 45:387–399, 1996.
6. Frost HM: The biology of fracture healing—an overview for clinicians. Part I, *Clin Orthop* 248:283, 1989.
7. Sandberg MM, Aro HT, Vurio EI: Gene expression during bone repair, *Clin Orthop* 289:292, 1993.
8. Brand RA, Rubin CT: Fracture healing. In Albright JH, Brand RA, editors: *The scientific basis of orthopaedics,* ed 2, Norwalk, Conn, 1987, Appleton and Lange.
9. Ross R, Raines EW, Bowen-Pope DF: The biology of platelet derived growth factor, *Cell* 46:115, 1986.
10. Guenther HL, Fleisch H, Sorgente N: Endothelial cells in culture synthesize—a potent bone cell active mitogen, *Endocrinology* 119:193, 1986.
11. Shenk RK: The biology of fracture repair. In *Skeletal trauma* vol. 1, Philadelphia, 1992, WB Saunders.
12. Mckibbin B: The biology of fracture healing in long bones, *J Bone Joint Surg* 60B:150, 1978.
13. Subburaman M, Baylink DJ: Bone growth factors, *Clin Orthop* 263:30, 1991.
14. West JL, Bradford DS, Olgilvie JW: Results of spinal arthrodesis with pedicle screw fixation, *J Bone Joint Surg* 73A:1179–1184, 1991.
15. Gamble JG: Structural components. In Brand JG, editor: *The musculoskeletal system, physiologic basics*, New York, 1988, Raven Press.
16. Urist MR, Delange RJ, Finerman GAM: Bone cell differentiation and growth factors, *Science* 220:680–686, 1983.
17. Boden SD, Schimandle JH, Hutton WC: Use of osteoconductive growth factor for lumbar spinal fusion, *Spine* 20:263–264, 1995.
18. Kirker-Head CA, et al: Longterm healing of bone using recombinant human bone morphogenic protein, *Clin Orthop* 318:222, 1995.
19. Shen V, et al: Fetal rat chondrocytes sequentially elaborate growth and differentiation promoting peptides during their development in vitro, *Endocrinology* 116:920, 1985.
20. Lavine LS, Grodzinsky AJ: Current concepts review—electrical stimulation of repair of bone, *J Bone Joint Surg* 69A:4, 1987.
21. Brighton CT, et al: A Multicenter study of treatment of nonunion with constant direct current, *J Bone Joint Surg* 63:2–13, 1981.
22. Brighton CT, Pollack SR: Treatment of recalicitrant nonunion with a capacatively coupled electric. A preliminary report, *J Bone Joint Surg* 67A:577–585, 1985.
23. Barker AT, et al: Pulsed magnetic field therapy for tibial nonunion. Interim results in a double-blind trial, *Lancet* 1:994–996, 1984.
24. Bassett CAL: The development and application of pulsed electromagnetic fields (PEMFs) for Ununited fractures and failed arthrodeses, *Orthop Clin* 15:61–87, 1984.
25. Tejano NA, Puno R, Ignacio JMF: The use of implantable direct current stimulation in multilevel spinal fusion without instrumentation. A prospective clinical and radiographic evaluation with longterm follow-up, *Spine* 21:1904–1908, 1996.
26. Kahanovitz N, Arnozcky SP: The efficacy of direct current electrical stimulation enhance canine spinal fusions, *Clin Orthop* 251:2, 1996.
27. Kane WS: Direct current electrical stimulation for spinal fusions, *Spine* 13:363–365, 1988.
28. Zdeblick TA: A Prospective randomized study of lumbar fusion, *Spine* 18:983–991, 1993.
29. Dekel S, Lenthall G, Francis MJO: Release of prostaglandins from bone and muscle after tibial fracture: an experimental study in rabbit, *J Bone Joint Surg* 63B:185, 1981.
30. O'Sullivan ME, Chao EYS, Kelly PJ: Current concepts review. The effects of fixation on fracture healing, *J Bone Joint Surg* 71A:306–310, 1989.
31. Gamble JG: Bone morphology and biology. In Gamble JG, editor: *The musculoskeletal system. Physiological basics*, New York, 1988, Raven Press.

32. Gazdag AR, et al: Alternatives to autogenous bone graft: efficacy and indications, *J Am Acad Orthop Surg* 3:1–8, 1995.
33. Loder RT: The influence of diabetes mellitus on the healing of closed fractures, *Clin Orthop* 232:210–216, 1988.
34. Kane T, et al: Spinal cord injury from civilian gunshot wounds: the rancho experience 1980–1988, *J Spinal Disord* 4(3):306–311, 1991.
35. Chao EYS, et al: The effect of rigidity on fracture healing in external fixation, *Clin Orthop* 241:24–35, 1989.

18

PSEUDARTHROSIS AS A COMPLICATION OF SPINAL FRACTURE

John M. Larsen

PSEUDARTHROSIS

DEFINITION

In the field of spinal surgery, the term *pseudarthrosis* refers to the failure of solid arthrodesis to occur following a surgical fusion attempt. It is defined as a false joint but is commonly understood to imply the lack of solid bony union. Generally, the diagnosis cannot be confirmed with certainty until a year after surgery, although the diagnosis may be suspected within 6 months of the index operation.

The first major work addressing pseudarthrosis was written by Cleveland and published in 1948.[1] He evaluated a large population of patients who had previously undergone posterior lumbar fusion surgery. Pseudarthrosis was diagnosed by the presence of pain, tenderness, lack of visible bony union on static radiographs, and visible vertebral motion on dynamic flexion and extension radiographs. It was noted that the incidence of pseudarthrosis increased dramatically as the number of vertebral levels treated increased. Cited causes for the development of pseudarthrosis included the use of too little bone and the use of cortical bone only.

Most notably, Cleveland identified pseudarthrosis in only 11% of patients when static radiographs alone were used. This figure climbed to 21% when dynamic flexion and extension radiographs included. Presently, the incidence of pseudarthrosis following the surgical treatment of spinal fractures varies widely. Similar to the experience of Cleveland, the reported incidence of pseudarthrosis varies significantly with the accuracy of the diagnostic methods used.

HISTOLOGY

Before considering the histology of pseudarthrosis, one must understand the process of fusion. Friedlaender has eloquently described the histology of bone graft incorporation.[2] Initially, a hematoma forms about the implanted bone, and the graft necroses stimulating an inflammatory response. Fibrocytes, blood vessels, and osteogenic precursor cells invade the graft resulting in the deposition of osteoid. As the fusion matures it is remodeled in accordance with Wolff's law.

The major contributions of the graft to the fusion process are termed *osteoconduction* and *osteoinduction*. Osteoconduction refers to the deposition of new bone on a framework supplied by the graft, while osteoinduction is the graft's ability to stimulate the host to invade the structure with osteogenic activity. Vascularized autograft has osteogenic action secondary to the transport of live bone cells and marrow.

When the graft is cortical bone, the invading vascular buds travel through existing haversian or Volkmann canals reducing the mass of the graft. Following resorption, new bone formation becomes more substantial and gradually returns the net bone mass, along with the mechanical strength, toward normal. Cancellous bone grafts, being more porous than cortical grafts, are revascularized more rapidly and may subsequently be incorporated to a greater degree. Any factor that interrupts this process places the patient at risk for pseudarthrosis. For example, inadequate vascularity of the adjacent soft tissues can limit the blood supply to the fusion mass and has been shown to hamper fusion.[3] Similarly, suboptimal decortication or immobilization of the motion segment results in greater rates of pseudarthrosis. Bone disease, malnutrition, certain pharmacologic agents, radiation treatment, and smoking are all positively associated with pseudarthrosis.

In 1993, Heggeness[4] reported histologic findings from biopsy material obtained from 35 patients undergoing pseudarthrosis repair. Biopsy material was obtained from the fusion mass, from areas of motion, and from the lumbar facet remnant. The soft tissue found between adjacent bony segments was predominantly fibrous. No tissue innervating the pseudarthrosis site was found. The bone immediately adjacent to the fibrous area was universally sclerotic. Microfractures of the cancellous bone overlying the opposed bone ends were present. These microfractures were believed to be possible sources of pain.

Further study is necessary to relate this data to the issues of pseudarthrosis causation and pain.

CLASSIFICATION

Heggeness in 1991 devised a classification of lumbar pseudarthrosis. Four distinct morphologic categories were described: atrophic, transverse, shingle, and complex. The transverse, shingle, and complex varieties were felt to be able to bear load, but the atrophic form appeared to have no load-bearing or load-sharing potential.

A striking association was noted between the atrophic pattern and the presence of a clearly recognizable facet joint. Haggeness reasoned that the intact facet joint provided significant stress shielding to the bone graft resulting in resorption according to Wolff's law. Similarly, implants may cause stress shielding. Of patients fused with internal fixation, 61% showed the atrophic pattern compared with only 38% of those patients fused without instrumentation.[5]

Logically, although unproved, it seems that patients with the atrophic form of pseudarthrosis should have more severe symptoms than those with the remaining three types, which are able to sustain loads. Further investigation should include correlation of the apparent load-bearing capacity and stability of the described pseudoarthritic morphologies with subjective pain complaints.

CLINICAL SIGNIFICANCE

The clinical significance of spinal pseudarthrosis has been debated for decades. While it is generally believed that pseudarthrosis can cause the chronic pain that patients sometimes experience following fusion surgeries, some do not believe this to be true. Surgeons who tend to discount the clinical significance of pseudarthrosis usually refer to the work of DePalma and Rothman.[6] In 1968, they selected a group of patients with radiographically proved lumbar pseudarthroses and compared them with a matched group whose lumbar fusion was radiographically solid. Each patient was evaluated for clinical course and subjective complaints. Little difference was found between the pseudarthrosis group and the solid fusion group regarding overall relief from symptomatology. They concluded that the presence of pseudarthrosis did not increase the morbidity of lumbar fusion nor compromise the long-term result of subjective relief from symptoms. It was hypothesized that pseudarthrosis represented a state of fibrous stabilization, which was essentially as effective as solid arthrodesis. Similar results have been reported by others.

There exists, however, a large body of work that supports the notion of pseudarthrosis being a condition that causes pain. Kim[7] retrospectively reviewed the results of the surgical treatment of 50 failed back surgery patients in 1989. He found that 81% of those patients who had successful repair of a pseudarthrosis achieved a satisfactory outcome while similar results occurred in only 23% of those whose pseudarthrosis repair was unsuccessful. Kim concluded that successful pseudarthrosis repair is the key to a high clinical success rate in revision surgery for failed back surgery syndrome.[7]

Turner[8] noted a significant positive relationship between solid arthrodesis and satisfactory outcomes in a literature review. Frymoyer[9] studied a group of 205 patients who had undergone fusion and required a second operation. He found that pseudarthrosis contributed to the need for reoperation in 78%.

The vast majority of literature, however, refers to the treatment of patients whose index operation was performed to treat a degenerative condition of the neck or low back. A large body of knowledge pertaining to the treatment of pseudarthrosis, which has arisen following the fusion of spinal fractures, does not exist. These two populations of patients are fundamentally different. Patients with degenerative spinal conditions requiring fusion surgery tend to be older, less active, and many times have issues other than spinal pathology contributing to the pain they experience. Examples of such issues include deconditioning, narcotic medication abuse, and medical-legal concerns. On the other hand, the spinal fracture population tends to be younger, more active, and healthier. The clinical presentation of this group of patients tend to be more straightforward. Although the chronic pain these patients sometimes experience following surgery may be complicated by other issues, it is not likely. I have found that the treatment of pseudarthrosis following fusion for spinal fractures likely leads to symptomatic relief.

To complicate this issue, there also exists a population of asymptomatic patients in whom pseudarthrosis is radiographically apparent. In this instance, it is possible that the stability provided by fibrous union, with or without, spinal fixation is sufficient to result in a good clinical outcome. In this second population, many asymptomatic patients develop symptoms if followed over long periods of time. Most surgeons have encountered patients who have persistent and severe pain despite unequivocal evidence of solid lumbar arthrodesis. In this population, physiologic sources of pain that are encountered most frequently include incomplete surgical decompression, adjacent injured disks, which were not addressed at surgery, and high profile or incorrectly applied internal fixation. Correction of these problems may require surgery.

If physiologic sources of pain are not identified, nonphysiologic sources of pain are treated. These can include narcotic dependence and psychosocial difficulties. Muscular deconditioning, if present, is treated with an appropriate strengthening regime.

Causation

Pseudarthrosis has a variety of causes. The rate of pseudarthrosis increases with the number of levels included in the fusion.[1] Pseudarthrosis occurs more often in revision fusion attempts than in primary surgery.

The condition of the host affects the fusion process. Advanced age, poor nutrition, and obesity have all been associated with an increase in the incidence of pseudarthrosis. Hematologic disorders may decrease the osteogenic potential of bone marrow and limit the fusion process. Raney and Kolb[10] have suggested that metabolic bone disease plays a significant role in pseudarthrosis. They found 35 patients with metabolic problems that might affect bone metabolism in a series of 66 patients with pseudarthrosis. They included excess use of alcohol or tobacco as metabolic abnormalities. Forty-seven of the 66 pseudarthroses healed after correction of the metabolic abnormality. In contrast, Schofferman[11] studied 47 patients with pseudarthrosis to evaluate the contribution of abnormalities in bone or mineral metabolism as a cause of pseudarthrosis. Based on his data, metabolic disorders were believed to play a role in a small percentage of patients, but most pseudarthroses were not believed to be due to metabolic factors.

The use of nonsteroidal antiinflammatory medication has been demonstrated to hamper fusion. Chemotherapeutic agents and the use of radiation in the treatment of malignancies adversely affects fusion formation. Emery demonstrated an increased risk of pseudarthrosis in thoracolumbar anterior interbody fusion patients when the postoperative irradiation delivered exceeded 4000 cg.[12]

Smoking has been implicated in pseudarthrosis as it interferes with bone metabolism, revascularization, and inhibits bone formation. Brown[13] studied a group of 100 patients who had undergone two level lumbar fusion. Equal numbers of smokers and nonsmokers were included. Pseudarthrosis was present in 40% of smokers, whereas only 8% of the nonsmokers developed pseudarthrosis.

Rogozinski[14] studied a group of 139 patients who had undergone fusion surgery and classified them as nonsmokers, preoperative smokers, and postoperative smokers. The nonsmokers and preoperative smokers achieved solid arthrodesis at a roughly equivalent rate around 85%. The postoperative smokers solidly fused at a rate less than 60%. Although smoking should cease prior to each and every fusion procedure, this is not always possible, especially in spinal fracture surgery. This information indicates that cessation of smoking following surgery may be effective in preventing pseudarthrosis.

The choice of graft material can influence the fusion rate. One of the best studies addressing this issue was reported by An in 1995.[15] Patients undergoing lumbar fusion with internal fixation had autograft placed on one side and either freeze-dried grafts or frozen allografts or a mixture of the two were used on the contralateral side. This study showed that autografts were clearly superior in producing solid bony arthrodesis. In another study reported during the same year, An[16] demonstrated that anterior cervical fusion with autograft was superior to freeze-dried allograft. These observations have been confirmed by others.

Cleveland et al.[1] described a relationship between pseudarthrosis and the primary lesion for which the fusion was performed. Patients in whom fusion was included in the treatment of disk herniations developed pseudarthrosis 11% of the time whereas 29% of those treated for arthritis experienced this complication. Those being treated for other conditions demonstrated pseudarthrosis at a rate intermediate to these two extremes. There are mechanical factors that influence fusion formation. Maximization of the surface area of the fusion leads to more consistent fusion formation.

Fusion is more likely to occur if the adjacent bones are stabilized rigidly. External braces or internal fixation accompany fusion surgery for this reason. Although the optimal modulus of elasticity for fusion is unknown, recent advances in lumbar internal fixation have resulted in increased stiffness of the constructs.

Zdeblick in 1993 published the results of a study comparing the fusion rate of patients fused without internal fixation, with semirigid pedicle screw fixation systems, and with rigid pedicle screw fixation systems.[11] The use of pedicle screw fixation led to a significantly higher rate of radiographic fusion than did surgery without internal fixation. The fusion rate also was higher with rigid pedicle screw systems compared with semirigid fixation.

Some believe that fusion is more likely if the graft is subject to compressive rather than tensile forces. It is thought that a bone graft placed in an area of tension is resorbed in accordance with Wolff's Is law. Close examination of Wolff's Is law does not support this notion. Wolff's law states that bone is laid down where stresses require its presence and bone is resorbed where stresses do not require it. It neither states nor implies that bone is built up when it is loaded in compression and adsorbed when it is loaded in tension. Bone is remodeled to accommodate tensile as well as compressive stresses.

Diagnosis

The late diagnosis of pseudarthrosis is rarely problematic. Patients complain of pain and demonstrate radiographic findings of hardware failure, loss of correction, or abnormal motion on dynamic radiographs. Steinmann found the criteria most useful in establishing the diagnosis of pseudarthrosis to include:

1. lack of trabecular bone continuity from one end of the fusion to the other
2. collapse of the graft height with a gap present between the vertebral end plate and the bone graft
3. shift in the position of the graft after expected healing was to have occurred
4. loss of fixation through dislodgment or fracture of the rods, screws, or hooks after expected healing was to have occurred
5. unexplained pain occurring in the area of the fusion

The early determination of pseudarthrosis is most difficult. The subjective complaints of patients with early pseudarthrosis vary from a complete absence of pain to constant, severe spinal or extremity pain. Treatment should be considered only when the subjective complaints are of sufficient intensity to warrant further surgery.

Physical findings generally include paraspinal tenderness and a restriction in the range of motion. Objective neurologic deficits may be observed in the presence of persistent neurologic compression or instability. Likewise, nerve tension signs may be positive.

The most accurate method of assessing the fusion mass is direct surgical exploration. It is not practical to operate on every patient in whom pseudarthrosis is suspected and thus, historically, radiographic findings have been the keystone in the preoperative assessment of pseudarthrosis.

Consistent radiographic demonstration of lumbar pseudarthrosis is most difficult. Reports in the literature have included the use of plain radiography; flexion and extension radiography; biplanar radiography; stereophotogrammetry; tomography; diskography; computed tomography (CT) using axial cuts, two dimensional reformations, and coronal techniques; bone scintigraphy; and magnetic resonance scanning (MRI).[18-24] Unfortunately, the results of radiographic assessment have been compared with those of direct surgical inspection only rarely. The best clinical information is gleaned from studies in which radiographic data has been confirmed by surgical investigation and the results of these will be briefly reviewed.

Plain radiographs were used to assess the competency of the fusion mass by Kant.[20] The radiographic findings for each of the 75 patients were compared with surgical results. A 68% correlation was noted.

Dawson retrospectively studied 198 patients who had undergone posterior fusion for scoliosis and were suspected to have a pseudarthrosis. The results of preoperative radiographs and tomograms were compared to the status of the fusion mass found at surgery. Standard radiographs and lateral tomograms were found to be uninterpretable 21% and 60% of the time, respectively. Anteroposterior tomograms, however, were interpretable in all but one patient and correlated with the surgical finding in 96% of patients.

The use of bone scintigraphy employing technetium (Tc) is based on the postulation that reactive bone should be present adjacent to the site of pseudarthrosis. Two investigations have compared the results of bone scintigraphy with those of surgical exploration. In a study of 11 patients, Hannon and Wetta[22] concluded that bone scintigraphy did not readily predict pseudarthrosis. McMaster and Merrick[23] performed routine bone scans following fusion in 110 patients. Their prediction of fusion included a 50% false-positive rate compared with surgical results. They noted that scans performed after 1 year seemed more accurate than those performed 6 months postoperatively.

Diskography has been used to investigate the presence of pseudarthrosis. Johnson correlated diskographic and surgical findings in a group of 24 patients in whom pseudarthrosis was suspected.[24] He concluded that the decision to perform revision surgery should not be made on the results of diskography alone.

Larsen studied a group of 25 patients who had previously undergone lumbar fusion using pedicle screw fixation and were suspected to have a pseudarthrosis.[19] Preoperative radiographs included plain films, dynamic lateral films, CT scanning, and bone scintigraphy. Each patient then underwent surgical exploration. The radiographic studies, when evaluated individually or collectively, failed to predict the surgical finding. It was concluded that in the presence of pedicle screw instrumentation, surgical exploration was the best diagnostic technique.

In summary, Dawson's 96% correlation of anteroposterior tomography with surgery is the sole demonstration of acceptable accuracy of a preoperative radiographic technique to predict the surgical assessment of the fusion mass.[21]

The surgical diagnosis of pseudarthrosis is technically demanding. The fusion must be meticulously dissected free of soft tissue. In posterolateral fusion masses, one must view the facet joint remnants. If the fusion is anterior, the vertebral bodies on either side of the graft must be clearly visualized. Internal fixation must be disconnected or removed. The fusion mass must be carefully inspected. Dynamic stress testing is accomplished by distracting the vertebrae on either side of the fusion. Cobb elevators can be used to depress various aspects of the fusion. Many times it is necessary to enter the spinal canal and use a curved curette placed in the lateral recess or foramen to dorsally stress the fusion mass. Any motion documented between vertebrae included in the previous fusion attempt signifies pseudarthrosis.

INCIDENCE

The incidence of pseudarthrosis following surgical fusion of spinal fractures varies substantially with the various fracture patterns encountered and surgical techniques employed. The reported incidence also varies considerably with the accuracy of the method used to detect it. In general, pseudarthrosis complicates the treatment of spinal fractures rarely. Fusion procedures for spinal fractures result in solid arthrodesis more often than similar procedures used to treat spinal deformity or degenerative disk conditions. With regard to spinal fractures, a well-conceived operation performed in a competent manner usually leads to solid arthrodesis.

Large series of cervical fractures and dislocations have been documented with good results following surgical fusion. Verbiest in 1969 and Bohlman in 1979 reported on large groups of patients operatively treated for fractures and dislocations of the cervical spine without a single failure of fusion.[25,26] Rogers reported on the surgical treatment of 39 unstable cervical fractures.[27] Spinous process wiring and posterior fusion was successful in all but two patients who had a failure of fusion.

In contrast, Stauffer noted persistent instability in all of the 16 patients suffering from cervical fracture-dislocations treated with primary anterior interbody fusion.[28] Each of these patients had disruption of the posterior ligaments. Stauffer conclude that this technique should not be performed alone in the face of posterior ligamentous disruption. Similarly, the incidence of pseudarthrosis following fusion of thoracolumbar fractures has been described by a variety of authors. The literature reflects vast experience treating unstable thoracic and lumbar injuries with internal fixation using rods with or without sleeves along with posterolateral fusion. Flesch in 1977 reported only one failure of fusion complicating the treatment of 40 patients undergoing Harrington instrumentation and fusion for unstable fractures of the thoracic and lumbar spine.[29] Yosipovitch in the same year noted solid fusion in 15 of 16 patients.[30] Dickson[31] found four patients with pseudarthrosis in his series of 95. Gertzbein[32] described 34 patients to achieve solid fusion out of 36 treated operatively with posterolateral fusion and rod fixation.

Edwards, in a series of 200 injuries treated with rods, found nonunions in only 2% of thoracic and upper lumbar injuries.[33] Each of the upper lumbar nonunions resulted from the surgeon's failure to extend the graft to the transverse or mammary processes, which are located well above the upper hooks. A much higher nonunion rate of 8% was found at the lumbosacral junction. After an extensive review of the literature, Edwards estimated that pseudarthrosis is reported in 4% of spinal injury patients with posterior fixation.

TREATMENT

When encountering a patient with pain and significant functional impairment, who has undergone prior fusion of a spinal fracture, a careful and thorough diagnostic evaluation must be undertaken. Only after the cause of a patient's persistent symptoms has been established unequivocally can there be any hope of successful treatment.

First, the rationale and technical details of the prior surgery should be carefully reviewed. Incomplete neurologic decompression with persistent radiculopathy or stenosis and technical difficulties with internal fixation are examples of possibly remediable postoperative pain. Obviously, a successful revision surgery must include correction of these problems.

Second, it is possible that pathology has arisen since the last surgery and is responsible for the patient's present symptoms. Recurrent disk herniation or instability or stenosis adjacent to a fusion mass are examples of these problems. Radiographic investigation of reasonable possibilities is appropriate. Third, nonsurgically treatable sources of pain such as deconditioning, medication abuse, or psychosocial problems should be evaluated carefully. If any of these problems are present, it is unlikely that further surgery will improve the patient's condition.

Finally, the possibility of pseudarthrosis must be considered. Many times this diagnosis is difficult to appreciate radiographically. In practice, the best method is the use of plain radiographs, motion radiographs, and anteroposterior tomography. Then, in an appropriately symptomatic patient in whom other reasonable causes of pain have been excluded, it is preferable to explore the fusion mass and, if nonunion is found, attempt to promote solid bony union. Again, it must be emphasized that successful pseudarthrosis repair leads to a successful surgical result only if the rational for the original surgery was sound and if other pathology reasonably responsible for the patient's pain is appropriately treated. Also, it must be candidly explained to the patient that the expectations of revision surgery do not match those of primary procedures. Revision surgery is associated with greater rates of complication and less favorable outcomes.

Additionally, prior to surgery, it is necessary to define and treat any systemic factors that could lead to the failure of fusion. The nutrition of the patient should be adequate and metabolic abnormalities should be corrected. Smoking should cease. The patient should not be exposed to nonsteroid antiinflammatory drugs (NSAIDS), steroids, chemotherapeutic drugs, or therapeutic radiation.

Nonsurgical options such as bracing and external electrical stimulation can be used in an attempt to treat nonunion. These methods are best used as adjuncts to surgical treatment and should not be relied upon alone.

The treatment of pseudarthrosis varies with the variety of clinical situations in which it is encountered. Failure of a primary posterior cervical fusion to heal solidly is a rare occurrence. Capen encountered two such patients in a series of 144 surgeries.[34] Both of these were treated with revision posterior wiring and bone grafting. Solid arthrodesis resulted in each instance. In such cases, while anterior interbody fusion with or without plating is an option, the author recommends that the initial revision procedure be posterior with fixation and grafting.

Anterior interbody fusion is rarely used alone to treat unstable cervical fractures. Should such a situation be encountered, the revision procedure should be performed posteriorly. Internal fixation should accompany revision grafting. Excellent results have been demonstrated by Farey[35] using triple wiring and by Lowery[36] using articular pillar plating.

When a patient has nonunion of a posterolateral thoracic or lumbar fusion without fixation, I prefer rigid internal fixation across the pseudarthrosis and regrafts the area. If at all possible, I use an autologous bone graft. In general, when performing revision surgery, bone graft substitutes are used only after the autologous donor sites have been exhausted.

When posterior fixation is in place, I strive to determine if the instrumentation is providing rigid fixation across the pseudoarthritic gap. Loose or broken fixation is revised and the area is regrafted. A less attractive option involves removal of the fixation and regrafting the nonunion site. This is combined with internal or external electrical stimulation and bracing.

Should a second posterior procedure fail to result in solid bony union, the author recommends anterior lumbar interbody fusion. In the rare case in which the posterior fixation is found to be functionally intact, I usually prefer to regraft the posterolateral area and then proceed directly to anterior lumbar interbody fusion.

When a failed anterior fusion is encountered, every effort is made to remedy the situation posteriorly. Rigid posterior segmental fixation is required along with primary or revision grafting in the posterolateral gutter. Although revision using anterior fixation and regrafting is an option, the potential complications that can be encountered make this a last resort.

SUMMARY

Prevention of pseudarthrosis is the most successful treatment. This begins with appropriate patient selection and presurgical reduction of risk factors. It extends to a well-planned procedure in which equal attention is given to bone-grafting technique and safe application of internal fixation. It ends with well-managed postoperative rehabilitation. This remains the key to cost control and successful outcomes.

REFERENCES

1. Cleveland M, Bosworth DM, Thompson F: Pseudarthrosis in the lumbosacral spine, *J Bone Joint Surg* 30A:302–312, 1948.
2. Friedlaender GE: Bone grafts, the basic science rationale for clinical applications, *J Bone Joint Surg* 69A:786–790, 1987.
3. Boden SD, Summer DR: Biologic factors affecting spinal fusion and bone regeneration, *Spine* 20:102S–112S, 1995.
4. Heggeness MH, Esses SI, Mody DR: A histologic study of lumbar pseudarthrosis, *Spine* 18:1016–1020, 1993.
5. Heggeness MH, Esses SI: Classification of pseudarthroses of the lumbar spine, *Spine* 16:S449–454, 1991.
6. DePalma AF, Rothman RH: The nature of pseudarthrosis, *Clin Orthop* 59:113–118, 1968.
7. Kim SS, Michelsen CB: Revision surgery for failed back surgery syndrome, *Spine* 17:957–960, 1992.
8. Turner JA, et al: Patient outcomes after lumbar spinal fusions, *JAMA* 268:907–911, 1992.
9. Frymoyer JW, et al: Failed lumbar disc surgery requiring a second operation, *Spine* 3:7–12, 1978.
10. Raney FL, Kolb DO: The effect of metabolic bone diseased on spinal fusion. In White AH, Rothman R, Ray CD, editors: *Lumbar spine surgery techniques and complications*, St. Louis, 1987, Mosby–Year Book.
11. Schofferman J, et al: Metabolic bone disease in lumbar pseudarthrosis, *Spine* 15(7):687–689, 1990.
12. Emery SN, et al: The fate of anterior vertebral grafts in patients irradiated for neoplasm, *Clin Orthop* 300:207–212, 1994.
13. Brown WC, Orme TJ, Richardson HD: The rate of pseudarthrosis (surgical nonunion) in patients who are smokers and patients who are nonsmokers: a comparison study, *Spine* 11:942–943, 1986.
14. Rogozinski C, Rogozinski A, Weiss H: Effect of cigarette smoking on instrumented lumbosacral fusion. Presented at the AAOS 1996 Annual Meeting, Orlando, FL, JBJS Feb. 24, 1996.
15. An HS, et al: Comparison between allograft plus demineralized bone matrix versus autograft in anterior cervical fusion, *Spine* 20(20):2211–2216, 1995.
16. Foley MJ, et al: Radiologic evaluation of surgical cervical spine fusion, *AJR* 138:79–89, 1982.

16. An HS, Lynch K, Toth J: Prospective comparion of autograft vs. allograft for adult posterolateral lumbar spine fusion: differences among freeze-dried, frozen, and mixed grafts, *J Spinal Disord* 8(2):131–135, 1995.
17. Zdeblick TA: A prospective, randomized study of lumbar fusion. Preliminary results, *Spine* 18:983–991, 1993.
18. Steinmann JC, Herkowitz HN: Pseudarthrosis of the spine, *Clin Orthop* 284:80–90, 1992.
19. Larsen JM, et al: Assessment of pseudarthrosis in pedicle screw fusion, *J Spinal Disord* 5:153–166, 1997.
20. Kant AP, et al: Evaluation of lumbar spine fusion. Plain radiographs versus direct surgical exploration and observation, *Spine* 20:2313–2317, 1995.
21. Dawson EG, Clader TJ, Bassett LW: A comparison of different methods used to diagnose following posterior spinal fusion for scoliosis, *J Bone Joint Surg* 67A:1153–1159, 1985.
22. Hannon KM, Wetta WJ: Failure of technetium bone scanning to detect pseudarthrosis in spinal fusion for scoliosis, *Clin Orthop* 123:42–44, 1977.
23. McMaster MJ, Merrick MV: The scintigraphic assessment of the scoliotic spine after fusion, *J Bone Joint Surg* 62A:6572, 1980.
24. Johnson RG, Macnab I: Localization of symptomatic lumbar pseudarthroses by use of discography, *Clin Orthop* 197:164–170, 1985.
25. Verbeist H: Anterolateral operations for fractures and dislocations in the middle and lower parts of the cervical spine, *J Bone Joint Surg* 51A(8):1489–1530, 1969.
26. Bohlman HH: Acute fractures and dislocations of the cervical spine, *J Bone Joint Surg* 61A(S):1119–1142, 1979.
27. Rogers WA: Fractures and dislocations of the cervical spine, *J Bone Joint Surg* 39A(2):341–376, 1957.
28. Stauffer ES, Kelly EG: Fracture-dislocations of the cervical spine, *J Bone Joint Surg* 59A(1):45–48, 1977.
29. Flesch JR, et al: Harrington instrumentation and spine fusion for unstable fracturedislocations of the thoracic and lumbar spine, *J Bone Joint Surg* 59A:143–153, 1977.
30. Yosipovitch Z, Robin GC, Makin M: Open reduction of unstable thoracolumbar spinal injuries and fixation with Harrington rods, *J Bone Joint Surg* 59A:1003–1015, 1977.
31. Dickson JH, Harrington PR, Erwin WD: Results of reduction and stabilization of the severely fractured thoracic and lumbar spine, *J Bone Joint Surg* 60A:799–805, 1978.
32. Gertzbein SD, Macmichael D, Tile M: Harrington instrumentation as a method of fixation in fractures of the spine, *J Bone Joint Surg* 64B:526–529, 1982.
33. Edwards CC, Levine AM: Complications associated with poster instrumentation in the treatment of thoracic and lumbar injuries. In Garfin SR, editor: *Complications of spine surgery*, Baltimore, 1989, Williams & Wilkins.
34. Capen DA, Garland DE, Waters RL: Stabilization of the cervical spine, a comparison of anterior and posterior fusion, *Clin Ortho* 196:229–237, 1985.
35. Farey ID, et al: Pseudarthrosis of the cervical spine after anterior arthrodesis, *J Bone Joint Surg* 72A:1171–1177, 1990.
36. Lowery GL, Swank ML, McDonough RF: surgical revision for failed anterior cervical fusions, Articular pillar plating or anterior revision? *Spine* 20:2436–2441, 1995.

19

PENETRATING SPINAL TRAUMA

Christopher O. Neubuerger
Gregory M. Yoshida

PENETRATING SPINAL INJURIES

EPIDEMIOLOGY

The incidence of penetrating injuries to the spine in the civilian population has been increasing steadily, especially in urban areas. The rate of low-velocity gunshot wounds has increased as the rate of stab wounds has decreased.[1] With few exceptions, these gunshot wounds result in spinal cord injury (SCI).[2,3] Between 1973 and 1981, 6,014 cases of SCI were reported to the National Spinal Cord Injury Data Research Center by the various regional SCI systems. Of these, 782 (13%) were the result of gunshots and 41 (0.7%) were the results of stab wounds.[4] In this series, gunshot wounds were the third leading cause of SCI after motor vehicle accidents (38%) and falls (16%). Since 1991, violence has become the second leading cause of SCI (30%), surpassing falls (20%). Here again, the increase in gunshot injuries are responsible; stab wounds have decreased slightly.[5] In Los Angeles County, an average of 48.3% of individuals receiving rehabilitation for SCI were gunshot victims.[6] In a prospective study of 148 patients with SCI from penetrating injuries admitted for rehabilitation in Los Angeles, 94% were men with an average age of 25 years.[7] The ethnic distribution was 47% black, 45% hispanic, 4% white, and 4% other. Of the 148 patients, 135 were the result of bullet injuries, 12 were due to stab injuries, and one involved abdominal penetration by a beam.

With the exception of South Africa, reports of stab wounds that result in SCI are rare. In 1977, Peacock[8] reported from South Africa that his series of 450 stab-wound patients comprised 25% of all SCI seen at his institution. In the Lipschitz series of 314 patients, only 6 were female; 90% occurred between the ages of 15 and 50.[9] A recent study from South Africa by Velmahos and coworkers[1] from 1988 to 1992 reported that SCI was caused by gunshot wounds in 35% (193) and stab wounds in 26% (143) of patients. In developed countries where guns are readily accessible, SCI caused by stabbing is relatively infrequent. In the period from 1980 to 1993, 1,763 individuals with SCI began and completed rehabilitation in the Regional Spinal Cord Injury Care System of Southern California. Intentional violence accounted for 810 cases (42.8%): gunshot wounds accounted for 760 cases (40.2%) and stab wounds 50 cases (2.6% overall or 6.2% of those due to violence).[10] Similarly, the National Spinal Cord Injury Statistical Center reports that only 1.1% of the 16,024 cases on file were caused by penetrating injuries other than gunshot wounds.[11]

INJURY CHARACTERISTICS

In stab wounds to the spinal cord, the instrument must directly cause intrinsic cord damage or vascular insult. A bullet or fragment does not have to contact the spinal cord to cause injury; damage may result from the concussive effects of the bullet.[12] Nevertheless, a bullet fragment completely traverses or remains inside the spinal canal in the majority of cases (Fig. 19-1). In a series of 245 patients admitted to Rancho Los Amigos Medical Center with SCI caused by gunshot wounds, 96 patients (37%) had large bullet fragments lodged within the spinal canal.[13]

WOUND BALLISTICS

The damage created by a bullet depends on the kinetic energy of the projectile.[12,14,15] Kinetic energy can be calculated by the formula $KE = 1/2\ MV^2$, where M equals mass of the projectile and V equals velocity. Increasing the bullet velocity, therefore, results in greater energy and greater wounding capacity than a similar proportional increase in the bullet mass. In addition, because a lighter bullet can be accelerated to a higher velocity by a given charge, high-velocity bullets are of a smaller caliber.

When a bullet hits the soft tissue of the body it becomes unstable. The angle of yaw may become so great that it tumbles and may be halted releasing all of its energy. A bullet that remains stable in the body may not be halted and in this case loses only 10% to

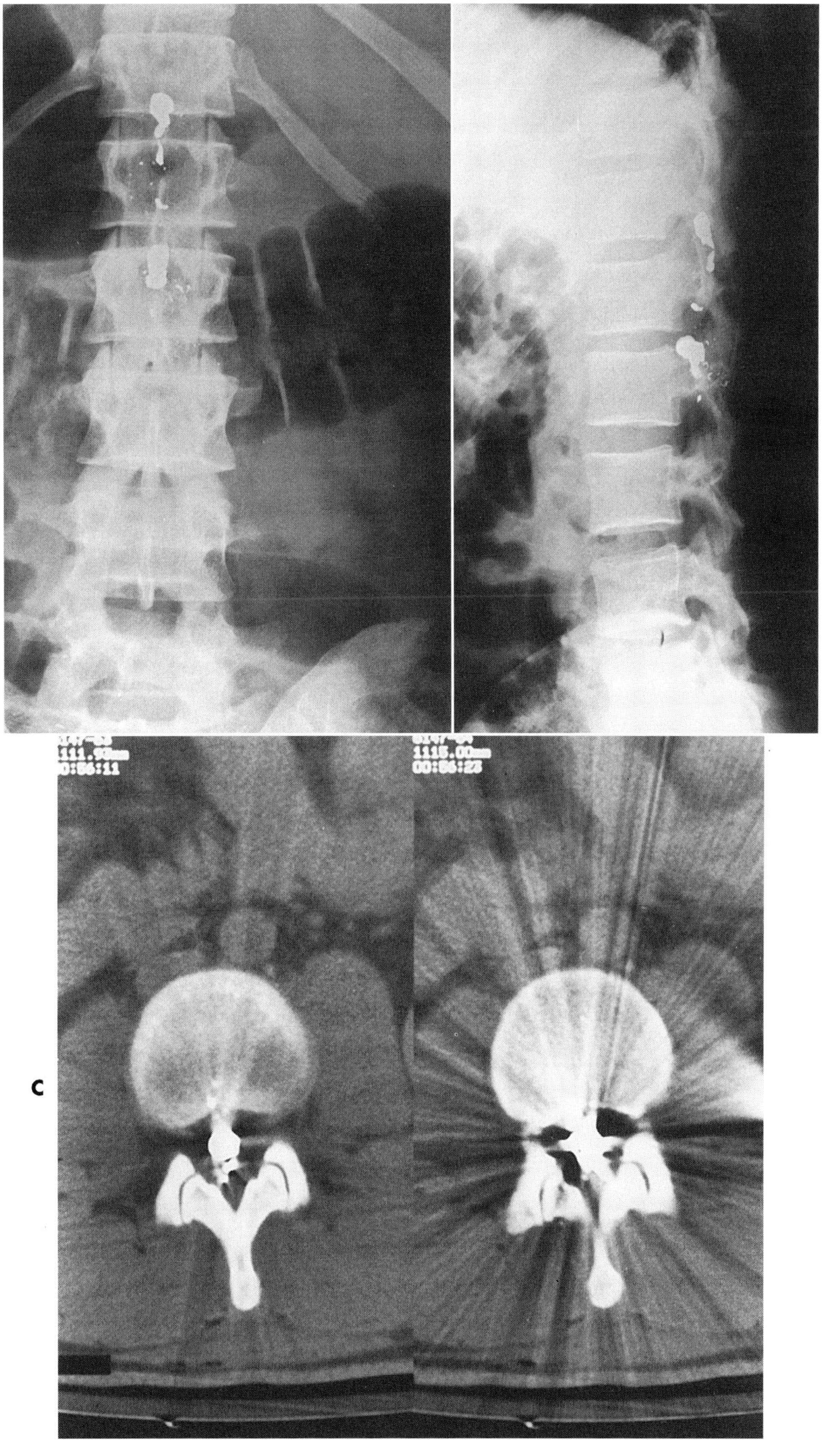

A B C

FIGURE 19-1

A and **B,** AP and lateral radiographs, **C,** CT scan revealing major bullet fragments retained in the spinal canal.

20% of its energy during penetration.[16] A low-velocity missile causes injury either by direct laceration and crushing of tissues in its path or by generating shock waves, which cause damage some distance from the wound track. Only high-velocity objects create temporary cavitation. High-velocity missiles release energy to the local tissues, which are violently accelerated forward and outward as secondary missiles. A large cavity at subatmospheric pressure and up to 40 times the diameter of the missile is created. Debris is sucked into the wound through entry and exit sites, leaving a large mass of grossly contaminated tissue. Bone may be fractured without actual contact being made. Blood vessels far from the direct path of the bullet may become thrombosed. Nerves may be overstretched.[16]

Most civilian gunshot wounds are from low-velocity weapons with muzzle speeds less than 1,000 ft/sec; high-velocity injuries to the spine usually result in death. In a prospective study from Rancho Los Amigos Medical Center, the most common type of gunshot injury was from medium-caliber bullets (.32–.38, including 9mm) followed by large caliber (.45) bullets.[17] The bullet size appeared to be related to the severity of neurologic injury; complete SCI occurred with 61% large, 55.2% medium, and 47.1% small bullets. In this study, more than twice as many patients (40%) were shot in the back as were shot in the front (19%). In addition, twice as may patients had left-sided entry wounds (27%) compared with right-sided entry wounds (14%). In 30% of cases, the bullet entered the spinal canal (see Fig. 19-1); 40% enter and pass through the canal, and another 30% do not enter the spinal canal. The locations of spinal injuries were cervical (20%), thoracic (50%), and thoracolumbar (30%).[17] Cervical injuries are becoming more common as intensive care has improved the tetraplegic's chance for survival. Several decades earlier these same patients would have died shortly after injury.[16]

STAB WOUNDS

Stab wounds of the spinal cord may be inflicted by knives, axes, ice picks, screwdrivers, bicycle spokes, or glass fragments.[18,19,20] Knives accounted for 84.2% in the Peacock series.[8] In the majority of cases (65.1%), the stab wound is single and part of a haphazard assault (Fig. 19-2 A and B).[8] In many cases, the victim does not know what weapon was used as he or she is surprised from the rear. Commonly, in thoracic stab injuries, the patient was bending over resulting in spreading of the lamina. In the thoracic spine, the stab wound is often in an upward direction or is deflected up by the lamina.[21]

The anatomy of the vertebral column is such that the blade tends to enter the gutter formed by the spinous process in the midline and transverse process laterally. The blade tends not to cross midline because lateral deviation is prevented by the backward projection of the transverse process.[8] Occasionally, the implement enters through an intervertebral foramen. In the cervical and lumbar regions, the stab is often horizontal or slightly downward.[21] In certain instances the lamina may be penetrated or fractured if the implement is sharp enough or if enough force is used (Fig. 19-2 C).[21] The site of skin entry often bears no clear relationship to the level of injury to the cord.

In stabbings, the cord may be injured either directly by the weapon or indriven bone fragments, through vascular damage, or through contrecoup concussion caused by the blade carrying the cord forward and traumatizing it against the walls of the bony canal.[19]

Lipschitz found the majority of spinal injuries from stab wounds were in the thoracic spine (74%), followed by the cervical spine (18%), and the lumbar spine (8%).[21] Peacock reported 63% of the stab wounds occurred in the thoracic spine, 30% in the cervical spine, and 7% in the lumbar spine.[8]

PATIENT EVALUATION

A patient with a gunshot wound or stab wound to the spine should undergo a standard trauma evaluation. Penetrating injuries to the anterior or anterolateral neck should be carefully evaluated for carotid injury and tracheal or esophogeal perforation. Tracheal, pharyngeal and esophogeal perforations have a high incidence of infection and subsequent streptococal osteomyelitis and should be thoroughly debrided with concomitant mucosal perforation repair.[21–27] In cervical stab injuries the brachial plexus is vulnerable.[21] Cardiac and pulmonary injuries may have grave consequences and are always a concern for the patient with penetrative thoracic spinal trauma; in one series of gunshot wounds, hemothorax occured in 35% of the patients.[28] In stab wound injuries between 5% and 15% had associated pneumothorax and/or hemothorax.[8,21] In the lumbar spine the abdominal viscera, kidney, descending aorta, and inferior vena cava can all be damaged by the bullet or blade, especially if the entry wound is anterior.[29,30,31] The diagnosis of intraabdominal injury is usually difficult as the patient does not complain of pain, and abdominal muscular rigidity may be absent. The diagnosis initially depends on shifting dullness, shock, gas under the diaphragm, diagnostic peritoneal lavage, and/or computed tomography (CT) scanning.[8]

In Lipschitz's series of 314 stab wounds of the spinal cord, there were two cases of osteomyelitis, two cases of chronic epidural granuloma, four cases of meningitis and nine cases of chronic cerebrospinal fluid leakage.[9,19,21] In this same series, 86 patients (34%) had associated extraspinal injuries.

A thorough neurologic examination should be performed and documented as soon as possible using

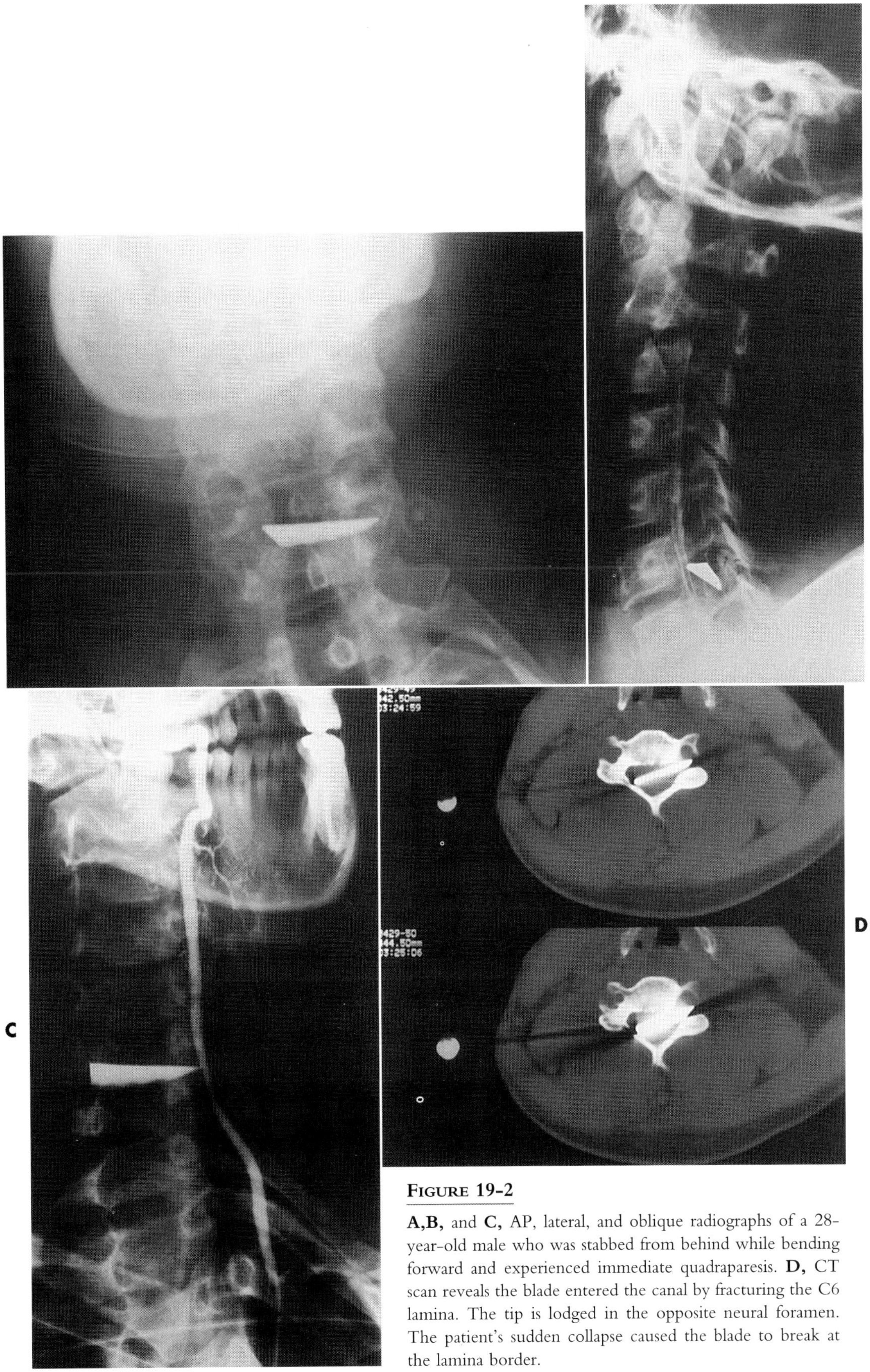

A B C D

FIGURE 19-2

A,B, and **C,** AP, lateral, and oblique radiographs of a 28-year-old male who was stabbed from behind while bending forward and experienced immediate quadraparesis. **D,** CT scan reveals the blade entered the canal by fracturing the C6 lamina. The tip is lodged in the opposite neural foramen. The patient's sudden collapse caused the blade to break at the lamina border.

the motor and sensory scales recommended by the American Spinal Injury Association.[32] If a neurologic deficit is found, intravenous steroid administration may be initiated within 8 hours. The current recommended dosing strategy for SCI is an initial bolus of 30 mg/kg of methylprednisone, followed by a continuous infusion of 5.4 mg/kg/hr for 23 hours.[33]

The role of steroids in penetrating cord injury is currently unclear. The National Acute Spinal Cord Injury Study II excluded all patients with penetrating injuries. A study by Prendergast and coworkers[34] found no benefit in administering methylprednisone in penetrating spinal injury patients and a potential harm of impaired host resistance to infection. Simpson and coworkers[35] also found no benefit to steroid administration in penetrating injuries; the 66 patients who received steroids accrued no neurologic benefit over the 94 patients who did not receive steroid administration. This study included 18 stab wound injuries. We recommend caution in selecting methylprednisone for gunshots or stab wounds until clear scientific benefit has been established.

Radiographic evaluation should begin with biplanar radiographs of the wound region to locate the spinal segments involved. In 2% of stabbing injuries the knife tip breaks off.[21] A fine-cut CT of the injured segment should then be obtained to determine the extent of bony destruction and the presence of bone, blade, or bullet in the canal.[36] These two studies usually provide all the information necessary to evaluate the spinal column after a gunshot or stab wound.

Spine Stability

Most gunshot wounds to the spine are stable, although little has been published to uphold this commonly held belief.[16,23,37] Meyer and coworkers[38] reported that of 1,300 spinal gunshot wounds, none demonstrated spinal instability. Gunshot wounds in children may be more likely to produce instability because of a greater amount of bony and soft tissue destruction.[23] Additionally, a greater number of gunshot wounds in children produce complete injuries; paralytic scoliosis below the lesion develops in nearly all patients as it does in other causes of paralysis and the immature skeleton.[39–44]

We have observed cases of both acute and chronic spinal instability after gunshot wounds to the lumbar spine.[45] In all cases, the bullet passed transversely fracturing both pedicles or facets. One patient underwent immediate posterior instrumentation and fusion for acute spinal instability. Another patient originally believed to have a stable injury complained of back pain and radicular symptoms 6 months after injury. Flexion and extension radiographs demonstrated spinal instability; fusion with instrumentation was necessary. We have not observed any instance of spinal instability if one pedicle and facet remained intact. This was proven biomechanically in a nonpenetrating injury setting by Raynor and coworkers[46] who demonstrated that if more than 50% of the facet joints remained intact at one cervical level, that level remained stable.

We also recently observed an instance of acute instability of the cervical spine from a close range gunshot wound to the neck (Fig. 19-3 A,B). Despite treatment in a halo and a delayed posterior spinal fusion, instability persisted at 6 months after injury. Subsequently, the patient underwent anterior fusion with strut grafting and reapplication of the halo (Fig. 19-3 C).

We have not observed any cases of thoracic spinal instability, nor have any been reported. Likewise, no cases of unstable stab wounds have been reported in the literature.

Although civilian gunshot wounds seldom result in instability, consideration must be given to the anatomic structures damaged by the bullet and the effect this damage has on the integrity of the spinal column. Stability can be automatically determined from careful evaluation of the plain radiographs and CT scan. The vast majority of injuries to the spine are stable and require only symptomatic treatment, which includes some type of supportive orthosis until symptoms subside. The majority of the spinal injuries are complete; therefore, for unstable injuries we recommend early operative stabilization via posterior spinal fusion with short segment fixation. This treatment allows for early movement by the patient and, in the case of a patient with a SCI, facilitates rehabilitation.[47] Anterior fusion and decompression are rarely necessary.

Neurologic Injury

In 70% of gunshot wound cases, the neurologic level is one level higher than the vertebral level; in 10% it is two levels higher, and in 20% the levels are equal.[17] Stab injuries may be two segments above or five segments below the exterior wound measured by the spinal column.[21]

Gunshot injuries causing paraplegia and tetraplegia are complete in 74% and 55% of cases, respectively.[48] In another report of the thoracic injuries, 70% are complete compared with 57.7% of the cervical and 33% of the lumbar injuries.[7] If the bullet passed through the canal, the injury is more likely to be complete.[48] In stab wounds 66% to 80% suffer an incomplete lesion, generally a form of the Brown-Sequard syndrome.[8,10,21]

Neurologic Recovery

One year after gunshot wounds, two thirds of complete injuries gain no additional function; 25% gain one level. Of incomplete injured patients two thirds also have no additional recovery 1 year after injury; the remaining patients' improvement varies, regaining function from one level to complete recovery.[17] Improvement varies by the region of the spine involved.

A C B

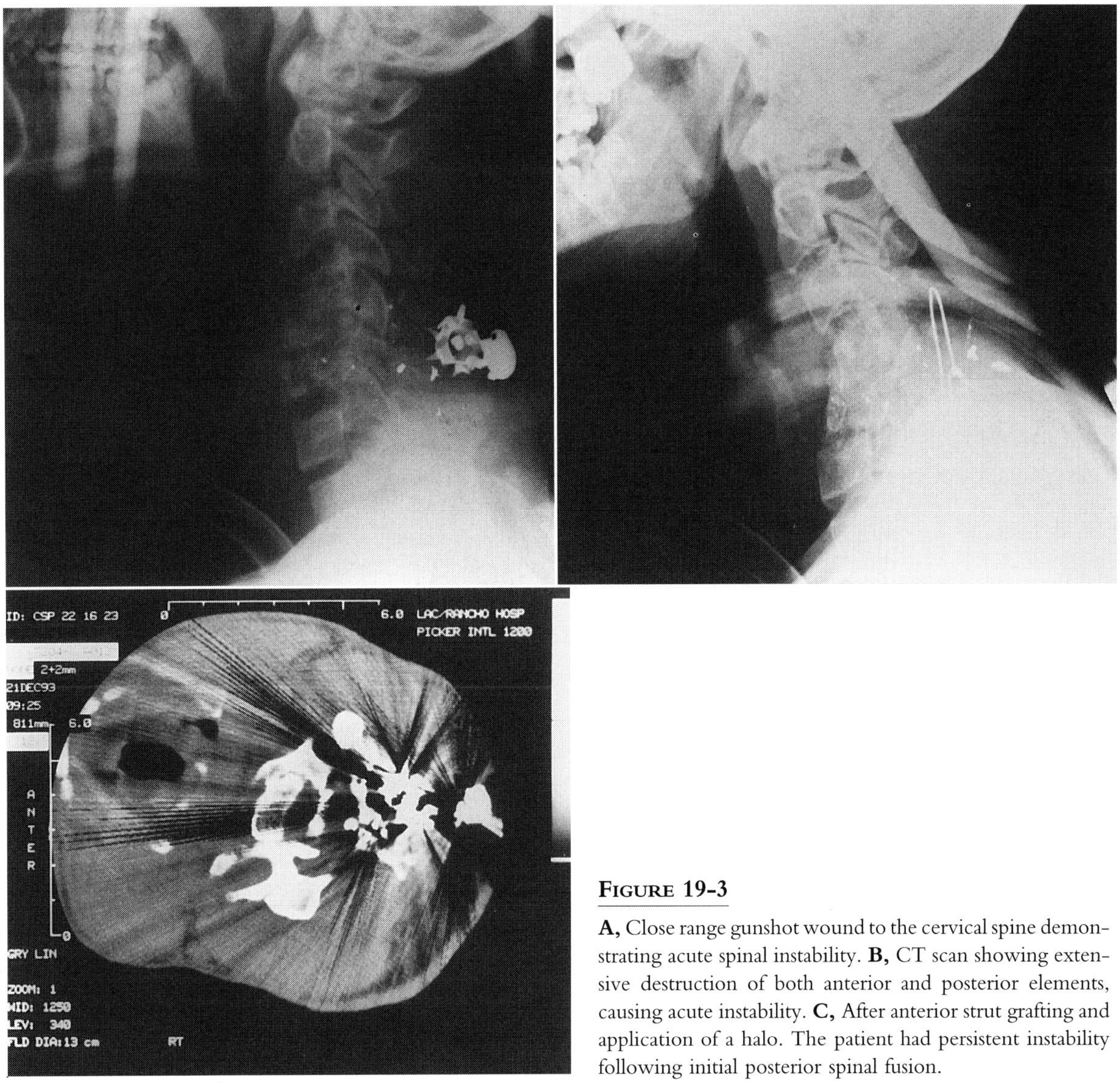

FIGURE 19-3

A, Close range gunshot wound to the cervical spine demonstrating acute spinal instability. **B,** CT scan showing extensive destruction of both anterior and posterior elements, causing acute instability. **C,** After anterior strut grafting and application of a halo. The patient had persistent instability following initial posterior spinal fusion.

Cervical injuries improve the most, followed by lumbar and thoracic injuries. As expected, complete injuries improve less at all levels than incomplete injuries.[17] Between 24% and 32% of all gunshot wound SCI patients were household or community ambulators 1 year after injury.[1,6]

The relatively high percentage of motor incomplete lesions following stab wounds accounts for the relatively favorable outcome compared with other causes of SCI. Incomplete Brown-Sequard injuries have a favorable prognosis for functional recovery. Lipschitz reported that in incomplete injuries more than half of all patients return to their former employment and 14% demonstrated total recovery.[21] Peacock stated that good or fair recovery was present in 83% of his patients.[8] After recovery, 44% to 66% of stab wound patients become household, if not community ambulators. Complete lesions, as with other mechanisms of injury have a poor prognosis for recovery.[8,10]

SURGICAL EVALUATION

ROLE OF DECOMPRESSION

Numerous reports discuss the role of surgery in gunshot wounds to the spine associated with SCI. Many of these, particularly those based on wartime experience, favor bullet removal through laminectomy as proper management.[49–60] Others advocate removal only for certain conditions, primarily progressive neurologic decline.[13,61–68] Those who favor removal indicate that this procedure prevents complications, which include meningitis, cerebrospinal fluid leak, lead toxicity, and late neurologic decline. Some consider laminectomy with or without bullet removal as a mandatory part of proper treatment of SCI.[69,70,71] Recent research indicates that neurologic recovery is not facilitated by laminectomy alone and that the complication rate increases with laminectomy.[35,61,62,65,66,69–73]

Reports on stab wounds have recommended retained foreign body removal because of case reports of delayed myelopathy. Others have advocated laminectomy to assess cord damage; we do not advocate laminectomy for this purpose.[1,35]

In Peacock's series, 20 cases (4.4%) had laminectomies.[8] These were performed for retained knife blades or to repair the uncommon persistent cerebrospinal fluid leak. They also considered persistent sepsis with an epidural abcess an indication for surgical exploration, but did not encounter this problem. These indications are identical to those espoused by Lipschitz.[19]

INDICATIONS FOR BULLET OR BLADE REMOVAL

Given a nondeteriorating neurologic status, the issue of when bullet or bone fragment removal from the spinal canal is indicated has not been completely resolved. Improved neurologic recovery and prevention of complications are theoretic reasons for bullet removal.

A collaborative study by the National Spinal Cord Injury Model Systems, which was sponsored by the National Institute on Disability and Rehabilitation Research, was undertaken in 1984 to assess the influence of bullet removal from the spinal canal on neurologic recovery.[17] The results of this study demonstrated that bullet removal from the thoracolumbar spine significantly improved neurologic recovery in both complete and incomplete injury (Fig. 19-4). Bullet removal did not statistically alter neurologic outcome in thoracic injuries. The sample size of cervical injuries was too small for statistical analysis.

In the cervical cord where one level may make the difference between an independent wheelchair ambulato and one who is dependent on bed-to-chair transfers, a patient with persistent compression of the spinal nerve exiting above the level of the lesion may benefit from surgical decompression.[23,74] Empiric but unproven support for this position could be extrapolated from Bohlman and coworkers' observation of neurologic improvement after late decompression from nonpenetrating causes.[74]

In 1975, Heiden[61] reported on 38 civilian patients sustaining cervical gunshot wounds. The 25 patients with complete SCI failed to improve regardless of

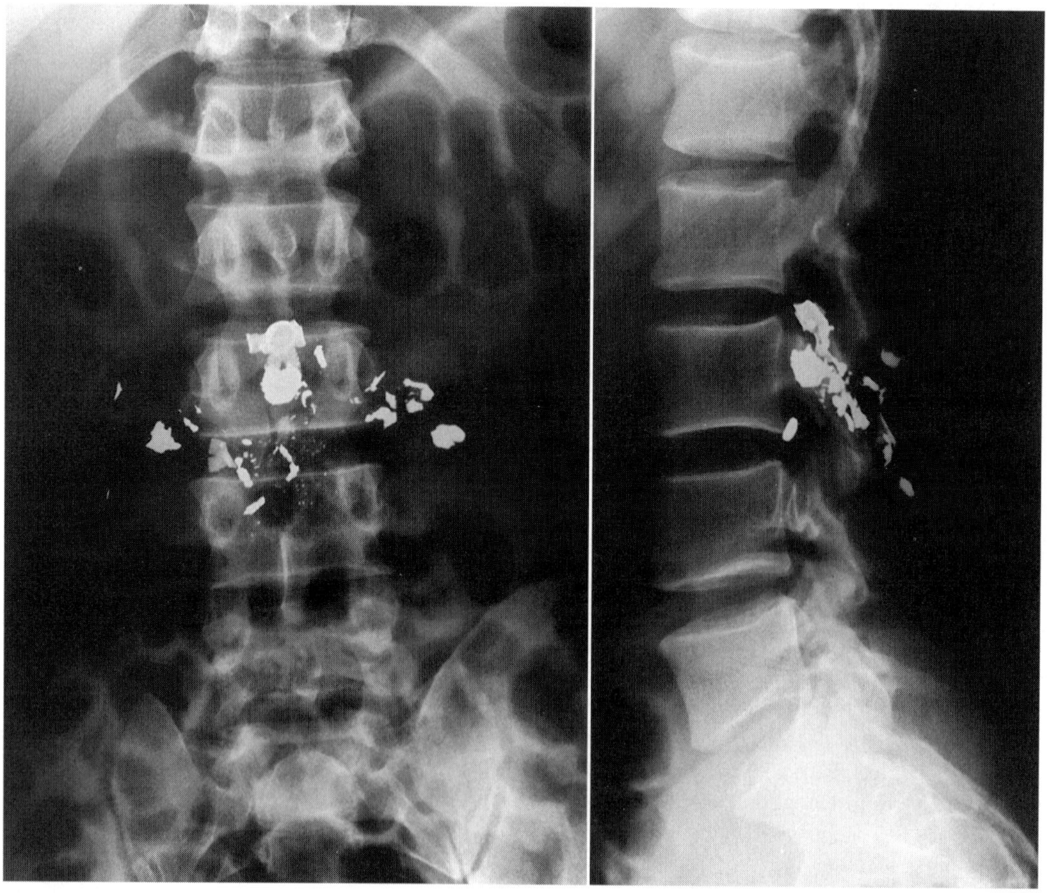

FIGURE 19-4

A and **B,** AP and lateral radiographs demonstrating retained bullet fragments at L3. The patient underwent removal of the intradural fragments and had significant neurological recovery.

whether surgery was performed. The 13 patients with incomplete injury improved regardless of decompression status. In the series of Kupcha and coworkers,[75] 75% of 28 patients with gunshot wounds to the cervical spine had complete injuries. Six of ten with intracanal bullets improved with or without laminectomy; 6 of 11 patients without retained bullets improved one level. Of the seven incomplete patients, two had laminectomies. One patient improved two levels and the other deteriorated one level. This demonstrated that decompressing and removing retained intracanal bullet fragments in the cervical spine conferred no benefit. Other authors echo this belief.[66,70,76–78] Complications of meningitis and instability were higher after decompression.

Venger and coworkers demonstrated that patients who were decompressed had a higher incidence of meningitis and wound infection than those treated conservatively.[79] Stauffer found a 10% incidence of complications consisting of cerebrospinal fluid fistula and wound infection in 101 patients undergoing laminectomy; six of these patients developed instability.[66]

The regional anatomy of the thoracic spinal cord contributes to increased susceptibility to injury. Tenuous collateral circulation to the spinal cord versus the cauda equina may account for the differences in the effect of bullet removal on neurologic recovery in the thoracic and thoracolumbar regions.[52,80] Above T12 in the thoracic and cervical spine, nerve roots exit the spinal canal just below the level from which they branch from the spinal cord; therefore, a bullet at this level can only compress nerve roots emanating from one neurologic level and the spinal cord. Conversely, in the thoracolumbar spine, the spinal cord expands at T10 forming the conus, which usually ends at the L1–L2 interspace and gives rise to the lumbar sacral roots (cauda equina).[71] These roots may descend many levels before exiting the spinal canal.[81] Therefore, a bullet within the spinal canal at or below T12 can compress multiple nerve roots that innervate the lower extremities, having a greater impact on American Spinal Injury Association (ASIA) motor scores. In addition, the cauda equina is composed of peripheral nerves, which have a greater potential for recovery after injury than the spinal cord proper, which has little or no recovery potential. Cord swelling is at a maximum 3 to 10 days after initial injury rendering the cord more susceptible to further damage. Consequently, when indicated, bullet removal should be performed within 48 hours of injury or 2 weeks after injury, unless the patient is losing further function.

Broken knife blades or glass should usually be removed to reduce the risk of delayed myelopathy.[69,82–88] LeBlanc and coworkers[89] reported that a patient who underwent reapproximation of severed nerve roots in the cauda equina after a stab wound improved neurologically.[84,89]

COMPLICATIONS

NEUROLOGIC DETERIORATION

Late neurologic deterioration has not been observed in more than 1,000 cases of SCI injury secondary to gunshot wounds monitored at Rancho Los Amigos Medical Center; however, rare instances of delayed neurologic change from retained bullets have been reported.[50,82,90–94] Likewise, delayed cases of neurologic decline have been reported with retained knife blades.[82–85] The symptoms were varied and the delay from injury to onset of neurologic symptoms ranged to 15 years. Symptoms can be caused by migration of a fragment within the canal and fibrous reactive tissue produced in response to fragments remaining in a disc space or vertebral body.[3,82,90–92] Excision of the fragments, the fibrous tissue, or both can improve symptoms. Patients with retained bullet fragments in the spinal canal should be observed for neurologic symptoms or neurologic loss, and the bullet or causative tissue should be excised if such symptoms develop.

INFECTION

Prevention of infection is commonly cited as a reason for bullet removal when the bullet perforates the alimentary canal before injuring the spine. Romanick and coworkers[31] reported on 20 cases of patients with low-velocity missile injuries to the spine with abdominal injuries. Of eight patients who sustained colon perforations before the bullet entered the spinal column, seven developed infection. Romanick and coworkers concluded that bullet removal is indicated when the alimentary canal is perforated. Most patients in this series received only 2 to 4 days intravenous antibiotic therapy.[31] Teams headed by Roffi and Kihter recently reviewed antibiotic treatment in patients with SCI associated with perforated abdominal viscera who did not undergo bullet removal.[29,30] The patients in the Roffi series received 7 to 14 days of broad-spectrum intravenous antibiotic agents and those in the Kihter series underwent irrigation of the missile track and a 48-hour course of antibiotic therapy. No spinal infections were seen in either series. Prophylactic removal of bullet fragment from the canal in civilian low-velocity cases is not recommended. In cases of high-velocity gunshot wounds, laminectomy, debridement, and removal of the bullet fragments may be appropriate.

PAIN

Pain is a common problem in patients with SCI, but seems more prevalent when the injury is from a gunshot wound. Meirowsky[59] and Kane and coworkers[95] have noted that "somatic pain" is worst in partial or peripheral nerve root lesions. Unfortunately, recent studies have concluded that the incidence of pain after injury was not affected by removal of the bullet and that after bullet removal, patients were more likely to develop deafferentation pain (often the most difficult type to treat).[17,96–98] Likewise, pain is only temporarily controlled after cordotomy and usually returns in a matter of months.[99]

LEAD TOXICITY

Lead toxicity resulting from bullets lodged in the spine is rare.[87,100,101] Lead from bullets is relatively insoluble and seldom causes systemic effects. Generally, bullets become encapsulated by poorly vascularized fibrous tissue that shields the bullets from body fluids.[100] If the fragment, however, is in contact with synovial fluid, such as a joint or pseudocapsule, symptoms of lead poisoning (abdominal pain, anemia, headaches, memory loss, and muscle weakness) may occur.[87,102,103] Chelation therapy with ethylenediaminetetraacetate (EDTA), D-penicillamine, or dimercaptol (BAL) should be initiated before bullet removal for better clinical results.[104]

TRAUMATIC FISTULA

Traumatic subarachnoid-pleural fistula after gunshot wounds has been reported.[105–110] This can be diagnosed in the patient with traumatic paraplegia and a persistent concomitant pleural effusion. The diagnosis is confirmed with myelography. Initial treatment should be conservative. Thoracentesis may be indicated for larger effusions; persistence or recurrence is an indication for surgical repair of the defect. Cerebrospinal fluid leakage occurs uncommonly after stab wounds and in almost all cases discontinues at 7 to 10 days. If the leakage is persistent, then repair is indicated. This occurred in 4% (18 cases) in the Peacock series.[8]

SYRINX

Posttraumatic syrinx may develop from ischemic necrosis of neural tissue or possibly from lysosomal destruction of the spinal cord.[111,112] A syrinx should be suspected in a patient with a stable SCI who suddenly develops progressive motor weakness, sensory loss, hyperhidrosis or increasing spasticity. Myelography or magnetic resonance imaging allows visualization of the cyst. Shunting of the cyst to the subarachnoid space may significantly improve symptoms.[113]

ARACHNOIDITIS

Focal arachnoiditis has been described as a late complication of penetrating injuries to the spine. Its occurrence has been reported years after a gunshot wound to the spine.[82,92,93] Irritation of the cauda equina is not directly produced by the foreign body itself; rather, it is the reactive formation of an extra- or intradural fibrotic mass that causes displacement, stretching, or constriction of the affected nerve roots. Alternatively, ischemia of the neural tissue may be the source of radicular pain and progressive neurogenic claudication. Surgical excision of the fibrotic mass may ameliorate the symptoms.[23]

SUMMARY

Penetrating injuries to the spine are becoming more prevelent, especially in urban areas. With gunshot injuries, neurologic injury can occur even if the projectile does not penetrate the spinal canal. The majority of stab wounds involve an incomplete Brown-Sequard lesion of the thoracic cord; most gunshot wounds injure the thoracic cord causing complete neurologic injury.

Initial treatment of penetrating SCI should consist of stabilizing the patient's medical condition followed by a careful neurologic examination. Spine stability can be determined from plain radiographs and a CT scan, with the overwhelming majority of injuries being stable.

Routine laminectomy has repeatedly been shown not to alter neurologic outcome and increases complication rates. Retained bullets rarely cause problems of delayed infection, late neurologic decline, or lead toxicity, eliminating the need for prophylactic bullet removal; however, in the thoracolumbar spine, removal of bullet fragments within the spinal canal has been shown to significantly improve neurologic recovery.

Retained sharp portions of knives, and other stabbing devices should be prophylactically removed in neurologically intact or incomplete patients as there are reports of delayed significant neurologic injury.

REFERENCES

1. Velmahos GC, et al: Changing profiles in spinal cord injuries and risk factors influencing recovery after penetrating injuries, *J Trauma* 38(3):334–337, 1995.
2. Fischer DK, et al: Shielding of the spinal cord by cervical and facial structures in penetrating trauma, *Neurochirurgia* 34(1):37, 1991.

3. Karim NO, et al: Spontaneous migration of a bullet in the spinal subarachnoid space causing delayed radicular symptoms, *Neurosurgery* 18(1):97, 1986.
4. Young JS, et al: *Spinal cord injury statistics: Experience of the Regional Spinal Injury Systems*, Phoenix, 1982, Good Samaritan Medical Center.
5. University of Alabama at Birmingham National Spinal Cord Injury Statistical Center: *Spinal cord injury facts and figures at a glance*, Birmingham, July 1996, The Center.
6. Waters RL, Sie IH, Adkins RH: Rehabilitation of the patient with a spinal cord injury, *Orthop Clin of North Am* 26(1):117, 1995.
7. Waters RL, et al: Profiles of spinal cord injury and neurologic recovery after gunshot injury, *Clin Orthop* 267:14–21, 1991.
8. Peacock WS, Shrosbee RB, Key AD: A review of 450 stabwounds to the spinal cord, *S Afr Med J* 51:961–964, 1977.
9. Lipschitz R: Associated injuries and complications of stab wounds of the spinal cord, *Paraplegia* 5:75–82, 1967.
10. Waters RL, et al: Motor recovery following spinal cord injury caused by stab wounds: a multicenter study, *Paraplegia* 33:98–101, 1995.
11. The University of Alabama at Birmingham, National Spinal Cord Injury Statistical Center: *Annual report for the Model Spinal Cord Injury Care Systems, Downey, California*, Birmingham, 1994, The Center.
12. de Muth WE, Jr: Bullet velocity and design as determinants of wounding capability: an experimental study, *J Trauma* 6(2):222, 1966.
13. Waters RL: Gunshot wounds to the spine: the effects of bullet fragments in the spinal canal, *J Am Paraplegia Soc* 7:30, 1984.
14. de Muth WE, Jr: Bullet velocity as applied to military rifle wounding capacity, *J Trauma* 9(1):27, 1969.
15. Hopkinson DA, Marshall TK: Firearm injuries, *Br J Surg* 54(5):344, 1967.
16. Gardner BP: Penetrative injuries: stabbings and gunshot wounds. In Frankel HL, editor: *Handbook of clinical neurology*, 1992, Elsevier Science Publishers B.V.
17. Waters RL, et al: The effects of removal of bullet fragments retained in the spinal canal. A collaborative study by the National Spinal Cord Injury Model Systems, *Spine* 16(8):934–939, 1991.
18. Guttman L: *Spinal cord injuries: Comprehensive management and research*, Oxford, 1973, Blackwell.
19. Lipschitz R, Block J: Stab wounds of the spinal cord, *Lancet* 2:169–172, 1962.
20. Nagoulitch I, Borne G, Belval J: Spinal cord wounds due to firearms and knives: comparative study of 50 cases, *Lyon Chir* 64:424–433, 1968.
21. Lipschitz R: Stab wounds of the spinal cord. In Vinken PJ, Bruyn GW, editors: *Handbook of clinical neurology*, Amsterdam. 1976, North Holland Publishing.
22. Fetterman BL, et al: Management of traumatic hypopharyngeal injuries, *Laryngoscope* 105:8–13, 1995.
23. Errico TJ, Bauer RD, Waugh T: *Spinal trauma*, Philadelphia, 1991, JB Lippincott.
24. Craig JB: Cervical spine osteomyelitis with delayed onset tetraparesis after penetrating wounds of the neck, *S Afr Med J* 69:197–199, 1986.
25. Pattisapu JV, Al-Mefty O: Gunshot wound to the odontoid process: a case report, *Spine* 12:1052–1054, 1987.
26. Schaefer SD, et al: The management of transpharyngeal gunshot wounds to the cervical spine, *Surg Gynecol Obstet* 152:27–29, 1981.
27. Schaefer SD, et al: Treatment of transpharyngeal missile wounds to the cervical spine, *Laryngoscope* 91:146–148, 1981.
28. Kane T, et al: Spinal cord injury from civilian gunshot wounds: The Rancho experience 1980–1988, *J Spinal Disord* 4(3):306–311, 1991.
29. Kihtir JT, et al: Management of transperitoneal gunshot wounds of the spine, *J Trauma* 31(12):1579, 1991.
30. Roffi RP, Waters RL, Adkins RH: Gunshot wounds to the spine associated with a perforated viscus, *Spine* 14:808, 1989.
31. Romanick GM, et al: Infection about the spine associated with low-velocity-missile injury to the abdomen, *J Bone Joint Surg* 67A:1195–1201, 1985.
32. American Spinal Injury Association: *Standards for neurological classification of spinal injury patients*. Chicago, 1989, The Association.
33. Bracken MB, et al: A randomized, controlled trial of methylprednisolone or naloxone in the treatment of acute spinal cord injury: results of the Second National Acute Spinal Cord Injury Study, *N Engl J Med* 322:1405, 1990.
34. Prendergast MR: Massive steroids do not reduce the zone of injury after penetrating spinal cord injury, *J Trauma* 37(4):576–580, 1994.
35. Simpson RK Jr, Venger BH, Narayan RK: Treatment of acute penetrating injuries of the spine: a retrospective analysis, *J Trauma* 29(1):42–46, 1989.
36. Plumley TF, Kilcoyne RF, Mack LA: Computed tomography in evaluation of gunshot wounds of the spine, *J Comp Assist Tomog* 7(2):310, 1983.
37. Yashon D: *Missile injuries of the spinal cord and cauda equina*, ed 2, Norwalk, 1986, Appleton Century Crofts.
38. Meyer PR et al: Symposium: management of fractures of the thoracolumbar spine, *Contemp Orthop* 27:90, 1988.
39. Betz RR, Mulcahey MJ: Spinal cord injury rehabilitation, In Weinstein SL, editor: *The pediatric spine: principles and practice*, New York, 1994, Raven Press.
40. Campbell J, Bonnett C: Spinal cord injury in children, *Clin Orthop* 112:114–123, 1975.
41. Dearolf WW III, et al: Scoliosis in pediatric spinal cord injury patients, *J Pediatr Orthop* 10:214–218, 1990.
42. Kilfoyle RM, Foley JJ, Norton PL: Spine and pelvic deformity following traumatic spinal cord injury in

childhood and adolescent paraplegia: a study of 104 cases, *J Bone Joint Surg* 47A:659–682, 1965.

43. Lancourt JE, Dickson JH, Carter RE: Paralytic spinal deformity following traumatic spinal cord injury in children and adolescents, *J Bone Joint Surg* 63A:47–53, 1981.
44. Mayfield JK, Erkkila JC, Winter RB: Spine deformity subsequent to acquired childhood spinal cord injury, *J Bone Joint Surg* 63A:1401–1411, 1981.
45. Davis HW, Rosen C, Zigler J: The effect of gunshot wounds on stability of the thoracolumbar spine in paraplegia (unpublished data), Rancho Los Amigos Medical Center, Downey, California.
46. Raynor R, Pugh J, Shapiro T: Cervical facetectomy and its effects on spine strength, *J Neurosurg* 63:278–282, 1985.
47. Rimoldi R, et al: The effect of surgical intervention on rehabilitation time in patients with thoracolumbar and lumbar spinal cord injuries, *Spine* 17(12):1443–1449, 1992.
48. Waters RL, et al: Injury pattern effect on motor recovery after traumatic spinal cord injury, *Arch Phys Med Rehab* 76:440, 1995.
49. Hagelstam L: Late laminectomey in traumatic paraplegia, *Acta Chir Scand* 110:218–226, 1955.
50. Matson DD: *The treatment of acute compound injuries of the spinal cord due to missiles*, Springfield, 1948, Charles C Thomas.
51. McCravey A: War wounds of the spinal cord: a plea for exploration of the spinal cord and cauda equina injuries, *JAMA* 129:152–153, 1945.
52. Nino HE, et al: Progressive sensory loss one year after bullet injury of spinal cord, *JAMA* 240:1173–1174, 1978.
53. Tinsley M: Compound injuries of the spinal cord, *J Neurosurg* 3:306–309, 1946.
54. Wannamaker GT: Spinal cord injuries: a review of the early treatment in 300 consecutive cases during the Korean conflict, *J Neurosurg* 11:517–524, 1954.
55. Haynes WG: Acute war wounds of the spinal cord. Analysis of 184 cases, *Am J Surg* 72:424–433, 1946.
56. Munro D: *The treatment of injuries to the nervous system*, Philadelphia, 1952, Saunders.
57. Scarff JE: Injuries of the vertebral column and spinal cord: In Brock S, editor: *Injuries of the brain and spinal cord and their coverings*, ed 4, New York, 1960, Springer Publishing.
58. Shroyer RN, Forston CH, Theodotu CB: Delayed neurological sequelae of a retained foreign body (lead bullet) in the intervertebral disc space, *J Bone Joint Surg* 42A:595–599, 1960.
59. Meirowsky AM: Penetrating wounds of the spinal canal, *Clin Orthop* 27:90–107, 1963.
60. Pool JL: Gunshot wounds of the spine: observations from an evacuation hospital, *Surg Gynecol Obstet* 81:617–622, 1945.
61. Heiden JS, et al: Penetrating gunshot wounds of the cervical spinal cord in civilians: review of 38 cases, *J Neurosurg* 42:575, 1975.
62. Guttman L: Surgical aspects of the treatment of traumatic paraplegia, *J Bone Joint Surg* 31B:399, 1949.
63. Kuhn WG, Jr: The care and rehabilitation of patients with injuries of the spinal cord and cauda equina: preliminary report on 113 cases, *J Neurosurg* 4:40, 1947.
64. Lucas JT, Ducker TB: Motor classification of spinal cord injuries with mobility, morbidity and recovery indices, *Am Surg* 45:151, 1979.
65. Morgan TH, Wharton GW, Austin GW: The results of laminectomy in patients with incomplete spinal cord injuries, *Paraplegia* 9:14–23, 1971.
66. Stauffer ES, Wood RW, Kelly EG: Gunshot wounds of the spine: the effect of laminectomy, *J Bone Joint Surg* 61(A):389–392, 1979.
67. Maniker AH, Gropper MR, Hunt D: Transoral gunshot wounds to the atlanto-axial complex: report of five cases, *J Trauma* 37(5):858–861, 1994.
68. Hammoud MA, Haddad FS, Moufarrij NA: Spinal cord missile injuries during the Lebanese civil war, *Surg Neurol* 43:432–442, 1995.
69. Comarr AE, Kauffman AA: A survey of the neurological results of 858 spinal cord injuries: a comparison of patients treated with and without laminectomy, *J Neurosurg* 13:95–106, 1956.
70. Covalt DA, et al: Early management of patients with spinal cord injury, *JAMA* 151:89–94, 1953.
71. Daniels JT: Fractures and dislocations of the spine in warfare, *Am J Surg* 72:414–423, 1946.
72. Austin GM: *The spinal cord: basic aspects and surgical considerations*, ed 2, Springfield, 1972, Charles C Thomas.
73. Carey PD: Neurosurgery and paraplegia, *Rehabilitation* (Jan-March):27–29, 1965.
74. Bohlman HH, Eismont FJ: Surgical techniques of anterior decompression and fusion for spinal cord injuries, *Clin Orthop* 154:57–67, 1981.
75. Kupcha PC, Howard SA, Cotler JM: Gunshot wounds to the cervical spine, *Spine* 15(10):1058–1063, 1990.
76. Davidoff LM: Spinal cord injuries, *Surg Clin North Am* 21:433–441, 1941.
77. Matson DD: Treatment of compound spine injuries in forward army hospitals, *J Neurosurg* 3:114–119, 1946.
78. Mayfield FH, Cazan GM: Spinal cord injuries: analysis of six cases showing subarachnoid block, *Am J Surg* 55:317–325, 1942.
79. Venger BH, Simpson RK, Narayan RK: Neurosurgical intervention in penetrating spinal trauma with associated visceral injury, *J Neurosurg* 70:514–518, 1989.
80. Lazorthes G: Arterial vascularization of the spinal cord: recent studies of the anastomotic substitution pathways, *J Neurosurg* 35:253–262, 1979.
81. Rauschning W: Detailed sectional anatomy of the spine. In Rothman SL, Glann WV, Jr, editors: *Multiplanar CT of the spine*, Baltimore, 1985, University Park Press.

82. Wu WO: Delayed effects of retained foreign bodies in the spine and spinal cord, *Surg Neurol* 25:214–218, 1986.
83. Baghi P, Sheptak PE: Penetrating spinal injury by a glass fragment: case report and review, *Neurosurgery* 11(3):419–422, 1982.
84. Jones, FD, Woosley RE: Delayed myelopathy secondary to retained intraspinal metallic fragment: case report, *J Neurosurg* 55:979–982, 1981.
85. Criado E, Oller D, Fulghum J: Delayed diagnosis of a foreign body in the spinal canal, *South Med J* 83(3):332–334, 1990.
86. Fung CF, Thomas HK: Delayed myelopathy after a stab wound with a retained intraspinal foreign body: case report, *J Trauma* 32(4):539–541, 1992.
87. Grogan DP, Bucholz RW: Acute lead intoxication from bullet in an intervertebral disc space, *J Bone Joint Surg* 63A:1180–1182, 1981.
88. Yashon D: *Stab wounds of the spinal cord*, ed 2, Norwalk, 1986, Appleton Century Croft.
89. LeBlanc HJ, Gray LW, Kline DG: Stab wounds of the cauda equina: case report, *J Neurosurg* 55:683–685, 1969.
90. Arasil E, Tascioglu AO: Spontaneous migration of an intracranial bullet to the cervical spinal canal causing Lhermitte's sign: a case report, *J Neurosurg* 56:158–159, 1982.
91. Soges LJ, Kinnebrew GH, Limcaco OG: Mobile intrathecal bullet causing delayed radicular symptoms, *AJNR* 9:610, 1988.
92. Staniforth P, Watt I: Extradural "plumboma." A rare cause of acquired spinal stenosis, *Br J Radiol* 55:772–774, 1982.
93. Amitani K, Tsuyuguchi Y, Hukuda S: Delayed cervical myelopathy caused by bomb shell fragment, *J Neurosurg* 44:626–627, 1976.
94. Karim NO: Spontaneous migration of a bullet in the spinal subarachnoid space causing delayed radicular symptoms, *Neurosurgery* 18:97–100, 1986.
95. Kane T, et al: Spinal cord injury from civilian gunshot wounds: the Rancho Experience 1980–88, *J Spine Disord* 4(3):306–311, 1991.
96. Richards JS, et al: Psycho-social aspects of chronic pain in spinal cord injury, *Pain* 8:355–366, 1980.
97. Richards JS, Stover SL, Jaworski T: Effect of bullet removal on subsequent pain in persons with spinal cord injury secondary to gunshot wound, *J Neurosurg* 73:401–404, 1990.
98. Davidoff G et al: Function-limiting dysesthetic pain syndrome among traumatic spinal cord injury patients: a cross-sectional study, *Pain* 29:39–48, 1987.
99. Freeman LW, Heimburger RF: Surgical relief of pain in paraplegic patients, *Arch Surg* 55:433–440, 1947.
100. Switz DM, Elmorshidy ME, Deyerle WM: Bullets, joints and lead intoxication. A remarkable and instructive case, *Arch Intern Med* 136:939–941, 1976.
101. Dillman RO, Crumb CK, Lidsky MJ: Lead poisoning from gunshot wound. Report of a case and review of the literature, *Am J Med* 66:509–514, 1979.
102. Leonard MH: The solution of lead by synovial fluid, *Clin Orthop* 64:255–261, 1969.
103. Linden MA et al: Lead poisonings from retained bullets. Pathogenesis, diagnosis and management, *Ann Surg* 195(3):305–313, 1982.
104. Graef JW, Lovejoy FH: Heavy metal poisoning, In Braunwald E, et al, editors: *Harrison's principles of internal medicine*, ed 11, New York, 1987, McGraw-Hill.
105. Beutel EW, et al: Subarachnoid-pleural fistula, *J Thorac Cardiovasc Surg* 80:21–24, 1980.
106. Bramwit DN, Schmelka DD: Traumatic subarachnoid-pleural fistula, 89:737–738, 1967.
107. Djergaian RS, et al: Subarachnoid-pleural fistula in traumatic paraplegia, *Arch Phys Med Rehab* 63:488–489, 1982.
108. Lovaas ME, Castillo RG, Deutschman MS: Traumatic subarachnoid-pleural fistula, *Neurosurgery* 17:650–652, 1985.
109. Milloy FJ, Correl NO, Langston HT: Persistent subarachnoid-pleural space fistula: report of a case, *JAMA* 169:1467, 1959.
110. Ozer, H, Barki Y, Bertran V: Traumatic arachnoidopleural fistula: report of a case, *J Can Assoc Radiol* 23:287–289, 1972.
111. Barnett HJM, Jousse AT, Ball MJ: Pathology and pathogenesis of progressive cystic myelopathy as a late sequela to spinal cord injury. In Barnett HJM, Foster JB, Hudgson P, editors: *Syringomyelia*, Philadelphia, 1973, WB Saunders.
112. Kao CC, Chang LW: The mechanism of spinal cord cavitation following spinal cord transection: Part 1. A correlated hiztochemical study, *J Neurosurg* 46:197–209, 1977.
113. Eismont FI, Green BA, Quencer RM: Post-traumatic spinal cord cyst, *J Bone Joint Surg* 66A:614–618, 1984.

20

SPINAL INJURIES IN THE ELDERLY

Jack E. Zigler
John E. Lankenau

The elderly population in the United States continues to grow at a higher rate than any other segment. From 1960 to 1990, the overage-65 segment has increased by 89% compared with growth of 39% for the total population. One person in eight is currently over the age of 65, and this ratio will increase to one in five by the year 2030. Individuals over the age of 85 represent the fastest-growing portion of the U.S. census.[1,2,3] The rapid growth of the geriatric segment is a consequence of an overall increase in life expectancy coupled with the aging of the post World War II baby boomers (Table 20-1).

As the older population segment continues to increase, spinal injury care of senior citizens will assume increasing importance. The number of patients requiring spine injury care is certain to increase. Operations on those 65 years of age and older have increased fivefold in the last decade. Eighty percent of lifetime health care costs occur in the last 6 months of life. Given the increasing focus on health care cost containment, medical care delivery to the aged population will come under increased scrutiny.

Very little has been published on the management of spinal injuries in the elderly. The mechanisms of injury, the regions of the spine affected, and the fracture patterns encountered are different in this subgroup. Merely assuming that the elderly should be treated the same as younger patients would be a disservice.

The goal of management of the older patient with spinal cord injury (SCI) is to maximize function and quality of life. With a relatively shorter anticipated lifespan, the elderly are naturally less concerned with absolute prolongation of survival than they are with maintaining or improving the quality of their remaining years. Although based on the same database, the elderly may make different health care decisions than their younger counterparts.

Because elderly patients do not generally tolerate prolonged immobilization, the underlying guiding principle of spinal injury management in the elderly is early mobilization. Any treatment option based on prolonged recumbency should be reconsidered.

GENERAL CONSIDERATIONS

The elderly population segment has a higher incidence of chronic illness than the population as a whole. Underlying medical diseases are often present which can profoundly affect the preoperative, intraoperative, and postoperative management of spinal injuries. The patient's overall medical condition, including pulmonary, cardiovascular, and renal status must be factored into the surgical decision-making process as well as any decision favoring nonsurgical treatment.

In general, spine injury in the elderly presents following lower energy trauma. The aforementioned underlying multisystem conditions make most high-energy trauma difficult for the elderly to survive. Most presenting spinal injuries are lower energy and, therefore, instability patterns tend to be less extreme; however, even with low-energy trauma, the treatment of this group requires many special considerations.

In general, the postoperative complication rate is related to the individual's state of health at the time of surgery, the quality of surgical procedure performed, and the postoperative medical management. Surgical mortality is significantly elevated in patients who have four or more preexisting serious medical conditions.[4] In particular, recent myocardial infarction and cerebral dysfunction appear to be important risk factors.

Based on data collected in the management of hip fractures in the elderly, postoperative mortality rates are lower when perioperative antibiotics and prophylaxis for deep venous thrombosis are used. Surgery within 24 hours of fracture has a higher mortality rate than surgery performed 2 to 5 days postfracture. Although the indications for emergent spinal surgery are rare in the general population, this data would indicate that medical stabilization of the patient, with correction of electrolyte imbalances and hypovolemia, may be even more important in the elderly population.

When deciding the appropriate course of action for any patient with a spinal injury, there are two primary objectives. The first is to preserve and maximize neurologic function, and the second is to achieve anatomic alignment and spinal stability. Stability must be assessed not only in the acute posttraumatic setting but frequently as a later problem if the initial treatment causes instability. In some situations, early surgical intervention may be the preferred option, even in the elderly patient. Prompt restoration of anatomic alignment is almost always preferred to maximize the potential for spinal cord recovery. Surgical canal decompression in the face of incomplete SCI can often lead to improved cord function.

Once the extent of the spinal injury and the patient's overall medical condition have been assessed, an appropriate management course can be determined. Acute traumatic cervical SCI in the elderly is associated with increased morbidity and mortality. Whether operative or nonoperative treatment options are chosen, older patients benefit from aggressive mobilization efforts. These promote improved respiratory function, lessened risk of medical complications due to recumbency, and provide for earlier and more effective rehabilitation.

EPIDEMIOLOGY

Traumatic SCI in the elderly is different from similar injury in the younger adult population in mechanism, gender distribution, anatomic location, and specific fracture patterns.

In the geriatric population, injuries most frequently result from falls rather than vehicular trauma or violence. Patients 65 years of age and older have a much higher incidence of SCI caused by minor trauma. One study demonstrated that 78% of cord injuries in the elderly were caused by falls in the home.[5] Impaired eyesight, balance, and muscle tone are frequent contributing factors to at-home fall accidents.

The distribution of SCI is evenly divided between men and women in the aged population. This contrasts with the 4:1 male predominance seen in the young. In one study, 13.7% of spinal column injuries in the study period occurred in patients over 65 years of age. Eighty-two percent of these injuries involved the cervical spine, with quadriplegia resulting in 52%. In patients without cord injury, 70% involved the occiput to C3 segments.[6] Odontoid fractures were the single most common cervical injury.[5]

Table 20-1. Average Life Expectancy of Elderly in the United States

Years	Survival	Life Expectancy
Males		
65	15.1	80.1
70	12.3	81.3
75	9.8	84.8
Females		
65	19.9	84.9
70	16.3	86.3
75	13.0	88.0
80	6.2	91.2

CERVICAL SPINE INJURIES

Although the cervical spine is the most common area of injury in the geriatric population, there have been few recommendations made regarding treatment of these injuries in the older patient. Most studies combine patients from a wide-age spectrum and often include only small numbers of patients over 65 years of age.

Cervical spine injuries can be divided into upper (C1–C3) and lower cervical levels. Each group accounts for about half of the cervical injuries observed in the elderly. Odontoid fractures account for 37% of all cervical fractures in patients over 65 years of age and are the most common upper cervical injury (Fig. 20-1). The incidence of odontoid fracture increases with age, and in patients over age 79 years of age are more common than all other fracture types combined.[7] The majority of odontoid fractures (69% to 85%) are

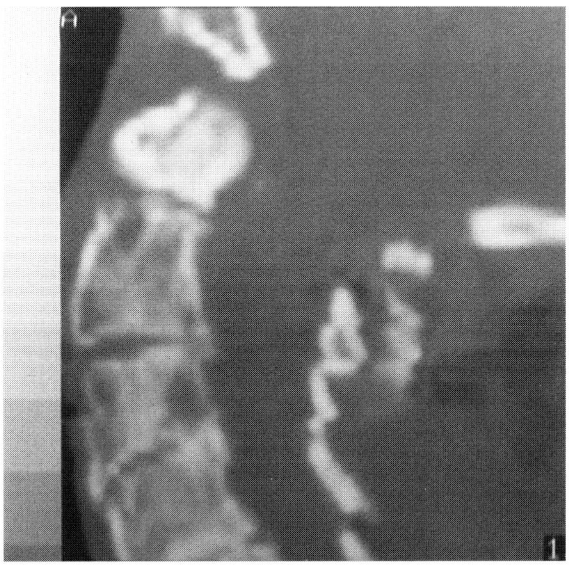

FIGURE 20-1

Odontoid fractures are common in the elderly, and most are type II.

type II fractures.[5,8,9,10] Displaced type II injuries are associated with a high rate of delayed or nonunion. These fractures also have the potential for late mechanical instability causing neurologic involvement. Greater than 80% of all odontoid fractures seen in elderly patients are displaced. The majority (88%) are displaced posteriorly, average displacement being 7 mm.[8] There is often a delay in the diagnosis of odontoid fractures in the elderly, because the fracture often occurs through osteopenic cancellous bone and may be poorly visualized on routine radiographs. Further, the low energy threshold required for odontoid fractures in osteopenic bone means that a high index of suspicion must be maintained to establish the diagnosis in timely fashion.[11] Initial failure to diagnose the injury can result in complications including neurologic injury.

Management of odontoid fractures is somewhat controversial. Most sources agree with nonoperative halo management for type III and nondisplaced type II fractures. Both operative and nonoperative management of displaced type II fractures have been advocated.[5,9,10,12,13] It is often difficult to achieve and maintain acceptable reduction of displaced fractures, resulting in a high rate of nonunion following nonoperative treatment of displaced type II fractures. Although nonunion has been reported in up to 40% of the fractures treated nonoperatively, a stable fibrous union often occurs.[8,10] This undoubtedly contributes to the surprisingly high rates of acceptable results in these fractures treated nonoperatively with rigid collar or halo-vest immobilization. Generalized age-related reduction of cervical motion also contributes to this success despite failure of fusion.

Early mobilization of elderly patients clearly reduces morbidity and mortality, regardless of treatment modality chosen.[8,12] Age, overall medical condition, and characteristics of the fracture should all be considered in deciding how to treat the displaced odontoid fracture in the older patient, but treatment plans based on prolonged recumbency should be avoided.

Subaxial cervical fractures in the elderly commonly involve unilateral or bilateral facet dislocations (Fig. 20-2) [5] Evaluation should include assessment of mechanical stability and the concern for prevention of neurologic compromise. In the majority of cases, the goal should be prompt reduction and adequate stabilization. Posterior cervical fusion should be considered in cases with pure ligamentous disruption, where the healing potential may be suboptimal. Even in cases of fracture-dislocation typically treated by closed reduction and 12 weeks immobilization in a halo vest in younger patients, strong consideration should be given to posterior cervical fusion in the elderly, allowing for immediate and better-tolerated mobilization in a collar.

Incomplete SCI in this population frequently result in a central cord syndrome.[14] Hyperextension of a cervical canal narrowed by degenerative osteophytosis

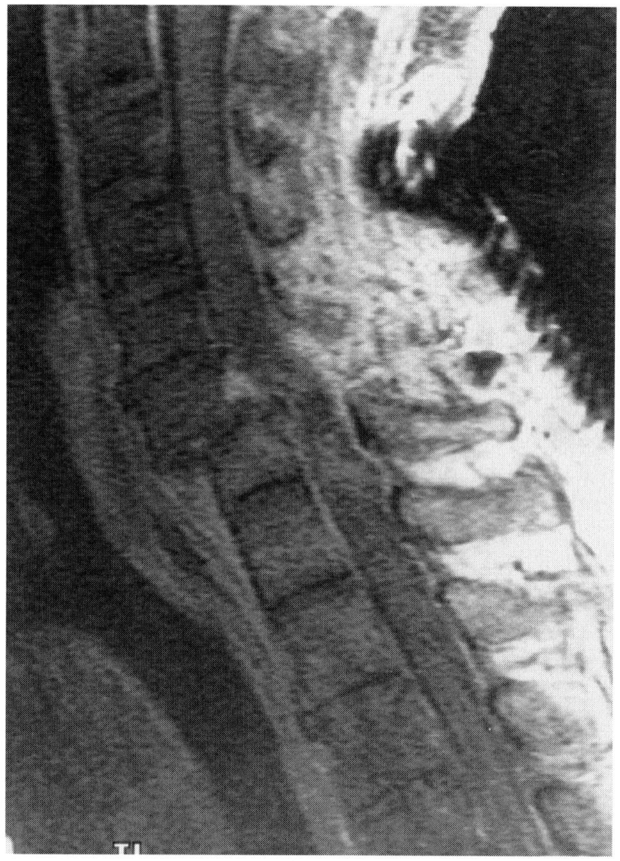

FIGURE 20-2

Lower cervical fractures (below C2) often result from flexion-distraction forces causing facet dislocations with significant spinal canal compromise. These fractures are acutely unstable, and posterior wiring and fusion is recommended in the elderly to avoid the need for a halo vest.

may lead to cord edema and a central hematomyelia that has a relatively good recovery potential overall. No studies have specifically followed the resolution of central cord syndrome in the elderly as a separate group. The role of early surgical decompression in this subgroup can, therefore, not be easily determined. Laminoplasty or anterior decompression, when appropriate, can assist in recovery, but central cord lesions have a natural tendency toward recovery without surgery. We prefer allowing maximum recovery before considering surgical intervention.

THORACIC AND LUMBAR SPINE INJURIES

Compression fractures are the most common injuries found in the thoracic and lumbar spines of the elderly. Osteoporosis, reducing both bone density and trabecullar morphology, may predispose the elderly to fracture following minimal trauma.[15] Twenty-five percent

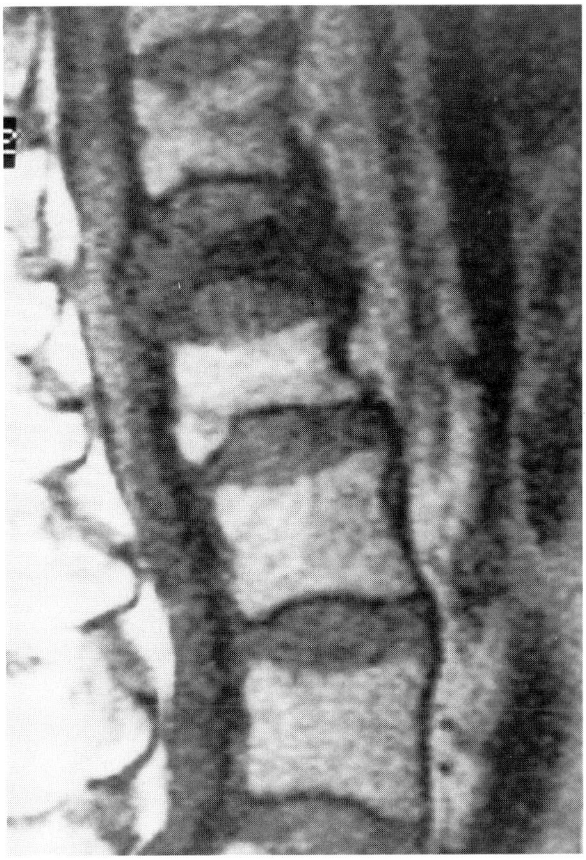

FIGURE 20-3

Osteoporotic compression fractures may rarely cause compression of the spinal cord, conus medullaris, or cauda equina. Surgical decompression may be required in that case.

of 85-year-old women and 13% of 85-year-old men have vertebral compression fractures.[16] This is probably an underestimate, because the study group in question did not include a representative sample of the more severely affected who live in assisted care environments.

Most patients with vertebral compression fractures are treated symptomatically. Surgical treatment is rarely indicated unless spinal cord or cauda equina compression results from either the initial fracture or a later kyphotic deformity (Fig. 20-3). Brace fitting and brace compliance for an elderly patient may be difficult. Lighter appliances with special padding for boney prominences may be necessary in some more debilitated or cachectic patients. Treatment typically consists of activity restriction, analgesics, physiotherapy, and bracing if tolerated. Metastatic disease or myeloma should be excluded as a cause of similar-appearing fractures following minimal trauma. Magnetic resonance imaging (MRI) is sometimes helpful in distinguishing between tumors and osteoporotic fractures.

TRAUMATIC SPINAL CORD INJURY IN THE ELDERLY

The aged suffer a significantly increased mortality rate following acute SCI. One study recently reported a 27% mortality rate in patients over 65 years of age with acute quadriplegia.[6] A second study reported no survivors of complete quadriplegia when onset occurred after 65 years of age.[17]

Central cord syndrome is the most common incomplete lesion found in the geriatric population.[14] Instability is not generally present. Surgical intervention is rarely necessary, because most patients recover ambulatory ability and bowel and bladder control. Surgical indications are individualized based on severity of injury, amount of canal stenosis, rapidity of improvement, and the overall condition of the patient.

SUMMARY

There are differences between elderly patients with spinal injuries and the younger population. Care for elderly patients with spinal trauma requires a comprehensive evaluation of each patient. Surgical decision making must consider the patient's overall medical condition and the mechanical and neurologic components of the injury. Geriatric patients do poorly with prolonged immobilization, and this must be considered in formulating a treatment plan. Early mobilization of the older patient should be of paramount concern when choosing the most appropriate treatment option. Bracing or surgery must take into account the physiologic and psychologic requirements of the elderly patient.

REFERENCES

1. Havlik RJ, et al: *Health statistics on older persons, United States, 1986.* Washington, DC, U.S. Public Health Service, 1987-66, US Health and Human Services Pub (DHS) 87–1409, Vital and Health Statistics. Series 3, No. 25, U.S. Government Printing Office.
2. Schneider EL, Gusalnik JM: The aging of America: impact on health care costs, *JAMA* 263:2335–2340, 1990.
3. Spencer G: Projections of the population of the United States by age, sex and race; 1988 to 2080. Current

Population Reports, Series P-25, No 1018, Washington, DC. 1989, US Bureau of the Census.

4. Kenzora JE, et al: Hip fracture mortality: relation to age, treatment, preoperative illness, time of surgery, and complications, *CORR* 186:45–56, 1984.
5. Lieberman IH, Webb JK: Cervical spine injuries in the elderly, *J Bone Joint Surg* 76B:877–881, 1994.
6. Spivak JM, et al: Cervical spine injuries in patients 65 and older, *Orthop Trans* 18:689, 1994.
7. Ryan MD, Henderson JJ: The epidemiology of fractures and fracture-dislocations of the cervical spine, *Injury* 23:38–40, 1992.
8. Hanigan WC, et al: Odontoid fractures in elderly patients, *J Neurosurg* 78:32–35, 1993.
9. Pepin JW, Bourne RB, Hawkins RJ: Odontoid fractures, with special reference to the elderly patient, *CORR* 193:178–183, 1985.
10. Ryan MD, Taylor TKF: Odontoid fractures in the elderly, *J Spinal Disord* 6:397–401, 1993.
11. Anderson LD, D'Alonzo RT: Fractures of the odontoid process of the atlas, *J Bone Joint Surg* 56A:1663–1674, 1974.
12. Bednar DA, Parikh J, Hummel J: Management of type II odontoid process fractures in geriatric patients; a prospective study of sequential cohorts with attention to survivorship, *J Spin Disord* 8:166–169, 1995.
13. Wang GJ, Nabie KN, Whitehill R: The nonsurgical management of odontoid fractures in adults, *Spine* 19:229–230, 1984.
14. Zigler JE, Capen DA, Rothman SLG: Spinal disease in the aged, *Clin Orthop* 316:70–79, 1995.
15. Snyder BD, et al: Role of trabecular morphology in the etiology of age-related vertebral fractures, *Orthop Trans* 17:453, 1992.
16. Johansson C, et al: Prevalence of vertebral fractures in 85 year-olds, *Acta Orthop Scand* 64:25–27, 1993.
17. Alander D, Andreyclik D, Stauffer ES: Early outcome in cervical spinal cord injured patients greater that 50 years of age, *Orthop Trans* 18:689, 1994.

21

MANAGEMENT OF LATE DEFORMITY AFTER SPINE TRAUMA

Scott E. Reeg
Oheneba Boachie–Adjei

Destabilizing fractures to the thoracic and lumbar spine are common injuries in our mechanized society. They are complex injuries for which acute treatment remains controversial and continues to evolve. There are many potentially serious complications resulting from unstable thoracic and lumbar fractures including late sagittal or coronal plane deformities. The thoracolumbar junction has unique anatomical properties, which predispose it to acute fracture and subsequent decompensation. The predominant posttraumatic deformity is angular kyphosis at the thoracolumbar junction. The cause of posttraumatic deformities is frequently multifactorial. Patient age, lifestyle, degree and level of neurologic deficit, and preexisting deformity all play a role. It is, however, the relative stability of the initial fracture and subsequent management that sets the stage for late spinal decompensation and deformity.[1,2] Neglected, inappropriate, and failed primary treatment of destabilizing injuries to the spine may fail to alter the natural history of such injuries to a significant degree allowing for the preservation of spinal alignment and stability.

Late deformities resulting from spinal fractures are disabling as a result of chronic pain, progression, and compression of neural elements; however, patients may benefit dramatically from reconstructive surgery to reestablish spinal alignment. The surgical management of these fractures and associated deformities have seen marked advancements in both instrumentation systems and surgical techniques. Despite these advancements, the surgical treatment presents an array of challenging issues to the reconstructive spine surgeon. Goals of surgery remain relief of pain, restoration of spinal alignment, decompression of neural tissues, and securing a solid arthrodesis. Surgical correction of these deformities requires a comprehensive evaluation of the patient and experience in executing the operative plan. Correction of three-dimensional deformities is technically demanding with potentially devastating complications.

PATHOMECHANICS

The thoracolumbar junction has unique anatomical features, which account for a biomechanical propensity for acute fractures and subsequent deformity.[3] Late deformity is a potential complication with any of the four major classes of fractures described by Denis. Each injury requires careful evaluation and an individualized treatment program. Following a destabilizing injury to the spine, errors in evaluation and treatment account for most late failures. Such treatment errors are often rooted in the clinicians misinterpretation of the severity of the initial injury and the failure to apply sound biomechanical principles to treatment strategies.

Deformity is defined as loss of normal sagittal or coronal alignment of the spinal column. In the sagittal plane, normal thoracic kyphosis measures 15° to 45° and normal lumbar lordosis ranges from 30° to 60°. The normal spine is straight in the coronal plane with the spinous process of C7 vertically aligned with the spinous process of S1. In addition, the body of C7 is vertically centered over the body of S1 on the lateral projection radiograph. Angular deformities are problematic as a source of pain and potential neural compression at the site of the fracture; however, of equal concern is the effect the deformity has on the overall balance of the spine. Any shift in the mechanical axis of the spine can further escalate the deformity with incapacitating symptoms and crippling consequences.

The thoracolumbar junction is the most common site for acute fractures and late posttraumatic deformity. There are a number of anatomic factors contributing to this. Most thoracic and lumbar fractures result from a combination of axial loading and flexion of the spine with varying degrees of vertebral body compression and tensile failure of the posterior ligamentous structures; however, translational and rotational forces may add to the complexity of these injuries. This is especially true at the thoracolumbar junction. The natural kyphosis of the thoracic spine and lordosis of the lumbar spine protect these regions to some degree with applied axial loads. The sagittal contour allows some of the forces to be transferred to soft tissues. At the thoracolumbar junction, however, the spine is essentially straight and axial loads are directed almost entirely through the vertebral bodies. In addition, there is a concentration of forces in this region as a result of disparity in stiffness between the thoracic spine and more mobile lumbar motion segments. Andriachi and coworkers[4] documented the stabilizing effects of the rib cage on the thoracic spine. With a fully intact rib cage, the flexion bending stiffness of the thoracic spine was increased by a factor of two and the lateral bending was increased by a factor of three. With ribs removed, there was much less stability documented. The thoracolumbar junction, with floating ribs at T11 and T12, lacks the stability of more cephalad levels in which the rib is supported both anteriorly to the sternum and posteriorly to the transverse process.

In contrast, the lumbar spine is much more mobile, and receives significant support from facet joints. Facets in the thoracic spine are sloping forward 30° to 40° in the frontal plane. In the lumbar spine, they are larger and vertically orientated and angled 45° in the sagittal plane. The facets are in sharp transition at the thoracolumbar junction. Oxland and coworkers[5] described orientation of the facets in this region and the effects on stability in flexion, extension, and rotation. The forward slope of facets in the upper thoracic spine is lost at T11 where they assume an almost vertical orientation. There is an abrupt reorientation in the sagittal plane of the facets at T11 and T12 levels. The sharp transition in geometry translated into abrupt changes in how one motion segment would respond to applied loads in comparison with another. This leaves T11 and T12 susceptible to rotational deformity and instability. The abrupt change in mechanical properties with applied loads predisposes this region to a concentration of forces and failure. The susceptibility to acute injuries also translates into a propensity for subsequent deformity.

The natural history of spinal fractures is often a direct extension of mechanism of injury and physiologic loads applied at that level. The principle deforming forces in the unstable spine are in the sagittal plane. The center of gravity over the thoracic spine lies anterior in most sitting and standing postures. At the thoracolumbar junction, the center of gravity passes through the vertebrae in transition to its posterior alignment in the lumbar spine. With any uncorrected or progressive kyphosis, the center of gravity is shifted anteriorly, further escalating the deforming forces.[3,6] Not all posttraumatic deformities, however, are in the sagittal plane. Although much less common, coronal and axial plane deformities can occur alone or in a combination with an angular kyphosis, creating a complex three-dimensional deformity.

Late deformity is a potential sequela with each of the major categories of spinal injuries described by Denis.[7] These include compression fractures, burst fractures, seat belt injuries, and fracture dislocations. Each is capable of producing late deformity with poorly selected, executed, or failed surgical or nonoperative treatment.

Compression fractures are the most common fracture in the thoracic and lumbar spine. They are generally stable injuries with axial failure of the anterior and preservation of the middle columns. They generally heal rapidly and require symptomatic treatment only. Despite having an intact middle column, however, severe compression may result in tensile failure of the posterior column. Failure to recognize and properly treat the posterior column disruption can result in a progressive angular kyphosis. In addition, several adjacent compression fractures may contribute to a significant sagittal plane deformity, which can progress with time. Each individual compression fracture may be stable with minimal kyphotic deformity. When combined with similar injuries at several adjacent levels, however, the summation of individual deformities may result in a significant sagittal plane imbalance with potential progression, chronic pain, and compression of neural elements.

Burst fractures by definition have axial failure of the anterior and middle columns with varying degrees of retropulsion of bone into the spinal canal. Traditionally, they are divided into stable and unstable fractures based on the integrity of the posterior column. With a loss of mechanical integrity of the anterior and middle columns, axial settling occurs through the fractured vertebral body. The potential angular kyphosis is a function of the relative comminution of the involved vertebral body and the integrity of the posterior osteoligamentous complex. Severe comminution of the vertebral body may progress into problematic kyphosis irrespective of the integrity of the posterior soft tissue elements. The same is also true for burst fractures that occur over several adjacent levels. Any given level may be moderately involved, however, when combined with similar injuries at adjacent levels, a significant deformity may result. If the posterior ligamentous structures remain intact, potential for problematic deformity is considerably less. The fractured vertebral body may settle somewhat as the patient is mobilized. Burst fractures settle 5° to 10° then stabilize from restraints in the posterior ligaments. Such fractures would likely heal leaving rigid kyphotic deformity that may be mild and well tolerated by the patient. The same injury combined with a severe posterior ligamentous disruption, could progress into extreme kyphosis if improperly treated.[7,8]

Seat belt injuries result from failure of all three columns in distraction. As a result of a lap belt in a motor vehicle accident, the fulcrum or axis of rotation is located anterior to the spine. Tissues fail from posterior to anterior starting with the spinous process or interspinous ligament. It then proceeds through the lamina, pedicles, and vertebral body or disk. Failure can occur through bone, soft tissue, or a combination of the two. There may be very little initial sagittal plane deformity, and initial plain radiographs may fail to show a fracture. Irrespective of injury pattern, these injuries are acutely unstable with a potential for progressive kyphosis if improperly treated. A pure osseous injury heals predictably if held reduced for an appropriate period of time; however, a pure ligamentous disruption may heal incompletely with scar tissue that is incapable of withstanding the high tensile loads generated within the posterior osteoligamentous complex. Despite aggressive bracing, the spine may be unstable to progressive angular kyphosis over time. Pure soft-tissue, seat-belt injuries are best treated with short segment posterior compression instrumentation. Distraction systems only worsen the deformity and fail to resist the forces propagating the deformity.

Flexion-distraction injuries are potentially unstable injuries with compression failure of the anterior column and tensile failure of the posterior column. The middle column remains intact and acts as a fulcrum. Failure to recognize injury to the posterior column may result in a misdiagnosis of the injury as a stable compression fracture. Inappropriate treatment may fail to prevent the progression of an angular kyphosis at the fracture site.

Coronal plane deformities are far less common following trauma. Denis burst fractures of type E, by definition have lateral compression on the anterior-posterior radiograph and the severity of which may result in a coronal plane deformity which may progress without proper treatment.[7] The injury with the greatest potential for multiplaner instability is the fracture dislocation. Fracture dislocations are highly unstable injuries resulting from any one or more likely a combination of axial loading, shear, or distractive forces. The initial recumbent radiographs may be misleading as spontaneous reduction of the dislocated or subluxed elements may have occurred. As with compression and burst fractures, a cursory review of the imaging studies may underestimate the degree of spinal instability. These injuries are extremely unstable and prone to severe angular deformities in all three planes. Patients with these types of injuries are often neurologically compromised and uniformly require posterior reduction, segmental fixation, and fusion. Fusion should extend over several motion segments above and below the fracture to stabilize the spine to a degree to allow for safe early mobilization without excessive bracing. Attempts at nonoperative treatment often fail to prevent a late deformity. In addition, pure posterior distraction or short-segment rod and hook constructs also are likely to fail.

Isolated anterior procedures in treatment of fracture dislocations also are prone to failure. The extreme instability can lead to failure or displacement of the anterior graft. An isolated anterior procedure with or without instrumentation may fail to stabilize the spine to allow for the safe early mobilization important to the recovery of these patients. Highly aggressive and extended bracing in the neurologically compromised patient is poorly tolerated. Prolonged bedrest, bracing, or anterior instrumentation may improve the chances for a successful arthrodesis; however, the zone of injury can extend over several adjacent motion segments allowing for a possible junctional deformity, despite a successful anterior arthrodesis. The failures resulting from isolated anterior procedures in the treatment of fracture dislocations can result in combined sagittal or coronal plane deformities.

Charcot arthropathy of the spine following a fracture with spinal cord injury (SCI) is a rare but additional source of late deformity. Angular deformities can develop in both the coronal and sagittal planes. The deformity generally develops below the level of SCT. Charcot changes are rare for fractures above the thoracolumbar junction. The essential feature is a loss of deep sensation in the spine below the level of a complete neurologic deficit. Initial changes are subtle and include facet joint enlargement, effusions, and thinning of the cartilage. Ligamentous laxity and subchondral fractures combine to produce disk degeneration with endplate sclerosis and spur formation. Progression occurs with gross subluxation of the vertebrae and formation of large hypertrophic osteophytes. There is often extensive heterotopic bone formation in the paravertebral tissues with a "parrot beak" appearance at the site of maximal instability.[9] A large pseudarthrosis develops with a possible ball-and-socket appearance of the spine on plain radiographs. The presence of a prior laminectomy may predispose and accelerate the entire process over a 1- or 2-year period of time.[10] Figure 21-1 shows the anterior and lateral radiographs of a 39-year-old paraplegic male 5 years after a T12 burst fracture, which left him neurologically complete. He was initially treated with distraction instrumentation using Edward rods and sleeves. Acceptable reduction was achieved and a solid arthrodesis was gained. As a result of his neurologic injury, however, he developed classic neuropathic changes between L3 and L4. He had centralized back pain and declining sitting balance. The progressive deformity proved problematic, necessitating surgical intervention.

In addition to mechanical failure of the vertebral body and posterior ligamentous complex, relative

A 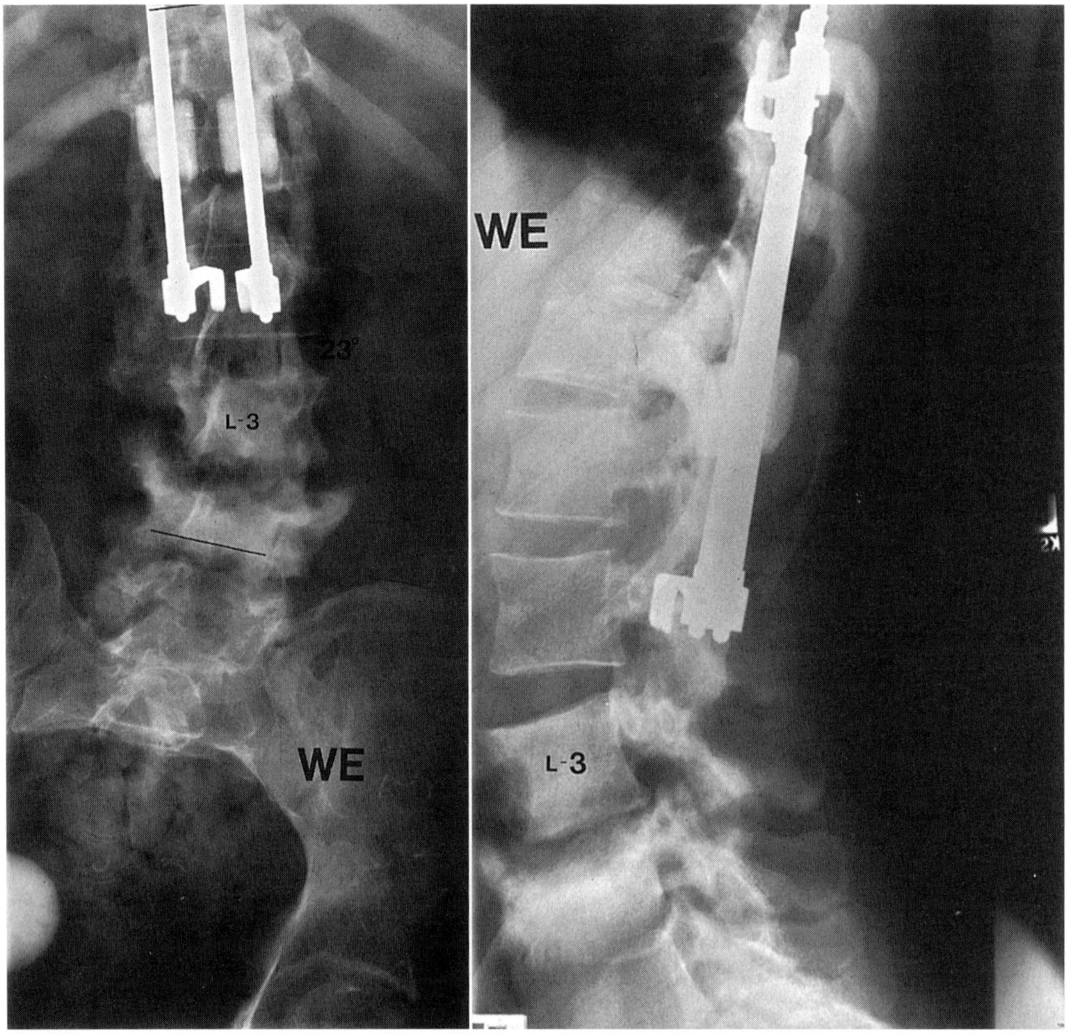 B

FIGURE 21-1

Anterior **A** and lateral **B** lumbar radiographs of a 39-year-old paraplegic male 5 years after a T12 burst fracture. He presented with back pain and declining sitting balance. Radiographs show a deformity at the L3-L4 level from instability consistent with a neuropathic spinal arthropathy.

integrity of adjacent disk spaces may also contribute to a progressive kyphosis. Burst fractures may extend into either or both adjacent disk spaces. Extension of the fracture into adjacent disk may disrupt the internal architecture, leaving it susceptible to collapse with application of physiologic loads; therefore, the relative kyphosis measured on initial supine radiographs may be underestimated. Intervertebral disk within the lumbar spine are larger and assume more of a role in the spinal alignment than disk in other areas of the spine. Andreychik and coworkers[11] attributed an increase in postoperative kyphosis without an increase in the percentage of vertebral body compression to structural failure of adjacent disk spaces resulting from the original injury. In addition, late degenerative disk collapse adjacent to or below a deformity can result in further sagittal imbalance and progression. As deformity progresses, additional disks can degenerate, adding on to the deformity further escalating deforming forces. Late secondary effects also include insufficiency fractures from osteoporosis and the compressive forces generated by a fixed sagittal imbalance.

Experts are still in disagreement regarding surgery in treating acute fractures to the thoracic and lumbar spine.[2,7,8,12,13,14] In addition, considerable variability exits in selecting anterior, posterior, or combined surgical approach. The goal of the initial treatment is to restore normal alignment to the unstable spine with internal or external support for such a period allowing for restoration of spinal stability through natural healing or surgical arthrodesis. Failure to gain adequate correction before initiating some form of external support results in a deformity that may progress or become symptomatic. Bedrest, hyperextension casting, and bracing are effective strategies in the management of unstable spine fractures; however, successful nonoperative treatment requires proper patient selection, fitting, and compliance with the appropriate device. Acute injuries with large deformities, poor potential for healing, severe canal compromise, and marked instability are prone to late deformity with nonoperative treatment. An additional source of late deformity is failure to appropriately monitor for progression following bedrest, bracing, or surgery. Early and frequent standing lateral radiographs are essential when the patient is mobilized into an upright or sitting posture. Views must be repeated at regular intervals to guard against progression. Otherwise, an opportunity could be missed to intervene with a more effective treatment program when the deformity remains flexible or moderate in size.

There are several potential errors in executing the surgical treatment of acute spine fractures that can predispose the patient to treatment failure and late deformity. Failure to adhere to biomechanical principles in the selection and application of anterior and posterior instrumentation systems has led to sagittal or coronal plane imbalance. In addition, postoperative complications in the form of infection or instrumentation failure can also account for late failure even with proper surgical techniques.

The disastrous effects of isolated laminectomies for neural element decompression in the management of acute spinal fractures is well documented. Isolated laminectomies without instrumentation and fusion further destabilize the spine resulting in severe angulation and worsening compression of the neural elements. A malignant kyphosis has been described with angular deformities exceeding 90° and complete spondyloptosis at the fracture site.[15] Malcolm and coworkers[1] reported on 48 patients with posttraumatic kyphosis. Half the patients had an isolated laminectomy with the original injury. The detrimental effects of isolated laminectomy was confirmed at all levels of the spine. At the thoracic level, resulting kyphosis was 15° higher for patients with isolated laminectomies compared to those without laminectomy. At the thoracolumbar junction, kyphosis was 54° and 41°, respectively, when 16 patients who had laminectomies alone were compared with the 13 patients who had not. The difference in kyphosis for patients who had or had not had laminectomies was 35° and 24° in the lumbar spine, respectively. Fortunately, greater recognition of the detrimental effects of isolated laminectomies in the treatment of neural deficits following trauma have led to fewer cases of acute fractures being treated in this way.

There are a number of potential pitfalls in the technical application of posterior instrumentation constructs, which can result in late deformity. Factors resulting in failure include a fusion that is too short. If the zone of injury extends beyond the intended arthrodesis, a junctional deformity can develop despite a successful fusion. This is especially true if the fusion ends at the apex of the normal thoracic kyphosis or an existing premorbid deformity. In addition, failure to gain correction of a kyphotic deformity with the instrumentation leaves the spine unbalanced and places the posterior bone graft in tension. This predisposes the patient to pseudarthrosis with hardware failure, chronic pain, and probable progression. If a solid arthrodesis is gained, the fixed spinal imbalance can still prove to be debilitating from chronic pain, progression, and compression of the neural elements. Additionally, short-segment posterior constructs lack the mechanical forces to fully realign the spine. When applied in the face of severe anterior comminution, short-segment constructs (i.e., one level above and one level below) are especially prone to failure. Such applications, often intended to preserve lumbar motion segments, require an anterior procedure to reestablish the anterior column with a structural graft.

Additional technical errors in posterior instrumentation systems include the application of distraction systems to unstable fractures in the lumbar spine. This is shown by late failures of Harrington instrumentation systems in the lumbar spine. Application of distraction forces to lumbar motion segments below L3 has resulted in the loss of normal lumbar lordosis. Although a solid arthrodesis often was achieved, the flat-back deformity has proved to be problematic.[16,17] Patients often would develop chronic pain from the muscular strain when attempting to maintain their sagittal balance. In addition, degenerative spondylosis and stenosis develop at the adjacent motion segments forced to hyperextend in response to the fixed deformity.

These patterns of deformity underscore a basic biomechanical principle of spinal stability. The preservation of spinal alignment necessitates a sound anterior column for load sharing and a functional posterior ligamentous complex functioning as a tension band. The foundation for proper treatment of destabilizing injuries to the spine is an accurate anatomic diagnosis of the fracture pattern. Understanding natural history of the injury anatomy permits proper treatment planning. Treatment algorithms that either positively or negatively affect the natural history can be initiated or avoided, respectively.

PATIENT EVALUATION

Patients presenting with a fixed or progressive spinal deformity are easily recognized by their posture and often incapacitating symptoms. This is especially true in patients injured from motor vehicle accidents, falls, or recreational sports. The preponderance of male patients reflects the higher incidence of spine trauma in men. The age at the time of reconstructive surgery is generally between 35 and 45 years. Roberson and Whiteside[6] found an average age of 37 in their series. Kostuik and Matsusaki[18] reported a mean age of 42 in their series of 37 patients. Individuals generally have debilitating pain, progression of their deformity, or persistent or new neurologic deficits.

The symptoms may be insidious in onset following a pain-free period, but often escalate to a level to produce a state of complete disability. As many as 70% to 90% of patients who have suffered a fracture to the thoracic or lumbar spine experience chronic pain at the level of the fracture no matter what the treatment or deformity. As many as 40% are limited in their function and 20% may be disabled.[7,13,19,20] With fixed deformity, patients can experience rapid decline in function and often present within the first 2 or 3 years after the injury. Malcolm and coworkers[1] reported a mean of 33 months from injury to reconstructive surgery. Kostuik and Matsusaki[18] reported a mean of 4.2 years in their 57 patients. Debilitating pain, generally categorized as mechanical or neurologic, is often the presenting symptom and leading indication for reconstructive surgery. It is important to differentiate among potential sources of pain, as the relative success of any surgical procedure likely hinges on the impact it has in relieving the patient's discomfort. Individuals with residual complete or incomplete neurologic deficits, however, are often less symptomatic. Isolating the source of pain benefits the surgical planning and improve the chances for success in relieving the symptoms. Doing so, however, can prove to be a challenge.

Rarely is there only a single source to account for the full constellation of symptoms in patients with a fixed spinal deformity. Significant insight can be gained by first localizing the site of the discomfort relative to the fracture deformity. Pain that occurs over the apex can have several sources. Persistent instability or fracture nonunion produces a localized aching pain over the apex that radiates out into the flanks, buttocks, or thighs. Instability was present as a symptom in 36% of patients in the series by Malcolm and coworkers.[1] Symptoms from local instability are more likely with a prior laminectomy, pseudarthrosis, or Charcot arthropathy.[10] Patients reported inability to control their trunk with flexion and painful crepitation with flexion and extension. With existing instrumentation, similar pain also could represent infection, pseudarthrosis, or pain relating directly to the hardware. In all these cases, the pain is often mechanical in nature with variable relief following rest.

Centralized mechanical pain above and below the deformity may be related to degenerative disk or facet arthrosis at adjacent levels. The deformity produces compensatory loads at adjacent motion segments leading to degeneration of the facets. Disk space collapse can occur along with the facet arthrosis producing lateral recess stenosis and symptoms of dynamic neurogenic claudication. In addition, compression fractures also can occur through the involved or adjacent levels as a result of the large flexion moment generated by the deformity and shift in the mechanical axis. Regional pain may result from pressure directly on the spinal cord or exiting nerve roots. The potential for neural compression is a function of the relative deformity and residual retropulsed bone within the canal.

A separate pattern of symptoms occurs in patients with significant sagittal or coronal imbalance, which is worth distinguishing from the more apical sources described earlier. Patients with significant sagittal imbalance often develop a sensation of chronic fatigue, pain, and spasms diffusely in the lumbar musculature when assuming an upright posture. This discomfort worsens throughout the day, but unlike the discomfort already described, consistent relief will generally be gained with recumbency. Paraspinal muscles undergo chronic fatigue from constant load of overcoming the sagittal deformity to maintain an upright posture and horizontal gaze.

There is conflicting data correlating the severity of kyphosis and the presence of chronic back pain. Kyphosis in the thoracic spine, however, is better tolerated than a similar curve at the thoracolumbar junction or lumbar spine. Farcy identified a threshold of 25° for probable symptoms at the thoracolumbar junction and 15° for the lumbar spine.[21] The lumbar spine tolerates less deformity as there are fewer motion segments available to help compensate for the deformity. Andreychik and coworkers[11] in their review of 55 burst fractures from L2 to L5, however, found no relationship between the magnitude of kyphosis and pain scores. Malcolm and coworkers reported similar observations to Farcy.[21] Subjective pain, therefore, is likely be a function of magnitude and location of deformity and the lifestyle of the patient. Heavy laborers or individuals who place greater demands on their back do not tolerate a given deformity as well as more sedentary individuals.

In addition to pain, patients also experience progression of deformity. The neurologically compromised patient often has less pain and is more likely to have complaints relating to a progressive deformity.[22] In the paraplegic patient, progression of deformity results in diminished sitting balance. Altered sitting balance interferes with arm swing and powering the wheelchair. Skin breakdown can occur over a gibbous deformity or bony prominence, such as the greater trochanter or ischial tuberosity. Progressive kyphosis pitches them forward in their chair, obligating their arms and hands to support the head and shoulders rather than performing necessary tasks. Patients with a neuropathic spine may develop an obstructive uropathy from compression of the ureters by hypertrophic bone formation in the paravertebral soft tissues. In the neurologically incomplete patient with weakness in the trunk and lower extremities, subtle progression of a deformity can overwhelm the compromised motor function to a degree that there is a decline in their ambulatory function. Patients also notice a decrease in height, change in posture, or alteration in how clothing fits.

In the series of 48 patients by Malcolm and coworkers[1] presenting signs and symptoms were pain in 94%, progression of kyphosis in 46%, and increasing neural deficits in 27%. A progressive angular kyphosis may result in new neurologic deficit or failure of an existing incomplete lesion to improve. Compression of neural elements within the canal is a function of angular kyphosis and retropulsed bone from the original injury. Both factors combine to drape the spinal cord or cauda equina over a rigid deformity. Retropulsed bone fragments have been shown to resorb with time.[23,24] Presence of an angular deformity with significant stresses directed across the deformity, however, may alter remodeling potential. In addition, segmental instability may result in hypertrophic changes within the end plates and facets at the level of the fracture, contributing to the relative stenosis within the canal.[10] Posttraumatic syrinx also can contribute to local compression with early decline or a failure to improve. Compensatory hyperextension of adjacent motion segments above or below the deformity can overload the facets with secondary spondylosis.

The nature of the neurologic deficit depends on the level of deformity. The spinal cord generally ends at the L1 and L2 disk space in most adults. Above the conus, upper motor neuron changes predominate. These would include long tract signs of diminished sensation and strength in the lower extremities with increasing spasticity. Bowel and bladder control can be compromised by lesions at any level. A postvoid residual or urodynamic studies may detect subtle changes in bladder function that are still unrecognized clinically. A change in bowel or bladder control is often the presenting complaint with compression at the level of the conus (T12–L1); however, a mixture of upper and motor neuron findings also may be present. Below L2, lower motor neuron changes predominate from pressure on the cauda equina with hyporeflexia, radiating pain, weakness, and sensory deficits within the lower extremities.

In addition to pain, progression, or neurologic dysfunction, other subjective complaints include pulmonary dysfunction and escalating fatigability. Patients report poor endurance with walking because of fatigue, shortness of breath, or leg weakness. They experience weight gain from the progressively sedentary lifestyle. A careful history helps differentiate among sources of pain and loss of function; however, preoperative evaluation and surgical planning also necessitate judicious use of diagnostic modalities including magnetic resonance imaging (MRI), computed tomography (CT), tomograms, dynamic plain radiographs, diskograms, and diagnostic injections and blocks.

Magnetic resonance imaging is a noninvasive means to image vertebral bodies for fractures, infection, and retropulsed fragments. It outlines the contour of the spinal canal to help define neural element compression. An MRI scan cannot be taken in the region of metal implants other than titanium. In addition, intervertebral disk are effectively imaged by MRI for signs of herniation or excessive degeneration at or adjacent to the level of fracture. Posttraumatic spinal cord deformation, spinal cord atrophy, or intramedulary syrinx also can be detected.

Computed axial tomography provides the most detailed imaging of injury patterns and quality of bone. When combined with myelography, CT can help define neural element compression when metal implants preclude the use of MRI. Bone quality within the body and pedicles obtained from the CT scan can prove beneficial in planning strategies for instrumentation. Tomograms may help in detecting pseudarthrosis or bony bridges and in planning spinal osteotomies. Technetium scans may detect signs of an infection or pseudarthrosis. Dynamic flexion and extension radiographs identify potential segmental instability. Diskography or selective blocks of nerve roots or facet joints adjacent to or at the level of the fracture also may help localize the source of pain and plan the surgical procedure. In cases in which pain was not clearly localized to the apex of the deformity, Kostuik and Matsusaki[18] performed diskograms in 17 of the 37 cases of posttraumatic kyphosis. Twelve of the 17 cases had positive findings at the level just caudal to the fracture whereas five cases had positive findings more than two levels below. They also report on success of regional facet blocks in localizing the source of pain in nonrevision cases.

Deformities are often complex with three-dimensional changes in the sagittal, coronal, and axial planes. In addition to the individual planer deformity, the relative balance of the spine also should be assessed, specifically, any truncal shift or translation of C7 with respect to S1. The spinous process of C7 should line up with S1 in the coronal image, and the body of C7 should be centered over the sacrum on the lateral image. The importance of the standing anterior-posterior and lateral long cassette radiographs cannot be overemphasized. Any sagittal or coronal deformity or imbalance should be assessed for flexibility with bending films and noted to be at, above, or below the level of the fixed deformity. Axial rotation is assessed at the apical vertebrae and may account for a rib prominence with significant cosmetic changes to the posterior chest. Lateral flexion and extension radiographs or supine lateral images using a bolster over the apex of the deformity assesses kyphosis for flexibility.

With the more common fixed sagittal deformity,

the patient is forced to hyperextend the motion segment above and below to maintain a horizontal gaze. If the spine lacks the mobility to overcome an advance angular kyphosis, a crouch gait develops. With time, hip flexion contractures develop. Severe hip flexion contractures may necessitate treatment before reconstructive surgery on the spine.

Coronal plane deformities are far less common following trauma but are potentially problematic. They often are combined with sagittal plane deformities making reconstruction more complicated. They also can progress producing truncal shift, chronic pain, and degenerative changes above and below the deformity. Pulmonary dysfunction can occur with advanced thoracic level coronal plane deformities; however, the deformity would have to be quit large and combined with late intrinsic chronic obstructive lung disease. Pure sagittal deformities in the thoracic spine are less likely to produce pulmonary dysfunction. The kyphosis generally expands the volume of chest cavity; however, lumbar kyphotic deformities with significant thoracic compensatory lordosis can significantly restrict residual lung volumes.

CLASSIFICATION

Denis and Burkus[25] outlined a system for classifying posttraumatic deformity based on the region of the spine involved, the neurologic status, and the presence of any deformity outside the region of the local kyphosis. They proposed three types with each type having three subtypes. This classification system proved beneficial to the authors in planning the surgical approach, type of instrumentation, and fusion techniques; however, it does not take into consideration the relative size of the angular deformity.

Type I deformities involve the thoracic spine above T11. Type I-A are without neurologic deficit and have no regional increase in kyphosis outside the local deformity. Type I-B are also neurologically intact but have an increased regional kyphosis as well. Type I-C have some neurologic deficit.

Type II deformities have the principle deformity at the thoracolumbar junction between T12 and L1. Type II-A have no adjacent thoracic kyphosis and no neurologic deficits. Type II-B deformities have an increase in the adjacent thoracic kyphosis and no neurologic deficit. Type III-C deformities have a neurologic deficit.

Type III deformities are in the lumbar spine from L2 to L4. These lesions may not have true measurable kyphosis but a relative loss of normal lumbar lordosis, which proves problematic. Type III-A are neurologically intact with local kyphosis or loss of lordosis only. Type III-B deformities have no neurologic deficits yet have an increased regional kyphosis. Type III-C deformities have a neurologic deficit.

TREATMENT

NONOPERATIVE

Nonsurgical treatment is appropriate for patients with mild deformities, minimal complaints, or if the patient is not a candidate to undergo a complex reconstructive procedure. Surgical correction of complex deformities necessitates a realistic appraisal of the physical, financial, social, and psychologic well-being of the patient. In addition, technical demands of the procedure should match the expertise of the available surgeon.[26]

The use of pain medication can be beneficial in the short-term to control symptoms but may prove problematic in the long-run. Use of narcotics for chronic pain conditions should be strongly discouraged. Extended use of nonsteroidal antiinflammatory drugs (NSAIDs) can have serious complications of renal insufficiency and gastrointestinal bleeding. Localized blocks offer temporary improvement but rarely provide any sustained symptomatic relief.

Bracing with a thoracic-lumbar-sacral orthosis (TLSO) may help delay or arrest progression of a deformity and improve apical pain. For pure sagittal plane deformity with instability in a single plane, a low-profile Jewitt brace may help control symptoms; however, deformities with instability in several planes require the more rigid TLSO. In addition, exercise programs that strengthen the musculature of the back may improve the endurance and fatigue pain to some degree; however, complete resolution of symptoms or stabilization of significant deformity is unlikely with nonoperative treatment.

SURGICAL INDICATIONS AND GOALS

Indications for surgical reconstruction in the patient with late deformity following spinal trauma include progression of the angular deformity. In addition, incapacitating pain attributable to deformity, segmental instability, pseudarthrosis, or adjacent spondylosis also can benefit from surgery. The final indication is a new or progressive neurologic deficit. Patients with incomplete neurologic deficits with significant residual neural compression have shown consistent improvement following delayed decompression in several reported series.[1,6,18,27] Thus, failure of an incomplete neurologic deficit to improve with residual neural compression warrants strong consideration for decompression and stabilization. Cosmetic concerns may contribute to a decision to pursue a reconstructive procedure; however, the potential for serious complications must be carefully considered before undertaking a procedure for this reason.

Goals of surgery are to reestablish a functional anterior and posterior column. A reduction in the angular deformity should occur with a restoration of spinal alignment and balance. Immediate stability should be gained to allow for early mobilization of the patient and promote a solid arthrodesis. Significant compression of neural element should be decompressed when a neurologic deficit exists. Finally, an attempt should be made to preserve motion segments whenever possible.

Factors to Consider

The principle factors in planning the surgical approach are location and size of the deformity and presence of a neurologic defect requiring decompression. The surgical strategies described below reflect the bias of the senior author to use the anterior approaches to improve correction, restore the anterior column, and decompress neural elements. Edwards, however, has developed surgical strategies for correcting late posttraumatic deformity almost exclusively through a posterior procedure.[12] This technique relies on viscoelastic stress relaxation of the contracted ligaments, callus, and scar. Three-point loading is applied with posterior hooks, rods, and sleeves. The sleeve size is sequentially increased until correction is gained. Gentle compression is applied following the realignment to further promote fusion. Success has been achieved with angular deformities in excess of 30° and as late as 10 years after the acute fracture. Patients with an anterior bony bridge necessitate limited release of the bar than posterior viscoelastic extension of the deformity.

Posterior instrumentation used in the treatment of kyphotic deformity is generally a compression construct. Multiple claws are employed across the apex to shorten the posterior column. As kyphosis is reduced, some limited anterior indirect decompression of the cord or roots can occur. Anterior procedures target neural compression directly and restore mechanical integrity of the anterior column through structural grafting. In addition, the key element in the anterior release for any kyphotic deformity is complete division of the anterior longitudinal ligament. Failure to do so, may compromise potential correction gained with the procedure.

In the neurologically complete patient with a fixed deformity, aggressive posterior reconstruction can be attempted with long segmental instrumentation and corrective osteotomies when needed. Anterior release and grafting can improve correction with large rigid coronal or sagittal plane deformities. Combined procedures also improve the rate of fusion with revision cases.

The presence of an existing pseudarthrosis and hardware often dictates the initial approach. Pure pseudarthrosis not requiring significant correction usually responds to compression instrumentation alone in the thoracic spine. The lumbar spine, however, usually requires an anterior and posterior procedure when revising for pseudarthrosis. Failed instrumentation and fusions, which remain rigid and in need of significant correction, often necessitate hardware removal with combined anterior and posterior osteotomies. It is also important to consider the possibility of an indolent infection as a source of failure and pseudarthrosis. If the preoperative work-up remains equivocal, tissue or fluid suspicious for infection at the time of hardware removal should prompt an intraoperative Gram stain and frozen section. Bacteria or neutrophils in excess of five per high-powered field should warrant strong consideration for hardware removal and staging the reinstrumentation following an extended period of appropriate antibiotics.

Indolent infection as a source of failure and pain is uncommon in nonrevision cases. One exception is the patient presenting with late deformity as a result of a gunshot injury. If the projectile penetrated the colon, failure to perform a formal irrigation and debridement with extended antibiotic therapy may result in chronic osteomyelitis of the spine. Romanick reviewed 20 patients treated with laparotomy for penetrating trauma. None received spinal irrigation and debridement or antibiotic therapy beyond 2 days. Sepsis was a complication in each of seven patients in which the colon was perforated. No infections occurred in those cases where the colon remained unviolated.[28]

Use of preoperative traction for posttraumatic deformity is rarely indicated. Late deformities following trauma are generally rigid. Longitudinal traction with rigid deformities is contraindicated. Applying traction across a rigid deformity can tension the neural tissue within the canal. Doing so at the level of a rigid angular deformity increases spinal cord or cauda equina compression and results in neurologic deterioration.

Additional factors that warrant consideration include the age and general health of the patient. There are significant risks from the prolonged anesthesia with potential hypotension. There is a potential for significant blood loss. Most patients should undergo preoperative autologous blood donation. Nutritional analysis also should be done to assess the need for a staged procedure and parenteral nutritional support. Patients with prior laminectomies may require an anterior and posterior procedure to improve the fusion rate. Consideration also should be given to combined anterior and posterior procedures for revision surgery, fusion to the pelvis, and long lumbar fusions. Spinal cord monitoring with a wake-up test should be used. Availability of autologous bone in revision cases warrants consideration for use of allograft bone or bone substitutes. Consideration also should be given to the potential need for custom implants.

OPERATIVE TREATMENT

THORACIC LEVEL DEFORMITIES (T2 TO T11)

For type I-A angular kyphotic deformities less than 15° with persistent apical pain or signs of progression warranting surgery, a posterior spinal fusion is indicated. If the sagittal balance of the spine is unaffected and there is no compensatory pain other than apical discomfort, a short posterior compression instrumentation and fusion suffices. Two factors may warrant a long posterior fusion. If the sagittal balance is compromised from excessive thoracic level kyphosis in addition to the mild angular kyphosis (type I-B), a long posterior compression instrumentation and fusion rebalances the spine and prevents compensatory lumbar hyperlordosis in most cases. In addition, in cases where there is a neurologic deficit and mild compression of the spinal cord over the angular deformity (type I-C), a long posterior compression instrumentation and fusion is indicated. The compression instrumentation with a multiple claw construct shortens the posterior column allowing for an indirect reduction as the cord migrates posteriorly. The canal can be imaged postoperatively to ensure decompression. Failure to achieve a complete decompression would necessitate a second-stage anterior procedure to decompress the canal and place a structural graft. With moderate or severe cord compression from retropulsed bone, indirect reduction is no longer indicated and a primary anterior procedure should be performed. A subsequent posterior fusion would than be indicated based on the use of anterior instrumentation, choice of graft, integrity of the posterior column, and the residual thoracic kyphosis. No matter what the approach, the goal is 40° or less of thoracic kyphosis from T2 to T12 following the reconstruction.

Short angular deformities with an apex above T11 which are larger than 15° to 20°, are potentially more complex. Again, the goal is a balanced spine with 40° or less of thoracic kyphosis. This improves the rate of fusion, helps control local symptoms, prevents adjacent degenerative changes, and eliminates the need for compensatory hyperlordosis and its ill effects. If the hyperextension lateral of the thoracic spine over a bolster reduces the total thoracic kyphosis to less than 50°, a long posterior compression instrumentation and fusion is indicated, regardless of the size of the fracture kyphosis. If there is cord compression, however, indirect reduction is unlikely with larger kyphotic deformities. This usually necessitates a primary anterior procedure to decompress the spinal cord directly and place a structural graft. If there is marginal correction of kyphosis during the anterior procedure or kyphotic changes adjacent to the short angular kyphosis on the preoperative lateral radiograph, an anterior release should be added and a second stage posterior instrumentation and fusion should be performed. The length of the posterior fusion is a function of the need for additional correction to reduce total thoracic kyphosis to 50°. A short construct suffices if the anterior procedure was successful in gaining correction yet some additional stability is necessary to allow for early mobility or obviate need for anterior instrumentation.

For very large angular kyphotic deformities above T11, complete anterior release with local cord decompression followed by a posterior compression construct of the thoracic spine may not gain adequate correction. The goal remains sagittal balance to allow for horizontal gaze. If a combined anterior and posterior procedure of the thoracic spine alone fails to gain correction necessary to do so, the posterior procedure should be extended into the lumbar spine. An eggshell decancellation procedure should be performed at L2 provided the preoperative MRI confirms the conus ends as the L1 and L2 disk space. The thoracic claw construct should extend down to lumbar segments where pedicle screw fixation is used. Fusion often extends to the L4 level. This leaves two motion segments open in the lumbar spine. Lumbar lordosis must be preserved during the instrumentation process. L3 is a guide to the rod bend in planning the apex of the induced lordosis. Anterior structural allografts also may be necessary to help restore lordosis. Preexisting spondylosis or segmental instability between L4 and the sacrum are always considerations in choosing levels for fusion. In addition, preoperative assessment of the hips for fixed contractures is essential when planning the correction of fixed sagittal plane deformities.

THORACOLUMBAR JUNCTION (T12 TO L2)

With small deformities, less than 15° to 20°, in which there is no neurologic deficit and a normal contour to the thoracic spine (40°) adjacent to it (type II-A), a posterior instrumentation or fusion can be performed when attempting to preserve lumbar motion segments. Indications for surgery include apical pain, pseudarthrosis, or progression. If there is neurologic deficit with residual canal compression in excess of 25% (type II-C), an anterior procedure is indicated. Direct decompression is performed and a structural graft is placed. A second-stage posterior procedure can be added if there is residual posterior column instability and a reluctance to use anterior instrumentation or prolonged bedrest.

Significantly larger angular deformities at the thoracolumbar junction require careful evaluation of symptoms and the relative alignment and balance of the thoracic spine. With significant thoracic kyphosis in addition to the local angular kyphosis (type II-B), the thoracic level deformity also must be addressed. The goal is always balanced correction with thoracic kyphosis of less than 50° from T2 across the thoracolumbar junction. If the thoracic level deformity is flexible above the fixed deformity at the thoracolumbar junction, a limited anterior release and decompression can be done with a structural anterior graft. This is followed by a second-stage posterior instrumentation and fusion incorporating the thoracic spine and the thoracolumbar junction (Fig. 21-2). The addition of structural grafts at the thoracolumbar junction may allow for preservation of lumbar motion segments. Again, we prefer pedicle screws in the lumbar spine. If the upper thoracic level deformity is rigid, a more extensive anterior release of the thoracic spine is required in addition to the neural decompression and local release. This may require apposing incisions to fully accomplish both tasks.

For complex three-dimensional deformities, surgical strategies are directed at restoring balance to the spine. Pure coronal deformity can be treated with a posterior instrumentation and fusion if adjacent segments are flexible. Osteotomies can be performed through an existing fusion mass to augment correction. With large deformities, revisions, or stiff adjacent motion segments and decompensation, combined anterior and posterior procedures should be considered. For highly complex deformities, apical vertebrectomy may be indicated.[29] Hardware removal, osteotomies, and reinstrumentation with segmental fixation offers the best chance for restoring balance and securing an arthrodesis in these complicated cases.

Success has been reported in correcting pure sagittal deformities at the thoracolumbar junction with an isolated anterior procedure using femoral neck allograft and vascularized rib strut grafts. McBride and Bradford[30] reported on their technique of treating posttraumatic kyphosis associated with a neurologic deficit. They treated six patients with a mean angular kyphosis of 38° (range, 20° to 83°) and canal encroachment ranging from 25% to 57%. All patients but one had a neurologic deficit. All deformities were at the thoracolumbar junction between T12 and L1. The time since the original injury ranged from 0.6 to 24 years. All patients were treated with thoracolumbar exposure through a tenth rib approach. The tenth rib was harvested as a vascularized pedicle graft. Vertebrectomy was performed at the site of the canal encroachment. Adjacent vertebrae were distracted and a femoral neck allograft was placed as a structural graft. The vascularized rib graft was placed within a trough cut into the lateral margin of the adjacent vertebrae and allograft. The mean postoperative correction in kyphosis was 63% or 26°. The vascularized rib graft was found to incorporate as early as 7 weeks. There were no pseudarthrosis and all neurologically incomplete patients improved. One case required early revision for graft displacement. This patient was neurologically complete and also had a wound infection and transient postoperative respiratory dysfunction. This technique necessitates a structurally sound posterior osteoligamentous complex. Marked instability requires the addition of anterior instrumentation or a second stage posterior instrumentation and fusion.

Irrespective of approach, potential pitfalls include ending a posterior construct at the apex of a thoracic kyphosis. In addition, sagittal decompensation recurs or persists with failure to use sound anterior structural grafts at the site of the angular deformity. Similarly, anterior structural grafts of femoral ring allograft or titanium implants should be used in the lumbar spine when long constructs incorporating the thoracic spine end at L4 or L5. The femoral ring allografts are packed with morselized autograft or allograft to aid incorporation. A cancellous screw with a washer placed at the margin of the femoral ring graft helps prevent early displacement. Failure to gain adequate correction is always a potential sources of late mechanical failure. Incomplete decompression of neural elements may compromise the neurologic recovery in the incomplete patient. In addition, posterior only procedures have a greater risk of under correcting any deformity.

LUMBAR SPINE (L2 TO L5)

Sagittal deformities in the lumbar spine are rarely kyphotic. They are more often a loss of normal lumbar lordosis from prior distraction instrumentation ending at L4 or L5. Although several osteotomies have been described, our preferred procedure is the eggshell decancellation procedure. This procedure shortens the spinal column with less risk of distraction to neural or vascular structures.[31,32,33] Ideally, it is performed at the apex of the deformity for maximal correction. As much as 40° of coronal deformity can be corrected through asymmetric decancellation and instrumentation. Fifty degrees of sagittal plane correction can be obtained. Segmental instrumentation with pedicle screws is used with posterolateral bone grafting.

The first spinal osteotomy for a kyphotic deformity was performed by Smith-Peterson in 1945.[34] The fulcrum lay at the anterior border of the foramina with correction through the disk space. Serious complications related to this technique prompted further investigation for effective techniques. The original eggshell decancellation procedure was described by Heinig and later popularized by Thomasen in 1983.[35] The approach is a standard posterior midline dissection with subperiosteal dissection over the intended fusion levels. Exposure is extended out to the transverse processes. Sites for pedicle fixation are identified and prepared with decortication and facetectomies. Pedicle screws

A B

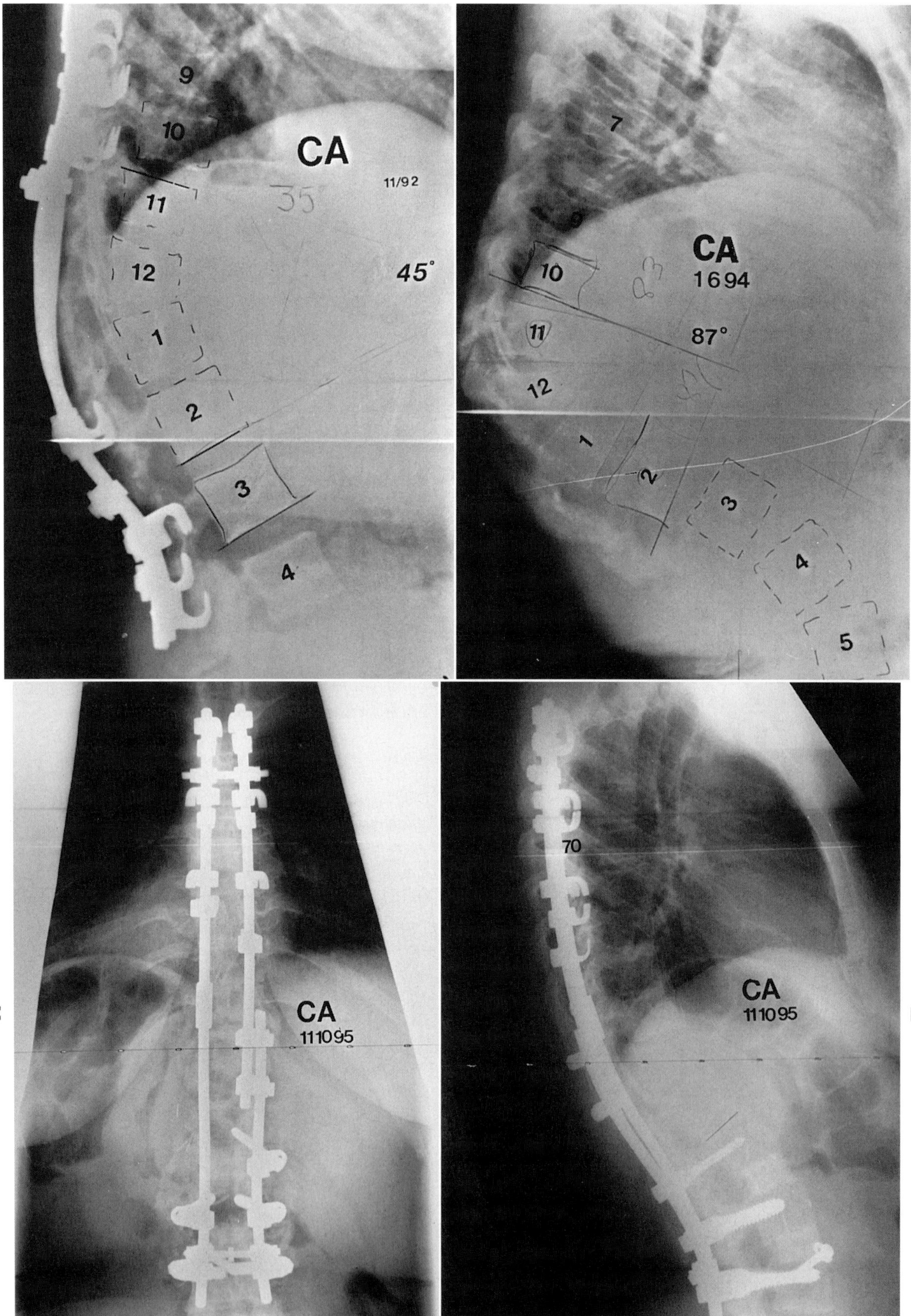

C D

Figure 21-2

For legend see opposite page.

FIGURE 21-2

A, Lateral radiograph of a 34-year-old female 10 years after an unstable T12 fracture. The T7 to L3 posterior instrumentation and fusion failed from under-correction as well as deep sepsis necessitating removal of the hardware. Despite bracing, she developed a progressive deformity at the thoracolumbar junction. **B**, Preoperative lateral radiograph showing an 87-degree angular kyphosis at the thoracolumbar junction. She was neurologically intact at the time of her revision. **C** and **D**, Postoperative anterior and posterior radiographs following a staged anterior and posterior reconstruction from T5 to L3. She underwent an anterior release with discectomies from T1 to L-3 with structural ring allografts at L1/2 and L2/3 followed by posterior osteotomies, instrumentation, and fusion. A four-rod cantilever construct was used with multiple claws above and pedicle screws below as foundations.

are placed in standard fashion two levels below and at least three levels above the intended site. Distal fixation may require extension to the pelvis with iliac screws or rods depending on the level of osteotomy and regional biomechanics at the lumbosacral junction. Proximal fixation is often supplemented with either thoracic level pedicle screws or laminar claws. The spinous process, lamina, facet, and pedicle are removed bilaterally at the intended level. The rods are sized and prebent. A four-rod construct often is used with parallel rods above and below, which are cantilevered down to close the osteotomy. With rods prepared, osteotomy is performed by drilling down through the pedicles with a high-speed burr. The dura must be retracted and free from the posterior margin of the body during decancellation. Potential for serious bleeding cannot be overemphasized. Communication between the surgeon and anesthesiologist is essential. The decancellation procedure should not be started until the patient is stable, fully volume resuscitated, and replacement blood products are readily available. In addition, proximal and distal instrumentation must be prepared and readily secured to allow expeditious closure of the osteotomy in the event of excessive bleeding. Bone wax, gel foam, and thrombin are used to control bleeding from exposed cancellous bone. The quantity of bone removed is a function of the intended correction. The osteotomy is closed with the cantilever effect and extension of the table. The rods are secured longitudinally. Nerve roots above and at the level of osteotomy share a common foramina created by the removal of the pedicle. Nerve roots and dura are carefully explored to ensure there is no bony impingement resulting from closure of the osteotomy. Autologous iliac graft is placed and generously supplemented with cancellous allograft if needed. An intraoperative lateral radiograph should ensure acceptable correction.

This procedure is effective for all type III lesions (Fig. 21-3). The posterior osteotomy, however, may necessitate an anterior procedure in cases where an extensive anterior bony bridge has developed or to improve the chances for fusion in revision cases or long constructs, which include the pelvis.

COMPLICATIONS

There are a number of potential complications, some minor, whereas others are potentially life threatening. The risk of a complication with a major reconstructive procedure can be as high as 100% in an elderly population. Medical complications include myocardial infarction, strokes, pulmonary emboli, renal insufficiency, and postoperative ileus. Deep vein thrombosis prophylaxis should be used. Pneumatic compression devices are effective in diminishing the risks of deep vein thrombosis without the risks of anticoagulation following spine surgery. Malnutrition also can occur and significantly increase the risk of infection and other complications. Use of total parenteral nutrition should be used with staged procedures or in large complex cases in which a prolonged ileus or intubation is anticipated. Patients should undergo preoperative nutritional evaluation several months prior to the anticipated surgery. Patients should be discouraged from dieting prior to the procedure and the procedure postponed if they demonstrate evidence of malnutrition during the preliminary evaluation.

Anterior thoracic spinal surgery can be complicated by chylothorax as a result of an injury to the thoracic duct. The patient may have a persistent pleural effusion, hemothorax, or pneumothorax in the postoperative recovery period. The diaphragm can dehisce or undergo delayed rupture following a thoracoabdominal exposure. The ureters and viscera are susceptible in retroperitoneal dissections as are segmental and great vessels. This is especially true with revision anterior lumbar exposures. In addition, risk of retrograde ejaculation exists with dissection over the anterior spine at the lumbosacral junction.

Ophthalmic complications can be devastating and irreversible. Ischemic optic neuritis has been associated with direct pressure on the globes, hypotension, air emboli, and prolonged surgery. The risk of dural tears and cerebral spinal fluid leaks are higher in revision cases.[36] Neural injury from direct or indirect forces to the spinal cord or nerve roots may result in motor paralysis, sensory deficits, chronic pain, or loss of bowel or bladder control.[37] Spinal cord monitoring should be used if available along with a Stagnara wake-up test. A motor electrode can be placed into the epidural space during the procedure to gain additional information when somatosensory evoked potentials are equivocal.

Excessive blood loss can be life threatening and a covariable with many other potential complications.

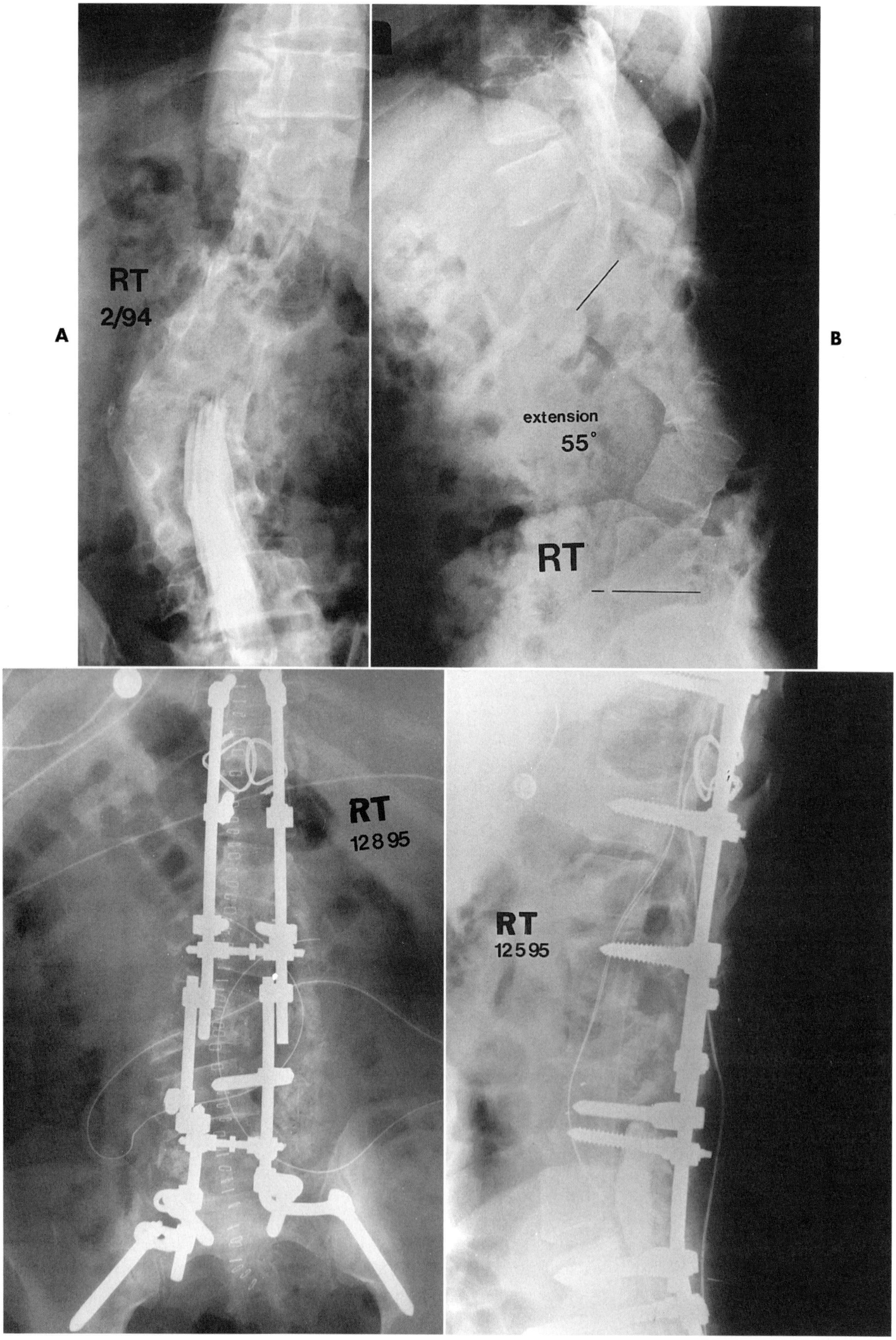

Figure 21-3

For legend see opposite page.

FIGURE 21-3

A, Preoperative AP and **B**, lateral radiographs of a 37-year-old male 20 years after a destabilizing lumbar spine fracture. He presented with increasing pain, weakness in his lower extremities, and a progressive deformity. He had 38° of scoliosis and 90° of kyphosis which corrected to 55° on hyperextension. A posterior instrumentation and fusion was undertaken utilizing an eggshell decancellation osteotomy at L3. Postoperative **(C)** AP and **(D)** lateral radiographs showing the substantial improvement in sagittal balance following the procedure.

Preoperative autologous donation should be used along with intraoperative blood salvage devices. Use of the cell saver can decrease the requirements for homologous transfusions; however, the cell saver necessitates judicious use of clotting factors to prevent dilutional coagulapathy. Fresh frozen plasma and platelets should be replaced routinely as the cell saver is used rather than waiting for coagulation parameters to become abnormal. Such coagulapathies often take hours to correct resulting in excessive perioperative blood losses.

The risk of pseudoarthrosis is raised with poor fixation or excessive residual kyphosis tensioning the bone graft. In addition, use of allograft alone significantly raises the risks for nonunion, especially in the lumbar spine. All revision surgery carries an increased risk of pseudarthrosis. Older patients, smokers, and obese patients may be predisposed to higher failure rates secondary to nonunion.[38] Such patients should be considered for implantable or external bone stimulators to improve the chance for successful arthrodesis.

The risk of deep wound infection varies but averages 8% for major spinal reconstructive procedures.[1,6,16,18,27] It is decreased significantly with appropriately timed prophylactic antibiotic therapy. Infection rates are higher in revisions, longer cases, nutritionally depleted, and posterior procedures. Infections are also higher in obese patients, smokers, elderly, and diabetic patients. Anterior procedures have a lower infection rate than posterior procedures. Any procedure using instrumentation also increases the risk of infection. When Galveston pelvic fixation is present, a deep wound infection can be complicated by pelvic osteomyelitis.

Complications relating specifically to use of hardware include mechanical failure resulting from poor bone quality. Preoperative bone mineral density and CT may help in recognizing such a predisposition. Overcorrection or inadequate anterior release may result in excessive force application and failure at the bone metal interface. In addition, over- or undercorrection may fail to restore acceptable balance to the spine. Subtle residual coronal plane imbalance often can be successfully managed with a shoe lift; however, moderate residual coronal or mild sagittal plane imbalance following extensive reconstructive surgery is poorly tolerated. This is especially true with long constructs into the lower lumbar segments or pelvis. Injury also can occur to vascular or visceral structures from pedicle screws, which penetrate the anterior vertebral body. Sublaminar wires, laminar hooks, and pedicle screws can injure the spinal cord or nerve roots directly.

SUMMARY

Destabilizing fractures to thoracolumbar spine are common injuries in which the treatment continues to evolve. Untreated fractures, lack of early recognition, and treatment errors are the foundation for late failure and deformity. The principle deformity is an angular kyphosis at the thoracolumbar junction. Angular deformities with sagittal imbalance are potentially debilitating from chronic pain, progression, or compression of neural elements. Reconstructive spinal surgery is a serious undertaking necessitating a thorough evaluation of the patient and careful planning and execution of the surgical procedure. Goals of surgery are to restore spinal balance, secure stable fixation, and decompress neural tissues. Successful outcomes are possible with diminished pain and improved function; however, such outcomes are not without risk of serious and potentially life-threatening complications.

REFERENCES

1. Malcolm BW, et al: Post-traumatic kyphosis: a review of forty-eight surgically treated patients, *J Bone Joint Surg* 63A:891–899, 1981.
2. Harms J, Stoltze D: The indications and principles of correction of post-traumatic deformities, *Eur Spine J* 1:142–151, 1992.
3. White AA, Panjabi MM, Thomas CL: The clinical biomechanics of kyphotic deformities, *Clin Orthop* 128:8–17, 1977.
4. Andriacchi T, et al: A model for studies of mechanical interactions between the human spine and rib cage, *J Biomech* 7:497–507, 1974.
5. Oxland TR, Lin R-M, Panjabi MM: Three-dimensional mechanical properties of the thoracolumbar junction, *J Orthop Res* 10:573–580, 1992.

6. Roberson JR, Whitesides TE Jr: Surgical reconstruction of late post-traumatic thoracolumbar kyphosis, *Spine* 10:307–312, 1985.
7. Denis F: The three column spine and its significance in the classification of acute thoracolumbar spinal injuries, *Spine* 8(8):817–831, 1983.
8. Weinstein JN, Collalto P, Lehmann TR: Thoracolumbar "burst" fractures treated conservatively: a long-term follow-up, *Spine* 13:33–38, 1988.
9. Holland H: Charcot's arthropathy of the spine. With a note on a case, *Br J Radiol* 25:267–269, 1952.
10. Sobel JW, Bohlman HH, Freehafer AA: Charcot's arthropathy following spinal cord injury, *J Bone Joint Surg Am* 67:771–776, 1985.
11. Andreychik DA, et al: Burst fractures of the second through fifth lumbar vertebrae, *J Bone Joint Surg* 78A(8):1156–1165, 1996.
12. Edwards CC, Rhyne A: Late treatment of posttraumatic kyphosis, *Semin Spine Surg* 2:63–69, 1990.
13. Jodoin A, et al: Unstable fractures of the thoracolumbar spine: a 10-year experience at Sacre Coeur Hospital, *J Trauma* 25:197–202, 1985.
14. Denis F, et al: Acute thoracolumbar burst fractures in the absence of neurologic deficit: a comparison between operative and non-operative treatment, *Clin Orthop* 189:142–149, 1984.
15. Whitesides TE Jr: Traumatic kyphosis of the thoracolumbar spine, *Clin Orthop* 128:78–92, 1977.
16. Kostuik JP, et al: Combined single stage anterior and posterior osteotomy for correction of iatrogenic lumbar kyphosis, *Spine* 13:257–266, 1988.
17. Lagrone MO, et al: Treatment of symptomatic flatback after spinal fusion, *J Bone Joint Surg* 70A:569–580, 1988.
18. Kostuik JP, Matsusaki H: Anterior stabilization, instrumentation, and decompression for post-traumatic kyphosis, *Spine* 14:379–386, 1989.
19. Young MH: Long-term consequences of stable fractures of the thoracic and lumbar vertebral bodies, *J Bone Joint Surg* 55B:295–300, 1973.
20. Nicoll EA: Fractures of the dorso-lumbar spine, *J Bone Joint Surg* 31A:376–394, 1949.
21. Farcy JC, Weidenbaum M, Glassman SD: Sagittal index in management of thoracolumbar burst fractures, *Spine* 15:958–965, 1990.
22. Place HM, et al: Stabilization of thoracic spine fractures resulting in complete paraplegia. A long-term retrospective analysis, *Spine* 19(15):1726–1730, 1994.
23. Edwards CC, et al: The fate of retropulsed bone following thoracolumbar burst fractures, *Orthop Trans* 13:32–33, 1989.
24. Fiddler MW: Remodeling of the spinal canal after burst fracture: A prospective study of two cases, *J Bone Joint Surg* 70B:730–732, 1988.
25. Denis F, Burkus J: Classification and treatment of post-traumatic kyphosis in the thoracic and lumbar spine, *Semin Spine Surg* 5(3):187–198, 1993.
26. Bradford DS, Tribus CB: Current concepts and management of patients with fixed decompensated spinal deformity, *Clin Orthop* 306:64–72, 1994.
27. Bradford DS, et al: Techniques for anterior spinal surgery for the management of kyphosis, *Clin Orthop* 128:129–139, 1977.
28. Romanick PC, et al: Infection about the spine associated with low-velocity missle injury to the abdomen, *J Bone Joint Surg* 67A:1195–1201, 1985.
29. Boachie-Adjei O, Bradford DS: Vertebral column resection and arthrodesis for complex spinal deformities, *J Spinal Disord* 4(2):193–202, 1991.
30. McBride GG, Bradford DS: Vertebral body replacement with femoral neck allograft and vascularized rib strut graft. A technique for treating post-traumatic kyphosis with neurologic deficit, *Spine* 8(4):406–415, 1983.
31. Weatherly C, Jaffray D, Terry A: Vascular complications associated with osteotomy in ankylosing spondylitis, *Spine* 13:43–46, 1988.
32. Thiranont N, Netrawichien P: Transpedicular decancellation closed wedge vertebral osteotomy for treatment of fixed flexion deformity of spine in ankylosing spondylitis, *Spine* 18(16):2517–2522, 1993.
33. Lehmer SM, et al: Posterior transvertebral osteotomy for adult thoracolumbar kyphosis, *Spine* 19(18):2060–2067, 1994.
34. Smith-Peterson MN, Larson CB, Aufranc OE: Osteotomy of the spine for correction of flexion deformity in rheumatoid arthritis, *J Bone Joint Surg* 27A:1–11, 1945.
35. Thomasen E: Vertebral osteotomy for correction of kyphosis in ankylosing spondylitis, *Clin Orthop* 194:142–152, 1985.
36. Chang K: Oligosegmental correction of post-traumatic thoracolumbar angular kyphosis, *Spine* 18(13):1909–1915, 1993.
37. Lonstein JE: Neurologic deficits secondary to spinal deformity. A review of the literature and report of 43 cases, *Spine* 5:331–355, 1980.
38. Brown CW, Orme TJ, Richardson HD: The rate of pseudarthrosis in patients who are smokers and patients who are nonsmokers: a comparison study, *Spine* 11:942–943, 1986.

22

NEUROSURGICAL PROCEDURES IN SPINE TRAUMA

Allan D.O. Levi
Volker K.H. Sonntag

EPIDEMIOLOGY

Spinal trauma continues to present a challenging spectrum of diseases for the surgeon to manage despite substantial improvements in emergency, diagnostic, and surgical care. When spinal trauma results in a spinal cord injury (SCI), the emotional and financial toll inflicted on individuals and their families is enormous. Typically, these injuries occur in males at the peak of their productive lives.[1] The incidence of SCI after trauma is approximately 10,000 new cases each year with a prevalence of 191,000.[2,3] The amount spent on the treatment of SCI in the United States is approximately 5.6 billion dollars each year and rises annually.[4] The cost of caring for the individual spinal cord–injured patient is directly related to the level at which the spinal cord is injured and to the patient's age, with the highest costs associated with the older quadriplegic patients who are dependent on respirators. Most spinal injuries result from high-speed motor vehicle accidents.[5] Falls, recreational injuries, violent crimes, and work-related injuries are other important contributors. Reducing the incidence of SCI through preventive programs clearly is the most effective method of reducing the devastation these injuries cause.

Advances in the emergency care of these patients include the recognition by emergency personnel that any trauma patient with multiple injuries could have a potential spinal column injury. Initial immobilization of the cervical spine with a hard collar and sandbags, transporting patients on backboards, and their rapid evacuation to level I trauma centers have improved the outcome of spinal injuries by reducing the risk of iatrogenic SCI in patients with unstable fractures. Also, the potential for causing secondary damage to the spinal cord can be reduced by adhering to a protocol of resuscitation that ensures adequate oxygenation and control of blood pressure to assure perfusion of oxygenated blood to the traumatized spinal cord.[6]

The ability to image the spinal column and the spinal cord after spinal trauma also has improved. Most notably, high-resolution computed tomography (CT) with uniplanar and three-dimensional reconstructions has largely replaced tomography in diagnosing fractures of the spinal elements. Similarly, magnetic resonance imaging (MRI) is a valuable, noninvasive tool in imaging the spine and related structures after an injury. Some of the most important advantages of MRI include the ability to image soft-tissue injuries including muscles and ligaments, to define the presence of a hematoma within the spinal canal or spinal cord, and, most importantly, to define the relationship of the fractured spinal column, the spinal cord, and the nerve roots in a noninvasive manner.

In the past 30 years, major advances in the surgical treatment of the fractured spinal column have occurred. Spinal surgeons are comfortable in using anterior approaches for the cervical spine and anterolateral and posterolateral approaches for the thoracolumbar spine. Some of the most notable advancements include the development of screw fixation systems for odontoid fractures and transarticular screws for atlantoaxial instability, a wide variety of anterior plating systems for the entire spinal column, and posterior instrumentation devices including lateral mass plates for the cervical spine, hook and claw systems for the thoracic spine, and pedicle screw fixation for the lower thoracic and lumbar spine. These constructs have provided immediate stabilization of the spine until bony fusion is achieved thus allowing patients to be mobilized earlier.

The concepts of primary and secondary SCI are important principles in understanding the pathophysiology and the role of pharmacotherapeutic agents in the emergent treatment of SCI. The primary injury mechanism results from a mechanical insult that occurs at the time of impact and includes acute compression, impaction, distraction, laceration, and shear.[7] Secondary injuries occur after the initial injury and account for some of the progressive pathologic changes associated with SCI.[7] A number of drugs have been tested in the laboratory, but only a few of these agents have progressed to clinical trials to evaluate their efficacy. Five randomized controlled trials of pharmacotherapy for acute SCI have been conducted, focusing on the therapeutic effect of either steroids or gangliosides.

In general a number of studies have shown improved neurologic recovery in animals with SCIs that have received either dexamethasone or methylprednisolone.[8–12] Steroid treatment initially held promise as a potential therapeutic agent for its putative role in reducing white matter edema and inflammation. Current evidence, however, suggests that the major mechanism of action is by reducing the effects of secondary injury and, in particular, the destructive effects of lipid peroxidation on cell membranes.[13] Other actions include improving spinal cord blood flow, enhancing the post-injury activity of Na^+/K^+ ATPase, and facilitating the recovery of extracellular calcium ion.[11,14]

The first North American Spinal Cord Injury Study (NASCIS I) examined low- (100 mg) and high- (1000 mg) dose methylprednisolone given for 10 days. Unfortunately this trial had no control group, and no significant difference in outcome was found except for an increased number of wound infections among patients in the high-dose group.[1] The second (NASCIS II) trial was a prospective, randomized, double-blinded, multicenter trial, which demonstrated improved neurologic outcomes after 6 weeks, 6 months, and 1 year in patients who had received a regimen of methylprednisolone, which included a bolus dose of 30 mg/kg followed by a maintenance dose of 5.4 mg/kg given for 23 hrs.[15] The improved outcomes associated with methylprednisolone were only observed if the drug was given within 8 hours of injury when compared with naloxone or a placebo. Although the results of this study can be criticized, the administration of this drug is believed to reduce the amount of secondary injury that occurs to the spinal cord and has become an important tool in the treatment of SCI in most North American centers.[16] A new clinical trial, NASCIS III, will compare the results of the NASCIS II protocol with a longer dosing regimen of methylprednisolone and with a 21-aminosteroid. The 21-aminosteroids (Lazaroids), a new class of steroids, are potent inhibitors of lipid peroxidation. They lack much of the glucocorticoid activity of many of the traditional steroid compounds.

Gangliosides are complex sialic acid–containing glycoshingolipids, which are present in high concentrations in neural membranes. These compounds are involved in a variety of cell surface phenomenon such as cell-substrate binding and receptor functions.[17] Basic research in the past 15 years has demonstrated that these compounds can (1) promote the survival of neurons in cell culture; (2) increase the number, length, and branching of neuronal processes in cell culture; and (3) improve functional recovery after a variety of traumatic and ischemic insults to the peripheral and central nervous systems. A limited number of animal studies have examined the role of gangliosides after SCI and have shown only a modest effect on the regeneration of serotinergic neurons.[18] A recent prospective, randomized, double-blind, single-center study found a beneficial effect in functional neurologic outcomes when the ganglioside GM_1 was administered within 72 hours of human SCI.[19] A multicenter trial is now being conducted to test both high and low concentrations of the drug.

DECOMPRESSION AFTER SPINAL CORD INJURY

INDICATIONS FOR SURGERY

There are several indications for surgery after spinal trauma. These include (1) deformity correction; (2) stabilization; and (3) the decompression of neurologic elements. In cervical fractures, some deformities can simply be corrected by the application of cervical traction, which is then followed by an external orthosis, such as halo immobilization or surgical stabilization to maintain the desired alignment.[20] Surgical approaches for deformity correction are necessary when a traumatic herniated disk is present and realignment of the spine without prior disk removal may result in further spinal cord compression or when locked or fractured facets preclude external reduction. Occasionally, late recognition of a cervical fracture can result in a maligned fusion. In thoracic and lumbar fractures, deformity correction often requires surgical intervention. At the time of surgery, various combinations of bone grafts and instrumentation can be used to maintain alignment. Failure to correct significant deformities can result in future neurologic compromise, abnormal posture, respiratory complications, or chronic pain.

Another important indication for surgery in spinal trauma is an unstable fracture. Unstable fractures result from the loss of the normal relationship between adjacent vertebrae so that under physiologic loading neurologic damage, progressive deformity, or intractable pain ensues. Major advances in surgical instrumentation in the past two decades have facilitated the stabilization of some of the most difficult spinal fractures.[21] One of the implicit advantages of immediate surgical stabilization is the possibility of early mobilization of the patient and the potential for reducing the complications associated with prolonged bedrest.[22]

HISTORICAL RESULTS

The decompression of neurological elements either by the realigning the spinal column or by elevating vertebral bone fragments or disk appears a logical approach to improve the neurologic outcome associated with spinal injuries. Yet the value of surgical decompression of neurologic elements in spinal trauma is rife with controversy. There are two major issues in the literature. First, does the decompression of injured neural tissue ultimately improve neurologic outcomes in patients with SCI? Second, how does the timing of surgery influence the analysis of such an effect? It is convenient to distinguish between functionally complete and incomplete neurologic injuries, because the potential for neurologic recovery associated with complete and incomplete injuries appears to be vastly different independent of any specific management decisions. Patients with no evidence of motor or sensory function below their SCI are considered to have functionally complete injuries. Patients with functionally incomplete injuries cover a wide range of neurologic dysfunction from no voluntary motor function below the level of injury but with some sensory modality preserved to only minimal neurologic dysfunction, which may allow them unlimited ambulation.

RESULTS OF DECOMPRESSION IN EXPERIMENTAL MODELS

An understanding of the potential benefits of surgically decompressing the spinal cord after spinal trauma should be derived from both laboratory and clinical research. There are a number of animal models for initiating and maintaining a predetermined level of spinal cord compression. In most instances, a laminectomy is performed, and a deforming force is applied to the spinal cord. The rate, force, and duration of compression are varied so that the degree of injury imparted to the spinal cord can be quantified. Several well-investigated models of injury include the weight-drop method developed by Allen during the early part of this century, the rapid inflation of extradural balloons, and the application of modified aneurysm clips.[23,24,25]

Although all of the models are imperfect simulations of human SCI, a few basic observations have consistently been found. The force of impact and the duration of compression both appear to be important predictors of neurologic recovery in several different animal models and types of injuries. Although in most studies the duration of compression is too short to be considered clinically significant, Guha and colleagues demonstrated a benefit from decompressing the spinal cord as long as 4 hours after injury in rats with mild injuries.[24,26,27] No benefit, however, appears to be derived from delayed decompression when large forces are used to compress the spinal cord. *This contrasts with clinical data that suggest recovery does occur with later decompression.* In summary, some experimental data support the claim that surgical decompression of the injured spinal cord, particularly with lesser injuries, improves neurologic outcome.

In an analysis of the older clinical literature, the diagnostic and therapeutic tools available to the surgeon for the management of patients with SCI have changed substantially in the past three decades. With the advent of CT and especially of MRI, surgeons can specifically assess the degree of neural compression in a patient. The adequacy of the decompression also can be evaluated. Before the 1970s, surgical procedures designed to decompress neural elements after spinal trauma were essentially limited to the performance of a laminectomy. This procedure is valuable only in those rare cases when a posteriorly projecting piece of bone or posteriorly located hematoma compresses the spinal cord. Morgan and coworkers[29] quelled the initial enthusiasm for decompressive laminectomies by demonstrating that most patients deteriorated or showed no neurological improvement afterward. A laminectomy also increases the risk of destabilizing the spine, thereby inducing a posttraumatic kyphotic deformity.[30]

EFFECT OF OPERATIVE DECOMPRESSION ON ULTIMATE NEUROLOGIC RECOVERY

Among contemporary series, a number of retrospective reports and case studies have confirmed that patients who sustain complete SCIs have only a small chance of neurologic recovery and that their potential to regain ambulation is less than 3%.[31–35] Variables that can confound an assessment for a complete injury include the presence of an associated head injury, alcohol or drug intoxication, multiple associated injuries, and spinal shock as demonstrated by the absence of a bulbocavernosus reflex on admission. Categorizing some of these patients as having complete injuries may account for some of the unexpected recoveries that have been reported.

The role of surgical decompression in patients with complete SCIs remains controversial. The number of patients who demonstrate significant neurologic improvement remains low with all treatment modalities, including both nonsurgical and surgical approaches. Consequently, it is impossible to ascribe a direct role to surgery in the occasional patient with a complete injury who improves functionally after surgical decompression. Heiden and colleagues,[33] for example, retrospectively analyzed 199 patients with complete cervical spine injuries, of which 61% underwent surgical decompression. No patients in the surgical group recovered ambulatory function. Of the 78 patients who were managed nonsurgically, however, two were ambulatory at a later follow-up examination. At the other end of the spectrum, in another retrospective series by Levi and coworkers,[34] 53 patients with complete injuries all were managed surgically on either an early (less than 24 hours) or a delayed basis (more than 24 hours). On later follow-up, 3.8% of the patients were ambulatory when both groups were combined.

TIMING OF DECOMPRESSIVE SURGERY

The timing of spinal cord decompression after trauma in patients with complete cord injuries is another unresolved issue. With certain cervical fracture-subluxations, the spinal cord can be decompressed rapidly using traction to realign the spine. Traction must be accompanied by serial radiographs and clinical examination of the patient. When this treatment was applied to a small series of patients examined retrospectively, the few patients with complete injuries who were reduced in a timely fashion were those who tended to achieve significant recoveries.[20] No significant difference in neurologic outcomes, however, was identified in a cohort of patients who underwent surgical decompression on either an early or delayed basis.[34] The former approach promoted earlier transfer to rehabilitation and consequently was less costly. Advocates of delayed surgery have suggested that early surgery results in an apparent increase in medical complications.[33,35] Duh and colleagues[36] support the opposite view and suggested a lower complication rate was associated with early surgery.

Finally as an offshoot of the NASCIS II trial, a retrospective review of neurologic outcome was analyzed with respect to performance and timing of surgery.[36] There was no significant difference in the neurologic outcomes of patients treated surgically or nonsurgically; however, when surgery was performed within 25 hours of injury or more than 200 hours after injury, neurologic recovery appeared to improve. The potential for provoking injury to the spinal cord by operating during the immediate phase of injury (1 to 8 days), which is associated with white matter edema and all the pathologic correlates of secondary injury, was suggested as the explanation for this finding.

Whether prompt surgical decompression ultimately results in functional improvement in patients with complete neurologic injuries will remain unanswered until a randomized, prospective, double-blind study is performed. Given the amalgamated knowledge from numerous retrospective studies, however, it appears that prompt surgical decompression of the spinal cord in patients with complete injuries benefits very few patients.

The role of decompressive surgery also is unclear in patients with incomplete injuries. A number of retrospective studies have suggested that decompression, even when delayed, can improve the degree of neurologic function in patients with incomplete injuries.[32,37–39] This finding is consistent with experimental studies that have documented improvement in rats with less severe SCIs after decompression.[27] Unlike many patients with functionally complete SCIs, many patients with incomplete injuries improve over time, even without surgical treatment, particularly those with syndromes such as acute central cervical SCIs or cruciate paralysis.[2,39,40,41] Thus, the improvement in incomplete injuries after surgery should not be inappropriately attributed to the surgery when, in fact, it reflects the natural history of the disease. Sorting out this dilemma could only be accomplished by designing a study on the role of decompressive surgery in incomplete injuries that contains a control group of untreated patients. Most surgeons in North America believe so strongly that decompressive surgery benefits incomplete injuries that a clinical trial including a nonoperated cohort of incomplete patients is unlikely.

But because the role of surgical decompression in incomplete SCIs has never undergone randomized, prospective, double-blind testing, rigorous evidence supporting this procedure is still lacking. However, many reports support the benefits of prompt surgical decompression after a variety of other central nervous system (CNS) insults, including mass lesions after traumatic brain injuries. The bulk of evidence suggests that decompression of the spinal cord in patients with incomplete injuries, either through external reduction using traction or operative decompression, is beneficial. This reasoning, combined with the other well-established indications for spinal surgery after trauma, dictates an operative approach for many patients with incomplete SCIs.

MANAGEMENT

Complete Injuries. The management of patients with traumatic injuries who initially have a neurologic deficit that then substantially improves or completely resolves by the time the patient is examined by the attending surgeon is particularly complex. A subset of patients with cervical SCIs presents with weakness or paralysis of the hands and arms with relative preservation of lower extremity strength. These patients can often be categorized under two clinical syndromes: (1) cruciate paralysis or (2) acute central cervical SCI depending on the level of the cervical cord injury.[2] In the first of these two syndromes, cruciate paralysis, most patients have sustained an upper cervical spine fracture. Acute central cervical SCI was first described by Schneider and coworkers,[39] and its clinical manifestations are similar if not identical to those of cruciate paralysis. The mechanism of injury in many cases is thought to result from hyperextension of the cervical spine and squeezing of the spinal cord in the anteroposterior plane by an inward bulging of the ligamentum flavum in an already narrowed spinal canal. In both instances, the natural history is associated with neurologic improvement.

Incomplete Injuries. A fracture associated with cruciate paralysis should be managed according to the presence or absence of instability because most patients lack significant compression at this level of the spinal cord after cervical traction. Patients with acute central cervical SCI often have a significant degree of cervical spinal stenosis but lack an overt fracture or instability. Surgeons should refrain from the temptation to decompress the cervical spinal cord, particularly in patients who continue to show spontaneous recovery. In patients with significant cervical spinal cord compression who have reached a plateau in neurologic recovery, who are exhibiting neurologic deterioration, or who have the potential to injure their cervical spine repetitively, one can make a logical argument for operative decompression.

Injuries Associated with Transient Neurologic Disturbances. Another complex management issue arises in patients, particularly athletes, who present with transient neurologic disturbances such as quadriparesis after sustaining a high-velocity impact injury to the cervical spine. Most of these individuals improve within 24 hours of injury, although some may take as long as 5 days to regain complete neurologic function.[42,43] Plain radiographs, CT scans, and dynamic radiographs often fail to disclose a fracture or overt instability. MRI, however, may confirm the presence of a spinal cord contusion, particularly on T2-weighted images. Often, a concomitant finding in these patients is that of single or multilevel cervical spinal stenosis.[43] Surgery is almost never indicated for these patients because they tend to make complete neurologic recoveries. The prevention of further injuries, however, often requires discontinuation of the contact sport in which the injury was sustained.[44]

Spinal Column Injuries in Neurologically Intact Patients. In patients who are neurologically intact after spinal trauma, the surgeon should be guided primarily by the principles of correcting deformities and repairing the instability associated with the vertebral injury. In general, the decompression of uninjured neurologic elements should not enter into the management strategy of a vertebral fracture. Although somewhat controversial, the current recommendations for surgery to treat burst fractures associated with compromise of the spinal canal but no neurologic deficit illustrate this point.

Denis and colleagues[45] retrospectively reviewed the management of a series of burst fractures at two institutions. A significant number of the nonoperated patients developed late neurologic deterioration, progressive kyphosis, and severe pain (17%–25%). Thus, some patients who were initially managed conservatively with bracing deteriorated and ultimately required surgery, consisting of decompressing a narrowed spinal canal followed by stabilization. The cohort of neurologically intact patients with burst fractures who were initially treated surgically had their fractures stabilized without decompression of the spinal canal. None of these patients deteriorated neurologically either during surgery or on follow-up.

A commonly cited indication for surgery for thoracolumbar burst fractures are those considered unstable and include fractures with an angular deformity greater than 30%, more than 50% of the spinal canal, or both.[46] The natural history of stenosis of the spinal canal associated with trauma is unknown. Bone, however, can remodel after the spinal column has been stabilized to the point that the diameter of the spinal canal can be restored.[47] In summary, the surgical management of burst fractures illustrates how stabilization of the spine alone in neurologically intact patients can prevent the onset of delayed neurologic deterioration.[45] This goal can be accomplished without directly decompressing nervous tissue but by preventing the onset of late deformity in combination with decompression of a pathologically narrowed canal through the process of bony remodeling.

DURAL REPAIR

ETIOLOGY OF POSTTRAUMATIC LEAKS

Dural tears are common after spinal trauma. The more severe the injury, the greater is the likelihood for a dural laceration.[48] Burst fractures associated with a laminar fracture are reported to have a high incidence of an associated dural laceration.[49] Centrally driven bone fragments can tear the dura and injure the neurologic elements. Removal of disk or bone fragments at a fracture site during a decompression procedure also can inadvertently tear the dura and is a well-recognized complication of spinal surgery. Finally, with the more widespread use of instrumentation to repair spine injuries, iatrogenic tears of the dura can result from the insertion of the wires, cables, or screws used to anchor a variety of hardware to the bony elements. Reoperation for spinal fractures has the highest risk for a dural tear because scar tissue obscures the normal anatomic tissue planes.

CLINICAL PRESENTATION

A spinal cerebrospinal fluid (CSF) fistula can lead to a number of complications, including (1) a dural-cutaneous fistula; (2) a pseudomeningocele; (3) meningitis; (4) traction of neurologic elements with subsequent neurologic deterioration; and (5) arachnoiditis. The clinical presentation of a dural-cutaneous fistula can manifest by the leakage of clear or blood-tinged fluid from an operative incision or within a surgically placed drain. Large volumes of fluid can be observed because the choroid plexus makes more than 20 mL of CSF each hour.[50] The patient may complain of a postural headache, which worsens when an upright posture is assumed and is relieved by a recumbent position. Typically, the diagnosis of a dural-cutaneous fistula is obvious. When a diagnosis is questionable, however, analysis of the fluid for J_2-transferrin, a component of CSF, can be useful.[51]

A pseudomeningocele occurs when CSF becomes encysted within the soft tissues surrounding the spine after a dural tear. The condition may manifest itself days to months after spinal trauma or a surgical procedure. A dural tear missed at surgery or failure to repair the dura in a watertight fashion can lead to a pseudomeningocele. MRI facilitates diagnosis because a cyst has the same signal characteristics of the CSF within the tissues surrounding the spine on both T1- and T2-weighted images (Fig. 22-1). The patient may be asymptomatic or may have a fluctuant, swollen, extremely tender wound and a postural headache. When nerve roots herniate through the dura-arachnoid defect, a painful radiculopathy also is present.[52]

The presence of a dural-cutaneous fistula increases the risk of an infectious organism entering the CNS and causing meningitis. The most common infectious organisms are *Staphylococcus* and *Streptococcus*, both common skin pathogens. The use of prophylactic antibiotics in the presence of a fistula only selects for a resistant organism. Infection may lead to arachnoiditis and subsequent neurologic deterioration.

The most practical classification of dural tears is according to their location (dorsal, lateral, and ventral). The site of the dural tear combined with the surgical approach to the spine determines the feasibility of obtaining a watertight closure. With a posterior approach, dorsally located tears are most accessible to direct repair. Laterally located tears can be reached by removing sufficient lamina to expose the lateral dura. In some cases, the dura can be opened in the midline so that a stitch anchored to muscle or fat can be fed medially to laterally so that the transplanted tissue obstructs the mouth of the lateral dural opening.[53] Ventral tears above the tip of the conus medullaris are the most difficult to repair by direct suture during a posterior approach. Consequently, indirect approaches to repair, including fibrin glues and lumbar drains, must be used (see next section). Dural tears below the conus medullaris and ventral to the nerve roots of the cauda equina often can be repaired by gently displacing the nerve roots to access the dural edges even with a posterior approach (i.e., a transdural repair).

DURAL REPAIR TECHNIQUES

Any method of dural repair should be safe, easy, cost effective, and predictably produce a watertight seal (Table 22-1). Magnification and excellent lighting can facilitate the closure. The operating microscope or the combination of loops and an overhead light is often useful. Sutures should be nonabsorbable and have a fine caliber (4-0 to 5-0). Needles with a small internal diameter and a slender needle driver facilitate closure. Both interrupted and noninterrupted suture techniques are acceptable (Fig. 22-2 A), and each has inherent advantages and disadvantages.

If the dural edges cannot be directly opposed, the interposition of graft material may be a useful adjunct (Fig. 22-2 B). The source of the graft can be obtained locally from the wound, for example, from the lumbodorsal fascia. Alternatively, the lateral thigh can be prepared to obtain a fascia lata graft. Dural substitutes also exist. Lyodura, a lyophilized cadaveric dura, is no longer used because many cases of Creutzfeldt-Jakob disease were reported after these grafts were used as dural substitutes.[54,55] Recently, the Food and Drug Administration approved bovine pericardium that has been cross-linked with glutaraldehyde (Duraguard) for use in humans as a dural substitute.

The goal of each dural repair is a watertight closure to prevent the egress of CSF from the subarachnoid space. Sometimes, a watertight dural closure is impossible to achieve. Consequently, an excellent fascial closure is equally important and prevents the formation of a duralcutaneous fistula. When the CSF can be localized to a subfascial plane, the wound often heals without forming a pseudomeningocele.

A few other techniques can reduce the risk of developing a CSF fistula when a dural tear cannot be closed directly. Fibrin sealants are one of the most successful tissue adhesives developed to date.[56] These glues are the most biocompatible and least toxic of several potential sealants tested and offer the surgeon a versatile tool to assist with dural repairs.[57] Their use has recently been approved in the United States, and they are popular

Box 22-1. General Guidelines for Repairing Dural Defects after Spinal Trauma

1. Use adequate lighting and magnification.
2. Clearly identify the boundaries of the dural tear.
3. Reintroduce any nerve roots entrapped within the dural opening into the dural tube.
4. Use a fine needle holder and a 4-0 to 5-0 nonabsorbable stitch to oppose the dural edges in a watertight fashion.
5. Ensure the adequacy of closure and rule out the presence of other tears by asking the anesthesiologist to apply a Valsalva maneuver.
6. Do not use an intramuscular drain in the wound that is under negative pressure.
7. Reoppose the fascia in a watertight fashion.
8. Maintain the patient flat in bed for the first 24 to 48 hours.

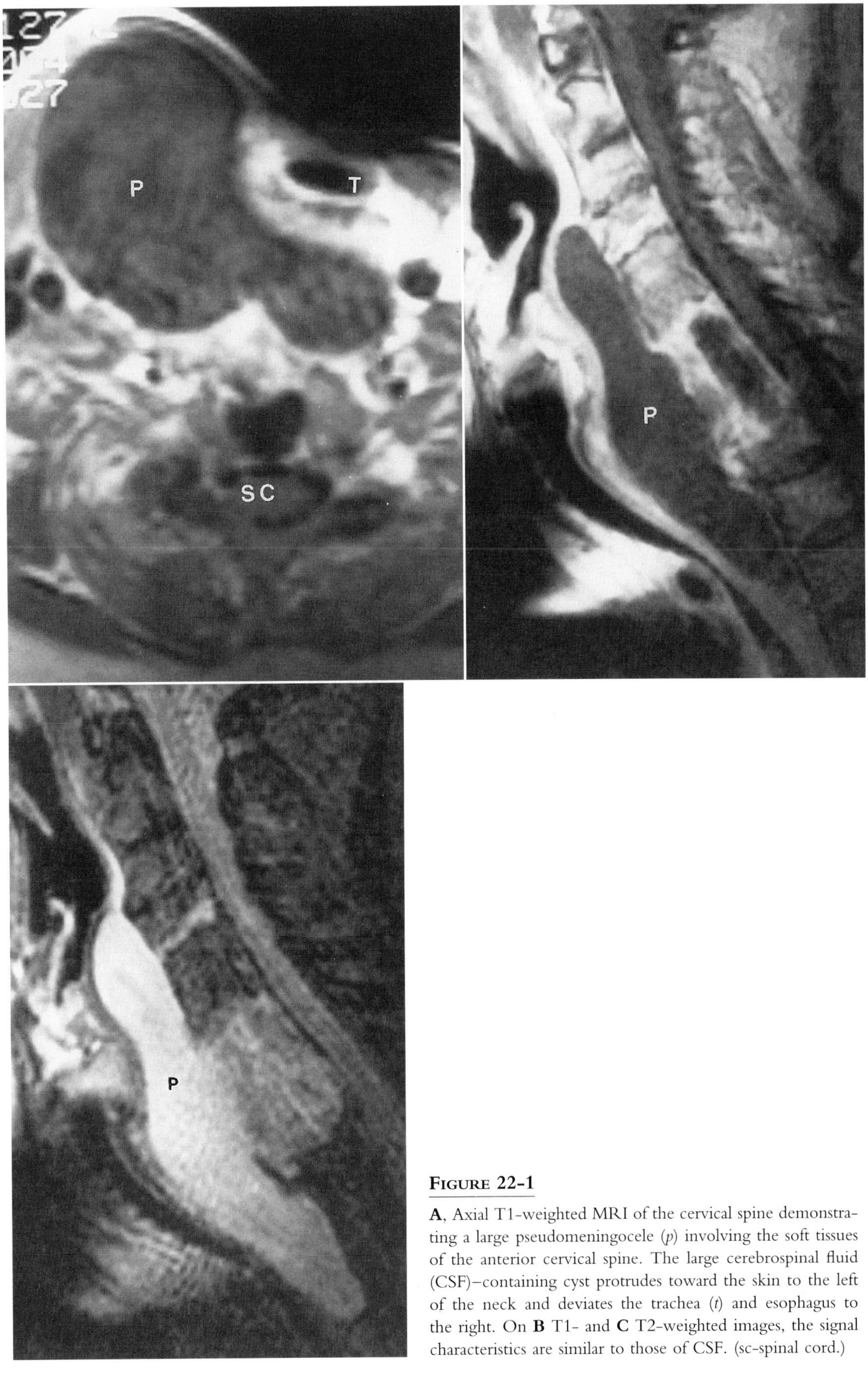

FIGURE 22-1

A, Axial T1-weighted MRI of the cervical spine demonstrating a large pseudomeningocele (*p*) involving the soft tissues of the anterior cervical spine. The large cerebrospinal fluid (CSF)–containing cyst protrudes toward the skin to the left of the neck and deviates the trachea (*t*) and esophagus to the right. On **B** T1- and **C** T2-weighted images, the signal characteristics are similar to those of CSF. (sc-spinal cord.)

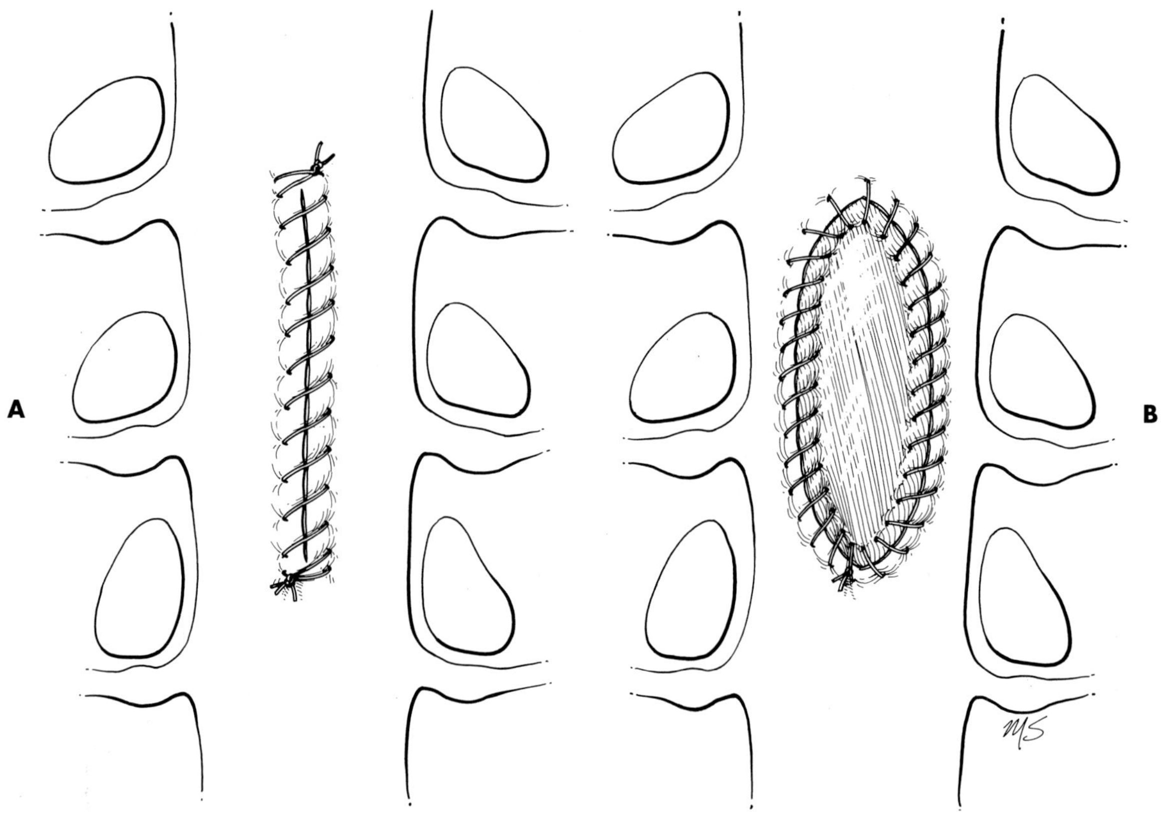

FIGURE 22-2

Illustration demonstrating the repair of **A** a midline dural tear and **B** a midline dural defect with a patch graft. (With permission of Barrow Neurological Institute.)

for multiple surgical uses in Canada and Europe. The sealants are derived from pooled blood products, which have been screened for the human immunodeficiency virus (HIV) and hepatitis B. Fibrinogen, normally converted to fibrin monomers by thrombin, is the main structural protein in serum responsible for clotting. The biological glues are delivered as separate components through syringes that empty through a common needle port. When the fibrinogen and factor XIII components are mixed with thrombin carried in a $CaCl_2$ solution, a fluid-tight adhesive mass forms. Tisseel (Immuno AG, Austria), in a two-component kit consisting of lyophilized pooled human fibrinogen/factor XIII and bovine thrombin, is the glue most commonly used in dural repairs in neurosurgery. It readily adheres to the surface of various tissues and is gradually resorbed in vivo by enzymatic and phagocytic pathways. Some evidence suggests that these glues can reduce postoperative epidural fibrosis.[58]

Few studies have systematically compared the efficacy of various methods of dural closure. In the immediate postoperative period, fibrin sealants appear to have a higher bonding strength compared with sutures, but sealants may lose tensile strength as the wound maturates.[59,60,61] Fibrin glue may be used by itself, particularly if the dural edges cannot be directly apposed, because of the location of the dural defect (e.g., a ventrally located dural tear during a posterior approach). Usually, however, fibrin glues are used as an adjunct to a suture repair to increase the tensile strength of the dural repair in the immediate postoperative period.[59]

Temporary drainage of CSF into the catheter and away from the healing incision allows the time needed for the wound to heal.[62,63] The subarachnoid space can be drained by a catheter as either a prophylactic measure or as a definitive treatment for a spinal CSF fistula. At the time of dural closure, a drain can be placed in the subarachnoid space. Diversion of CSF flow through the catheter for 4 or 5 days allows the dura, fascia, and skin closure to mature. The track left by removing the drain can then be closed with a simple suture on the skin. If a dural-cutaneous fistula is identified after surgery, a catheter can be placed into the subarachnoid space by a Touhy needle. Continuous passage of CSF over the apposed tissue layers prevents maturation of a surgical incision, resulting in the development of a fistula. When the fistula is located over a lumbar incision, a lateral needle entrance combined with fluoroscopic guidance permits the catheter to be placed safely away from the draining incision.

The drain must be monitored closely for continuous

drainage of CSF (approximately 20 mL/hr) because blockage or dislodgment of the catheter reestablishes CSF drainage from the wound. If CSF drainage from the wound persists despite the above measures, surgical reexploration of the site and a more definitive closure with grafts or the creation of local flaps are required. Certain dural tears can be managed only by introducing a permanent drain into the lumbar subarachnoid space or the lateral ventricular system. The drainage catheter is then tunneled subcutaneously and empties into the peritoneal cavity.

POSTTRAUMATIC SYRINGOMYELIA

INCIDENCE

Syringomyelia is characterized by a cystic cavitation of the spinal cord. The word *syrinx* is derived from the Greek and means tube or pipe. A syrinx can have many potential causes, which traditionally have been divided into communicating and noncommunicating forms (Table 22-1).[64] The communicating forms of syringomyelia have been attributed to a communication between the fourth ventricle and the central canal of the spinal cord through the obex of the medulla. Recent evidence, however, has questioned the existence of this communication.[65] When a syrinx is lined solely by ependyma, it represents a pathologic dilatation of the central canal and may be more aptly termed *hydromyelia*.[66]

Table 22-2. Syringomyelia

Noncommunicating Forms	Communicating Forms
Posttraumatic	Chiari malformations
Arachnoiditis	Basilar impression
Vascular	
Tumor	

PATHOPHYSIOLOGY/PATHOLOGY

A posttraumatic syrinx is a form of noncommunicating syringomyelia from spinal trauma. In general, the more severe the injury, the greater is the likelihood of developing a syrinx.[67,68] The development of a posttraumatic syrinx after a vertebral fracture in the absence of a preexisting neurologic deficit is rare. The most common pathologic change after a traumatic SCI is a central area of hemorrhagic necrosis and spinal cord infarction.[69,70] Over time, the liquefaction of the hematoma can evolve into a cystic lesion. The cavitation usually begins at the level of the vertebral fracture in the relatively avascular plane between the dorsal columns and the central gray matter.[71,72] The area surrounding the syrinx shows a prominent layer of glial tissue with a moderate amount of reactive gliosis.[69,73] The surrounding white matter tracts may be compressed, and the cavity usually contains CSF-like fluid with a high protein content. Another important pathologic feature of posttraumatic syrinxes is the presence of septae. The presence of these walls within the cyst can lead to compartmentalization and make direct drainage of the cyst more challenging. A syndrome of progressive posttraumatic myelomalacic myelopathy (PPMM) is characterized by the lack of a confluent cyst.[74] Rather, it is associated with multiple microcysts, reactive astrocytosis, and thickening of the piaarachnoid. This entity may present with a clinical picture and radiographic images similar to posttraumatic syringomyelia but represents a precursor of the larger confluent cysts.

The exact pathogenesis for the initiation and growth of posttraumatic cysts remains controversial. Cavitation of the spinal cord after trauma is a common pathologic change as evidenced by MRI studies and pathologic series.[69,71,75,76] Spinal arachnoiditis often is observed in SCI and may be an important contributing factor for the expansion of the syrinx. Even in the absence of trauma, spinal arachnoiditis can cause a syrinx to form.[77] In spinal trauma, these local areas of scarring (arachnoiditis) may tether the spinal cord to the dural tube and thus impair the circulation of CSF around the spinal cord. A pressure dissociation between the upper and lower compartments of the subarachnoid space may form as a consequence of this tethering. Transmission of distensile pressure pulse waves within the epidural veins during coughing and sneezing can, in concert with the pressure dissociation, cause the syrinx to expand within the spinal cord.[70] The initial influx of CSF may be derived from the Virchow-Robin spaces or the dorsal root entry zone and can enter the syrinx by transmural fluid migration.[78,79]

DIAGNOSIS

All patients with spinal cord cavitations after a SCI are at risk of developing clinical symptoms and signs as a consequence of their syrinx. The onset of these symptoms can vary from many months to several decades after the initial injury.[80] The percentage of patients with SCIs who develop symptoms from a posttraumatic syrinx ranges from 0.3% to 3.2%.[68,81] Since the original description by Barnett, the perceived incidence of posttraumatic syringomyelia has been increasing.[77] The key factors contributing to this apparent rise include an improvement in the ability of physicians to recognize the disorder, longer patient survival times that increase the opportunity to develop this delayed complication, and improved imaging of the spinal cord. Using MRI criteria, Backe and associates have estimated the incidence of syringomyelia in the spinal–cord–injured patient to be as high as 51%.[75] Although these investigators noted a higher incidence of a syrinx in patients with spasticity, none of their patients had an ascending myelopathy. This report underlines the importance of correlating a patient's history and physical examination with imaging studies to determine the correct management.

The most common presentation is that of a patient with a stable deficit after a SCI who develops a delayed onset of pain and neurologic deterioration years after the initial injury. The most common single manifestation of posttraumatic syrinx is pain. Classically, the pain is described as a dysesthetic burning type of pain, but it may be dull and aching. The most common location for pain is at the site of the previous injury, and it may radiate cephalad. In patients with incomplete injuries, the pain may radiate inferiorly into the arms or legs. The next most common manifestation is a progressive sensory disturbance, which may present as an ascending sensory loss in a patient with a complete injury or as a dissociated suspended sensory loss manifested by a decrease in pain sensation with preservation of light touch or joint position sense.[68] Increasing motor weakness is a frequent accompaniment but is rarely the sole clinical feature.[82] The weakness may present with upper (spasticity) or lower motor neuron findings (decreased deep tendon reflexes, muscle wasting). Although ulnar neuropathy does occur in wheelchair-bound patients, the diagnosis of a posttraumatic syrinx should not be overlooked in patients who develop wasting of C8-T1 innervated muscles. Progressive scoliosis or the development of neuropathic joints is the musculoskeletal changes associated with syringomyelia. Autonomic disturbances can include a Horner's syndrome, hyperhidrosis, or increased autonomic dysreflexia. Cephalad dissection of the syrinx into the brainstem is termed *syringobulbia*. This condition may be associated with multiple cranial nerve (CN) palsies, usually of CNs V, XI, and XII.

The work-up of posttraumatic syringomyelia must include plain radiographs and CT scans to rule out other causes for progressive neurologic deterioration after an injury. The differential diagnosis includes spinal column instability or residual spinal cord compression from bony elements or disk material. The gold standard for diagnosing posttraumatic syringomyelia is MRI. Sagittal (Figs. 22-3 A,B) and axial T1- and T2-weighted images can accurately delineate the rostral and caudal extent of the syrinx. The relationship of the syrinx to the spinal subarachnoid space and the overlying bones also can be determined. Gadolinium enhancement is absent in posttraumatic syringomyelia. The syrinx may appear as only a focal enlargement of the spinal cord limited to the injury level, or it may extend several levels above and below the epicenter of the patient's SCI. In a recent study, the mean length of posttraumatic syrinx was 14 vertebral levels.[80] In PPMM, the intramedullary signal intensity on T1-weighted images tend not to be as low as CSF and the "syrinx" has irregular margins. Tethering of the spinal cord to the adjacent dura with areas of local or diffuse arachnoiditis is a feature common of posttraumatic syrinxes and PPMM.

MANAGEMENT

An alternative diagnostic investigation includes administration of intrathecal water-soluble contrast agents followed by delayed imaging (4 to 24 hrs) of the syrinx.[83] The delay in imaging permits the contrast agent to diffuse into the cyst, which can then be detected by CT (Fig. 22-3 C). The invasiveness of the procedure and the inferior quality of the images make this technique only a second best modality of investigation. Spinal instrumentation can create large amounts of artifact on MRIs thus obscuring the anatomy of the spinal cord and syrinx. Myelography followed by a delayed CT can assist with treatment planning in these difficult cases. Hopefully, nonferromagnetic spinal implants will reduce this problem in the future. Intraoperative ultrasonography is another valuable tool for imaging a spinal cord syrinx. After the laminectomy is performed, a pool of irrigation fluid is placed over the dura and the ultrasound probe can then image the syrinx through the dura mater in both the sagittal and axial planes. The information can be used to determine the optimum site for entering the syrinx and the adequacy of internal decompression after cyst drainage. Intraoperative ultrasonography is more sensitive than MRI in detecting septations within the syrinx.[84] In cases of PPMM, the ultrasound is invaluable for confirming the lack of a confluent cyst and obviates the need for incising the spinal cord in an attempt to decompress the syrinx.[74]

The natural history of posttraumatic syringomyelia is poorly understood and can be quite variable. Most modern surgical series have documented improvement in symptomatic patients who undergo an internal decompression of their syrinx.[80,85,86] Options include shunting the syrinx to the subarachnoid space or to either the pleural or peritoneal cavities via a valveless tube.[80,85,86,87] Insertion of a T tube into the syrinx may facilitate the retention of the tube within the collapsed cyst cavity. Suturing the tube to the pia mater with an 8-0 nylon suture and to the dura in cases of syringoperitoneal or syringopleural shunts also prevents tube migration. Avoiding the areas of arachnoiditis facilitates insertion of the tube and reduces the incidence of subsequent scarring, which can block the tube.[80] An-

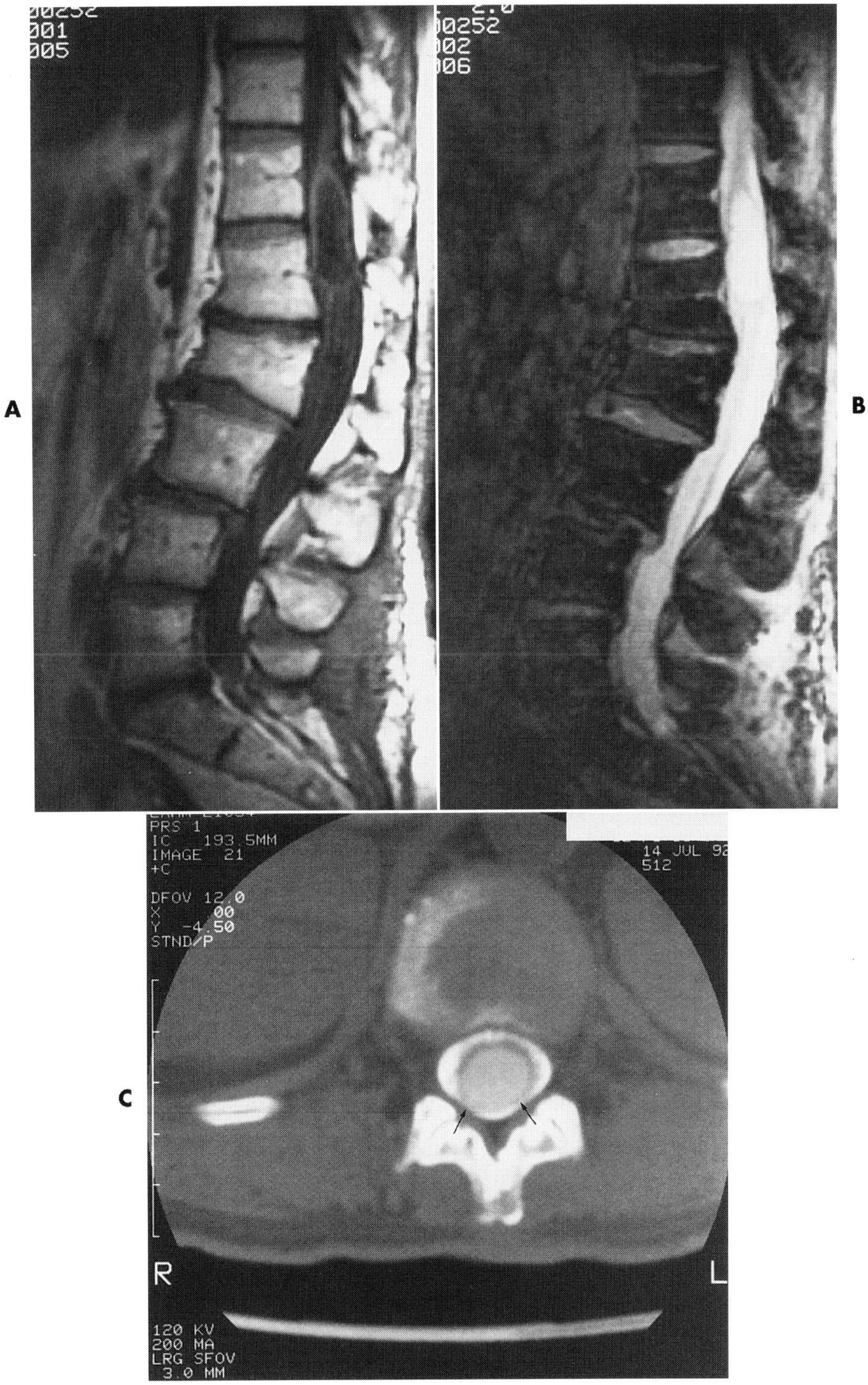

FIGURE 22-3

A Sagittal T1-weighted image of the lumbosacral cord and cauda equina demonstrating a posttraumatic syrinx of the conus medullaris extending from the midbody of T12 to L1. **B** T2-weighted image demonstrating that the signal within the syrinx is similar to CSF. **C** Axial postmyelographic CT scan of the same patient showing myelographic dye within the syrinx and tethering of the dorsal cord to the dura (*arrows*).

other surgical option includes untethering the spinal cord from the dura by lysing arachnoid adhesions and fenestrating the cyst through a single opening or through multiple openings in the case of a multiloculated syrinx. The addition of an expansile duraplasty can recreate the CSF pathways through the subarachnoid spaces and prevent the reformation of the syrinx. Other reported techniques include spinal cord transection at the level of the syrinx in plegic patients, myelopediculotomy, which consists of multiple fenestrations through the cyst wall using a laser, and the use of a neuroendoscope to breakdown septae within an established syrinx.[73,67,88]

Postoperative MRI can help determine if the syrinx has been decompressed. There appears to be a good correlation between syrinx decompression and improvement of symptoms.[82,89,90] Improvements in pain and motor strength are more common than reversal of sensory loss in the early postoperative period.[68,87,91] The long-term outcome for the surgical treatment of posttraumatic syringomyelia is still poorly understood. In patients treated with a shunting procedure, shunt obstruction associated with reaccumulation of fluid within the syrinx is a well-recognized complication.[80,87] Shunt migration also has been reported. Retethering of the spinal cord after lysis of arachnoid adhesions and duraplasty also is possible in cases associated with progressive arachnoiditis.[68] Although a 100% improvement rate has been reported in one series of 11 patients,[80] 50% improvement and 25% stabilization rates appear more realistic with long-term follow-up.[82,85,87]

SUMMARY

Despite the advances in the diagnosis and treatment of spinal fractures over the past three decades, a number of questions remain about the most appropriate management of patients with traumatic spinal fractures. Only a few aspects of the surgical management of spine trauma have been examined in this chapter, and a number of issues still need to be resolved. Technologic advances in spinal instrumentation and pharmacotherapeutics will continue into the twenty-first century. It will be critical that neurosurgeons and orthopedic surgeons work together to test the efficacy and cost effectiveness of some of the newer treatment modalities because the best possible treatment and cost containment will both be part of the management equation in the future. Outcome assessment should be at the forefront of all new ideas. Only through a critical and open-minded analysis of our treatment strategies will we improve the outcome of patients whose lives are too often devastated by spinal trauma.

REFERENCES

1. Bracken MB, et al: Efficacy of methylprednisolone in acute spinal cord injury, *JAMA* 251:45–52, 1984.
2. Levi ADO, Tator CH, Bunge RP: Clinical syndromes which result in disproportionate weakness of the upper versus the lower extremities after cervical spinal cord injury, *Neurosurgery* 38:179–185, 1996.
3. Harvey C, et al: New estimates of traumatic SCI prevalence: a survey-based approach, *Paraplegia* 28:537–544, 1990.
4. Berkowitz M: Assessing the socioeconomic impact of improved treatment of head and spinal cord injuries, *J Emerg Med* 11:63–67, 1993.
5. Traynelis VC, et al: Traumatic atlanto-occipital dislocation. Case report, *J Neurosurg* 65:863–870, 1986.
6. Young W: Secondary CNS injury, *J Neurotrauma* 5:219–221, 1988.
7. Tator CH, Fehlings MG: Review of the secondary injury theory of acute spinal cord trauma with emphasis on vascular mechanisms, *J Neurosurg* 75:15–26, 1991.
8. Braughler JM, Hall ED: Correlation of methylprednisolone levels in cat spinal cord with its effect on $(Na^+ + K^+)$-ATPase, lipid peroxidation, and alpha motor neuron function, *J Neurosurg* 56:838–844, 1982.
9. Ducker TB, Hamit HF: Experimental treatments of acute spinal cord injury, *J Neurosurg* 30:693–697, 1969.
10. Green BA, Kahn T, Klose KJ: A comparative study of steroid therapy in acute experimental spinal cord injury, *Surg Neurol* 13:91–97, 1980.
11. Young W, Flamm ES: Effect of high dose corticosteroid therapy on blood flow, evoked potentials, and extracellular calcium in experimental spinal injury, *J Neurosurg* 55:209–219, 1982.
12. Hansebout RP: A comprehensive review of methods of improving cord recovery after acute spinal cord injury. In Tator CH, editors: *Early management of acute spinal cord injury,* New York, 1982, Raven Press.
13. Hall ED, et al: Biochemistry and pharmacology of lipid antioxidants in acute brain and spinal cord injury, *J Neurotrauma* 9:S425–S442, 1992.
14. Lewin MG, Hansebout RR, Pappius HM: Chemical characteristics of traumatic spinal cord edema in cats. Effects of steroids on potassium depletion, *J Neurosurg* 40:65–75, 1974.
15. Bracken MB, et al: A randomized, trial of methylprednisolone or naloxone in the treatment of acute spinal cord injury. Results of the Second National Acute Spinal Cord Injury Study, *N Engl J Med* 322:1405–1411, 1990.
16. Shapiro SA: Methylprednisolone for spinal cord injury. Letter to the editor, *J Neurosurg* 77:324–327, 1992.
17. Rodden FA, Wiegandt H, Bauer BL: Gangliosides: the relevance of current research to neurosurgery, *J Neurosurg* 74:606–619, 1991.
18. Commissiong JW, Toffano G: The effect of GM_1 gan-

glioside on coerulospinal, noradrenergic, adult neurons and on fetal monoaminergic neurons transplanted into the transected spinal cord of the adult rat, *Brain Res* 380:205–215, 1986.

19. Geisler FH, Dorsey FC, Coleman WP: Recovery of motor function after spinal cord injury. A randomized placebo-control trial with GM_1 ganglioside, *N Engl J Med* 324:1829–1838, 1991.
20. Hadley MN, et al: Facet fracture-dislocation injuries of the cervical spine, *Neurosurgery* 31:661–666, 1992.
21. Paramore CG, Sonntag VKH: Advances in spinal instrumentation, *Jpn J Neurosurg (Tokyo)* 4:111–120, 1995.
22. Wilberger J: Diagnosis and management of spinal cord trauma, *J Neurotrauma* 8:521–530, 1991.
23. Allen AR: Remarks on the histopathological changes in the spinal cord due to impact. An experimental study, *J Nerv Ment Dis* 41:141–147, 1914.
24. Tarlov IM, Klinger H: Spinal cord compression studies. Time limits for recovery after acute compression in dogs, *Arch Neurol Psychiatry* 71:271–290, 1954.
25. Rivlin AS, Tator CH: Effect of duration of acute spinal cord compression in a new acute cord injury model in the rat, *Surg Neurol* 10:39–43, 1978.
26. Dolan EJ, Tator CH, Endrenyi L: The value of decompression after acute experimental spinal cord compression injury, *J Neurosurg* 53:749–755, 1980.
27. Guha A, et al: Decompression of the spinal cord improves recovery after experimental spinal cord compression injury, *Paraplegia* 25:324–329, 1987.
28. Morgan TH, Wharton GW, Austin GN: The results of laminectomy in patients with incomplete spinal cord injuries, *Paraplegia* 9:14–23, 1971.
29. Covalt DA, et al: Early management of patients with spinal cord injury, *JAMA* 151:89–94, 1953.
30. Malcolm BW, et al: Post-traumatic kyphosis: a review of 48 surgically treated patients, *J Bone Joint Surg* 63A:891–899, 1981.
31. Hansebout RR, Kuchner EF, Romero-Sierra C: Effects of local hypothermia and of steroids upon recovery from experimental spinal cord injury, *Surg Neurol* 4:531–535, 1975.
32. Benzel EC, Larson SJ: Functional recovery after decompressive operation of thoracic and lumbar spine fractures, *Neurosurgery* 19:772–778, 1986.
33. Heiden J, et al: Management of cervical spinal cord trauma in Southern California, *J Neurosurg* 43:732–736, 1975.
34. Levi L, et al: Anterior decompression in cervical spine trauma: does the timing of surgery affect the outcome, *Neurosurgery* 29:216–222, 1991.
35. Marshall LF, et al: Deterioration following spinal cord injury. A multicenter study, *J Neurosurg* 66:400–404, 1987.
36. Duh M, et al: The effectiveness of surgery on the treatment of acute spinal cord injury and its relation to pharmacological treatment, *Neurosurgery* 35:240–249, 1994.
37. Benzel EC, Larson SJ: Functional recovery after decompressive spine operation for cervical spine fractures, *Neurosurgery* 20:742–746, 1987.
38. Bohlman HH, Anderson P: Anterior decompression and arthrodesis of the cervical spine: long-term motor improvement. Part I. Improvement in incomplete quadriparesis, *J Bone Joint Surg* 74A:671–682, 1992.
39. Schneider RC, Cherry G, Pantek H: The syndrome of acute central cervical spinal cord injury, with special reference to the mechanisms involved in hyperextension injuries of cervical spine, *J Neurosurg* 11:546–577, 1954.
40. Brakmaan R: Some neurological and neurosurgical aspects of injuries of the lower cervical spine, *Acta Neurochir (Wien)* 22:245–260, 1970.
41. Dickman CA, et al: Cruciate paralysis: A clinical and radiographic analysis of injuries to the cervicomedullary junction, *J Neurosurg* 73:850–858, 1990.
42. Zwimpfer TJ, Bernstein M: Spinal cord concussion, *J Neurosurg* 72:894–900, 1990.
43. Bailes JE, et al: Management of athletic injuries of the cervical spine and spinal cord, *Neurosurgery* 29:491–497, 1991.
44. Torg JS, et al: Neurapraxia of the cervical spinal cord with transient quadraplegia, *J Bone Joint Surg* 68A:1354–1370, 1986.
45. Denis F, et al: Acute thoracolumbar burst fractures in the absence of neurological deficit, *Clin Orthop* 189:142–149, 1984.
46. McAfee PC, Yuan H, Lasda NA: The unstable burst fracture, *Spine* 7:365–373, 1982.
47. Rea GL, Miller CA: *Spinal trauma: current evaluation and management,* Park Ridge, 1993, American Association of Neurological Surgeons.
48. Pau A, Silvestro C, Carta F: Can lacerations of the thoraco-lumbar dura be predicted on the basis of radiological patterns of the spinal fractures, *Acta Neurochir (Wien)* 129:186–187, 1994.
49. Camissa FP, Eismont FJ, Green BA: Dural lacerations occurring with burst fractures and associated laminar fractures, *J Bone Joint Surg* 71A:1044–1052, 1989.
50. Greenberg MS: *Handbook of neurosurgery,* ed 3, Lakeland, 1994, Greenberg Graphics.
51. Ryall RG, Peacock MK, Simpson DA: Usefulness of B_2 transferrin assay in the detection of cerebrospinal fluid leaks following head injury, *J Neurosurg* 77:737–739, 1992.
52. Kaar GF, Briggs M, Bashir SH: Thecal repair in post-surgical pseudomeningocele, *Br J Neurosurg* 8:703–708, 1994.
53. Mayfield FH, Kurokawa K: Watertight closure of spinal dura mater. Technical note, *J Neurosurg* 43:639–640, 1975.
54. Martinez-Lage JF, et al: Pediatric Creutzfeldt-Jakob dis-

ease: probable transmission by a dural graft, *Childs Nerv Syst* 9:239–242, 1993.

55. Thadani V, et al: Creutzfeldt-Jakob disease probably acquired from a cadaveric dura mater graft, *J Neurosurg* 69:766–769, 1988.
56. Rossitch EJ, Wilkins RH: The use of fibrin glue in neurosurgery. In Wilkins RH, Rengachary SS, editors: *Neurosurgery Update I,* New York, 1991, McGraw-Hill.
57. Sierra DH: Fibrin sealant adhesive systems: a review of their chemistry, material properties, and clinical applications, *J Biomater Appl* 7:309–351, 1993.
58. Vacquero J, et al: Effect of fibrin glue on post-laminectomy scar formation, *Acta Neurochir (Wien)* 120:159–163, 1993.
59. Cain JE, Dryer FD, Barton BR: Evaluation of dural closure techniques, suture methods, fibrin adhesive sealant, and cyanoacrylate polymer, *Spine* 13:720–725, 1988.
60. Cain JE, et al: Quantification of leakage pressures after durotomy repairs in the canine, *Spine* 15:969–970, 1990.
61. Jorgensen PH, et al: Mechanical strength in rat skin incisional wounds treated with fibrin sealant, *J Surg Res* 42:237–241, 1987.
62. Kitchel SH, Eismont FJ, Green BA: Closed sub-arachnoid drainage for management of cerebrospinal fluid leakage, *J Bone Joint Surg (Am)* 71A:984–987, 1989.
63. McCallum J, Maroon JC, Janetta PF: Treatment of postoperative cerebrospinal fluid fistula by subarachnoid drainage, *J Neurosurg* 42:434–447, 1975.
64. Barnett HJM, Jousse AT: Post-traumatic syringomyelia (cystic myelopathy). In Vinken PJ, Bruyn CH, editors: *Injuries of the spine and spinal cord. Vol. 26, Handbook of clinical neurology,* Amsterdam, 1976, North Holland Publishing.
65. Oldfield EH, et al: Pathophysiology of syringomyelia associated with Chiari I malformation of the cerebellar tonsils. Implications for diagnosis and treatment, *J Neurosurg* 80:3–15, 1994.
66. Madsen PW, Yezierski RP, Holets VR: Syringomyelia: Clinical observations and experimental studies, *J Neurotrauma* 11:241–254, 1994.
67. Edgar R, Quail P: Progressive post-traumatic cystic and non-cystic myelopathy, *Br J Neurosurg* 8:7–22, 1994.
68. Rossier AB, et al: Post-traumatic cervical syringomyelia. Incidence, clinical presentation, electrophysiological studies, syrinx proteins, and results of conservative and operative treatment, *Brain* 108:439–461, 1985.
69. Bunge RP, et al: Observations on the pathology of human spinal cord injury. In Seil FJ, editor: *Advances in neurology, vol. 59,* New York, 1993, Raven.
70. Williams B, et al: Syringomyelia as a sequel to traumatic paraplegia, *Paraplegia* 19:67–80, 1981.
71. Squier MV, Lehr RP: Post-traumatic syringomyelia, *J Neurol Neurosurg Psychiatry* 57:1095–1098, 1994.
72. Williams B: Post-traumatic syringomyelia, an update, *Paraplegia* 28:296–313, 1990.
73. Durward QJ, et al: Selective spinal cordectomy: clinicopathological correlation, *J Neurosurg* 56:359–367, 1982.
74. Falcone S, et al: Progressive post-traumatic myelomalacic myelopathy: Imaging and clinical features, *AJNR* 15:747–754, 1994.
75. Backe HA, et al: Post-traumatic spinal cord cysts evaluated by magnetic resonance imaging, *Paraplegia* 29:607–612, 1991.
76. Wozniewicz B, et al: Pathopysiological mechanism of traumatic cavitations of the spinal cord, *Paraplegia* 21:312–317, 1983.
77. Barnett HJM: Syringomyelia associated with spinal arachnoiditis. In Barnett HJM, Foster JB, Hudgson P, editors: *Syringomyelia,* London, 1973, W.B. Saunders.
78. Ball MJ, Dayan AD: Pathogenesis of syringomyelia, *Lancet* 2:799–801, 1972.
79. Williams B: Pathogenesis of post-traumatic syringomyelia (editorial), *Br J Neurosurg* 6:517–520, 1992.
80. Hida K, et al: Posttraumatic syringomyelia: its characteristic magnetic resonance imaging findings and surgical management, *Neurosurgery* 35:886–891, 1994.
81. Umbach I, Heilporn A: Review article: post-spinal cord injury syringomyelia, *Paraplegia* 29:219–221, 1991.
82. Biyani A, El Masry WG: Post-traumatic syringomyelia: a review of the literature, *Paraplegia* 32:723–731, 1994.
83. Lyons BM, et al: The diagnosis and management of post-traumatic syringomyelia, *Paraplegia* 25:340–350, 1987.
84. Gebarski SS, et al: Posttraumatic progressive myelopathy, *Radiology* 157:378–385, 1985.
85. Tator CH, Meguro K, Rowed DW: Treatment of syringomyelia with a syringosubarachnoid shunt, *Can J Neurol Sci* 15:48–57, 1988.
86. Wiarat L, et al: Mean term follow-up of a series of post-traumatic syringomyelia patients after syringo-periotoneal shunting, *Paraplegia* 33:241–245, 1995.
87. Barbaro NM, et al: Surgical treatment of syringomyelia. Favorable results with syringoperitoneal shunting, *J Neurosurg* 61:531–538, 1984.
88. Huewel N, et al: Neuroendoscopic technique for the operative treatment of septated syringomyelia, *Acta Neurochir (Wien)* 54:59–62, 1992.
89. Levy R, Rosenblatt S, Russell E: Percutaneous drainage and serial magnetic resonance imaging in the diagnosis of symptomatic posttraumatic syringomyelia. Case report and review of the literature, *Neurosurgery* 29:429–434, 1991.
90. Pillay PK, et al: Surgical management of syringomyelia: a five year experience in the era of magnetic resonance imaging, *Neurol Res* 13:3–9, 1991.
91. Vernon JD, Silver JR, Symon L: Posttraumatic syringomyelia: the results of surgery, *Paraplegia* 21:37–46, 1983.

23

THE SPINAL CORD AND ITS REACTION TO TRAUMATIC INJURY: IMPLICATIONS FOR THE TIMING OF SURGICAL INTERVENTION

David L. Kramer
Todd J. Albert

Most often when orthopedic surgeons discuss spinal cord injury (SCI) the emphasis is on vertebral fracture patterns, mechanism of injury, and definitions of stability. The purpose of this chapter is to focus more on the spinal cord itself to better understand its reaction to traumatic injury. By understanding the pathophysiology of SCI, the surgeon is better prepared to manage those factors that affect the course of the resultant neurologic deficit.

An estimated 30 new SCIs occur per million population each year in the United States. Fifty percent of these injuries are complete SCIs and more than two thirds occur in the region of the cervical spine. This translates to an overall prevalence of 906 patients with SCIs per million population.[1] According to the National Spinal Cord Injury database, the majority of these patients are between the ages of 15 and 20. Males are four times as likely to sustain a severe SCI compared to females. Nearly half of all SCIs are sustained as a result of motor vehicle accidents. Falls from a height account for a 20.8%, while penetrating injury including gunshot wounds or stabbings account for nearly 15%. Sports related injuries account for 14% of all SCI.[2]

With regard to neurologic level, Thomas in 1982 reported that approximately 28% of all patients with SCI are incomplete quadriplegics. Twenty-six percent are complete paraplegics while 24% are complete quadriplegics.[3] These percentages are actually in decline as a result of improved management in the field. One aspect of SCI that is not usually apparent is that a decrease in life expectancy is associated with increased age or increased magnitude of neurologic deficit at the time of injury. For instance, a 20-year-old patient who is a complete quadriplegic may have an estimated 20-year life expectancy, while a 60-year-old patient with the same injury has only a 1.9-year life expectancy. Similarly, the 20-year-old patient who is an incomplete paraplegic may have a 33-year life expectancy, while a patient of the same age who is a complete quadriplegic may only have an estimated 20-year life expectancy. Within the first month of SCI, mortality is most often associated with pulmonary embolus, septicemia, and pneumonia.

Philosophical differences have existed between the orthopedic and neurosurgical management of SCI. The orthopedic literature has focused primarily on defining what constitutes vertebral column stability and how best to surgically restore it. The literature on the management of SCI lacks well-designed, prospective studies, and as such is quite confusing. Most of these studies include small numbers of patients with limited follow-up. In many of these studies, the prospective neurologic status of the patient's is unclear, and relatively few consistent grading systems are employed. The interval between the injury and the intervention also varied from study to study. The role of stabilization seems well accepted in the orthopedic literature as it is believed to prevent further cord damage and provides the optimal environment for recovery. The role of decompression with respect to the timing of surgery, however, remains somewhat fatalistic and unclear, as pathologic changes that occur during the initial insult have previously been considered irreversible.

HISTORY

The first natural history study on SCI was reported by Sir Ludwig Guttman in 1963.[4] He reported the 20-year experience of the National Spinal Injury Center at the Stokes Mandiville Hospital in England. One hundred forty-two patients with cervical spine injuries were followed for 20 years during which approximately 50% of the patients had some neurologic improvement with nonoperative treatment. Improvement was defined as any increase in grade of strength or return of nerve root function. In 1969, Frankel reported the natural history data from the same institution after following 123 patients with complete SCI's.[5] Over time, 34% of the patients had some degree of functional recovery, while 2% experienced some degree of deterioration. It was unclear whether these patients deteriorated as the result of intervention or as the result of the natural progression of their injury. In a prospective study of 283 patients with SCIs Marshall later defined the incidence of neurologic deterioration. He noted that approximately 5% of patients deteriorated during the acute management phase of their treatment. The majority of these patients deteriorated as a result of a specific event such as surgery, traction, halo application, or striker frame rotation.[6]

In 1971, Bosch and Stauffer reported the natural history of various SCI patterns. They noted that in 60 patients with incomplete spinal cord lesions, 90% of those patients with Brown-Sequard syndrome experienced improvement, 50% of those with a central cord syndrome experienced improvement, and only 16% of those with an anterior cord syndrome experienced improvement.[7] When they looked at patients with complete injury patterns, they found that as many as 80% can expect to recover at least one nerve root level after a complete spinal cord lesion. The only consistently poor results with respect to the recovery of nerve root function was in those patients who had unreduced dislocated facets. Over the next decade, Stauffer went on to further describe several observations regarding the natural history of SCI.[8] Some of these include the following:

1. Complete lesions do not recover motor control.
2. Complete lesions recover one nerve root level of function.
3. Partial lesions recover partially.
4. Less injury allows greater recovery.
5. Patients with a Brown-Sequard syndrome have a higher rate of recovery compared with patients with a central cord syndrome, who in turn had better prognoses than patients with an anterior cord syndrome.
6. Reduction of dislocated facets facilitates neurologic recovery regardless of the time interval to reduction.

PATHOPHYSIOLOGY

It has been well documented that mechanical injury rarely transects the spinal cord even when the SCI is complete. This raises the question as to what changes occur in the structure of the spinal cord that makes the resultant neurologic deficit irreversible. This question was first addressed by Allen in 1911 when he described the phenomenon of posttraumatic autodestruction.[9] Using a weight dropped from a height to impart an SCI in a dog, Allen performed postinjury myelotomies to remove the hematomyelia and found subsequent improvement in neurologic function. From this, he concluded that there existed some biochemical factor in the necrotic hemorrhage that perpetuated the injury over time. This observation led to the development of the concept of primary versus secondary mechanisms of SCI. Primary injury mechanisms traditionally have been considered mechanical phenomenon, and most often include acute compression or impact, distraction, laceration, or sheer injuries.

In a prospective study examining the effects of primary injury mechanisms, Delamarter inflicted a compressive injury to the spinal cord in a dog using a band constriction technique.[10] In this model, a 50% constriction was applied to the spinal cord at the L4 level using a nylon band. Initially, this resulted in paraplegia in all dogs studied. The dogs were then divided into five groups each undergoing release of the constriction at various times from immediately through 1 week. Only those dogs who had release of the constriction band within 1 hour had return of motor function as demonstrated by the ability to walk, as well as by the return of bowel or bladder function. All dogs subjected to greater than 6 hours of spinal compression had no recovery of motor function or bowel and bladder function. The spinal cords of the dogs were then subjected to histologic exam.

While those spinal cords subjected to 1 hour or less of constriction experienced variable degrees of Wallerian degeneration and demyelination, those spinal cords subjected to greater than 6 hours had evidence of severe necrosis extending 2 cm cephalad to the level of the constriction. Caudal to the level of the constriction, there was loss of cellular architecture, axonotmesis, and increased fibrosis. In addition to primary mechanisms of injury, several secondary mechanisms of injury have been proposed. These include vascular insults to the spinal cord sustained by hypotension associated with neurogenic shock, hemorrhage, and decreased blood flow as a result of vasospasm and thrombosis. Electrolyte changes include increased intracellular calcium and increased extracellular potassium. Biochemical changes include neurotransmitter accumulation (noradrenaline, dopamine, and glutamate), free radical production, and lipid peroxidation. Secondary spinal cord edema also has been associated with progressive damage to the spinal cord. In 1991, Tator described a posttraumatic ischemic cascade in which hemorrhage and edema resulted in axonal and neuronal necrosis. This was followed by demyelination, aseptic degeneration, and ultimately infarction of the central portion of the spinal cord.[11] This cascade reflects similar pathologic changes previously observed by Allen in 1914 after using his weight-drop technique on the spinal cords of dogs.[12] Allen demonstrated that within 15 minutes after the acute compression, microhemorrhages developed within the gray matter, while edema occurred in the white matter. By 2 hours, there was increased hemorrhage in the gray matter. At 4 hours post injury, axial degeneration ensued and myelin sheaths were disrupted. Central cord necrosis could be identified within 1 to 2 days after acute injury.

By defining these secondary mechanisms of SCI, specific treatment interventions directed at each component of the ischemic cascade may be proposed. Volume expansion increases blood pressure and can thereby rapidly improve spinal cord profusion. Opiate antagonists, such as naloxone, improve blood pressure and spinal cord blood flow. Calcium channel blockers, including nimodipine, which exerts selective action on cerebral vasculature, prevents the intracellular influx of calcium responsible for toxic cell death. These calcium channel blockers also dilate blood vessels increasing spinal cord blood flow.

Based on these observations, with respect to the pathophysiology of SCI, certain conclusions can be made. First, the initial contusion is not solely responsible for the pathologic changes observed histologically in SCI. Progressive cellular degeneration seems to interfere with the ability to regenerate. The degree of demyelination is proportional to the duration of compression; if the decompression can occur within 1 hour, the spinal cord would have the best chance for recovery. Decompression beyond 6 hours of compression may preclude the recovery of function. As Delamarter stated, "Although the time available for intervention is short, there is a period when complete injury may be partially reversible."[10] Although ischemia, with or without compression, is related to loss of neurologic function, degree of pathologic change is related to the duration of compression.

CLOSED MANAGEMENT

Early administration of pharmacologic agents such as high-dose methylprednisolone has been shown to alter the course of neurologic recovery. Bracken reported in 1992 that methylprednisolone administered in a loading dose of 30 mg/kg over 15 minutes followed by a maintenance dose of 5.4 mg/kg/hr over the subsequent 23 hours improved neurologic recovery rate compared to naloxone or placebo if the methylprednisolone was administered within 8 hours after injury.[13] When administered beyond 8 hours, either methylprednisolone or naloxone resulted in a worse outcome when compared with placebo administration alone.[14] Methylprednisolone exerts its effect by inhibiting lipid peroxidation while increasing spinal cord blood flow, extracellular calcium, and overall cell metabolism. Closed reduction of cervical spine dislocations have been considered the earliest method of neurologic decompression. Cotler in 1987 reported results of early high-weight closed reduction of patients with unilateral and bilateral facet dislocations.[15] In his group of 24 patients, 9 of 10 patients with incomplete SCI improved at least one Frankel grade. Those reductions attempted within 24 hours were far more successful. Nearly half of the unreducable dislocations were those that were attempted after an average of 12 days. He recommended that patients with unilateral facet dislocations should undergo early closed reduction. If this procedure were done successfully, elective open reduction with internal fixation should be performed. When a bilateral facet dislocation with a neurologic deficit was identified, urgent reduction was recommended. If the surgeon was only able to convert the bilateral facet dislocation into a unilateral facet dislocation, early posterior open reduction and internal fixation should be carried out. If the patient with the bilateral facet dislocation and neurologic deficit is unreducable, the patient should be brought to the operating room for an immediate posterior open reduction with internal fixation. Findings from the Regional Spinal Cord Injury Center of the Delaware Valley suggested that urgent reduction of flexion distraction injuries (under 8 hours) improved recovery. These studies suggest that high-weight closed reductions were safe and effective in improving neurologic function if the patient was awake and cooperative.

The criticism of acute closed reductions of cervical dislocations stems from a documented incidence of herniated cervical discs as high as 54% in those patients with facet dislocations.[16] The concern is that the spinal canal volume is lessened by the disk herniation and that during the reduction, the cord is brought under direct compression by the disk herniation. In our institution, we have not observed any cases of neurologic deterioration associated with closed reduction when the patient was awake and cooperative. We believe that, if the patient is indeed awake and cooperative and has a documented neurologic deficit, obtaining an MRI scan before an attempt at closed reduction delays the decompressive effects of an early reduction and adds additional risk to the patient incurred during transport. An MRI scan should be obtained before reduction if the patient is unconscious, uncooperative, or if the *first* attempt at closed reduction is unsuccessful.

SURGICAL INTERVENTION

The controversy regarding early surgical intervention arises from the question of whether or not improvement or deterioration in the postoperative period is the result of surgery, or if it reflects the natural course of the injury. As such, surgical intervention has been controversial and is usually reserved for those patients with incomplete SCI. Early surgical intervention had traditionally been associated with a high rate of complication. Verbiest in 1962 reported results of nine patients with complete quadriplegia who underwent early anterior decompression to remove anterior bone fragments creating compression on the spinal cord.[17] Although four patients had some improvement in upper extremity strength, five patients died within 3 weeks. Verbiest therefore, abandoned surgery within the acute phase of SCI. Other studies have suggested that early intervention might be detrimental as well. Herbison described a period of initial spontaneous worsening after SCI and advocated delaying surgery until this period was over. This concept was partially based on the work of Tator and Fehlings with their description of the secondary mechanism of injury. Herbison noted that 27% of SCI patients had initial worsening within the first 72 hours when followed with serial neurologic examinations. These changes were noted to peak at approximately 1 week. In 1987, Marshall reviewed the outcome of 134 patients with SCI who underwent surgical intervention at various intervals from the time of injury.[6] Overall, 3% of the 134 patients experienced some degree of neurologic worsening. Interestingly, all patients with neurologic worsening had their operation within 5 days of their injury. Similarly, in a review of 1,031 patients with SCI treated at the Thomas Jefferson University Hospital, 2% experienced deterioration overall. None of the patients operated on after 5 days of injury experienced neurologic deterioration.[18] In 1982, Bohlman and Anderson studied a cohort of patients with complete quadriplegia who underwent late surgical decompression with anterior cervical discectomies and fusions.[19] In this group of patients, the average time from injury to surgical intervention was 15 months. At an average follow-up of 5 years, "root return" was noted to be at least one level in 18 patients, and at least two to three grades of improvement in six patients. Two levels of neurologic recovery were noted in seven patients. From this study, the authors concluded that the time to surgery was not the crucial factor contributing to functional recovery.

In summary, those advocates of delayed surgical intervention feel that true "early" intervention may not be practical. Delaying surgery until the patient has reached a neurologic plateau is preferable and allows the surgeon to carry out a well-planned procedure on a medically stable patient. According to Bohlman's work, many patients have experienced some degree of neurologic recovery even after late decompression.

Recently, with the advent of improved stabilization techniques and implants, renewed interest in early surgical intervention has surfaced. Advocates for early intervention suggest that the surgeon can maximize the environment for neurologic recovery by providing immediate decompression while simultaneously restoring alignment and stability. Early intervention may also allow earlier mobilization, thereby avoiding the systemic and psychiatric complications associated with prolonged immobilization. This would allow earlier transfer to rehabilitation facilities with an associated decrease in overall medical expenditure.

Wilberger demonstrated that systemic complications in patients with SCIs do indeed decrease if surgery is performed within 24 hours of injury.[20] The incidence of pneumonia has been shown to decrease from 21% to 10%, while the rate of decubiti decreases from 16% to 10%.

If one considers the findings by Bracken regarding the early administration of methylprednisolone with an associated improvement in neurologic recovery rates, then one must suspect that there does exist a therapeutic window during which surgical intervention also may affect the course of the neurologic deficit. This concept of a therapeutic window is consistent with the findings of Delamarter, who, as previously discussed, demonstrated that decompression of constricted spinal cords within 6 hours of injury provided for the ultimate complete return of motor and bowel and bladder function.

In a recent prospective randomized blinded trial looking at the effects of urgent surgical decompression with or without methylprednisolone, Rabinowitz and colleagues demonstrated that early decompression within 6 hours, with or without methylprednisolone, resulted in significantly better neurologic function than with methylprednisolone alone.[21] Whether or not methylprednisolone administration improves outcome when combined with decompression remains unclear.

Other studies have been somewhat more ambivalent. Levi and coworkers compared the outcomes of 103 patients with SCIs treated in under 24 hours compared with those treated surgically after 24 hours.[22] They noted that most patients undergoing surgical intervention within 24 hours experienced no difference in mortality, motor improvement, respiratory care, or duration of hospitalization. From this they concluded that there was no statistical difference in outcome between early and delayed surgery. There were no increased complications associated with early surgery. In conclusion, they advocated early surgery simply because it was easier to care for the stabilized patients and was subsequently easier to transfer them to their rehabilitation facilities.

In summary, advocates for early surgical intervention suggest that fewer systemic complications are experienced by the patient and that earlier transfer to rehabilitation may be possible. With recent improvements in surgical technique, early intervention is not only safer but may be better for possible neurologic improvement. Lastly, studies advocating the use of methylprednisolone within 8 hours of injury suggest that there may indeed exist an early therapeutic window during which time surgical intervention may provide for improved neurologic recovery. Surgery within 6 hours of injury, realistically is impossible in all but a select few patients with minimal multisystem trauma who have the injury close enough to an emergency center where diagnosis and surgical team assembly can take place.

SUMMARY

The surgical approach to the patient with SCI requires an understanding of primary versus secondary mechanisms of injury. Primary mechanisms of injury include mechanical trauma such as compression and may exert their effects in a time-dependent fashion. Secondary mechanisms of injury may be vascular in origin and may result in an ischemic cascade of injury at the cellular level within the spinal cord. Subsequent biochemical, electrolyte, and inflammatory changes may contribute to the propagation of the SCI. Like the primary mechanisms of injury, these secondary mechanisms exert their effects in a time-dependent fashion as well. In the decision-making process regarding surgical intervention, the surgeon must first ensure that the patient is medically stabilized. He must then thoughtfully evaluate the mechanism and extent of the SCI. Attention should then turn to decompression of the spinal cord, whether through early closed reduction or through early or delayed surgical intervention after which some form of mechanical stability to the spine is restored. Advocates for early, aggressive surgical intervention suggest that fewer systemic complications are sustained by the patient. Further, there may exist an early, albeit short, therapeutic window during which the neurologic deficit may be partially or even completely reversible. Advocates for delayed surgical intervention suggest that true early surgery within the theoretic therapeutic window of 6 to 8 hours may not be realistic. Accordingly, surgery after a neurologic plateau is reached may be safer. Delayed surgery allows the surgeon to carry out a well-planned procedure in a medically stable patient. Several studies show patients with SCIs have variable degrees of recovery even after late decompression.

REFERENCES

1. DeVivo MJ, et al: 1980 Prevalence of spinal cord injury: a re-estimation employing life table techniques, *Arch Neurol* 37:707–708, 1980.
2. *Accident Facts,* Chicago, 1983, National Safety Council.
3. Thomas JP: 1982 Inaugural lecture of the G. Heiner Sell distinguished lectureship. Presented at the Eighth Annual Scientific Meeting of the American Spinal Injury Association, New York, April 9, 1982.
4. Guttmann L: Early management of the paraplegic, symposium on spinal injuries, *J Roy Coll Surg* 1963.
5. Frankel IIL, et al: The value of postural reduction in the initial management of closed injuries of the spine with paraplegia and tetraplegia. Part I, *Paraplegia* 7:179–192, 1969.
6. Marshall LF, et al: Deterioration following spinal cord injury: a multi center study, *J Neurosurg* 66:400–404, 1987.
7. Bosch A, Stauffer ES, Nickel VL: Incomplete traumatic quadriplegia: a ten year review, *JAMA* 216:473–478, 1971.
8. Stauffer ES: Neurologic recovery following injuries to the cervical spinal cord and nerve roots, *Spine* 9(5):532–534, 1984.
9. Allen AR: Surgery of experimental lesion of spinal cord equivalent to crush injury of fracture dislocation of spinal column. A preliminary report, *JAMA* 57:878–880, 1991.
10. Delamarter RB, Sherman J, Carr JB: Pathophysiology of spinal cord injury. Recovery after immediate and delayed decompression, *J Bone Joint Surg* 77A:1042–1049, 1995.
11. Tator CH, Fehlings MG: Review of the secondary theory of acute spinal cord trauma with emphasis on vascular mechanisms, *J Neurosurg* 75:15–26, 1991.
12. Allen AR: Remarks on the histopathological changes in the spinal cord due to impact. An experimental study, *J Nerv Merit Dis* 41:141–147, 1914.
13. Bracken MB, et al: A randomized, controlled trial of methylprednisolone or naloxone in the treatment of acute spinal cord injury. Results of the second National Acute Spinal Cord Injury Study, *N Engl J Med* 322:1405–1411, 1990.
14. Bracken MB, et al: Methylprednisolone or naloxone treatment after acute spinal cord injury: 1-year follow-up data, *J Neurosurg* 76:23–31, 1992.
15. Cotler HB, et al: Closed reduction of cervical spine dislocations, *Clin Orthop* 214:185–199, 1987.
16. Eismont F: Extrusion of an intervertebral disc associated with traumatic subluxation or dislocation of cervical facets, *J Bone Joint Surg* 73A(10):1555–1560, 1991.
17. Verbiest H: Anterior operative approach in cases of spinal-cord compression by old irreducible displacement or fresh fracture of cervical spine. Contribution to operative repair of deformed vertebral bodies, *J Neurosurg* 19:389–400, 1962.
18. Farmer J, et al: Neurologic deterioration following cervical spinal cord injury, *Orthop Trans* 19(2):308, 1995.
19. Bohlman HH, Anderson PA: Anterior decompression and arthrodesis of the cervical spine: Long-term motor improvement, *J Bone Joint Surg* 74A:671–682, 1992.
20. Wilberger J: Diagnosis and management of spinal cord trauma, *J Neurotrauma* 8(suppl):S21–S28, 1991.
21. Rabinowitz RS, Currier BL, Jimenez MA: The effect of urgent decompression and methylprednisolone, and methylprednisolone alone on the outcome of spinal cord injury: a blinded, prospective, randomized trial in beagles, Presented at NASS, 1995.
22. Levi L, et al: Anterior decompression in cervical spine trauma: does the timing of surgery affect the outcome?, *Neurosurgery* 29(2):216–222, 1991.

24

RECOVERY AND FUNCTIONAL OUTCOME IN SPINAL TRAUMA

Christopher P. Silveri
Jerome M. Cotler

Spinal cord injury (SCI) occurs swiftly and unmercifully; a solitary moment in time with resultant lifelong ramifications. It has been estimated that more than 200,000 Americans have sustained traumatic injury to the spinal cord and currently live with their disability.[1] Historically, such an event results in a complete loss of function, immobility, and early mortality from the complications of recumbency. Lack of medical sophistication and knowledge through the early 20th century resulted in futile efforts to stabilize the trauma patient and allow for recovery. For those fortunate to survive the initial event, little hope existed for long-term function. Since the post–World War I era, great advances have been made in the treatment of all aspects of the severely injured patient and have led to the development and improvement of rehabilitation services. Cushing has been cited as noting a dismal outcome for soldiers with SCI sustained during World War I with an 80% mortality within weeks.[2] Since that time, efforts have been made in improving prehospital care, cardiorespiratory resuscitation, antibiotic treatment, and the use of coordinated interdisciplinary teams of professionals to care for the numerous complexities of the medical, surgical, psychosocial, and rehabilitative aspects of such patients. With these advantages came increased survival and greater dependence on hospital personnel and outpatient rehabilitation facility requirements. Specific treatment centers were developed to manage the chronically injured patient after acute hospitalization was no longer needed. These centers promote an organized system of individual care with the technical support, medical assistance, and a wide range of physical and occupational therapy programs to maximize recovery and resume a productive, meaningful life. This comprehensive rehabilitation system as suggested by DeVivo allows for more than half of the patients to achieve independence, self care, and mobility on level surfaces.[3,6] Although only half of these patients return to gainful employment, this modern era of rehabilitation has allowed virtually 95% to return to the community.

Over the past 20 years the incidence of SCI remains at approximately 10,000 per year. With improved long-term survival, this continues to escalate the social and economic burden to society. This is all too important in the age of managed care and cost analysis. Over the past few decades, motor vehicle accidents and falls have comprised the two leading causes of SCI accounting for more than 65% of all cases.[4,5] Men are most often affected at an average age of between 19.7 and 31 years.[6] Given such a youthful population, it is critical that some form of education and rehabilitation exists to facilitate their return in some capacity to everyday life and return them to the workforce.

THE TEAM

Yarkony stated "collaboration, not isolation is the key to enhanced rehabilitation success."[7] The multidisciplinary approach to the care of these patients has almost singlehandedly offered the greatest potential for recovery. Each member of the team brings a sense of purpose, energy, and knowledge to encourage patient outlook and physical improvement. Such an approach offers the greatest amount of protection from complications and specialized talent to solve the many complex problems of the spine-injured patient. The rehabilitation team consists of physicians of rehabilitation medicine, orthopedic and neurosurgical surgeons, nurses, physical and occupational therapists, social workers, and, often, psychologists. Several other consultants are used quite often in medicine, plastic surgery, general surgery, and urology to assist with complicated cases.

Often neglected in these discussions is the fact that the potential for recovery and rehabilitation *begins* at the moment treatment is initiated. Prehospital and emergency care is vital to the eventual patient outcome. Associated with SCI are other skeletal, cardiac, respiratory, visceral, or head injuries, which complicate the acute care in 50% of cases.[8] The potential morbidity rises even further when one considers 15% of these patients have a second noncontiguous spine fracture, which is often neglected.[9] The evaluation and stabilization of the spine-injured patient begins in the field with the emergency medical technicians. Proper attention to immobilization principles and transport minimizes further injury. These actions, however, have only been subject to scrutiny for the past two decades with the development of the Emergency Medical Services System Act of 1973 and other legislation. Efforts to improve emergency methods and educate field personnel resulted from reports of a high (26%) incidence of neurologic demise during transport to local hospitals.[10] In another series, Bohlman noted missed cervical spinal injuries in one third of cases reported in 1979.[11] Since these reports, however, iatrogenic injury, whether its in the field or in the hospital, has been greatly diminished because of better awareness and education. Whether caused by intoxication, disorientation, head trauma, or life-threatening system injuries, the potential to miss these injuries still exists and a high index of suspicion is required both in the field and by all emergency hospital personnel.

The acute care of the trauma patient begins with the ABCs of cardiorespiratory resuscitation. When spinal injury is suspected, however, orthopedic and neurosurgical consultation becomes necessary to maintain order in what often appears a chaotic life-saving environment. Protection of the neck and spine is critical to preserving neurologic function and is possible while cardiopulmonary resuscitation (CPR) and other life-saving measures are taken. Once stabilized, continued emphasis on spinal alignment is mandatory during transport, logrolling, and subsequent evaluations.

The neurologic evaluation has been standardized and must be evaluated and recorded at several points during the initial emergency hospitalization. It is recorded with careful attention to both sensory and motor function to accurately identify a level of neurologic injury. Subsequent evaluations must be consistent and performed in equivalent detail so subtle neurologic deterioration from malposition, hypotension, or edema are appreciated and acted upon swiftly. Muscle strength is determined on a point scale from 0 to 5. Paralysis is recorded as 0; evidence of muscle firing by contractions is given 1 point. Two points are assigned for movement without gravity resistance; 3 points for function against gravity; and 4 points are given for active motor function against moderate resistance. Normal motor strength is given 5 points. Although the skeletal level involved is determined by the level of greatest bony injury, the motor level is determined by that level with bilateral motor function of 3 out of 5 or greater. The sensory examination is recorded in a similar fashion with 2 points for normal sensation, 1 for impaired function, and 0 for absent sensory activity. These also are noted on a dermatomal chart to indicate the sensory level. Once these motor and sensory scores are recorded, guidelines have been established by the American Spinal Injury Association (ASIA) to assign an overall neurologic impairment rating, which standardizes and facilitate prognostic assessment[12]. An ASIA A classification represents complete SCI with no motor or sensory activity present distal to the level of injury. An ASIA B lesion represents an incomplete injury with preservation of some degree of sensory activity distal to the injury but with absent motor function. An ASIA C level is noted when sensory function and motor function are present distal to the injury and the motor grade is less than or equal to 3 out of 5. An ASIA D is present when motor grade is greater than 3 out of 5, and a normal neurologic examination is assigned an ASIA E grade.

Motor or sensory function below the level of injury indicates an incomplete injury pattern and recovery of function remains possible. Neurologic testing includes sacral and sphincter testing, because this area represents the lowest portion of the spinal cord and, if present, carries an improved prognosis. Spinal shock is manifested by total neurologic absence and usually resolves by 24 to 48 hours. During this time, it is impossible to determine the extent of neural injury. It is currently unclear as to the mechanism of this occurrence. With the return of distal reflex arc activity within the anterior horn cells of the cord, spinal shock has resolved and determination of complete versus incomplete lesions can be accurately assessed. With a bulbocavernosus reflex present, lack of sacral sensory or motor sparing indicates a complete cord injury and the worst prognosis. Incomplete lesions, when diagnosed, have the greatest potential for improvement. These have been classically divided into syndromes based on the neuroanatomical location of maximal injury within the cord (Table 24-1). The worst prognoses are associated with anterior cord syndrome. Motor loss, pain, and temperature sensitivity loss are related to injury to the anterior and anterolateral areas of the cord. Retropulsion of bone posteriorly into the canal, injury to the anterior spinal artery, and herniated nucleus pulposis all can contribute to this entity.

The central cord syndrome is the most commonly encountered pattern of injury and is frequently seen in the elderly or in patients with congenital cervical spinal stenosis. Severe extension forces cause compromise of the cord by a pincer mechanism with osteophytes and disk acting anteriorly and posteriorly by infolding of the hypertrophic ligamentum flavum. This results in injury and edema to the central cord with the area of insult diminishing radially outward producing greater upper extremity deficits than lower extremity.

Table 24-1. Incomplete SCI Syndromes

Name	Cause	Outcome	Prognosis
Anterior cord syndrome	Retropulsed bone-disk Anterior spinal artery injury	Motor loss Pain-temperature loss	Worst
Central cord syndrome (most common)	Advanced age Extension-Pincer mechanism Hyperflexion	Motor loss Upper ext > lower ext	Fair lower extremity recovery Poor upper extremity recovery Spasticity lower extremity
Brown-Sequard syndrome (unusual)	Penetrating injury Unilateral	Ipsilateral motor loss Contralateral sensory loss	Good recovery
Posterior cord syndrome (rare)	Posterior column injury	Motor intact or variable loss Decreased sensation and proprioception Pain intact	Unclear
Conus medularis syndrome	Injury to terminal cord L1-L2 (sacral anterior horn dysfunction; cells)	Bowel/bladder Perianal sensory deficits	Poor bowel/bladder Root escape
Cauda equina syndrome	Lower motor neuron injury to LS root	Variable motor and sensory loss	Good recovery

Neurologic recovery is variable with fair improvement in lower extremity function usually exceeding that of the upper extremity. Profound disability of hand and upper extremity function may remain with often improved but spastic lower extremities.

Unilateral lesions usually are linked to penetrating injuries such as gunshot wounds and knife wounds and are in reality not common. Known as Brown-Sequard injuries, one side of the cord is damaged resulting in loss of ipsilateral motor function and contralateral sensory function. The prognosis for recovery is typically quite good.

The last area of cord injury is the posterior cord syndrome, which is extremely rare. Theoretically it results in sensory dysfunction below the level of the injury without motor loss. Highly unusual, it is impossible to typify its prognosis.

The conus medullaris syndrome is a lesion at the end of the cord in which the sacral horn cells are located. Usually posterior to the L1-L2 interval, injury here produces bowel and bladder dysfunction, sacral and perianal sensory changes, and poor rectal tone. Poor prognosis is usually the case with little return of bowel and bladder function. Lower extremity function, however, often is preserved because of root escape. This occurs when the lumbar roots have already exited their anterior horn cells and have become more durable, peripheral type nerve roots at the level of injury. Surrounding the conus, they often are minimally injured when the conus has sustained a permanent injury. Also, the bulbocavernosus reflex, being a lower motor neuron reflex at this level, may be permanently disrupted complicating the issue of spinal shock.

Cauda equina syndrome describes injuries to the nerve roots below the level of the conus. Without upper motor neuron involvement at this level, the lumbosacral roots are durable and withstand great forces recovering as would a peripheral nerve. Lower motor neuron injury results in motor loss, sensory deficits, and loss of distal reflexes. The prognosis is excellent and aggressive surgical decompression often results in further recovery.

ACUTE PHASE CARE

The goals of treatment in the acute phase of SCI parallel those of the rehabilitation team. The objectives are to maximize and protect neural function, obtain and maintain stability, both skeletal and medical, potentiate neurologic recovery and prepare the patient for the rehabilitation process and assimilation back into society. Once the hemodynamic function of the trauma patient is normalized, efforts must focus on evaluating and treating spinal instability. This is either accomplished by nonoperative or operative means. Spinal alignment must be assessed and obtained if gross displacement or angulation is present. Individual fracture patterns will be discussed in other chapters, however several principles are worth mentioning here. Spinal stability is important for two reasons: First, persistent bony instability causes neural instability and continued injury to the spinal cord or roots; and second, rapid reduction and decompression of the neural elements should be achieved as soon as possible to maximize recovery. Animal studies suggest that decompression of the cord compression within 6 hours is statistically beneficial, with best results seen within 1 hour.[13] Urgent decompression of the spinal cord, however, does not mean early, rapid operative decompression. Several clinical studies have shown deleterious effects of surgical intervention performed too early in the course of treatment.[14,15]

The orthopedic surgeon has three other methods for enhancing neurologic recovery. The first critical step involves emergent decompression of the neural elements by means of closed reduction. Advocated at the Regional Spinal Cord Injury Center of Delaware Valley (RSCICDV), closed reduction techniques have been successfully used to obtain prompt reduction of a dislocated spine. Reduction is then followed by maintenance of traction for alignment or conversion to halo orthosis in most cases.[16,17] This is best performed within 2 to 3 hours of presentation to the emergency room. The patient is placed supine on the Stryker frame (Stryker Corp., Kalamazoo, MI) and Gardner-Wells tongs (Zimmer, Inc., Warsaw, IN) are applied to the cranium. Steel tongs are used in case high-weight reductions are necessary. To participate in a closed reduction technique, the patient must be awake and cooperative and able to respond to repeated neurologic testing. The only reports of neurologic demise in the literature seen with closed reduction techniques are those with patients under general anesthesia.[18] Dedicated radiology personnel are needed to obtain serial lateral radiographs after each 10-pound increment is added at 10- to 15-minute intervals until reduction is obtained. With prompt reduction, the surgeon's second opportunity to augment neurologic recovery is to efficiently immobilize the patient in the reduced position. This diminishes further neurologic injury, edema, and hematoma. Halo immobilization is easily converted from the Gardner-Wells tong traction once reduction is achieved. Repeat radiographs are then assessed to confirm maintenance of reduction. If unable to maintain reduction or use a halo immobilization orthosis, maintenance in traction is safely accomplished by placing the patient in a rotating bed to avoid pulmonary and skin complications. Thoracolumbar fracture dislocations are treated in a similar manner, either by supine postural reduction on a similar bed or by cranial tong bifemoral skeletal traction to maintain longitudinal traction on the reduced spine before surgical stabilization. The potential for redisplacement exists despite traction or halo immobilization, and strict communication is necessary between physician, nursing, and therapy staff to avoid such problems. Certain positions and some range-of-motion activities may be contraindicated and should be made clear to the floor staff. Neurologic level should be addressed and described so subtle changes can be noted by each nursing shift and communicated to the physician. A decrease in motor score may be a sign of loss of stability and steps must be taken quickly to reverse this decline.

The surgeon has one last method to potentiate neurologic recovery, and it involves the use of steroid therapy to minimize the deleterious effects of injury between the neuronal hypoxemia and cellular dysfunction. The administration of methyl prednisolone within 8 hours of SCI is now the standard of care in all trauma centers.[19] The dose is 30 mg/kg given over 15 minutes, followed by 5.4 mg/kg/hr × 24 hours. Contraindications to its use include diabetes, infection, open fracture, pregnancy and children less than 13 years of age. Its mechanism of action is not actually known, but it likely involves modulation of cellular membrane function, inhibition of lipid peroxidation, and hydrolysis at the injury site and reduction of edema and inflammatory reaction. Other medical therapies have been tried with variable success, however, have not yet become standard of care in most centers.

After evaluation, hemodynamic resuscitation, radiograph assessment, spinal reduction, and stabilization, the patient with SCI enters a period of time of great psychologic anguish and physical immobility. To complicate matters, the patient also becomes at risk for several acute-phase complications of recumbency. At this time, nursing care becomes a critical part of rehabilitation. Although the rotating bed and special mattresses assist in diminishing skin complications, it is only through aggressive positioning, logrolling, and screening that one prevents the formation of sacral and other pressure point decubiti. Important areas to monitor, aside from the usual sacral and buttock areas, include the halo-vest pressure points, occipital protuberance areas, scapulae, heels, and under the dorsal gibbous of thoracolumbar spine fractures. This is especially true when bolsters are placed at the area of gibbous for postural closed reduction manipulation.

Before long-term counseling and psychologic support, the nurse is the professional with the most initial contact facilitating the patient's difficult transition into a life of impairment. Compassion, kindness, gentle encouragement with hope and understanding helps the patient take the first and most difficult steps in accepting the injury and limitations of his or her lifestyle. It is at this point that the patient and the family need to appreciate the long-term goals expected of the patient and the degree of recovery anticipated.

As with most trauma patients, associated injuries are frequently experienced with skeletal injuries to the upper and lower extremities occurring in 9.5% of cases.[4] Similar to the principles of the multiple trauma patient, every effort is made for rapid, rigid internal fixation of such fractures to offer early immobilization and joint range of motion. Skin insensitivity and complications of prolonged recumbency preclude the use of skin or skeletal traction of long-bone injuries unless medical condition contraindicates surgery. Proper attention to long-bone injury assists the overall rehabilitation process. Transfers, assistive device use and ambulation all require upper and lower extremity function to the best of their neurologic capability. Weight-bearing injuries require standard intervals for healing and, unless treated urgently, the overall patient rehabilitation program is delayed. This exacerbate problems of recumbency and delays discharge to active intensive therapy units and eventual entrance back into society. To be admitted to a SCI rehabilitation facility the spine, the extremities, and all medical conditions must be fully stabilized.

Chronic Phase

After the initial injury stabilization and nonoperative or operative definitive treatment has been rendered, the patient enters the chronic phase of SCI rehabilitation. During this time, several changes occur both neurologically and those relating to bodily functions. The patient is at risk for early and late complications related to paralysis, immobility, sensory deficits, altered metabolism, and altered hemodynamic and respiratory function.

Recovery of neurologic function is the focus of all patients and practitioners in this setting. Often subtle improvements in motor root function are detected, however, rarely involving dramatic reversal of cord injury. Anticipation of neurologic improvement must proceed with cautious optimism. This is best handled by both family and patient if proper information and explanations are provided by the rehabilitation team. Recovery can occur and is identified by the improvements in neurologic function at the zone of injury or return of upper motor neuron activity distal to this zone. Improvements typically are seen in complete lesions where lower motor neuron function activity improves at the precise level of cord injury. Confined to a few segments, unilateral or bilateral improvements to functional levels of deltoid (C5), or biceps and wrist extension functions (C6) can be seen following a C5 quadriplegia for instance. Although the degree of these changes is impossible to anticipate, frequent neurologic examinations are vital to detect and specifically rehabilitate new muscle groups to improve overall functional status. Some degree of improvement in neurologic activity typically occurs after SCI, even in complete lesions, at the zone of injury. Such recovery has been documented in cervical injuries with improvements in upper extremity muscle strength occurring for as long as 2 years.[20] Review of 150 complete C4, C5, and C6 injuries revealed that patients with some muscle strength in the segment below the intact level showed 80% to 90% recovered strength to a grade of 4 or 5 within 4 to 6 months. In cases of no muscle strength from the segment below the intact level, only 25% to 35% showed recovery within 4 to 6 months; however, late improvement occurs after discharge from the rehabilitation facility. The significance of this statement is evidence of the managed care pressure to limit the length of inpatient rehabilitation stay. Although the exact mechanism of neural repair is not known, it involves some degree of peripheral sprouting of motor terminals.[21] This coupled with return of normal neural conduction (diminished neurapraxia) accounts for considerable motor improvement. According to Ditunno, long tract recovery is much less predictable and likely caused by some remyelinization and possible central sprouting.[20]

Incomplete cervical lesions tend to recover sooner than complete lesions, both at and distal to the site of injury. Patients with ASIA A injuries who remain that way for longer than 1 week usually do not recover useful neurologic function (ASIA D level) below the level of the zone of partial preservation. This is an area of partially innervated segments below the level of complete cord dysfunction. Most often such cases of dramatic improvement are related to misdiagnosis of an incomplete lesion for a complete lesion. Finalizing the prognosis during a period of spinal shock or concomitant head injury also may confound the neurologic picture.

Patients, however, with any signs of voluntary movement distal to the injury level, especially in the lower extremities, show useful motor recovery (ASIA D) in 80% of cases.[22] Recent data from Thomas Jefferson University Hospital showed that eventual walking could be predicted on the basis of initial and follow-up tests of motor strength in the quadriceps. Patients with some quadriceps function whose muscle grade improved to a grade of 3 or higher by 2 months postinjury had excellent prognosis for becoming a household or community ambulator by 1 year. Those who did not improve until after the 2-month mark showed less recovery.[23]

Exact prediction of recovery is not the goal of the rehabilitation team, and this should be deemphasized. It is important, however, to be cognizant of and respond to patient interpretation of perceived improvement with neurologic evaluation performed on a regular basis to confirm each advance and to adjust the physical and occupational rehabilitation accordingly. Neurologic decline, however, is not common and, if noted, warrants serious investigation to its etiology. Several situations could result in late neurologic demise including spinal instability, progressive deformity, cystic degeneration of the spinal cord, or tethered cord syndrome. Immediate treatment is imperative whenever possible. Referral to an acute facility may be required.

SECONDARY PROBLEMS

DECUBITUS ULCERATION

Loss of sensation below the level of injury poses great risk for skin breakdown in the patient with SCI. Pressure sores are the most common complication in this population. The incidence ranges from 10% to 25%; however, specialized rehabilitation centers can diminish risk to less than 5%.[24] Most often sores occur at the sacrum with this area accounting for 55% of all cases.[4]

The most common etiologic factors are prolonged pressure and shear with shifting of tissues producing a loss of blood flow to the skin surface. Risk begins during the first few hours of injury when many patients remain on hard spine boards awaiting evaluation in the emergency room. Prolonged immobility especially in patients who are critically ill who require ventilatory support, or require prolonged skeletal spinal traction are at greatest risk for sacral and heel decubiti. Even with the advent of rotating beds, such as the Roto Rest bed (Kinetic Concepts, Inc., San Antonio, TX), constant attention is required to identify and respond to potential skin irritations. If not checked during each shift on a daily basis, pressure from a thoracolumbar fracture gibbous or ankylosing spondylitis, for instance, may form over the midthoracic spine complicating potential surgical intervention. Any site of skin breakdown, for that matter, produces considerable infectious risk and significant hospital resources for conservative care or surgical debridement of those wounds.

Prevention is the only suitable goal for the rehabilitation team. This requires eliminating shear forces and markedly diminishing the time a patient stays in one dependent position. In the acute setting, this means nursing care is responsible for logrolling every 1 to 2 hours if a rotating bed is not available, and adequately padding any area of bony prominence or point of contact with the bed. Family and friends also take part in maintaining a constant vigil for skin irritation. Decubitus screening must be performed daily by the rounding physicians as well usually inspecting all areas at high risk. This ensures multiple levels of safety as improvement in medical and neurologic condition is achieved. Once mobilization is possible, the patient should be out of bed as much as possible. Despite using cushions, weight shifting programs designed for pressure relief every 15 to 30 minutes are extremely necessary in the wheelchair-bound individual with ischium pressure relief at least 1 minute per side.[25] The goal of any rehabilitation program is to lengthen slowly the time between logrolling or weight shifting to eventually allow for full nights sleep without logrolling and sitting for 1 to 2 hours without the risk of skin breakdown over the ischium.

Medical condition, skin texture, and durability vary with each patient and individual treatment program. Medical management also plays a preventive role. Nutrition, vitamin supplements, avoidance of anemia, local dressing measures to protect skin at risk, bio-occlusive dressings for existing skin breakdown, and prevention of fecal or urine contamination and skin maceration collectively maximize skin integrity and reverse the initial stages of skin breakdown. Small areas of ulceration may respond over time to removal of the pressure. With larger lesions, however, debridement may be the only means of determining the extent of damage. Underlying osteomyelitis can be difficult to diagnose as it interferes with the healing process. A magnetic resonance image (MRI) scan is useful to determine the depth of involvement.[26] Deep ulcerations require multiple debridement and eventual muscle flap coverage, all of which prolong the rehabilitation time. Several complications can and do occur despite surgical intervention and can be fatal. Local infection, abscess formation, sepsis, amputation, and death are all possible complications of decubiti. Prevention and patient and family education are the best lines of defense against this difficult problem.

UROLOGIC MANIFESTATIONS

Bladder dysfunction occurs commonly in patients with SCI. A delicate balance exists between urine retention and micturition with the bladder and urethral sphincter working in harmony toward opposite goals. Complete SCI, in essence, isolates the urinary system from voluntary cortical proprioception and control, and from the involuntary centers controlling detrussor function and coordinated sphincter relaxation. Incontinence occurs if the bladder sphincter is unable to hold back the pressure of a filled bladder, and retention occurs if the bladder is unable to fully empty. The volume of residual urine should be always less than 100 mL. With purely upper motor neuron lesions, patients may have a local reflex of bladder contraction but lose the ability to relax their urethral sphincter so reflex voiding occurs but only at high sphincter pressures (bladder-sphincter dyssynergia). This results in high intravesicular pressure. A flaccid bladder on the other hand, because of a sacral anterior horn or conus lesion or a cauda equina lesion, voids only as a result of overflow with large postvoid residuals. Both scenarios pose risk to the upper collecting systems by pressure-related injury and as well as infection both in the bladder and with extension superiorly resulting in pyelonephritis.[27] High-pressure reflex voiding results in injury to the upper collection system and increases risk of bladder infection.[28] Overflow voiding poses a direct threat of urinary tract infection secondary to the high residual urinary retention and concomitant increased bacterial count.

To micturate or expel urine, one must be able to sense bladder filling, and when voiding is desired detrussor function contracts the bladder and the external urethral sphincter then must relax. Appreciation of these stages is critical in the management of bladder dysfunction after SCI. Often the most difficult problem is controlling the sphincter function.

Awareness of bladder fullness, if impaired, can be taught by regular palpation of the suprapubic area; however, no exogenous means are known to relax sphincter function on demand in patients with SCIs. High-pressure reflex voiding is sometimes improved by α-adrenergic blocking agents and antispasmodic agents to relax the sphincter mechanism.[3,29] External collecting systems are necessary and become less advantageous for the female patient. Intermittent catheterization is used by both males and females and in both types of bladder dysfunction. This avoids the possibility of overdistention if done at regular intervals. When bladder paralysis exists, voiding can be augmented by intraabdominal valsalva maneuvers; however, this doesn't always work well, and residual urine may remain excessive.[30]

Indwelling catheters are most commonly used in the acute care setting to manage fluid balance. Although long-term use of indwelling catheters is not the best form of treatment, in quadriplegics who are unable to perform self-catheterization it may remain practical, outweighing the long-term complications of bladder carcinoma and bacterial colonization.[31] If used, maintenance of high-volume urine output helps dilute bacterial titers, diminishing sediment and the possibility of catheter obstruction. If these techniques are necessary, many people prefer to choose a suprapubic catheter as another long-term option; however, this has complications of leakage and recurrent bladder stones. Intermittent catheterization regularly empties the bladder and avoids the problems associated with overdistention. This is best used if return of function is possible. It is best performed every 4 to 6 hours or when the bladder is full to resist infection and high-pressure injury. Annual bladder evaluations with a cystogram to rule out stones, as well as evaluate bladder function, along with screening of kidney function with nuclear scans should also be performed. Abnormal bladder dynamics unfortunately lead to the high incidence (an estimated 20%) of urinary tract infections after SCI.[32] Urinary tract infection is likely the most common complication seen in the first year following SCI. Although less common in recent years, septicemia from a urinary tract infection still remains a potential risk and can certainly be a cause of death in this population.[33] Fever and chills, when present in these patients, are clear indications of occult urinary tract infection until proven otherwise. Bacturia, however, without clinical signs and symptoms remains common indicating colonization, and acute treatment is not advocated.[34] By declaration of a recent research consensus when bacturia is accompanied by tissue invasion and tissue response with signs and symptoms, then by definition a urinary tract infection is present. Pyuria in patients without ability to note the classic symptoms also indicates potential impending morbidity and treatment is indicated. If high fever is associated with urinary tract infection, careful evaluation of both upper and lower collecting symptoms is necessary.

BOWEL FUNCTION

The bowel function of patients with SCI is significantly impaired (Table 24-2). Sphincter muscle control is affected with the primary cause being the inability to control inner sphincter relaxation to allow for elimination. This is often manifested by impaction, constipation, and incontinence. Early in the course of rehabilitation, bowel training to stimulate patterned movements may not be possible because of posttraumatic ileus or abdominal injury, which complicates the initial hospitalization.[35] As soon as possible, however, a program is set up to train the distal bowel to proceed with elimination. Dietary habits are kept regular, fluid intake encouraged, daily exercise and stool softeners, suppositories and timed evacuation are used to develop a routine of every-other-day independent bowel movements. Anal stimulation of the external sphincter aids in relaxation of the stronger inner sphincter and allows the bowel to empty. Care is taken to minimize narcotic use, because this delays bowel activity. Aggressive laxative or enema use is avoided because the effects are brief and not conducive to developing a simple gentle pattern of defecation. Especially in the high quadriplegic, constipation may cause bowel distention and affect the already compromised diaphragmatic excursion and limit title volume. In some cases, this could lead to respiratory distress, atelectasis, or pneumonia.

There is no doubt that bowel dysfunction along with bladder impairment creates patient concern and social handicaps far worse than lower extremity weakness. Interpersonal relationships, self-steem, and the ability to assimilate back into society are dependent on maintaining personal hygiene habits. A strict bowel regimen is possible and allows freedom from anxiety and embarrassment and greater independence in life.

SPASTICITY

When an individual injures his or her spinal cord, many of the inhibitory cortical signals used to regulate movement, reflexes, and coordination are lost. As a result, spasticity is almost ubiquitous in those with an SCI. Defined as a velocity-dependent increase in stretch reflexes, it becomes one of the most disabling aspects of the chronic rehabilitation effort. Paradoxically, patients with incomplete lesions actually exhibit more severe spasticity than complete counterparts. The pathophysiology is unknown; however, it may involve the formation of new synapses by motor neurons that have lost supraspinal input.[36] Usually absent in the initial postinjury period, development is insidious with nearly 75% of all patients with SCI becoming spastic by 1 year.[37] Precipitating factors of spasticity include pain stimulus, illness, and often signs of an impending urinary tract infection. Muscle contractions can be violent or relatively benign without much disruption in functional status. Treatment is indicated only if such activity does interfere with the rehabilitation process. Family and patient education can remove much of the anxiety about spasticity and actually calm episodes. With training, the patient may use mild spasticity to their advantage; as in assisting with standing or shifting in bed.[3]

Treatment includes a stretching program to diminish the stretch reflex and prevent contractures.[38] Medical intervention begins with Baclofen as the drug of

Table 24-2. Pathophysiology, Manifestations, and Management of Common Complications in Patients with Spinal Cord Injuries

Complication	Pathophysiology	Manifestations	Management*
Cardiac disease[†]	Decreased energy requirements; decreased glucose tolerance; adversely affected lipid values	Heart failure; ischemic heart disease; cardiac-related death	Modification of diet; exercise; possibly functional electrical stimulation
Pneumonia[‡]	Impaired cough due to intercostal and abdominal paralysis; decreased vital capacity	Fever; cough; respiratory failure; obtundation	Physical measures such as assisted cough, postural drainage, chest physical therapy, and incentive spirometry; maintenance of proper hydration; vaccination against influenza virus and pneumococcus
Musculoskeletal pain	Overuse of upper limbs to bear weight	Rotator-cuff disease; bicipital tendinitis; carpal tunnel syndrome	Training in modified or assisted transfers; NSAIDs; local injections; splinting and avoidance of weight bearing on extended wrists for carpal tunnel syndrome; use of a power-driven wheelchair
Deficient bowel control	Lack of cerebral control over anal sphincter	Impaction and incontinence	Clearance of impaction by use of cathartic agents; establishment of 3 : 2 : 1 regimen with a stool softener (docusate sodium, 100 mg orally 3 times a day), colonic stimulant (senna tablets, 2 orally each day 8 hours before bowel routine), and rapidly acting rectal stimulant (bisacodyl enema, 1 each day after a meal) to trigger the routine
Spinal cord pain	Deafferentation (poorly understood)	Burning, numb, tingling, or other noxious sensation below the level of injury	Consideration of possible primary exacerbating factor, such as posttraumatic cystic degeneration; treatment of secondary exacerbating factors, including depression; patient education; restoration of normal sleep pattern and activity level; antidepressant, anticonvulsant, and neuroleptic medications; neurosurgery

Continued

Table 24-2 CONT. Pathophysiology, Manifestations, and Management of Common Complications in Patients with Spinal Cord Injuries—cont'd

Complication	Pathophysiology	Manifestations	Management*
Autonomic hyperreflexia	Noxious stimulus below the level of injury resulting in sympathetic activity not moderated by supraspinal centers; occurs with injuries above the splanchnic outflow (T6)	Hypertension, diaphoresis, and severe headache; possibly seizures and intracerebral hemorrhage	With patient in sitting position, quick check for cause, such as a blocked catheter or tight clothing; sublingual nifedipine, parenteral antihypertensive agents (not β-adrenergic blockers); spinal anesthesia; for prophylaxis, α-adrenergic blockers, such as terazosin, and other medications, such as guanethidine and mecamylamine

From Ditunno JF Jr, Formal CS: Chronic spinal cord injury; *N Engl J Med* 330:550, 1994.
* NSAIDs denotes nonsteroidal antiinflammatory drugs.
† Cardiac disease is a leading cause of death in patients with spinal cord injuries, and the risk of death from this cause is at least as high in such patients as it is in the general population.
‡ The risk of death from pneumonia in patients with spinal cord injuries is more than 10 times higher than the risk in the general population.

choice.[36] Its mechanism to potentiate the inhibitory affects of gamma-aminobutyric acid (GABA) on reflex arcs. Several side effects exist, the most dangerous of which appears to be withdrawal seizures upon abrupt cessation of the baclofen. Otherwise, it is rare to exhibit delirium or seizure activity when taking the medicine, and early sedative effects usually diminish with continued use. Usually, dosages increase gradually to approximately 200 mg/day in divided doses. Other sedatives such as diazepam or other benzodiazepams also have beneficial effects on GABA; however, dependence on the sedative action and eventual tolerance interferes with their long-term effectiveness.

Dantrolene can also be used to interfere with the excitation-contraction coupling mechanism.[36] Initial dosage begins with 25 mg/day and reaches its maximum dose at approximately 100 mg four times a day. Hepatitis is a potential side effect, so careful monitoring of liver function tests is advised. Clonidine is also helpful, acting centrally through α to receptor activity depressing the motor neurons.[39] Dosages usually are 0.05 mg orally twice a day up to a maximum dose of 0.1 mg four times a day.

Unfortunately, severe cases do not always respond to medical therapy. In such instances, surgical intervention is possible. Dorsal rhizotomy or myotomy diminishes spasticity; however, they require destruction of neural elements. Less severe intervention would involve placement of epidural spinal cord stimulators or a subarachnoid baclofen pump.[40,41] These have shown some degree of success. Spasticity relief, however, is not predictable with these surgical techniques.

AUTONOMIC DYSREFLEXIA

Autonomic dysreflexia, or hyperreflexia, is a potentially life-threatening problem, which affects some patients during their rehabilitation. Its cause is not well described, but in response to a variable stimulus, the body exhibits a systemic sympathetic surge unresponsive to reflex vagal activity. Patients with injuries above T6 are at risk for this syndrome because their lesion is above the original of the sympathetic outflow tracks. There have been some scattered reports, however, of such activity in patients with injuries below this level.[42] It is manifested by hypertension and diaphoresis, headaches with potential for seizure activity, and intercerebral hemorrhage. Differential diagnosis includes catocholemine-producing tumors, such as pheochromocytoma, or pregnancy-induced toxemia. Incidence has been estimated to be between 45% and 85% of susceptible individuals.[43]

Occurring in both incomplete and complete lesions, onset of dysreflexia may indicate an underlying irritation or infectious process such as a urinary tract infection, bladder distention from an occluded catheter, or fecal impaction, and these should be investigated. Severe hypertension is the usual cause of morbidity.[44]

Treatment includes removing the inciting event, relieving a bladder obstruction by catheterization, establishing flow in a blocked urinary catheter, disimpacting the patient, and removing tight clothing. In acute cases antihypertensive medical management is also necessary, such as subcutaneous nitrates, calcium channel blockers, and nitroprusside. Prophylactic treatment can be used if repeated episodes are related to a bowel or bladder program. To avoid the problem, α-adrenergic blocking agents or ganglionic blockers can be administered.

POSTTRAUMATIC CYSTIC MYELOPATHY

The incidence of cystic myelopathy varies between 0.3% and 3%; however, it is more common in thoracic or thoracolumbar lesions, rather than cervical lesions. One percent of quadriplegics exhibit posttraumatic syringomyelia, whereas 1% to 2% of paraplegics do so.[45,46] The cause of this cystic cavitation of the spinal cord has not been clearly established. Possible causes include resorption of traumatic hematomyelia, softening or resorption of previously injured neural tissue, or occlusion of the ventricular outlet for cerebral spinal fluid (CSF) in the brain.[47–50] Variable in onset, it generally appears in the first year or two; however, it may develop earlier within months or later within decades. It occurs in equal frequency with incomplete or complete lesions. It presents with pain, sensory or motor loss, scoliosis, dissociated sensory loss (loss of pain sensation but preservation of tactile sensation), spinothalamic tract lesion, and neurogenic arthropathy, especially of the upper extremities.[51] An MRI scan demonstrates the lesion well, and it is the test of choice, able to distinguish between fluid and spinal cord tissue on the T1- and T2-weighted images. Clear visualization of the extent of the syrinx is possible from the brain down to the filum terminale. Postmyelogram computed tomography (CT) scans have also clarified the diagnosis of these lesions. Contrast dye concentrates within the cavity and shows up on the axial images as a ring within the cord. Plain radiographs are negative unless late structural changes, such as kyphosis or scoliosis, occur.

Treatment consists of diverting the accumulation of spinal fluid within the cord. This is accomplished by placing a stent to allow drainage into the subarachnoid space, pleural space, or peritoneal cavity. Although shunt complications, such as malfunctional or infection, do exist, individuals obtain significant relief of symptoms after the diversion. Progressive pain and neurologic deficit as well as increased pressure from the CSF are common indications for surgery.

EXTREMITY COMPLICATIONS

In the acute and long-term setting, deep venous thrombosis (DVT) remains a constant risk for patients with SCI. During the first 4 to 6 weeks postinjury, despite mobilization, the patient remains at risk for leg DVT, and pneumatic compression devices should remain in place. Although the morbidity does diminish because of heightened awareness and more aggressive preventative measures, there still remains a risk of fatal pulmonary embolism. Reports indicate its incidence is between 2% and 16% in the first 2 to 3 months of the SCI.[43] Diagnosis remains clinical initially with constant vigilance and screening for calf tenderness, asymmetric swelling of the lower extremities, and fever, although calf symptoms may not always be reliable. When DVT is suspected, the duplex ultrasound is the best method for diagnosing the proximal venous obstruction. Smaller calf veins do not show as well, but experienced technicians can produce real time images in iliac, femoral, popliteal, and some larger calf veins. Venogram, although the gold standard, is difficult, uncomfortable, and considerably invasive.

Prevention is the key to the problem. Early stabilization allows for aggressive mobilization with upper and lower extremity joint range of motion. When unable to get the patient out of bed, passive range of motion may be of some benefit. A great deal of time has been devoted to the medical prophylaxis for DVT in this population and has included Coumadin, adjusted dose heparin, subcutaneous heparin, and low-molecular-weight heparin such as Lovenox. Limiting factors, however, exist and all relate to the potential bleeding complications of such anticoagulants. Iliac crest hematoma at the bone-graft site can increase the risk of infection, and drainage and neural compression secondary to a postoperative hematoma at the site of the laminectomy can cause neurologic deficits and cauda equina syndrome in some cases. Careful attention must also be paid to the elderly population who are at risk for intracranial bleeding. Large drops in hematocrit also can result from subdural hematomas and intraabdominal bleeding from peptic ulcer and other diseases. Noninvasive techniques, however, have proved to be advantageous and have not posed the significant risks of bleeding. Electrical stimulation of the legs to produce muscle contractions resulting in a pumping action on the veins has been reported to be of benefit.[52] The most commonly used regimen, however, remains the pneumatic compression devices on the lower extremities augmented by subcutaneous heparin of 5000 units twice a day. This is because of its practicality and ease of administration. Laboratory screening is not necessary during follow-up. Clearly, a DVT prophylactic regimen must be established by all participating physicians on the rehabilitation team, especially in the acute setting with the use of prophylactic dose–adjusted heparin or other anticoagulants specified by the surgical team, for they have the greatest knowledge of the potential complications resulting from their surgery.

HETEROTOPIC OSSIFICATION

Heterotopic ossification has long been associated with brain injury, with severe disability resulting from joint ankylosis. In patients with SCI, heterotopic ossification may occur in 30% to 50% of patients; however, few (less than 5%) have significant contractures, which result in disability in sitting and transfers.[53] Most often it occurs about the hip; however, knees, shoulders, and elbows can be affected.[54] It may occur more frequently in complete lesions.[55] Generally, it develops within 4 months of injury and can be diagnosed on bone scan before plain radiograph identification.[56] It remains unclear why some patients develop heterotopic ossification and others do not. In patients with elective total-hip replacement or patients with acetabular fractures, clinical use of radiation therapy and indomethacin has been successful in decreasing the incidence, especially in those prone to its formation (patients with severe degenerative joint disease or previous heterotopic ossification formation).[57,58] Such studies, however, have not been conclusive in patients with SCI. Given the younger average age of these patients, care must be taken when considering radiation treatment for prevention given the possibility of radiation-induced sarcomatous changes occuring. The treatment of evolving heterotopic ossification relies on inhibiting further crystalline growth of hydroxyapatite. Etidronate disodium (Didronel) has been successfully used in some patients with SCI. When used prophylactically it has been associated with less bone formation, although the overall incidence of heterotopic ossification remains the same.[59] Dosage begins 3 weeks postinjury and continues for 12 weeks beginning at 20 mg/kg for the first 2 weeks and then followed by 10 mg/kg for the remaining 10 weeks.[60]

If ankylosis should occur, care should be taken when attempting surgical reconstruction. Attempts to restore range of motion may involve significant blood loss and recurrence of the heterotopic ossification. Neurovascular compromise is the most suitable indication for resection aside from disabling joint immobility. Serial bone scans should be assessed to plan surgery at a time after the heterotopic ossification has matured to avoid recurrence.[61] Resection should be limited to that which restores some function; entire resection leads to excessive blood loss and morbidity.

SEXUAL FUNCTION

The majority of patients both male and female wish to remain sexually active after SCI.[62] This becomes a significant issue for the rehabilitation team. Much more research has been conducted in the male patient, so the pathophysiology is more understood than in the female population. The majority of men with complete lesions at the cervical or thoracic level above the thoracolumbar junction experience reflex erections capable of permitting intercourse. These are mediated by the sacral parasympathetic system and functions unless disabled by lower motor neuron injury. Men with complete injuries are infertile, and unable to produce ejaculate, although incomplete injuries have been shown to allow for some ejaculation in approximately 32% of cases.[63] Ejaculation is also generally more common with the more caudal lesions. In these cases, men are also more likely to have psychogenic erections and less frequent reflex stimulation. Even in complete lower motor neuron injuries, the psychogenic pathway still exists through the sympathetic system.

Despite the presence of erections, their duration or ability to penetrate may still be insufficient. Potency can be improved by an implanted penile prosthesis or vacuum constriction devices or assisted by topical or injected medicines. Electroejaculation techniques and other methods of semen retrieval also exist and can be used to produce insemination.[64]

The female reproductive and sexual physiology has been much less investigated. Early in the course of the rehabilitation process, women exhibit amenorrhea, which could last several months. Eventually, however, normal menstruation returns in the regular pattern reconstituting fertility. The female patient with SCI has difficulty, however, with the sensation of sexual intercourse, the ability to reach orgasm, and the lubrication response to sexual activities. Participation, however, can be enjoyable if counseled properly by therapists and could lead to successful pregnancy. The state of pregnancy unfortunately has several side effects on the female with SCI, which should be anticipated. The side effects are mainly stimulation of autonomic hyperreflexia and spasticity. Also, during the latter portion of the pregnancy, inability to feel the descent, contracture, and delivery of the child can be a risk for an unsupervised premature delivery. Pregnancy such as these are complicated both for the mother and child and require attentive team-oriented counseling and supervision during the prenatal and postnatal periods. Once delivered, the stress and challenge of caring for the newborn is added to the already difficult lifestyle of the patient with a SCI.[65]

AGING

Rehabilitation allows the patient with SCI to lead a fulfilled life despite the limitations. The life expectancy for these people, however, is slightly lower than that of the general population. During the initial 12 years postinjury, the survival rate is estimated to be less than 88% of expected normal values.[6] Common potential complications of SCI are responsible for the higher morbidity, including sepsis from urinary tract infection, pulmonary emboli, pneumonia, and decubiti.

Improvements in the life span of these individuals would result from efforts to prevent and improve treatment of these problems. Also, in the older patient with SCI the recovery process begins to place greater demands on the individual now without the reserve to handle the additional burden. Age-related loss of strength is not as well tolerated in these people who rely on movements that expend greater amounts of energy just to perform activities of daily living. Concentrated use of upper extremities in manual wheelchair use or during transfers can lead to overuse syndromes in the arms or shoulders, rotator cuff tendinitis, and carpal tunnel syndrome. These chronic musculoskeletal complaints can be managed by training with assisted transfers, nonsteroidal antiinflammatory medicines (NSAIOs), local injections, avoiding irritating activities, and a power-driven wheelchair. The aging process also places stress on the cardiorespiratory function of the patients. Decreased energy requirements exist in the spine-injured patient and with this comes a decreased tolerance to glucose and lipid metabolism. As a result, with aging these patients generally exhibit limited cardiovascular and metabolic reserve.[68] Patients with quadriplegia have reduced maximal heart rates, reduced stroke volume, and the resultant diminished cardiac output. Left ventricular atrophy has also been noted in quadriplegics because of immobilization and chronic vasomotor paralysis. Wheelchair exercise and weight training for the upper extremities improves overall endurance, but the elderly may not have the muscle mass to increase cardiovascular fitness. Functional electrical stimulation can contract paralyzed muscles repetitively, which increases muscle mass and reduces venous pooling in the extremities. As a result, cardiac output is also improved. Thermoregulatory mechanisms, however, may be deficient as well in these patients so caution is necessary to avoid spasm, overheating, and hypertension.

Pulmonary function is also diminished and can be a leading cause of death in long-term quadriplegics.[33] Early in the course of treatment, respiratory complications are common and result from poor ventilatory capacity from weak intercostal and abdominal muscles. Lesions at or above C3 interrupt phrenic nerve function and result in a ventilator dependent patient. At C4 early ventilation may be necessary, but, often once accessory muscle use is maximized, patients can become independent of the ventilator and breathe autonomously. Atelectasis, however, remains common (80%) even in patients with lesions at C4-C5. With lower lesions, however, the incidence is substantially less.[67] Impaired cough reflex and decreased vital capacity increase the potential for pneumonia especially in the early postinjury period when many patients remain recumbent. The quadriplegic patient initially uses only diaphragmatic muscle activity to develop a 1- to 1.5-liter vital capacity. Over the ensuing 4 to 5 months with proper breathing exercise and pulmonary toilet, vital capacity can increase approximately 1000 mL.[68]

Table 24-3. Expected Level of Function

Motor Level	Functional Activity
Occ–C3	Ventilator dependent; mouth-head controlled wheelchair
C4	Initially ventilator dependent; improved accessory muscle use for variable independent respiration
C5	Deltoid function ± biceps allows for independent activity with adaptive equipment; electric wheelchair with arm control
C6	Biceps and wrist extensors allows for increased hand function with adaptive equipment; may use manual wheelchair or electric with hand control
C7	Triceps, wrist flexion, and finger extension allow for increased upper extremity weight-bearing in transfers; operation of manual wheelchair
C8	Intrinsic and finger flexor function added to independence of ADLs; fine dexterity
T1-T10	High paraplegia; independent in manual chair; exercise ambulation with KAFO and assistance only
T11-T12	Improved ambulation and standing with long-leg KAFOs; assistive device
L1-L2	Iliopsoas aids in household ambulation with KAFOs and assistive device
L3-L4	Quadriceps control allows for coordinated ambulation in community with KAFOs
L4-L5	No longer requires KAFO. Ambulation with ankle-foot orthoses and assistive device
L5-S1	Community ambulation with or without orthoses ± bowel or bladder dysfunction

ADL = activity of daily living; KAFO = knee-ankle-foot orthosis.

This remains, however, an average of only 50% of normal in most cases, so deficits clearly exist.

SUMMARY

Expectations of independence after SCIs remains the greatest source of excitement and disappointment for patients and families. Prediction of the eventual outcome is not always possible; however, usually the motor function present early on dictates their overall activity level. Rehabilitation centers will and should participate in all levels of patient disability, because to a great degree all levels can show improvement. This, of course, requires special attention and dedication to education of the disabled patients and their families to maximize their independence and avoid future medical complications.

To summarize each level is far from accurate because patients and degrees of injury result in different degrees of recovery. Several generalizations, however, are possible (Table 24-3).

In a patient with an injury to C1 through C4, total dependence on others for care, transfers, and mobility is present. Wheelchair activity gives them their only degree of independence with either head, mouth, or computerized controls. Attention is paid to maximizing cushion support of their chairs because a great deal of time is spent in this position, and the potential for ischium breakdown is high. Rehabilitation centers need to spend significant effort with these patients because they require specialized equipment, ventilatory support, and concentrated efforts to minimize pulmonary complications common in this population. Patients with lower tetraplegia from C4 to C8 can be partially independent with adaptive equipment or totally independent; they usually require someone to aid in transfers: Manual wheelchairs are used for greatest independence over short distances, but motorized chairs are required for outdoor use. Specifically, the C5 quadriplegic enjoys the benefits of deltoid and some biceps function. Specialized orthoses that stabilize elbow extension and wrist position allow the patient to participate more fully in activities of daily living. These include feeding, grooming, oral hygiene, and wheelchair operation via a hand control. With the lesion at the C6 level, wrist extension is possible, which opens a world of activities associated with hand usage. With wrist extension intact, this motion can be harnessed by a wrist-driven flexion hinge splint. Other orthoses augment the finger flexion tenodesis and opponens capability for greater ability to write, feed, groom, upper extremity dressing, self-catheterization, and assisting in lower extremity dressing.

Return of the C7 and C8 function improves all hand function, and these patients can be expected to have full use of a manual wheelchair, transfer themselves to a car, and have independent seating with functioning triceps musculature. This level of activity also allows for attempts at ambulation with arm assistive devices and specialized walkers. Activities of daily living are independent at this level, and handling objects is possible with the improved finger dexterity and fine motor skills.

Paraplegics with lesions from T1 down are, of course, totally independent. A part of their rehabilitation should include sports activities appropriate for the level of the patient with wheelchair adaptation. Normal hand function is expected and ambulation should be possible with various hip-knee-ankle-foot orthoses (HKAFOs) in children and KAFOs in adults. Reciprocating gait orthoses have recently been devised to allow for a more normal gait.[69] Although gait appears more normal, the energy expenditure is higher and less efficient than with the standard, light-weight KAFOs. Despite the enthusiasm and significant rehabilitation efforts made to develop a pattern of walking in these patients, many never continue in the community. Most feel wheelchairs require less effort and are more functional out in the community without the danger of injury or appearing awkward. Gait training, important for exercise and therapy, is subject to the patient's own bias once discharged from the rehabilitation facility.

Most important in the overall discussion of functional outcome after SCI is the emphasis on the team approach towards managing all problems associated with the injury. Considerable medical, psychosocial, musculoskeletal, and sexual dysfunction can and will occur in all levels of SCI. The appropriate specialty personnel should anticipate this. Both acute and long-term complications occur jeopardizing the overall life expectancy and functional outcome of these individuals. Rehabilitation is a lifelong process, but with the appropriate education of both the patient and the family, goals can be achieved leading the patient back to the workplace as a productive member of society.

REFERENCES

1. DeVivo MJ, et al: Prevalence of spinal cord injury. A reestimation employing life table techniques, *Arch Neurol* 37:707–708, 1980.
2. Cushing H: Organization and activities of the neurological service American expeditionary forces. In Ireland MW editor: *The medical department of the United States Army in the World War,* Washington, 1927, US Government Printing Office.

3. Ditunno JF Jr, Formal CS: Chronic spinal cord injury, *N Engl J Med* 330:550–556, 1994.
4. Stover SL, Fine PR: Spinal cord injury: the facts and figures, Birmingham, 1986, University of Alabama.
5. Anderson DW, McLaurin RL: The national head and spinal cord injury survey, *J Neurosurg* 53:S1–S43, 1980.
6. DeVivo JM, et al: Spinal cord injury: rehabilitation adds life to years, *West J Med* 143:602–606, 1991.
7. Yarkony GM: Overview of spinal cord injury rehab in the acute phase, the rehabilitation team and classification of spinal cord lesion. In Yarkony GM, editor: *Spinal cord injury: medical management and rehabilitation*, Gaithersburg, 1994, Aspen Publishers.
8. Cohen M: Initial resuscitation of the patient with spinal cord injury, *Trauma Q* 9:38–43, 1993.
9. Vaccaro AR, et al: Noncontiguous injuries of the spine, *J Spin Disord* 5:320–329, 1992.
10. Toscano J: Prevention of neurological deterioration before admission to a spinal cord injury unit, *Paraplegia* 26:143–150, 1988.
11. Bohlman HH: Acute fractures and dislocations of the cervical spine. An analysis of 300 hospitalized patients and review of the literature, *J Bone Joint Surg* 61A:1119–1142, 1979.
12. American Spinal Injury Association: *Standards for neurological and functional classification of spinal cord injury*, rev ed, Chicago, 1992, The Association.
13. Delamarter RS, Sherman J, Carr JB: Pathophysiology of spinal cord injury, *J Bone Joint Surg* 77A:1042–1049, 1995.
14. Marshall LF, et al: Deterioration following spinal cord injury, *J Neurosurg* 66:400–404, 1987.
15. Heiden JS, et al: Management of cervical spinal cord trauma in Southern California, *J Neurosurg* 43:732–736, 1975.
16. Star AM, et al: Immediate closed reduction of cervical spine dislocations using traction, *Spine* 15:1068–1072, 1990.
17. Rizzolo SJ, Vaccaro AR, Cotler JM: Cervical spine trauma, *Spine* 19:2288–2298, 1994.
18. Eismont FJ, Arena MJ, Green BA: Extrusion of an intervertebral disc association with traumatic subluxation and dislocation of cervical facets, *J Bone Joint Surg* 73A:1555–1560, 1991.
19. Bracken MB, Shepard MJ, Collins WF: A randomized controlled trial of methylprednisolone or naloxone in the treatment of acute spinal cord injury: results of the Second National Acute Spinal Cord Injury Study. *N Engl J Med* 322:1405–1411, 1990.
20. Ditunno JF, et al: Motor recovery of the upper extremities in traumatic quadriplegia. A multicenter study, *Arch Phys Med Rehabil* 73:431–436, 1992.
21. Marino RJ, Herbison GJ, Ditunno JF: Peripheral sprouting in the zone of partial preservation in motor complete spinal cord injury. *J Am Paraplegia Soc* 15:122–130, 1992.
22. Folman Y, Masri WS: Spinal cord injury: prognostic indicators, *Injury* 20:92–93, 1989.
23. Crozier KS, et al: Spinal cord injury: prognosis for ambulation based on quadriceps recovery, *Paraplegia* 30:762–767, 1992.
24. Heinemann AW: Functional outcome following spinal cord injury: a comparison of specialized spinal cord injury center vs general hospital short-term care, *Arch Neurol* 46:1098–1102, 1989.
25. Staas WE Jr, Cioschi HM: Pressure sores—a multifaceted approach to prevention and treatment, *West J Med* 154:539–544, 1991.
26. Morrisson WB, Schweitzer ME, Bock GW: Diagnosis of osteomyelitis. Utilization fat suppressed contrast enhanced MR imaging, *Radiology* 189:251–257, 1993.
27. Chancellor MB, Kellhdma P: Urodynamic evaluation of patients following spinal cord injury, *Sem Urol* 10:83–94, 1992.
28. Hinman F Jr: Obstruction: back pressure or residual volume and laminar flow, *J Urol* 105:702–708, 1971.
29. Wyndaelle JJ: Pharmacotherapy for urinary bladder dysfunction in spinal cord injury patients, *Paraplegia* 28:146–150, 1990.
30. Cardenas DD: Neurogenic bladder. *Phys Med Rehabil Clin North Am* 3:75–763, 1992.
31. Dewire DM: A comparison of the urological complications associated with long term management of quads with or without chronic indwelling urinary catheters, *J Urol* 147:1069–1071, 1992.
32. Whiteneck GG, et al: Mortality, morbidity, and psychosocial outcome of persons spinal cord injured more than 20 years ago, *Paraplegia* 30:617–630, 1992.
33. Devior MJ, Black EJ, Stover SL: Causes of death during the first 12 years after SCI. *Arch Phys Med Rehab* 74: 248–254, 1993.
34. National Institute on Disability and Rehab: Research consensus statement: the prevention and management of urinary tract infections among people with spinal cord injuries, *J Am Paraplegia Soc* 15:194–204, 1992.
35. Gore RM, Mintzer RA, Calenoff L: Gastrointestinal complications of spinal cord injury, *Spine* 6:538–544, 1981.
36. Young RR, Delwaide PJ: Spasticity, *N Engl J Med* 304:28–33, 1981.
37. Maynard FM, Karunas RS, Waring WP III: Epidemiology of spasticity following traumatic spinal cord injury, *Arch Phys Med Rehab* 71:566–569, 1990.
38. Meritt JL: Management of spasticity in spinal cord injury, *Mayo Clin Proc* 56:614–622, 1981.
39. Donovan WH, et al: Clonidine effect on spasticity: a clinical trial. *Arch Phys Med Rehabil* 69:193–194, 1988.
40. Barolat G: Epidural spinal cord stimulation in the management of spasms and spasticity in spinal cord injury, *Neurosurg State Art Rev* 4:365–370, 1989.
41. Perr RD: Intrathecal baclofen for spasticity of spinal origin, *J Neurosurg* 77:236–240, 1992.
42. Gimovsky ML, et al: Management of autonomic hyper-

reflexia associated with a low thoracic spinal cord lesion, *Obstet Gynecol* 153:223–224, 1981.

43. Yarkony GM: Medical and physical complications of spinal cord injury. In Yarkony GM, editor: *Spinal cord injury: medical management and rehabilitation*, Gaithersburg, 1994, Aspen Publishers.
44. Kursh ED, et al: Complications of autonomic dysreflexia, *J Urol* 118:70–72, 1977.
45. Scher AT: Syringomyelia secondary to paraplegia due to fractures of the thoracic spine, *S Afr Med J* 50:1406–1408, 1976.
46. Vernon JD: Post traumatic syringomyelia, *Paraplegia* 20:339–364, 1982.
47. Lazar RL: Post traumatic syringomyelia. In Yarkony GM, editor: *Spinal cord injury: medical management and rehabilitation,* Gaithersburg, 1994, Aspen Publishers.
48. Feigin I, Ogata J, Budzilovich G: Syringomyelia: the role of edema in its pathogenesis, *J Neuropathol Exp Neurol* 30:216–232, 1971.
49. Gardner WJ: Hydrodynamic mechanism of syringomyelia. Its relationship to myelocele, *J Neurol Neurosurg Psychiatry* 28:247–259, 1965.
50. Williams B: Hypothesis: the distending force in the production of communicating syringomyelia, *Lancet* 2:189–193, 1969.
51. Rhoads CE, et al: Diagnosis of post traumatic syringomyelia presenting as a neuropathic joint, *Clin Orthop* 180:182–187, 1983.
52. Katz RT: Functional electric stimulation to enhance systemic fibrinolytic activity in spinal cord injured patients, *Arch Phys Med Rehab* 68:423–426, 1987.
53. Vernier L, Ditunno JF: Heterotopic ossification in the paraplegia patient, *Arch Phys Med Rehab* 52:475–479, 1971.
54. Tibone J, et al: Heterotopic ossification around the hip in spinal cord injured patients, *J Bone Joint Surg* 60A:769–775, 1978.
55. Nicholas JJ: Ectopic bone formation in patients with spinal cord injury, *Arch Phys Med Rehab* 54:354–359, 1973.
56. Orzel JA, Rudd TG: Heterotopic bone formation: clinical laboratory and imaging correlation, *J Nucl Med* 16:125–132, 1985.
57. Ayers DC, Evarts CM, Parkinson: The prevention of heterotopic ossification in high risk patients by low dose radiation therapy after total hip arthroplasty, *J Bone Joint Surg* 68A:1423–1430, 1986.
58. McLaren AC: Prophylaxis with indomethicin for heterotopic bone, *J Bone Joint Surg* 72A:245–247, 1990.
59. Stover SL, Niemann KM, Miller JM III: Disodium etidronate in the prevention of postoperative recurrence of heterotopic ossification in spinal cord injury patients, *J Bone Joint Surg* 58A:683–688, 1976.
60. Stover SL: Heterotopic ossification after spinal cord injury. In Block RF, Bausbaum M, editors: *Management of spinal cord injuries*, Baltimore, 1989, Williams & Wilkins.
61. Tanaka T, et al: Quantitative assessment of paraosteo-arthropathy and its maturation on serial radionuclide bone images, *Radiology* 123:217–221, 1977.
62. Sipisky ML, Alexander CJ: Sexual function and dysfunction after spinal cord injury, *Phys Med Rehab Clin North Am* 3:811–828, 1992.
63. Higgins GE: Sexual response in spinal cord injured adults, a review of the literature, *Arch Sex Behav* 8:173–196, 1979.
64. Linsenmeyer T, Wilmot CB, Anderson RU: The effects of electroejaculation procedure on sperm motility, *Paraplegia* 27:465–469, 1989.
65. Greenspan JS, Paul RH: Paraplegia and quadriplegia. Special considerations during pregnancy and labor and delivery, *Am J Obstet Gynecol* 155:738–741, 1986.
66. Naso F: Cardiovascular problems in patients with spinal cord injury. In Staas WE, Ditunno JF, editor: *Phys Med Rehab Clin North Am* 3:741–750, 1992.
67. Fishburn MJ, Marino RJ, Ditunno JF: Atelectasis and pneumonia in acute spinal cord injury, *Arch Phys Med Rehab* 71:197–200, 1990.
68. Carter RE: Intermittent catheterization: a small warning, *Emerg Med* 6:274–275, 1974.
69. Douglas R: The LSU reciprocation gait orthosis, *Orthopedics* 6:834–839, 1983.

25

REHABILITATION AND COMPREHENSIVE CARE OF THE PERSON WITH SPINAL CORD INJURY

Kristjan T. Ragnarsson
Adam B. Stein
Steven Kirshblum

Spinal cord injury (SCI) is a clinical condition of catastrophic magnitude to the individual afflicted and of great cost to society. During the twentieth century, remarkable progress has been made toward effectively preventing and managing the numerous medical complications of SCI, and, as a result, the life expectancy of persons with SCI has increased significantly. Early provision of comprehensive rehabilitation services has helped persons with SCI to regain at least limited self-care and mobility skills, which usually permits them to live at home, get around with assistive devices, and seek reintegration into their communities. Unfortunately, progress toward finding a cure for this condition has been slow. Scientific observations in the laboratory have not translated into significant new clinical interventions, and the neurologic consequences of a complete SCI, in general, are considered permanent. As the annual incidence of SCI has remained unchanged in most countries, life expectancy has increased, consequently a gradual increase in the prevalence and the importance of this condition as a health issue for society has occurred.

Only during the past half century have persons with SCI been given hope for survival. The earliest reference to SCI was made approximately 5,000 years ago by an unknown Egyptian physician in the so-called Edwin Smith Papyrus as "an ailment not to be treated."[1] Admiral Nelson, Commander of the British Navy at the Battle of Trafalgar in 1805, when felled by a French sniper's bullet was diagnosed by the ship's surgeon as having SCI and was informed, "My Lord, unhappily for our country nothing can be done for you."[1] Prior to World War II, life expectancy of persons with SCI was rarely greater than 2 years; most such persons succumbing from septic infections, renal failure, and pressure sores. With the advent of antibiotics and improved therapeutic techniques, life expectancy has markedly improved.

Perhaps the most significant development in the care of persons with SCI has been the establishment of comprehensive interdisciplinary health service systems, where physicians and other health care workers with expertise in SCI management work together as a team and with the person with SCI to maximize his or her potential by preventing medical complications from occurring, by restoring maximum self-sufficiency and mobility as permitted by the extent of the disability, and by facilitating community reintegration. The first move to such specialized care occurred during World War II in Great Britain, when persons with SCI were gathered in special care units at government hospitals. Such a unit at Mandeville in Aylesbury, England, grew in influence under the leadership of Sir Ludwig Guttmann and, in 1951, was designated as a national SCI center, providing comprehensive management and rehabilitation of persons with both acute and chronic SCI in Great Britain.

Simultaneously in the United States, the concepts of rehabilitation medicine were being formulated by Howard A. Rusk and adapted in the management of persons with physical disability. Special SCI programs were established. The first was a 10-bed SCI unit at Boston University Hospital under the directorship of Donald Munro and with sponsorship of the Liberty Mutual Insurance Company. Shortly thereafter the Veterans Administration (VA) sponsored six SCI units, the best known of which was at the VA Hospital at Long Beach, California, directed by Ernest Bors. It soon became clinically evident that if the best available care was provided from the onset of SCI and for as long as the disability lasted, outcomes were significantly improved. This observation has led to the establishment of numerous SCI Model Systems of Care, which since 1973 have been designated and partly funded by the U.S. Department of Education, National Institute of Disability and Rehabilitation Research. The Na-

The preparation of this manuscript was supported by grant number H 133 N50008 from the National Institute of Disability and Rehabilitation Research, U.S. Department of Education.

tional Spinal Cord Injury Data Research Center (NSCIDRC) was established in 1975 and since then has captured data from an estimated 15% of all new SCI cases in the United States. Since its inception, 21 federally funded Model SCI Care Systems have contributed data to the NSCIDRC on more than 15,000 persons with SCI. These data have been regularly analyzed and published, most recently in 1995.[2]

According to the NSCIDRC data analysis, significant changes in the care and rehabilitation of persons with SCI have occurred since its inception, most remarkably, reduced length of stay in hospitals and rehabilitation centers and consequently reduction in hospital charges, decreased rate of hospital readmissions, increased gain in function per day of hospitalization, improved survival rates, and heightened interests by health professionals to improve the care of persons with SCI.[3] Most recently, several medical and nonmedical developments have been noted that predictably affect the delivery of SCI care and rehabilitation.[4] First, the leading causes of SCI are gradually changing from unintentional injury to intentional injury. Consequently, the profile of persons with SCI has changed, as many victims of violence have neither conventional families nor conventional social support structures in their communities. The third major trend relates to new approaches of health care delivery that are being implemented across the United States. Many insurance policies now restrict access to high-quality acute rehabilitation programs for persons with disabling conditions, limit their lengths of stays at hospitals and rehabilitation centers, and provide little resources for outpatient, home, and long-term follow-up services.

MODEL SYSTEMS OF CARE

An SCI is a condition of relatively low incidence but of high cost. It results in a physiologic dysfunction of multiple organ systems and, therefore, places persons with SCI at a high risk for medical complications, particularly during the acute phase of the condition. If the early medical complications of SCI can be prevented, the rehabilitation course is facilitated, institutional length of stay is shortened, functional gains are greater, human suffering is reduced, and the total cost of medical care is decreased. The number and severity of complications often appear to be inversely related to the quality of care available at the hospitals that provide early care and subsequently refer patients for rehabilitation. These observations have been validated by studies that document the cost benefits of designated trauma centers.[5,6,7] Unfortunately, many people who sustain catastrophic and disabling injuries receive fragmented medical, surgical, rehabilitative, and follow-up care. Because their care is often poorly integrated, there are unnecessary delays at the interphases between each level of care. To meet these deficiencies, categorical SCI treatment programs have been developed in many countries, often referred to as systems of care. There are four essential components of each such system of care: emergency medical services (EMS), acute care, SCI rehabilitation, and follow-up clinical care. The effectiveness of such a system of care is enhanced by appropriate leadership and management, usually consisting of a physician who has specialized training and experience in the comprehensive management of patients with SCI and by an allied health rehabilitation professional, who serves as a coordinator of services, particularly during the vocational and placement phases.[8]

In addition to the four main components of a system of care, a substantial number of patients with SCI is necessary for each system to operate successfully. Preferably, a minimum of 50 new annual patients with spinal cord disorders, traumatic or nontraumatic, must be admitted into such a system to maintain professional expertise among the staff and to make the different components of the program effective. Additionally, each system must actively be involved in preventing injuries to the central nervous system (CNS). Different clinical components of an SCI Care System are organized to work together in harmony so that optimal management of the disability is provided from the onset and throughout the life of the person disabled by SCI.

EMERGENCY MEDICAL SERVICES

Regional EMS is the first essential component of a SCI system of care. All EMS technicians are trained to promptly identify individuals with SCI, provide proper spinal support, and stabilize respiratory and cardiovascular functions. After spinal stability is provided, prompt evacuation from the scene of injury and transportation in well-equipped ambulances to a designated level I trauma center, preferably one that specializes in the treatment of SCI, facilitates early specific diagnosis and ensures optimal treatment.

ACUTE CARE

Acute care should be provided at a designated specialized level I trauma center with a state-of-the-art emergency department and all supportive traumatology, surgical and medical services, and consultants who have interest and expertise in the care of persons with SCI. The diagnostic evaluation must be promptly completed and definitive medical-surgical care initiated. All patients with SCI should be evaluated within 48 hours of admission by a physiatrist with expertise in comprehensive SCI management. A specific disability diagnosis must be made, treatment plans must be formulated, and rehabilitation interventions must be started.

COMPREHENSIVE REHABILITATION SERVICES

Most patients with SCI require admission to an acute inpatient rehabilitation service, and this should be done as soon as the spine has been stabilized and the medical condition does not require continued monitoring and interventions in the intensive care unit (ICU). This may occur within the first week after SCI. Under direction of the physiatrist, the SCI interdisciplinary rehabilitation team becomes involved in the care of the patient. Team conferences are held weekly to increase the teams ability to address a variety of clinical problems, judge progress, and plan for discharge. Even before the major goals of SCI rehabilitation have been reached, institutional discharge may be achieved and the rehabilitation continued on an outpatient basis.

COMPREHENSIVE LIFELONG FOLLOW-UP SERVICES

Outpatient rehabilitation programs and follow-up services for persons with SCI must be as comprehensive and well coordinated as those provided on the inpatient service. As inpatient lengths of stays have been getting shorter, there has been less time during this phase to help the patient and the family to adjust emotionally to the disability and to anticipate and address the different social, vocational, and recreational obstacles in the community. The outpatient rehabilitation programs for individuals with SCI who have become self-sufficient and mobility independent should have as their main focus psychologic, social, vocational, and recreational goals for optimal community reintegration.

PREVENTION OF INJURIES

Each system of care not only should be designed to prevent development of secondary medical complications but additionally must also be committed to establishing primary prevention programs, that is, preventing injuries from occurring. A strategic plan for prevention of injuries involves both governmental and individual efforts, which may be divided into three different components.[9]

1. Education of persons at risk by reinforcing safe behavior and increasing use of self-protective measures (e.g., using safety belts and helmets)
2. Adoption of legislation (e.g., safety belt and helmet laws, tests for intoxication, and lowering of speed limits)
3. Modification of the environment (i.e., safety features in automobiles, highways, and stairwells)

Most systems of care have adopted *"Think First,"* which is a prevention program established by the American Association for Neurological Surgeons and the Congress of Neurological Surgeons to prevent injuries to the head and spine. The program consists of an educational program, which describes personal vulnerability and the consequences of excessive risk taking behavior. The program is presented to middle and high school students who are deemed particularly at risk.

EPIDEMIOLOGY

Numerous studies have been conducted on the epidemiology of SCI, but the most extensive data have been collected by the Model SCI Systems since 1973 and stored and analyzed by the NSCIDRC.[10-14] The epidemiology figures presented below are derived from this source.[15]

INCIDENCE

Excluding deaths at the scene of injury, the annual incidence of SCI in the United States is estimated to be between 30 and 40 new cases per million population. Estimated incidence varies somewhat from state to state for several possible reasons, and figures from other countries are often quite different. Based on the U.S. 1992 Census population of 254 million people, there should be between 8,000 and 10,000 new cases of traumatic SCI each year.

PREVALENCE

Several methods have been employed to estimate the total number of persons with SCI alive in the United States.[15-20] As life expectancy has improved, the prevalence of this condition has increased and is variably estimated to be somewhere between 183,000 and 230,000 persons.[15]

AGE AT INJURY

SCI occurs most often in teenagers and young adults, with 60% of such injuries occurring in persons between 16 and 30 years of age and another 21% occurring in those between 31 and 45 years of age.[15] The mean age at injury, which currently is 30.7 years according to NSCIDRC data, has risen slowly since 1973, in part because of the increased median age of the general population but also because of the almost doubling of the proportion of persons who are older than 60 years of age and who are suffering SCI, that is, from 4.5% for the 1973 to 1977 period to 8.5% since 1990.[15]

GENDER AND ETHNICITY

Virtually all demographic data reveal that 80% of all persons suffering SCI are male. With respect to racial composition, significant change has been noted during the past 20 years. According to the NSCIDRC data, comparing ethnicity of persons who sustained SCI between 1973 and 1977 to those injured between 1990 and 1992, Caucasians were 76.9% versus 56.3%, respectively; African Americans, 14% versus 29.9%; Hispanics 6.2% versus 11.2%; and Asians 0.8% versus 1.6%. Racial trends in the general population of the United States are not sufficient to account for this change.

EDUCATIONAL, OCCUPATIONAL, AND MARITAL STATUS

At the time of injury, most persons with SCI are at least high school graduates (59.3%) and are employed (59.6%). Some are still in school (18.5%), but 14.3% were unemployed. The majority are single at the time of injury, and less than one-third are married (30.6%).[15]

ETIOLOGY

Since the inception of a SCI model system program and data collection in 1973, almost half of the persons enrolled were injured in motor vehicle crashes (44.5%), followed by falls (18.1%), acts of violence (16.6%), and recreational sports activities (12.7%). This pattern varies somewhat according to the age group studied; however, noteworthy trends in the causes of SCI have been observed since 1990. The proportion of SCI caused by motor vehicle crashes has declined to 38.1% and those caused by recreational sports to 8.8%, whereas SCI caused by acts of violence has increased to 25.1% and fall-related injuries to 20.2%. Considering these different causes for SCI, it is understandable that SCI is most common during the summer months and on weekends.

NEUROLOGIC LEVEL AND EXTENT OF INJURY

Most studies show that a slight majority of persons with SCI have tetraplegia. In recent years, a slightly higher proportion of persons with paraplegia has been noted. This may be partly explained by a rising incidence of gunshot wounds as a cause of SCI, since such wounds usually result in paraplegia. Another explanation may be a decline in sports-related injuries that generally result in tetraplegia.[15] For many years, neurologically incomplete injuries (51.7%) have slightly outnumbered complete injuries (48.3%). Trends over the last 20 years indicate a rising proportion of persons with neurologically incomplete paraplegia and a diminishing proportion of those with complete tetraplegia.

ASSOCIATED INJURIES

A major trauma capable of causing SCI is often accompanied by associated injuries to other body parts and organ systems, which may lengthen the initial hospitalization and negatively affect rehabilitation outcome. The most common associated injuries include fractures (29.3%), loss of consciousness (28.2%), pneumohemothorax (17.8%), and traumatic brain injury affecting cognitive or emotional functioning (11.5%).[15]

NEUROLOGIC AND FUNCTIONAL ASSESSMENT OF SPINAL CORD INJURY

Diagnostic evaluation of the person with spinal injury using different imaging and electrodiagnostic studies is discussed in detail by other authors in this book. A careful and detailed examination of the person with SCI is of great clinical importance and should include a general systematic assessment of all body systems to discover associated injuries and preexisting conditions, which can influence treatment strategies and outcomes, and the neurologic examination, which may predict chances of recovery and functional potential.

Until recently, clinicians and researchers disagreed on accurate definitions of the neurologic and functional deficits of SCI, therefore, it was difficult to measure clinically and scientifically the outcome of different treatments. To address this issue, 49 leading physicians in the field of SCI care from 16 different countries responded in 1969 to a questionnaire mailed to them to establish an international agreement on neurologic terminology for SCI and to compare their opinions on the best time to accurately make a neurologic prognosis following SCI. Their recommendations were published, but clearly there was little consensus.[21] In 1982, the American Spinal Injury Association (ASIA) first developed and published a booklet *Standards for Neurological Classification of SCI* to serve as helpful guidelines for clinicians, but at first this was a rather primitive and controversial effort. These standards were further developed and refined for the next 10 years, involving experts from many professional organizations in the United States, including clinicians and researchers.[22] These standards have now been endorsed by the leading national and international organizations of professionals involved in SCI research and care and are referred to as the International Standards for Neurological and Functional Classification of Spinal Cord Injury.[23] To teach clinicians and researchers how to use the International Standards correctly, an instructional manual and three video tapes have been produced. These standards provide basic definitions of the most common terms used by clinicians in the assessment of SCI and describe the neurologic examination, how motor and sensory scores are obtained, how impairment is classified, how function is measured, and how the different clinical SCI syndromes are defined.

BASIC DEFINITIONS

Tetraplegia, now preferred to the term *quadriplegia*, is defined as impairment or loss of motor or sensory function in the cervical segments of the spinal cord because of damage of neural elements within the spinal canal. Tetraplegia results in impairment of function in the arms, trunk, legs, and pelvic organs. It does not include brachial plexus lesions or injury to the peripheral nerves outside the neural canal.

The term *paraplegia* is defined as impairment or loss of motor or sensory function in the thoracic, lumbar, or sacral segments of the cord (but not in the cervical segments), secondary to damage of the neural elements within the spinal canal. With paraplegia, neurologic function in the upper extremities is spared, but depending on the level of injury, the trunk, legs, and pelvic organs may be involved. Paraplegia refers to cauda equina and conus medullaris injuries but not to lumbar-sacral plexus lesions or injuries to peripheral nerves outside the neural canal.

The terms *quadriparesis*, or *tetraparesis*, and *paraparesis* are discouraged because they describe incomplete lesions imprecisely. The ASIA Impairment Scale provides a much more precise approach to describe incomplete lesions. *Dermatome* is defined as the area of the skin that is innervated by the sensory axons within each segmental nerve, that is, within each nerve root. *Myotome* is the collection of muscle fibers innervated by the motor axons within each segmental nerve, that is, within each nerve root.

The *neurologic level* is defined as the most caudal segment of the spinal cord with normal sensory and motor function on both sides of the body. It is true that the lowest segments with normal neurologic function are often different on the right or the left side of the body and in terms of sensory and motor function. To establish the accurate neurologic level, it may, therefore, be necessary on occasion to identify four different neurologic segments, for example, right sensory, left sensory, right motor, and left motor. In such cases, it is strongly recommended that each of these segments be separately recorded and that a single level not be used, because such can be quite misleading. *Sensory level* is defined as the most caudal segment of the spinal cord with normal sensation on both sides of the body. The *motor level* is defined as the most caudal segment of the spinal cord with normal motor function on both sides. Exact sensory and motor levels are determined by the neurologic examination. A *skeletal level* of injury is defined as the spinal level at which by radiographic examination the greatest vertebral damage is found, that is, where imaging studies show the worst fracture or fracture-dislocation. Fracture classification standards are currently under development.

Sensory and motor scores for SCI are defined as the numerical summary scores that reflect the degree of neurologic impairment associated with SCI.

Incomplete injury is defined as partial preservation of sensory or motor functions below the neurological level, and such preservation must include the lowest sacral segment. Sacral sensation includes sensation at the anal-mucocutaneous junction and deep anal sensation. The corresponding criterion for motor function is the presence of voluntary contraction of the external anal sphincter on digital examination. This definition of incomplete SCI was recently included in the International Standards at the insistence of neurologic surgeons. According to such definition, a patient with cervical SCI can have sensory and motor function in the trunk or even in the legs, but unless sacral neurologic function is present, the injury must be classified as complete with a large zone of partial preservation. *Complete injury* is defined as absence of sensory and motor functions in the lowest sacral segment.

The *zone of partial preservation* (ZPP) is an important concept and relates to complete lesions only. The ZPP is defined as the dermatomes and myotomes caudal to the neurologic level that remain partially innervated. When some impaired sensory or motor function is found below the lowest normal segment, the exact number of segments affected should be recorded for both sides as the ZPP.

THE NEUROLOGIC EXAMINATION

The neurologic examination of the person with SCI has two main components, that is, the sensory and motor, both of which have certain required and optional elements. The required elements include determination of the exact sensory, motor, and neurologic levels, generation of sensory and motor scores, and determination of the completeness of the SCI. The optional elements involve aspects of the neurological examination that may better describe the patients clinical condition but are not important for numerical scoring.

Often the patient's clinical condition may prevent the completion of an accurate neurological examination, for example, when a patient is comatose from an associated traumatic brain injury, has neurological impairment from injuries to the brachial or lumbosacral plexi, or has a limb immobilized because of a fracture. When the patient with SCI is not fully testable for any reason, the examiner should record "NT" instead of a numerical score. An accurate score should be deferred until the patient is fully testable. All motor and sensory scores should be entered on a large chart, which can be included as a standard form in the medical records. When performing the *sensory examination*, it is required that sensitivity to both pin prick and light touch be tested in each of the 28 dermatomes on both the right and the left sides of the body. Each dermatome should be scored on the three-point scale, that is, absent sensation is zero (0), impaired is 1 (impaired is defined as partial or altered sensation, including hyperesthesia), and normal is 2. If accurate testing is not possible "NT" should be entered. Testing for pinprick sensation is usually performed with a disposable safety pin, using both the sharp and the dull end of the pin for contrast. The normal sensation of the face is used as a reference point. Inability to feel any touch or inability to distinguish between dull and sharp sensation is graded as 0. Sharpness, different from normal, is graded as 1. Light touch is then tested with cotton. To perform the sensory examination and develop a sensory score, certain anatomic key points for 28 dermatomes are tested on each side of the body for sensitivity and scored. The score is entered on the summary chart. The optional elements of the sensory examination are also important, and it is strongly recommended that these be evaluated and entered into the medical record. These include proprioception, that is joint position and vibration, heat and cold, and deep pressure sensations.

The required elements of the *motor examination* consists of testing ten key muscles on each side of the body, five in the upper limbs and five in the lower limbs. Each muscle should be examined in a rostral-caudal sequence, starting above at the C5 innervated muscles (elbow flexors), and finishing below with ankle plantar flexors (S1). All muscles are tested with the patient in supine position, which is different from the standard neurologic examination. Each muscle is graded on a six-point scale from 0 to 5 (Table 25-1). Although it is well known that most muscles are innervated by more than one nerve root/segment, for the purpose of simplification, certain muscles to be tested have been chosen because of their consistency for being innervated primarily by the segments indicated and for their ease of testing in a clinical situation where the patient must be lying in the supine position. In addition to these key muscles, the external anal sphincter should be tested by a digital examination and sensing a voluntary contraction. Care must be taken not to confuse a reflex contraction of the anal sphincter with a voluntary contraction. The optional muscles that should be tested during the motor examination include the diaphragm by observation, breathing patterns, ability to cough, measurement of vital capacity, or by radiographic fluoroscopy, and the deltoid and the lateral hamstring muscles. Strength of these muscles is rated as absent, weak, or normal, but they are not included in the ASIA motor score.

Motor scores for each muscle tested and the *sensory scores* of each neurologic segment are entered on the form and added to create a total score. The maximum total motor score would be 50 on each side for a total of 100. Maximum sensory score would be 56 on each side for both light touch and pinprick, with a total of 112 maximum score for each side. Additional information to be entered on the form includes the neurological level, whether the cord lesion is neurologically complete or incomplete, and if there is a zone of partial preservation.

An important part of the international standards is the *ASIA Impairment Scale*, which is a modification of a scale originally developed by Frankel in the late 1960s.[24] The scale describes five different severities of SCI (Table 25-2).

The Clinical Syndromes of Spinal Cord Injury

Different clinical syndromes of SCI are frequently referred to by clinicians and in the literature, and include central cord, Brown-Sequard, anterior cord, conus medullaris, and cauda equina. In general these syndromes do not accurately describe the extent of the

Table 25-1. ASIA Motor Score (Possible Total Score of 100)

Grade on Right	Level	Muscle	Level	Grade on Left
0 to 5	C5	Deltoid and/or biceps	C5	0 to 5
0 to 5	C6	Wrist extensors	C6	0 to 5
0 to 5	C7	Triceps	C7	0 to 5
0 to 5	C8	Flexor profundus	C8	0 to 5
0 to 5	T1	Hand intrinsics	T1	0 to 5
0 to 5	L2	Iliopsoas	L2	0 to 5
0 to 5	L3	Quadriceps	L3	0 to 5
0 to 5	L4	Ankle dorsiflexors	L4	0 to 5
0 to 5	L5	Extensor hallucis longus	L5	0 to 5
0 to 5	S1	Gastrocnemius/Soleus	S1	0 to 5
0 to 50 total				0 to 50 total

neurological deficit. Nonetheless, they are important to define (see Table 25-2).

THE FUNCTIONAL EVALUATION

To fully describe the impact of SCI on a person and to monitor functional progress associated with rehabilitation interventions, it is necessary to use descriptive terms and to use a standard measure of the activities of daily living (ADL). The World Health Organization (WHO) has defined three terms that are frequently used when functional deficits are discussed, that is, impairment, disability, and handicap.[25] *Impairment* is "any loss or abnormality of psychologic, physical or anatomic structure of function," such as, paralysis. *Disability* is "any restriction or lack (resulting from an impairment) of ability to perform an activity in the manner within the range considered normal for a human being," for example, paralysis resulting in inability to walk. *Handicap* is "a disadvantage for a given individual, resulting from an impairment or disability that limits or prevents the fulfillment of a role that is normal (depending on age, gender and social and cultural factors) for that individual," such as paralyzed and unable to walk and, therefore, cannot meet the requirements of the job and return to work.

Table 25-2. ASIA Impairment Scale

A = Complete: No motor or sensory function is preserved in the sacral segments S4-S5.

B = Incomplete: Sensory but not motor function is preserved below the neurologic level and includes the sacral segments S4-S5.

C = Incomplete: Motor function is preserved below the neurologic level, and more than half of key muscles below the neurological level have a muscle grade less than 3.

D = Incomplete: Motor function is preserved below the neurological level, and at least half of key muscles below the neurologic level have a muscle grade of 3 or more.

E = Normal: motor and sensory function is normal

Clinical Syndromes

Central Cord
Brown-Sequard
Anterior Cord
Conus Medullaris
Cauda Equina

The most widely used functional assessment instrument in the United States is the Functional Independence Measure (FIM) (Table 25-3).[26] This scale is currently used at more than 1,000 rehabilitation centers in the United States and is rapidly gaining acceptance internationally. Since 1992, the scale has been a part of the "International Standards." The FIM focuses on six functions: (1) self-care; (2) sphincter control of bladder and bowel; (3) mobility, especially transfer mobility; (4) locomotion; (5) communication; and (6) social recognition, each with several subfunctions for a total of 18 functions. Each of these 18 functions is evaluated using a seven-point scale with respect to independence or dependence. The highest score of 7 is given for complete independence in which a task is performed in a timely and safe manner without any helper. Six is scored for modified independence when

Table 25–3. Functional Independence Measure (FIM)

LEVELS	
7 Complete Independence (Timely, Safely) 6 Modified Independence (Device)	NO HELPER
Modified Dependence 5 Supervision 4 Minimal Assist (Subject = 75%+) 3 Moderate Assist (Subject = 50%+) Complete Dependence 2 Maximal Assist (Subject = 25%+) 1 Total Assist (Subject = 0%+)	HELPER

	ADMIT	DISCHG	FOL-UP
Self Care			
A. Eating			
B. Grooming			
C. Bathing			
D. Dressing-Upper Body			
E. Dressing-Lower Body			
F. Toileting			
Sphincter Control			
G. Bladder Management			
H. Bowel Management			
Mobility			
Transfer:			
I. Bed, Chair, Wheelchair			
J. Toilet			
K. Tub, Shower			
Locomotion			
L. Walk/wheel Chair	W C	W C	W C
M. Stairs			
Communication			
N. Comprehension	A V V N	A V V N	A V V N
O. Expression			
Social Cognition			
P. Social Interaction			
Q. Problem Solving			
R. Memory			
Total FIM			

NOTE: Leave no blanks: enter 1 if patient not testable due to risk.

Table 25-4. Potential Functional Outcomes for Persons with Neurologically Complete Spinal Cord Injury (Cervical)

Activity	C3-C4	C5	C6	C7	C8-T1
Feeding	May be able	Ind. with equipment after set up	Ind. with equipment	Ind.	Ind.
Grooming	Dep.	With equipment after set up	Ind. with equipment	Ind. with equipment	Ind.
Upper extremity dressing	Dep.	Assists	Ind.	Ind.	Ind.
Lower extremity dressing	Dep.	Dep.	Assists	May be Ind. with equipment	Ind.
Bathing	Dep.	Dep.	Ind. with equipment	Ind. with equipment	Ind.
Bed mobility	Dep.	Assists	Ind. with equipment	Ind.	Ind.
Weight shifts	Ind. in power Dep. in manual	Assists	Ind.	Ind.	Ind.
Transfers	Dep.	Assists	? with transfer board	Ind. with or without board except floor transfers	Ind.
Wheelchair propulsion	Ind. with power	Ind. in power; short distances in manual with lugs indoors	Ind. for manual with lugs on plastic rims indoors	Ind. for except curbs	Ind.
Driving	Unable	Unable	Specially adapted van	Car with hand controls or adapted van	Car with hand control or adapted van
Bowel/bladder	Dep.	Dep.	Ind. for bowel Assists for bladder	Ind.	Ind.

Dep. = dependent; Ind. = independent.

the patient may require an assistive device but requires no personal help. A score of 5 is defined as modified dependence for which the person requires the supervision of another person for safety. A score of 4 means that the person requires minimal assistance and is able to perform the activity without help 75% of the time or more. A score of 3 means that the person requires moderate assistance of another person less than 50% of the time. A score of 2 means that the person requires maximal assistance but is still able to perform 25% to 50% of the effort required in the activity. Total assistance with the subject able to perform 0% to 25% of the effort required is scored as 1.

The sum of all items represents the total FIM score, which projects cost of the disability in terms of safety and a person's dependence on others and on technological devices. The FIM was developed for the disabled population in general and not specifically for persons with SCI. It is reliable and valid as an instrument, although it has not yet been tested for SCI specifically. The FIM is simple to use, reflects well the important functional issues, and is widely considered the best instrument available to measure function. It does require staff training for conformity and accuracy.

On admission to the rehabilitation service, each member of the rehabilitation team performs a discipline-specific assessment of the patients capabilities in each of the six functional areas, and the numerical score is entered on the form. The functional assessment using the FIM is updated at each team conference. The score is used as a measure of the patients progress and of the effectiveness of the rehabilitation program. For most people with SCI, the functional goals are quite predictable. In general, the lower the cord lesion, the more muscles remain under voluntary control and greater is the potential for function. Detailed charts that predict the obtainable goal for each level of complete SCI are available (Table 25-4 and 25-5).[27]

Table 25-5. Potential Functional Outcomes for Persons with Neurologically Complete Spinal Cord Injury (Thoracic and Lumbar)

Activity	T2–T10	T11–L2	L3–S3
ADL (Grooming, feeding, dressing, bathing)	Ind.	Ind.	Ind.
Bowel/bladder	Ind.	Ind.	Ind.
Transfers	Ind.	Ind.	Ind.
Ambulation	Exercise only with orthoses	Possible indoors with orthoses	Community ambulation
Orthoses	KAFO, bilateral forearm crutches or walker	KAFO/AFO, forearm crutches.	AFO, canes/crutches

ADL = activities of daily living; Ind. = independent; KAFO = knee, ankle, foot orthosis.

ACUTE MANAGEMENT

A detailed description of acute management of SCI is found in other chapters of this book and subsequently in this chapter, but a brief overview of this important phase may be helpful to the reader. Acute management of a person with SCI may determine the eventual outcome, that is survival, health, and function. Early recognition of potential SCI by emergency personnel is usually not difficult except in the unconscious victim. All unconscious victims of trauma should be considered to have both brain injury and SCI until proved otherwise. Several observations, however, may be helpful to indicate the presence of SCI. A restless patient may not be moving all parts of the body spontaneously. Painful stimulus may fail to evoke a response below a given neurologic level. Clinical observations of diaphragmatic breathing, absence of deep tendon reflexes, presence of priapism or spinal deformity may indicate an SCI.

Primary goals of acute SCI care should be saving the individual's life, minimizing the neurologic damage, stabilizing the spine, and preventing secondary medical complications. First, the medical condition must be stabilized by securing adequate respiration, blood pressure, heart rate, etc. As early as possible, drugs should be administered to minimize the neurologic damage. The recognition that progressive tissue damage occurs within the spinal cord for some time after the initial trauma has encouraged researchers and clinicians to employ different interventions during this period, that is, hypothermia, hyperbaric oxygen, postelectromagnetic fields, and a variety of drugs. A multicenter controlled trial has demonstrated that treatment with high-dose methylprednisolone within 8 hours of injury results in significant gains in motor and sensory scores.[28] This treatment is now well-accepted by clinicians, although it has not yet been approved by the Food and Drug Administration (FDA). Spinal stabilization is initially secured by emergency personnel by placing the patient supine on a spinal board with straps, immobilizing the entire spine from the skull to the sacrum. Application of cervical collars only is considered to be inadequate and may give a false sense of security. Spinal traction should not be applied until the specific diagnosis of spinal injury is firmly established, that is, after completion of proper imaging studies of the entire spine. After the medical condition and the spine have been stabilized and steroids have been given, the diagnostic evaluation must be completed with proper imaging and electrodiagnostic and laboratory studies. If spinal stability and decompression of the nervous tissue can not be obtained by nonsurgical means, a surgical operation is indicated and should be done as soon as possible. Medical complications are obviously best prevented, but should they arise, they must be treated promptly and effectively to decrease institutional length of stay and to improve outcomes.

Secondary medical complications following SCI may develop even in the finest institutions, but, by and large, the incidence of these complications appears to be inversely related to the quality of care and the expertise available, that is, the better the care the less likely these complications are to occur. Premorbid clinical conditions may make the patient with acute SCI more vulnerable for developing complications. Preexisting conditions are more likely to occur in older individuals than in the young. Similarly, injuries sustained to body parts other than the spine also make the treatment more difficult and development of secondary medical complications more likely. Frequent associated injuries include traumatic brain injury, contusion of the lungs and abdominal organs, rupture of major blood vessels, and fractures of the long bones of the extremities. Inexperience of staff in the treatment of persons with injuries to the central nervous system (CNS) also increases the likelihood of complications. A trauma center that cares for patients with acute SCI not only must have a spinal surgeon available but also medical and nursing staff with expertise in SCI care.

Respiratory insufficiency during acute SCI may occur for several reasons. Paralysis of some or all of the respiratory muscles develops with high SCI. Patients with cord injuries at or above C3 are not able to breathe on their own and require mechanic ventilation. Cord injuries below the C3 neurologic level may also require mechanical ventilation for a period of time. Patients with complete cervical SCI at C4 or below, that is, all patients with complete tetraplegia, depend on the diaphragm for breathing as all the intercostal and abdominal muscles are denervated. These patients are, therefore, unable to cough and secretions can easily accumulate in the respiratory tract. In many patients with tetraplegia, the diaphragm may only be partially innervated with corresponding reduction in pulmonary function test values. Injuries to the chest, such as rib fractures, hemopneumothorax, and lung contusions are commonly associated with thoracic SCI and may result in temporary respiratory insufficiency. Aspiration, atelectasis, and pneumonia are commonly present in persons with high-level SCI and are generally interrelated. Aspiration may occur very early after the SCI, particularly if the injury happens soon after a meal or if the SCI was the result of a diving injury. In general, the older the patient, the higher the neurologic level, and the more complete the neurologic lesion, the more likely these conditions are to develop.[29] Preexisting respiratory conditions clearly make the patient with SCI more vulnerable to develop respiratory complications, that is, history of cigarette smoking, chronic obstructive pulmonary disease, bronchial asthma, intrinsic lung disease, and marked obesity.

Good respiratory care during acute SCI is mandatory to prevent complications from arising and to secure effective treatment of any potential respiratory complications. Insertion of a nasogastric tube immediately following SCI, preferably at the site of injury, minimizes the chances of aspiration during ambulance transportation, emergency room care, and diagnostic evaluation. Airway must be secured by whatever means necessary, although utmost care during intubation must be taken when a cervical spine fracture is suspected. Oxygen should be administered liberally during acute SCI. Respiratory functions must be monitored carefully by taking chest radiographs as often as needed, assessing arterial blood gases, particularly for increased PCO_2 and decreased PO_2 and by performing simple pulmonary function tests such as an assessment of vital capacity at the bedside.

An active prophylactic respiratory therapy program must be started as soon as possible following SCI. Intermittent positive pressure breathing with saline, sodium bicarbonate, and/or bronchodilators, as individually indicated, should be provided for persons with high SCI. Postural drainage should be encouraged by placing the patient regularly in the Trendelenburg and reverse Trendelenburg positions and side-lying positions. Because the cough is weak in persons with high-level SCI as a result of paralyzed chest and abdominal muscles, assistive coughing is provided by manually pressing on the abdomen or by use of an insufflator/exsufflator machine. As soon as possible, active chest exercise program should begin to increase the strength of the diaphragm and other innervated accessory respiratory muscles. The diaphragm may decondition rapidly during mechanical ventilation and may not be able to sustain adequate pulmonary function immediately following its discontinuation. Mechanical ventilation, which may be provided either by intubation or by tracheostomy, is usually indicated when (1) the vital capacity decreases to 1,000 ml or less, (2) when arterial blood gasses become increasingly abnormal, that is, PCO_2 rises and PO_2 falls; and (3) when atelectasis occurs frequently and when chest radiographs show consolidation. Tidal volumes for patients with SCI on mechanical ventilation are generally kept higher than normally provided for nonparalyzed persons on ventilators, or at least 20 mL per kilogram of body weight. Weaning off the ventilator can begin when their respiratory status has been stabilized. Weaning is best accomplished by progressively increasing time off the ventilator, rather than by reducing intermittent mandatory tidal volume. Suctioning of the pharynx and trachea should be done regularly and as needed. When atelectasis and pneumonia occurs, antibiotics should be promptly administered intravenously.

Cardiovascular complications occur during acute SCI and of these *deep venous thrombosis* (DVT) is the most common. Its incidence has been found to vary between 30% and 60% depending on the diagnostic methods used and on the efficacy of the prophylactic treatment. Recent data from the Model Systems of Care indicate that the incidence of DVT may be decreasing (13.6%), perhaps as a result of effective prophylaxis.[29] The main etiologic factors for DVT in patients with SCI are decreased venous return from the paralyzed limbs and increased coagulability of the blood. *Pulmonary embolism* (PE) is a relatively frequent complication and a leading cause of death during acute SCI. It occurs in approximately 4% of persons with SCI, and this incidence does not seem to be decreasing.[29] *Cardiac dysrhythmia*, primarily bradycardia, occurs frequently in persons with high-level SCI, that is, those with tetraplegia, and in persons with paraplegia and neurologic level above T5 because of inadequate supraspinal control of the sympathetic nervous system and unopposed vagal tone. *Hypotension* during acute SCI may be the result of hypovolemia caused by severe hemorrhage or inadequate administration of fluids. Orthostasis caused by impaired sympathetic activity and inadequate vasoconstriction also may produce hypotension. *Cardiopulmonary arrest* occurs in approximately 5% of patients with acute SCI.[29] Especially at risk are older individuals, patients with tetraplegia, and those with complete neurologic lesions. Prophylactic treatment of DVT primarily consists of anticoagulation with subcutaneous heparin, which should be rapidly administered after SCI in the absence of contraindications, such as, active bleeding, evidence of traumatic brain injury, or coagulopathy. Traditional prophylactic treatment has consisted of administration of low-dose unfractioned heparin subcutaneously, that is, 5,000 units two or three times daily, but recent studies have shown that low-molecular-weight heparin may be safer and more effective for persons with SCI and other forms of major trauma.[30–33] Some form of external compression of the lower limbs is also customary, that is, elastic bandages or pneumatic pumps. To diagnose DVT promptly, nurses should perform a clinical assessment on each patient two or three times per day, observing such signs as increased circumference of the lower limbs, alteration in venous blood flow, discomfort, and low grade fever of unknown origin.[34] Placement of a vena cava filter is indicated for patients with SCI when anticoagulation fails or is contraindicated when recurrent pulmonary embolism occurs despite anticoagulation. In addition to clinical observation, certain laboratory tests may be necessary to diagnose DVT. Venography is still considered to provide the most accurate information but is cumbersome to perform and the contrast material can be quite irritating. Many clinicians, therefore, choose to perform Doppler sonography or, less often, impedance plethysmography or 1-125 labeled fibrinogen uptake scan. The duration of prophylactic treatment for DVT should be individually determined based on the clinical needs, perceived risk, and neurologic and functional status, but is usually 3 months or less.

When the diagnosis of DVT and/or pulmonary embolism is confirmed, treatment is begun immediately by administration of intravenous (IV) heparin and adjusting the doses daily according to the activated partial thromboplastin time (APTT). Sodium warfarin administration is started within a few days, and the heparin can usually be discontinued within 7 or 10 days when the prothrombin time has reached a level of 1.5 to 2.0 times the control value or the International Normalized Ratio (INR) is between 2.0 and 3.0.[29,35] Anticoagulation treatment for DVT without PE is usually continued for 3 months or for 6 months if PE occurs.

Bradycardia due to unopposed vagal influence on the heart during acute SCI usually does not require treatment unless the heart rate falls below 44 beats per minute. Anticholinergic agents, such as atropine, or adrenergic drug, such as norepinephrine, may have to be used intermittently in an IV drip as needed. Caution should be shown to avoid vagal stimulation by such maneuvers as prolonged tracheal suctioning. When bradycardia is profound and sustained despite precaution and drug treatment, a cardiac pacemaker may be required, at least temporarily, to regulate the heart beat. Autonomic dysreflexia is usually not a clinical problem during the acute phase of SCI but can become a vexing problem later, when the patient comes out of spinal shock.

Urologic dysfunction is noted immediately after SCI. Bladder sensation is lost and the detrusor muscle does not contract. The patient, therefore, experiences urinary retention and only evacuates urine by overflow incontinence when the bladder pressure rises and volume exceeds at least 500 ml of urine. A Foley catheter must, therefore, be promptly inserted to ensure adequate evacuation. Retention of urine, or presence of foreign bodies in the bladder, including the catheter, may lead to urinary tract infections, which can be recurrent. Intermittent catheterization is, therefore, recommended as early as possible, provided that the nursing staff is adequate and well-trained. Hematuria is common during the acute phase of SCI, sometimes because of a pelvic fracture and injury to the urethra or bladder, but otherwise hematuria may result from traumatic catheterization or urinary tract infection.

Gastrointestinal problems are relatively common with acute SCI. Virtually all patients experience paralytic ileus during the early phases of spinal shock, but this condition rarely lasts longer than 2 to 5 days. Peptic ulcer, esophagitis, and gastrointestinal (GI) hemorrhage may occur, but prophylactic treatment is effective with administration of histamine H_2-receptor antagonist and adequate nutritional support.[36] Pancreatic dysfunction with elevation of serum amylase frequently occurs, particularly with injury to the abdomen. Constipation and diarrhea are not major clinical problems during the acute phase of SCI, but both can be difficult to manage during the subacute and chronic phases.

The initial management of gastrointestinal dysfunctions in acute SCI, involves inserting a nasogastric tube, which should be left in situ for drainage, either by gravity or by low suction, until good bowel sounds have returned. Because abdominal distention indicating bowel obstruction may occur, abdominal girth should be assessed daily. Intravenous feedings should be continued until bowel sounds have appeared. Besides fluids and electrolytes, the average size adult male should receive at least 3,000 calories per day to secure adequate nutrition. Similar to other major trauma, the caloric requirements of persons with acute SCI are increased. When bowel sounds have returned, ordinarily within 1 week of the SCI, enteral feedings may begin, either by the nasogastric tube or orally, depending on the patients ability to chew, swallow, and tolerate oral feedings. Occasionally, parenteral hyperalimentation may be required. H_2-receptor antagonists should be given routinely to prevent peptic ulcers and GI bleeding, and hemoglobin and hematocrit should be monitored regularly. Because most patients with SCI lose both the urge to defecate and control voluntarily the anal sphincter, a bowel program to regulate evacuation of stools should begin as soon as bowel sounds return and the patient is receiving nasogastric or oral feedings. Stool softeners and laxatives are then prescribed and a suppository is administered to initiate evacuation.

Pressure ulcers occur during acute SCI unless a rigorous prophylaxis is maintained. Such ulcers most commonly develop on the sacrum and the heels.[37] Pressure ulcers can seriously delay the onset of rehabilitation therapies, lengthen the total hospitalization, and make the ultimate adjustment to the disability far more difficult. To prevent development of pressure ulcers, the patient with SCI must be turned and the skin must be completely inspected every 2 hours, beginning in the emergency room and continuing through the ICU, surgical suites, and different nursing wards. Prophylaxis involves use of special mattresses, air fluidized beds, kinetic beds, and securing adequate nutrition, but these do not provide complete protection nor do they eliminate the need for skin inspection. Medical complications, such as infections and malnutrition, make the patient with SCI more susceptible to develop pressure ulcers, and such complications are, therefore, best prevented or effectively treated.

Contractures of muscle and joints can develop quickly as a result of immobilization, paralysis, and increased muscle tone. Joint contractures are particularly prevalent in the upper limbs of persons with tetraplegia.[38] Spasticity and heterotopic ossification are conditions that are rarely seen during the acute care of persons with SCI but later become contributing factors to the development of joint contractures. Prevention of contractures involve proper bed positioning, regular turning and changing of position, splinting of key joints and passive range of motion and stretching exercises by nurses and therapists.

SPINAL ORTHOSES

External supports are commonly used to protect the painful or unstable spine during healing. Numerous designs of spinal orthoses are available, providing different degrees of support to different segments of the spine. Few, if any, spinal orthoses provide complete immobilization of the spine, but in general, the longer and better fitting the orthosis is, the greater is its effectiveness. When an orthosis is used to protect the spine during healing of a fracture or a surgical fusion, it ordinarily must be worn for 10 to 12 weeks. Wearing of spinal orthoses for lengthy periods of time may lead to emotional dependency and to disuse muscle weakness, and atrophy. It must, therefore, be made clear at the beginning that the spinal orthosis is only a temporary device which must be eliminated when the therapeutic goals have been reached. If clinically possible, the patient should be instructed to perform certain neck and trunk exercises and practice good body mechanics while wearing the spinal orthosis to decrease its deconditioning effects on the body.

Two main biomechanical principles are employed in the design of most spinal orthoses; that is, the orthosis must either provide counteractive horizontal forces through use of the three-point pressure system, or it must create a longitudinal traction-distraction force. When choosing a spinal orthosis, it is important to first determine its desirable function and the specific treatment objectives. Different orthoses restrict spinal motions in different ways and to different degrees. Some primarily limit flexion and extension, while others restrict lateral flexion or rotation. Other designs provide unloading of the spinal segments through longitudinal traction.

Among clinicians, different nondescriptive eponyms are frequently used for orthotic devices. To reduce confusion, a systemic nomenclature for orthotic devices was developed in 1973 in which orthoses are named according to the body segments involved. Consequently, spinal orthoses are classified as cervical orthoses (CO), head cervical orthoses (HCO), cervical thoracic orthoses (CTO), thoracolumbosacral orthoses (TLSO), lumbosacral orthoses (LSO), and cervical thoracolumbosacral orthoses (CTLSO). Spinal orthoses may be further classified as rigid, semirigid or flexible, and, depending on the prescription indications, as corrective or supportive.

CERVICAL AND CERVICAL THORACIC ORTHOSES

Three basic types of COs and CTOs are available: (1) collars; (2) poster appliances; (3) and custom molded orthoses. Most of these restrict flexion and extension to a greater extent than rotation and lateral flexion. The simplest CO are *soft cervical collars* made of cloth or foam rubber. These are usually comfortable to wear and restrict neck motion primarily through sensory feedback rather than by mechanical restriction. Prefabricated rigid cervical collars are made of various plastic materials in different designs to provide greater support and restriction, for example, the Philadelphia or Miami collars. *Poster cervical appliances* usually consist of chin and occipital pieces that are connected by two to four adjustable metal uprights to sternal and back plates. Such devices provide greater restriction of neck motions than collars. The *sternal occipital mandibular immobilizer (SOMI)* is lightweight and usually comfortable. It can be applied and fitted easily and provides substantial restriction of motion in the mid to low cervical region.

Maximum immobilization of the cervical spine is obtained by application of head, cervical, thoracic orthoses (HCTOs), the best known of which are the rigid

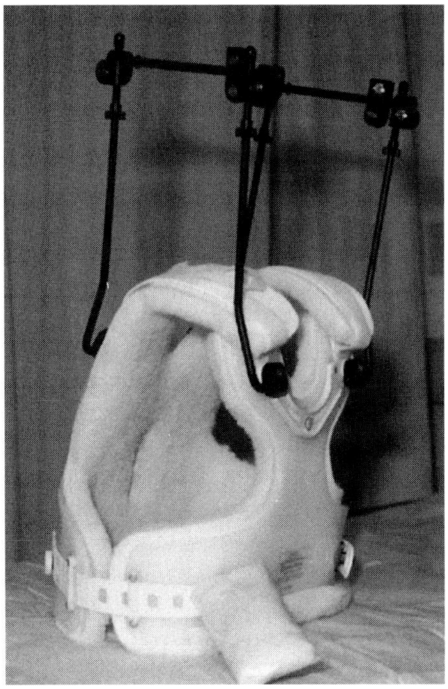

FIGURE 25-1

Halo vest (From Goldberg B, Hsu JD, editors: *Atlas of orthoses and assistive devices,* 3/e St. Louis, 1997, Mosby–Year Book, p. 254.)

halo orthosis (Figure 25-1) and the semirigid *Minerva orthosis.* The Minerva orthosis is usually a custom molded total contact appliance made of plastic materials, which are shaped over a positive body cast. It encloses the upper part of the trunk, the neck, and the back of the head and may have a band around the forehead. It provides excellent restriction of lateral and rotational neck motions and limits flexion and extension.

During the acute phase of cervical SCI, a halo orthosis is frequently applied for external support following a period of cervical traction or after surgical spinal fusion. Cervical traction by Gardner Wells tongs or by a halo ring should not be applied until a specific diagnosis of the cervical spinal injury has been established. Cervical traction often is indicated initially before application of a halo orthosis to reduce facet dislocations. Traction also may be applied temporarily to provide external stabilization for burst, odontoid, Jefferson, and hangman's fractures. Such traction is optimally provided by tongs made of titanium, which are MRI compatible, but stainless steel tongs may be required when heavy traction force is applied. When traction is used to reduce dislocations of the cervical spine, the patient must be kept awake and the neurologic condition carefully monitored by examination and by somatosensory evoked potentials. The spinal alignment should be assessed by a series of lateral radiographs. If the neurologic condition deteriorates, traction should be discontinued immediately and an MRI scan obtained to visualize any potential herniated disk material.

Although the halo orthosis provides the maximum restriction of flexion and extension of the potentially unstable cervical spine, it does not guarantee maintenance of alignment and ultimate fusion. The halo orthosis consists of a halo ring, a vest, and upright posters. The ring should be made of lightweight MRI-compatible metal, be large enough to provide 1 cm clearance around the head, and be open posteriorly to ease application and give access to the upper cervical spine. The ring is placed approximately 1 cm above the ears and is tilted so its anterior part is slightly higher than the posterior, thus placing the neck in slight extension. Four pins are placed, under local anesthesia, to attach the ring to the head, two anterolaterally on the forehead and two posteriorly. The anterior pins are placed approximately 1 cm above the upper and lateral half of the orbital rim but below the equator of the cranium. Special care must be taken not to insert the pin into the frontal sinus, the temporalis muscle, or the supraorbital nerve. The posterior pins are placed directly opposite to the anterior pins, carefully avoiding injuring the occipital nerves. The opposing pins are tightened alternatively with increments of 2 inches-pounds, usually to a total torque of 6 to 8 inches-pounds in a young adult. For children and elderly persons, the torque should be considerably less, between 2 and 5 inches-pounds. Because loosening of the pins may occur, they need to be retightened within 24 hours of the ring application and periodically thereafter. Excessive pin tightening may result in intracranial penetration with dural or even cerebral puncture. To prevent infection, the pin sites must be cleaned twice daily with normal saline solution. The halo vest is made of prefabricated plastic material and lined with sheepskin or a soft fabric. It must fit the body well to prevent pressure sores and loss of spinal reduction. The vest is usually made of two pieces, one posterior and one anterior. The posterior piece is usually applied first by logrolling the patient or by raising the trunk to approximately 30° while supporting the head and the neck firmly. Afterward, the upright posters, usually four in number, are attached to connect the halo ring to the vest and the specially made linkages are tightened. Once the halo orthosis has been securely applied, the patient can usually get out of bed and participate in physical activities, either ambulatory or in a wheelchair.

THORACOLUMBOSACRAL ORTHOSES

Immobilization of the thoracic spine by simple orthotic means is difficult, and the literature on such efforts is sparse. In general, a CTLSO is necessary to limit motion in the upper half of the thoracic spine, but a well-constructed TLSO can provide adequate protection for the lower thoracic spine. It is fortunate that an intact rib cage provides relative stability and minimizes displacement of a fracture in the upper thoracic spine, because this part of the spine is difficult to immobilize by simple orthoses. Effective immobilization of the lumbar spine, especially its lower part and the lumbosacral junction, is difficult to achieve by orthotic means although frequently attempted. The function of most LSOs is to remind the user to restrict movements, to support the abdomen, to reduce some of the load on the lumbosacral spine, to provide some movement restriction of the upper lumbar and thoracolumbar spine by three-point fixation, and to reduce excessive lumbar lordosis to provide a straighter and more comfortable lower back.[39,40] To achieve maximum external immobilization, a molded rigid pelvic girdle, or better, a hip spica, is required inferiorly, and the orthosis then must extend upward to the thoracolumbar region. In general, a hip spica is not well tolerated and its efficacy has been disputed.[41]

Flexible LSO or TLSO corsets made of different fabrics with adjustable sets of braces or straps are relatively ineffective in mechanically restricting motion but are usually comfortable and effective in reducing pain for various painful back disorders when spinal stability is not in question. When greater restriction of spinal motions is needed, a variety of prefabricated, adjustable, and more rigid orthoses are available, that is, Knight-spinal LSO, Knight-Taylor TLSO, and Jewett TLSO. These orthoses effectively reduce gross motion and provide trunk support, but they are inadequate for treatment of unstable spinal fractures. The Jewett TLSO (Figure 25-2) is frequently used after surgical stabilization of fractures at the thoracolumbar junction. This prefabricated, adjustable orthosis uses a three-point pressure system in which pressure is applied anteriorly on the sternum above and on the pelvis or pubic bone below, by means of pads attached to a firm metal frame. Posteriorly, pressure is applied over the lower thoracic and upper lumbar spine by a pad that is attached to the anterior metal frame by a adjustable straps. The Jewett TLSO provides, therefore, no abdominal muscle support and limits only flexion. It is lightweight but may be uncomfortable because the corrective forces are spread over a relatively small area.

The most rigid design is a custom molded total contact TLSO, sometimes referred to as a spinal or body jacket (Figure 25-3). It is prescribed for maximum restriction of flexion, extension, and rotation. This orthosis is usually made of plastic materials, although lightweight plaster cast also may be used. The orthosis is usually bivalved, and the anterior and the posterior halves are connected by Velcro straps. The jacket is molded to firmly fit the pelvis below. Above it may extend to the manubrium of the sternum anteriorly

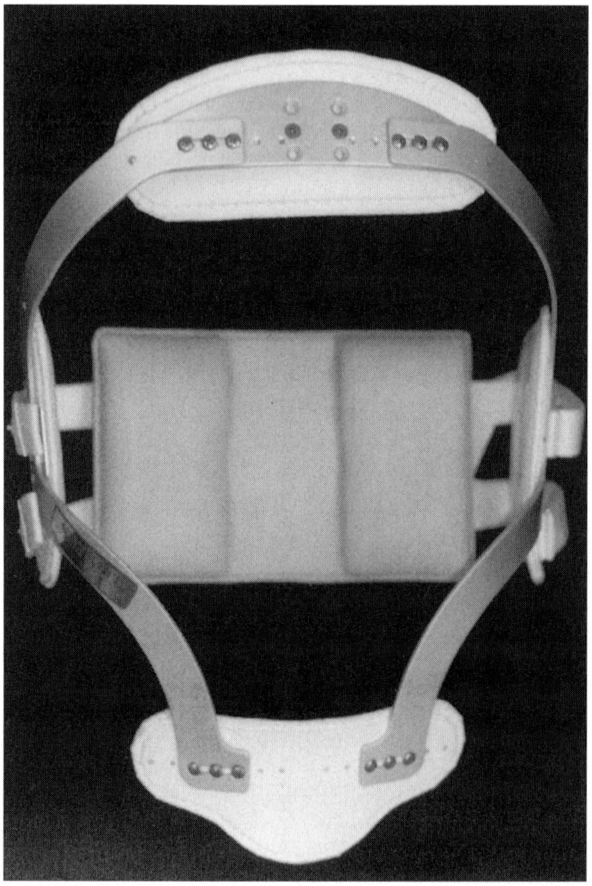

Figure 25-2

Jewett brace. (From Goldberg B, Hsu JD, editors: *Atlas of orthoses and assistive devices,* ed 3, St. Louis, 1997, Mosby–Year Book, p. 255.)

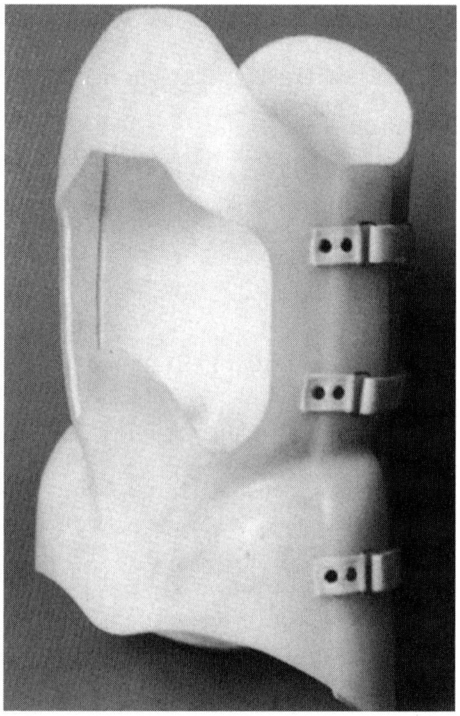

Figure 25-3

Custom molded total contact TLSO (spinal jacket). (From Goldberg B, Hsu JD, editors: *Atlas of orthoses and assistive devices,* ed 3, St. Louis, 1997, Mosby–Year Book, p. 503.)

and posteriorly to the midportion of the scapula. A cervical extension may be attached to provide restriction of motion of the upper thoracic and cervical spine. A rigid, total contact TLSO is particularly indicated for unstable fractures of the spine when surgical stabilization is not indicated or when the adequacy of the surgical stabilization is in question. Because of the total contact, this orthosis tends to be warm and somewhat uncomfortable. A Knight-Taylor TLSO with pectoral extensions may be used as an alternative to this orthosis.

REHABILITATION AND FUNCTIONAL OUTCOMES IN SPINAL CORD INJURY

The goal of SCI rehabilitation is to maximize the medical, physical, emotional, educational, vocational, recreational, and social function of the person with SCI. The extent to which this is possible is dependent on the age of the individual, preexisting and current medical condition, neurologic impairment, the resources available, the person's motivation, and the support of family and friends. There are many factors that predict functional outcome (see Chapter 24), but of particular significance is the neurologic level of injury (NLI), which determines the presence of the key muscle groups. The motor level, if different from the sensory level, is more consistent with ultimate function.[42] Tables 25-4 and 25-5 summarize anticipated functional goals for the key neurologic levels of injury.

These functional goals, however, are generalized and a significant variability in individual outcomes exists despite similar levels of injury. The treatment team should be guided by these long-term functional goals, and the rehabilitation program should be individualized to meet each person's strengths, weaknesses, social situation, etc. When monitoring the progress toward the functional goals, it is important to reassess the patients needs and capabilities, understand the limiting factors, and be ready to modify the rehabilitation program to help the patient meet the individual expectations. The predicted functional goals may not be attainable due to both physical and emotional factors, such as older age, excessive weight, premorbid clinical condition, lack of endurance, severe spasticity, and depression.

The rehabilitation program is not simply a recipe to achieve these goals but a comprehensive team approach, which uses the patients neurologic status as a starting point and the outlined goals as the long-term objective. Each functional skill that may be obtainable is further divided into different components, which are addressed separately to properly achieve the ultimate function. Each factor that may adversely affect the progress must be taken into account. The patient should be aware of the goals early to ensure active participation and total involvement in the program becoming an active consumer of medical rehabilitation services.

Physical activities and exercises that are prescribed include passive range-of-motion (ROM) exercises for all four extremities at least twice daily. Strengthening exercises for all muscle groups with partial or full innervation is very important, because of the great demand spared muscles now must endure. Mat activities are begun, focusing on training for balance, strength, and endurance for reaching, sitting, and transferring. These activities are helpful for mobility skills such as, turning in bed, transfers, basic wheelchair propulsion, and advanced wheelchair techniques. Community-level wheelchair mobility includes the ability to negotiate uneven surfaces such as riding on rough terrain, to ascend and descend ramps and curbs, to perform wheelies, to ride escalators, and to transfer from floor to wheelchair. The lower the neurologic level, the more tasks the SCI patient is expected to master. Training in ADL uses orthotics and other assistive devices.

Functional outcome for persons with SCI may vary from independence in all ADL to complete dependence; but, even if dependent, most are capable of instructing caregivers, recognizing clinical problems, and preventing complications.

C1–C4 LEVEL

Persons with such a high level of injury are dependent in most self-care activities and mobility. They should, however, be taught how to instruct others in providing pulmonary care such as assisted coughing techniques and use of ventilator when required, performing passive ROM exercises, assisting with ADL, positioning properly in bed and wheelchair, and setting up environmental control units (ECU) or other technologic aides. Mechanical lifts are often helpful in transferring, and these patients should be independent in the use of powered wheelchairs by breath (sip and puff), mouth stick, tongue, or chin control mechanisms. These patients should also be independent in the use of computers and ECUs. The ECUs are electronic scanning and switching devices, which allow independent operation of electrical appliances, such as the television, radio, lights, and telephone. The ECUs are controlled by different switches, identical to those for powered wheelchairs, but they may also be controlled by voice activation. The cost of ECU systems depends primarily on the number of appliances that they control and may range up to several thousands of dollars. Some patients with C4 NLI may be able to use a mobile arm support (MAS) to assist in feeding. Mobile arm supports, sometimes, referred to as balanced forearm orthoses, may enable patients whose deltoid strength is at least poor (grade 2/5) to achieve limited shoulder flexion and by practice to increase the strength and endurance of this motion. Additionally, the MAS allows performance of functional activities involving the head such as feeding, hygiene, and grooming. When the deltoid and biceps muscles have strength of a fair plus (3+/5) rating and adequate endurance, the MAS is no longer needed.

Equipment required for patients at this level include a manual wheelchair, a powered wheelchair with a back-reclining mechanism, a sliding board, a mechanical lift, wrist-hand orthoses, an electric hospital bed with rails, and urologic supplies. For ventilator dependent patients, a portable ventilator, respiratory equipment, and a vent tray on the wheelchair may be needed. Environmental control units, page turners, emergency call systems, and speaker telephones also would benefit patients with high-level injuries. See Table 25-6 for equipment recommendations.

C5 Level

The C5 patient gains the key muscle group of the biceps (elbow flexors) and also functional mobility of the deltoid. This should allow the patient to be partially independent in functional skills such as feeding with splints. An MAS may be necessary initially; however, the patient should become strong enough to perform

Table 25-6. Suggested Equipment for a Person with Complete Tetraplegia

	C1–C4	C5	C6	C7	C8–T1
Orthotics					
Mobile arm support	X	?	—	—	—
Resting hand orthosis	X	X	X	—	—
Long opponens orthosis	X	X	—	—	—
Spiral orthosis	—	X	X	—	—
Powered tenodesis orthosis	—	X	—	—	—
Wrist driven tenodesis orthosis	—	—	X	—	—
Rachet tenodesis orthosis	—	X	—	—	—
Short opponens orthosis	—	—	X	X	—
Lumbrical bar	—	—	—	—	X
Mobility					
Trans-aid lift (Hoyer lift)	X	X	X	—	—
Transfer board	X	X	X	X	X
Powered W/C with tilt recline	X	?	—	—	—
Powered wheelchair	X	X	?	?	?
Manual wheelchair	X	X	X	X	X
Feeding					
Adapted utensils	X	X	—	—	—
Universal cuff	X	X	X	X	—
Utensils with built-up handles			X		
Grooming & Dressing					
ADL splints (wash mitt, razor holders)	—	X	X	—	—
Dressing equipment (pant loops, sock aide, dressing stick, long shoe horn)	—	—	X	X	—
Gooseneck mirror	X	X	X	X	X
Communication					
Environmental control unit	X	X	?	—	—
Computer	X	X	X	X	—
Book holder	X	X	X	X	—
Bathing					
Grab bars	—	—	X	X	?
Reclining shower commode	X	—	—	—	—
Tub seat/shower chair	—	X	X	X	X
Hand-held spray attachment	—	—	X	X	X
Beds					
Full electric hospital bed	X	X	X	X	—
Full specialized mattress	X	X	X	?	—
Overlay mattress	—	—	?	X	—

X = Usually required; ? = Sometimes required; — = Usually not required these activities independently. Elbow flexion allows the patient to perform some mobility skills such as propelling a manual wheelchair on flat smooth surfaces. The wheelchair may require rim projections or a plastic coated handrim with a glove to help better propel the wheelchair. A universal cuff is often useful for the patient in many tasks including feeding, writing, or typing. A universal cuff fits around the palm of the hand and has a pocket for inserting utensils. Changing of the utensils allows the patient to perform different functional activities including brushing teeth, writing, typing, feeding, and performing hygiene and grooming activities. In addition a ratchet splint may be used. Many types of utensils can be attached to this or a long opponens orthosis. Although the C5 patient is usually independent in ADL after setup, including brushing teeth, washing face, applying makeup, shaving, and combing hair, dressing usually requires assistance, especially of the lower extremities. Because the C5 patient does not have use of either wrist or finger muscles, adaptive equipment is needed for most functional activities. Possible tendon transfers can allow the patient to become somewhat more functional. These patients must prevent elbow flexion and forearm supination contractures caused by the unopposed biceps activity. Stretching should, therefore, be performed and continued throughout the rehabilitation program in both the acute and chronic phases of care. Assistance is required throughout most of the day.

Anticipated equipment includes a lightweight wheelchair, powered wheelchair for longer distance mobility use, a transfer board, an MAS early in the postrehabilitation period, universal cuff with long opponens splints, adaptive equipment for feeding and grooming, and a hospital bed.

C6 Level

Additional functional muscles in the C6 patient are the extensor carpi radialis and forearm pronators. Active wrist extension can result in tenodesis, which is the opposition of the thumb and index finger occurring with finger flexion, as the tendons are stretched when the wrist is extended. Tenodesis orthoses are available and can assist with this action. Although these orthoses are rarely used, they can be used as a training device until the patient's fingers and wrist extensors assume enough strength. To enhance functional tenodesis, maintenance of correct hand and wrist position is extremely important. To maintain functional finger tightness necessary for optimal tenodesis, one must avoid stretching the finger flexors and losing the tenodesis action. Patients with C6 NLI most commonly use a short opponens orthosis with slots for different utensils. These patients can generally feed themselves and can assist in their upper extremity dressing and can perform oral and facial hygiene. Pull-over garments are usually preferable to buttoned shirts because of the difficulty in manipulating buttons and snaps. Clothing modifications including Velcro closures are helpful in allowing higher level SCI patients to be independent in upper extremity dressing. Some C6 patients can perform their own catheterizations with a catheter holder, but most require assistance. In addition, they have difficulty applying a condom catheter.

Transfers are now possible using loops and a transfer (sliding) board, and the patient can propel a manual wheelchair with plastic coated rims. A power wheelchair may still be required for long distances. These patients should be able to drive an adapted van with hand controls. The addition of a lift in the van may allow the patient to be fully independent in driving.

C7, C8, and T1 Levels

At the C7 level the elbow extensors, finger extensors and wrist flexors are functional. These further assist the patient in becoming independent in transfer activities and ADL. The level C7 is considered the key level in becoming independent in most activities. Patients at this level should be independent in transfers with a transfer board and eventually with lateral transfers, hygiene, feeding, bowel, bladder care, and upper extremity dressing. Many patients may also become independent in lower extremity dressing. Additionally at the C8 level, control of long finger flexors allows the patient to have improved hand and finger function. Patients at this level should be independent with a manual wheelchair although there are some C7 patients who may benefit for vocational purposes in having a powered wheelchair. A power add-on unit may be a good compromise. Patients at these levels usually do not require a van and are able to drive a car with hand controls. Many C7 patients become independent enough in all activities such that they can live alone with only occasional assistance.

T2–T6 Levels

One cannot accurately assign specific outcomes based on specific thoracic levels of injury, but these patients can be grouped into high- and low-level paraplegia. At the T1 level and below, hand function is normal and the intercostals muscles are functional. Patients with thoracic level injuries should be independent in ADL and basic mobility skills at the wheelchair level. These patients also should be independent with bowel and bladder care. The higher the level of the thoracic injury the less trunk control the patient has. Teaching advanced wheelchair activities to high-level patients is important. This allows patients to be more independent and also allows them to purchase less equipment such as a tub bench. Functional community ambulation for a complete high-level paraplegic is uncommon and should not be an initial goal of a rehabilitation program.

Bladder management is usually by intermittent catheterization, but anticholinergic medications are often required. Males may opt to reflexively void, but urodynamics should be performed to document the pressures of the sphincters and within the bladder.

T7–T12 Levels

Additional functional muscles at these levels include the abdominal and paraspinal muscles. These patients should be independent in all the above activities. The lower the level of injury, the greater the trunk control and the greater ability to perform advanced wheelchair techniques. In addition, patients with lower levels of injury can participate more with bilateral lower-extremity orthoses for ambulation as an exercise. Patients with both upper and lower thoracic level lesions usually do not ambulate in the community.[43,44] Although patients may use orthoses for a short time after the injury for exercise, because of the high energy requirements most patients give them up. There are some benefits to having these patients exercise with orthoses at these levels of injury including psychologic, improvement of the bowel program, decreased spasticity and potentially decreasing bone-mineral loss. Prescriptions for KAFOs for these patients, therefore, should not be discouraged for highly motivated individuals.

There are different types of orthoses available for ambulation including standard KAFOs, the Craig-Scott variant, reciprocal gait orthoses (RGO), the Parastep system, and the advanced reciprocal gait orthoses. The KAFO has an upper and lower thigh band, drop locks, and a double-action ankle joint. They are either plastic molded or steel; both can be inserted into a shoe. The Craig-Scott variant has a patellar tendon strap, a bail lock at the knee, and a rigid ankle support. It is lighter in weight as the lower thigh and calf band closures are eliminated.

Lumbar Paraplegia

The lower the level of injury, the greater opportunity for the patient to be independent in ambulation. To be a community ambulator, one should have functional bilateral hip flexors and at least one knee extensor, greater than a 3/5 manual muscle testing score, and a maximum bracing for community ambulation of one long leg KAFO and one ankle foot orthosis (AFO). The greater the muscle strength and the less bracing that is necessary, the more functional the patient can become for greater distances. These patients, unless there is concomitant injury, should be independent in all previously mentioned activities.

L1–L3 Levels

Additional functional muscles at these levels include the hip flexors and part of the quadriceps. With bilateral KAFOs the patient can walk for short distances, but a wheelchair is still required. Bladder elimination is usually by intermittent catheterization. Bowel evacuation may be by reflex stimulation but at times is by abdominal pressure and occasional manual disimpaction.

L3-L4 Levels

Usually AFOs are required for ambulation as well as canes or crutches, especially if the hip abductors, extensors, or ankle plantarflexors are weak. A wheelchair may not be necessary for these patients. For bladder management, these patients often have an areflexic detrusor (bladder wall) and lax sphincter muscles and, therefore, may void by Valsalva maneuvers if postvoiding residual urine volumes (PVRs) are within an acceptable range. Males may use a condom catheter, and both males and females may use an absorbent pad to protect their skin and clothes if there is any incontinence. The anal sphincter may also be flaccid, so that straining with the use of abdominal muscles may allow for an effective form of bowel elimination. Suppositories are often ineffective because of the inability to induce reflex emptying.

L5 and Below

These patients should be independent in all previously mentioned activities, including community ambulation, unless there are other associated problems and complications.

NEUROGENIC BLADDER

Although no longer among the leading causes of death for individuals with SCI, neurogenic bladder dysfunction remains a major management problem. Successful management involves minimizing complications to the kidneys and bladder while providing an acceptable means of urine collection and deposit.

Neuroanatomy

Normal micturition involves a complex interplay of the urinary bladder, the external urethral sphincter, and the nervous system. The bladder is innervated by the autonomic nervous system. Parasympathetic innervation is via the pelvic nerves whose cell bodies are in the S2–S4 spinal cord segments. Parasympathetic stimulation produces contraction of the urinary bladder with opening of the bladder neck and a tendency for urination to occur.[45] Sympathetic innervation is by the hypogastric nerves whose cell bodies lie in the T11–L2 cord segments. While the bladder has both α and β receptors, β receptors predominate in the body of the bladder while the α receptors predominate in the vicinity of the bladder neck. Sympathetic stimulation produces a relaxation of the bladder's body with narrowing of the bladder neck, a condition that inhibits urination.

The external urethral sphincter is innervated by the somatic nervous system through the pudendal nerve whose cell bodies lie in the S2–S4 spinal cord segments. Stimulation of the pudendal nerve results in a tightening of the external sphincter resulting in an inhibition of voiding.

Coordination of normal voiding is felt to occur at the level of the pons.[45] Suprapontine input to the pontine micturition center is inhibitory in nature allowing for normal bladder capacity and urine storage until voiding is permitted to occur.

In persons with SCI, coordination between bladder and sphincter is lost (detrusor sphincter dyssynergia) with both acting reflexively, generally with frequent spontaneous urination at abnormally low bladder volumes (hyperreflexic neurogenic bladder). If the injury involves the conus medullaris and/or cauda equina, however, the bladder and sphincter are denervated and a condition of urinary retention with overflow incontinence results (areflexic neurogenic bladder).

EVALUATION

Prevention of morbidity to the urinary tract of a person with SCI depends on proper evaluation and management. Evaluation should be both anatomic and physiologic. Based on the level and completeness of the injury and observations of the patients voiding pattern along with a careful rectal examination, the clinician should be able to formulate a working concept of the individual's bladder function. Initial management may be based on this concept, but urodynamic testing verifies the clinical hypothesis and provides quantitative data with regard to intravesical pressures and volumes. It also can be used to demonstrate and quantify the response to specific bladder management strategies and medications. During the urodynamic evaluation, the bladder is filled with either gas or water while the external sphincter activity is recorded either by needle or surface electrode.[46,47] As the catheter used has a pressure measuring device, a pressure-volume recording is generated. Along with this physiologic data, an imaging study of the bladder and the upper urinary tracts is recommended at the initiation of treatment and yearly thereafter. Imaging testing options include sonography, intravenous pyelography, excretory cystography, and renal scintigraphy, but many favor renal and bladder sonography because it is noninvasive, free of adverse effects, and sensitive in detecting upper tract pathology including calculi and hydronephrosis.

MANAGEMENT

The goal of management of the neurogenic bladder is to achieve an acceptable method of bladder drainage while preventing complications that may be typically associated with this condition, that is, infection, stone formation, hydronephrosis, and bladder-associated autonomic dysreflexia.

During the immediate postinjury period, an indwelling catheter is generally used. During this period of spinal shock, urinary retention is the rule as the bladder is areflexic. An indwelling catheter provides adequate bladder drainage and allows constant measurement of urine output when the person with SCI may be hemodynamically unstable owing to blood loss or autonomic instability.

Once the patient leaves the intensive care unit, a more thoughtful approach to bladder management begins. The major factors to consider include the gender of the patient and the NLI. Intermittent catheterization is generally believed to be the best option for long-term bladder management if voluntary control of micturition cannot be regained. Intermittent catheterization has physiologic advantages, as it allows for bladder filling and periodic emptying, and has been shown to be associated with fewer complications than long-term indwelling catheters.[48] Intermittent catheterization is usually performed four times per day but may need to be performed as often as six times per day. Patients are gradually advised to limit their fluid intake to approximately 2 liters per day with the desired volumes not to exceed 500 mL per catheterization. Some believe that nonsterile (clean) technique is equally as effective as sterile technique in terms of preventing urinary tract infection after hospital discharge.[49,50] Intermittent catheterization, however, is not a good option for every patient with SCI. A person with C1–C5 tetraplegia is unable to perform this procedure independently and usually is better off with another method of management.

Reflex voiding is an option for the male patient who develops a hyperreflexic bladder. A condom-type catheter is applied and connected by tubing to a receptacle. When the bladder contracts, voiding occurs. This type of voiding can be augmented by suprapubic tapping to trigger the reflex bladder contraction. Unfortunately, reflex voiding in SCI is often associated with detrusor-sphincter dyssynergia (DSD) and elevated voiding pressures, thereby placing the person at risk for vesicoureteral reflux and hydronephrosis. As the elevated intravesical pressures are often clinically silent, persons with reflex voiding should undergo urologic evaluations regularly to measure their pressures and detect the presence of reflux. Autonomic dysreflexia, which may occur with voiding, is usually a sign of DSD and elevated bladder pressures. In contrast to males, reflex voiding is a poor option for females as there is no useful external collection device available to act as a receptacle.

Bladder drainage by an indwelling Foley catheter is an option for females with hyperreflexic bladders and for males unable to perform self–intermittent catheterization or tolerate condom devices, either because of skin breakdown from the condom catheter or inability to obtain a secure fit. Use of indwelling catheters is associated with a high rate of urinary infection, and stone formation. These catheters do not allow for physiologic bladder filling, are damaging to the urethra, interfere with sexual performance, and are associated with an increased incidence of bladder cancer, therefore, indwelling catheter use is generally discouraged.[51]

At the time of hospital discharge, intermittent catheterization is the most common method of bladder management for both men and women, but with time, there is a change toward use of indwelling catheters for women and either reflex voiding or indwelling catheters, often in the form of suprapubic cystostomy, for men.[2]

Pharmacologic Management

Various medications are useful adjuncts in bladder management. *Anticholinergic agents* for example, oxybutinin, propantheline, hyoscyamine, and imipramine, act to relax the detrusor muscle and prevent reflex voiding. These agents are generally used toward achieving the goal of bladder continence for persons using intermittent catheterization. Side effects of these drugs include dry mouth, blurry vision, constipation, and palpitations. *Alpha-1 adrenergic blockers* (prazosin, terazosin) may be used to reduce bladder outlet resistance in DSD, which seems to occur at the level of the bladder neck rather than at the external sphincter.[52,53] The principal side effect of these agents is hypotension. *Sympathomimetics* (ephedrine, pseudephedrine) may be useful in the treatment of overflow and stress incontinence. In SCI, stress incontinence principally occurs in individuals with areflexic bladder and denervated sphincters usually caused by conus medullaris or cauda equina injuries. Although not consistently effective, they should be tried prior to consideration of more invasive treatments. Palpitations and difficulty sleeping are the most common side effects.

Antispasticity agents that act at the level of the spinal cord (baclofen and diazepam) may be used for treatment of external sphincter spasticity associated with DSD. Often, patients with DSD also have significant extremity or trunk spasticity and may be using these medications primarily to treat these conditions. Botulinum toxin injected directly into the external sphincter improves urodynamic parameters in the presence of DSD.[54]

Surgical Management

The most common surgical procedure currently used in the bladder management of SCI patients is suprapubic cystotomy. Its use becomes more frequent as time from injury increases such that by 10 years postinjury, it is used by more than 25% of men and nearly 10% of women as their method of bladder management. The procedure is technically simple to perform, and it is reversible. As with a Foley catheter, urine drains passively to an appropriate receptacle. This method may be used temporarily in the event of severe urethral or bladder damage during the acute postinjury phase, but during the chronic phase of SCI, suprapubic cystostomy also can be a useful temporary treatment for autonomic dysreflexia caused by bladder conditions.

Transurethral external sphincterotomy has been used for many years to treat symptomatic DSD in men in whom its efficacy has been estimated to be between 70% and 90%.[55] When unsuccessful, a repeat procedure is necessary. Currently, this procedure is declining in popularity as it is irreversible and leads to permanent incontinence. Recently, use of a sphincter stent prosthesis (Urolume) has been demonstrated to be an attractive alternative to external sphincterotomy.[56] This prosthetic device is a tubular wire mesh placed intraurethrally at the level of the external urethra, but it may be removed later if indicated. Balloon dilation of the external sphincter has also been used in the management of DSD.[57]

To improve bladder capacity and to permit successful intermittent catheterization in either males or females, who cannot be made continent with medications, augmentation cystoplasty may be used. The procedure involves incising the hyperreflexic bladder in a clam-shell fashion and harvesting a portion of the patients intestine, which is used to create a low-pressure, high-capacity reservoir.[58,59] Following this procedure, the patient may catheterize the bladder as previously mentioned. For certain clinical conditions, such as intractable skin breakdown, the augmentation cystoplasty may be combined with bladder neck closure and creation of a continent stoma in the abdominal wall.[60] For a woman with severe adductor spasticity of the lower extremities, such stoma may be much easier to catheterize than the urethra. Augmentation cystoplasty is a major surgical procedure with potentially significant morbidity including dehiscence of the native bladder-intestinal interface. For this reason, autoaugmentation by detrusor myomectomy has been developed. Its goals are the same as the traditional augmentation, but it is a smaller, safer procedure, as no bowel is used. The detrusor muscle is essentially removed from the mucosa, which is left intact and subsequently evaginated creating a lower-pressure, higher-capacity reservoir.[61] Long-term effectiveness of this procedure is unknown.

Urinary Tract Complications

Urinary tract infections (UTIs) are a nearly ubiquitous complication of SCI. Although the need to clinically treat an obvious UTI is not in question, there is considerable disagreement as to what constitutes a UTI. Patients with neurogenic bladder dysfunction often have significant bacteriuria, especially when the bladder management involves some type of appliance. Frequent treatment with antibiotics for asymptomatic UTIs may lead to highly resistant pathogens. Symptoms of UTI in individuals with SCI include fever, spontaneous voiding between catheterizations, increased spasticity, hematuria, autonomic dysreflexia, malaise, and vague abdominal discomfort. The urine may become increasingly malodorous and cloudy. Bacterial colonization can lead to epididymitis, orchitis, and prostatism in men. Although UTIs are common in persons with SCI, the clinician must resist concluding that every illness or vague symptom represents a UTI, but rather examine carefully other organ systems when there is an acute illness.

Urinary tract calculi are common in persons with SCI and may be present in the bladder, ureters, or kidneys. Presence of bacteria, sediment, and catheters are major reasons for the development of urinary tract stones, but in acute SCI hypercalciuria is also a significant factor. Urinary tract stones should be suspected in the presence of hematuria, recurrent UTIs, or unexplained autonomic dysreflexia. The diagnosis is made by imaging studies or when the stone passes. The treatment is removal of the stones, but the method of removal depends on the location and size of the stone.

Renal failure was formerly the most common cause of mortality in persons with SCI, but currently it is not even among the top 10.[2] Improved surveillance treatment of DSD and effective treatment of UTIs may be the primary reasons for this decline.

GASTROINTESTINAL DISTURBANCES

Virtually the entire length of the GI tract is affected by SCI. As noted earlier in this chapter, initially after injury there is gastric atony and paralytic ileus present. Oral feeding should, therefore, not begin until after bowel sounds are present. Abdominal complaints in persons with SCI are difficult to diagnose because of their limited ability to localize pain, but as discussed later, the clinician should have a high index of suspicion, carefully examine the patient, and order necessary diagnostic tests if the patient has worsening vague abdominal complaints without apparent cause.

Superior mesenteric artery (SMA) syndrome is a known cause of abdominal distention, discomfort, and recurrent emesis in persons with tetraplegia. It may be caused by obstruction in the distal part of the duodenum as it passes behind the SMA and in front of the lumbar spine and aorta. Symptoms often appear in immobilized patients who have lost significant amount of weight and retroperitoneal fat. The symptoms are usually worse when in the supine position, or in body casts. An upper GI series reveals an abrupt cessation of barium in the third part of duodenum. Treatment may include sitting upright or resting in the left lateral decubitus position after meals, ample nourishment to restore weight, and application of a lumbosacral corset to push the abdominal contents upward. Surgical intervention is only rarely necessary. *Cholecystitis or cholelithiasis* is the most common cause of emergency abdominal surgery in persons with SCI.[62] Gallstone disease has been reported to be common in persons with SCI as indicated by autopsy results that showed a three times higher incidence of gallstones compared to normal control.[63]

The most frequent GI problem after SCI is altered bowel elimination.[64] It has been reported that 27% of persons with chronic SCI have complaints relating to bowel elimination, hemorrhoids, abdominal distention, and autonomic dysreflexia caused by rectal impaction. Factors contributing to such symptoms include altered colonic compliance, impaired transit time, and poor dietary intake. The key to preventing such problems is the use of an effective bowel program, which allows the patient to have control over the time and frequency of their bowel elimination. The combination of oral medications (stool softeners, bulk formers, oral stimulants), suppositories, and digital stimulation is usually effective to secure effective elimination of stools. An ineffective bowel evacuation program may adversely affect most aspects of the patients life and the pursuit of physical, psychologic, social, vocational, and sexual goals.[65]

AUTONOMIC DYSREFLEXIA

Autonomic dysreflexia (AD), also known as autonomic hyperreflexia or sympathetic crisis, is a syndrome virtually unique to individuals with SCI. The syndrome may occur in any individual with SCI and neurologic level at or above T6.[66] Autonomic dysreflexia is a medical emergency because of severe hypertension and bradycardia. In addition to these symptoms, the syndrome may include a pounding headache, sweating and flushing above the level of injury, nasal congestion, piloerection, chest pain, and visual blurring.

The syndrome is caused by a noxious stimulus below the level of injury that the afflicted individual is unaware of because of his or her lack of sensation. These noxious stimuli most often reside in the urinary bladder, with overdistention being the predominant cause. Any noxious stimulus, however, may precipitate the syndrome whether it be the presence of detrusor-sphincter dyssynergia, an impacted rectum, or an ingrown toe nail.

Acute management is geared toward removing the inciting stimulus, which typically produces rapid resolution of the symptoms. Effective treatment, therefore, may include drainage of the bladder, disimpaction of fecal material from the rectum or resection of the ingrown nail. On the other hand, pharmacologic or surgical management may be required to treat AD related to a recurring condition such as detrusor-sphincter dyssynergia with α-blocking agents and external sphincterotomy.

ETIOLOGY

Most of the time, the inciting stimulus producing AD is located in the urinary tract.[67] Although overdistention of the urinary bladder is the most common cause, there are numerous other causes, including detrusor-sphincter dyssynergia, cystitis, epididymitis/orchitis, or stones. Autonomic dysreflexia can result because of malfunction of the collection or drainage devices, such as blockage of an indwelling catheter, kinking of an external catheter, or maximal filling of a collection bag. At times, an overly tight external catheter can produce constriction of the urethra with obstruction to urine flow. Finally, AD may occur in diagnostic procedures or therapeutic intervention, such as a urodynamic study, cystoscopy, or vibratory stimulation of the penis in an attempt to produce ejaculation.

The second most common site for inciting AD is the lower intestinal tract, with the principal precipitating event being distention of the rectum with impacted fecal material.[67] If fecal impaction is not present, AD may be caused by perirectal fissures or abscesses, inflamed hemorrhoids, or irritating suppositories or enemas. As with the urinary tract, diagnostic procedures, such as sigmoidoscopy, or therapeutic endeavors, such as electroejaculation with a rectal probe, may lead to AD. Finally, acute abdominal pathology, such as a ruptured appendix, may produce significant clinical signs and symptoms of AD.[68]

Some of the other possible inciting causes of AD include skin irritations, such as pressure ulcers, ingrown toe nails, or sunburns. Sexual intercourse may be interrupted by signs or symptoms of AD. Obstetricians need to be aware of AD because uterine contractions during labor and delivery may incite AD. Nasal decongestants with sympathomimetic properties, such as pseudoephedrine, may cause or worsen AD, and, in general, nasal congestion in SCI patients susceptible to AD should not be treated with these products.[69]

In summary, the causes of episodic AD are numerous and varied. Virtually any noxious stimulus can produce the syndrome. In most cases, the cause can be found quickly and alleviated. Awareness of the syndrome and its causes is vital to patient and caregiver education.

PATHOPHYSIOLOGY

Kurnick, in 1956, described the pathophysiology of AD.[70] He postulated that noxious stimulation is transmitted afferently in a normal fashion to the spinal cord. Supraspinal transmissions of these efferent impulses via the spinothalamic tracts is blocked by the cord lesion. The sympathetic chain, on the other hand, is intact. It is reflexly stimulated by the ascending afferent impulses and responds with a release of norepinephrine. Norepinephrine produces the characteristic hypertension through splanchic vasoconstriction in persons with SCI above T6. The reflex hypertension is sensed by baroreceptors located in the aortic arch and carotid sinus. To counteract the severe hypertension, the baroreceptors stimulate activity of the vagus nerve, which directly accounts for the parasympathetic aspects of the AD syndrome. These include bradycardia, flushing and sweating above the level of injury, visual blurring, and nasal congestion. The sympathetic features, in addition to the hypertension and related headache, include pallor and piloerection below the level of injury. Autonomic dysreflexia does not occur in spinal shock during which reflex activity below the level of injury is absent. Further, for AD to occur, the spinal cord distal to the level of injury must be intact.

CLINICAL PRESENTATION

As noted, AD occurs in SCI patients with NLI at or above T6. The incidence of this syndrome is 30% to 85% of persons with high SCI.[69] Presumably, some individuals experience the full blown form of the syndrome, whereas others may have minor or partial manifestations with brief, self-limiting symptoms. An example of this might be a person who experiences feelings of warmth and chest tightness during reflex urination, which ceases when urination is complete. In this example, the presence of detrusor-sphincter dyssynergia causes the symptoms, which subside upon completed urination and intravesical pressure reduction.

The most common and most serious clinical sign of AD is rapidly developing systolic and diastolic hypertension. Although normal blood pressure in a person with high SCI is typically in the 90/60 range, pressures double and triple that have been reported.[71] Such hypertension has led to cerebral hemorrhages and seizures, retinal hemorrhages, coma, and death.[72,73,74]

Most of the time, episodes of AD include pounding headache, sweating, and cutaneous vasodilatation, but there are a variety of other signs and symptoms.[75] Subjectively, the patient may note nasal congestion, gooseflesh, paresthesias, chest heaviness or tightness, and a desire to urinate.[76] They may feel anxious and listless and have a sense of acute distress.[69] Objectively, in addition to the hypertension and sweating, bradycardia frequently occurs. Tachycardia, although less common than bradycardia, also may occur.[67] Other arrhythmias, have been reported, including atrial fibrillation, atrioventricular block, and asystole.[77,78,79] Examination of the eyes may show mydiriasis, conjunctival congestion, and occasionally Horners syndrome.[81]

MANAGEMENT

The acute management of AD is directed at removing the inciting stimulus. With proper education and preparation of the professional staff, the patient, and the caregiver, AD can usually be resolved quickly and with no significant adverse outcome. After sitting the patient up to induce orthostatic hypotension, the blood pressure is measured, if possible. If a sphygmomanometer is unavailable, the presence of a pounding headache must be interpreted as a sign of hypertension. Tight clothing or straps are loosened. As the lower urinary tract is most often responsible for the precipitating stimulus, the bladder is checked for distention and emptied by catheterization. If an indwelling catheter is present, the catheter must be evaluated for patency. If such a catheter is blocked, it is either flushed or replaced. If a condom catheter is used, it and the connector tubing are checked for twisting or kinking. The drainage bag is checked for maximal filling.

If these steps fail to resolve the symptoms, the rectum is checked for impaction. If available, an anesthetic lubricant such as Xylocaine is used to assist with gentle disimpaction. Some clinicians feel that the anesthetic gel should be inserted into the rectum and allowed to remain there for 10 to 15 minutes before disimpaction.[82]

If evaluation and treatment of bladder and bowel conditions do not resolve the hypertension, a more extensive examination is performed. Specifically, the skin is checked for pressure ulcers, ingrown toenails, swelling, and erythema. Any identified stimulus is treated, when possible. If immediate treatment is not possible, as in the case of a severely inflamed joint, medical attention is immediately sought. Pharmacotherapy is indicated to control hypertension if the conservative measures enumerated do not resolve the episode. Several medications that act rapidly are available to produce, at least temporarily, a reduction in blood pressure. These agents are often kept in the patient's home or in the SCI unit of a hospital for immediate use. The most common of these is probably nifedipine, a calcium channel blocker, which dilates the coronary and peripheral arteries. This results in a reduction of blood pressure and reflex tachycardia.[83] Ten milligrams of nifedipine can be administered orally (bite and swallow). Nitroglycerine, a vasodilator that is taken sublingually, can be used instead of nifedipine for rapid reduction of hypertension. Mecamylamine, a nonspecific ganglion blocker, is taken orally but may take 30 minutes until the onset of activity. Its usual dose is 2.5 mg. Various IV medications may be used once professional medical treatment is obtained. Some of these agents are nitropresside (a venodilator), hydralazine (an arterial dilator), and diazoxide (a ganglion blocker). Fortunately, it is rare that IV treatment is required to control severe hypertension associated with AD.

Pharmacologic treatment of AD also may be required when episodes recur frequently, as in detrusor-sphincter dyssynergia, which sometimes occurs every time a patient voids reflexively. In such a case, pharmacologic management is geared toward either reducing the outlet resistance or reducing the force of the bladder contraction. To accomplish the former, α-1-antagonist agents are often preferred.[84] Terazosin, a well-tolerated α-1-blocker, is an example of this class of drugs. Compared to prazosin, terazosin has a lower incidence of first-dose hypotension and may be given once a day at bedtime. Prazosin is typically prescribed two to three times daily. Phenoxybenzamine, a nonspecific α-blocker, has a long history of usage in this clinical scenario. Although effective, many clinicians are wary of this agent because of its reported carcinogenicity.[85,86] Alternatively, anticholinergic agents, such as oxybutynin, propantheline and hyoscyamine, are used to decrease detrusor hyperreflexia and through this action reduce the degree of intravesical hypertension that can cause an episode of AD.

Mecamylamine can be used for prophylaxis of AD. When used for this purpose, it is begun at a dosage of 2.5 mg two to three times daily, but it can be used at higher dose. It has a potent hypotensive effect and may be difficult for the individual with high SCI to tolerate. Mecamylamine is also effective in treating autonomic sweating in persons with SCI. Surgical management has a role in control of AD, especially in the treatment of detrusor-sphincter dyssynergia–induced dysreflexia.[87] Surgical procedures that diminish the effects of dyssynergia include external sphincterotomy, suprapubic cystostomy, placement of a sphincter-stent prosthesis, balloon dilation of the external sphincter, and bladder augmentation. These procedures are discussed in the Neurogenic Bladder section of this chapter. Other examples of surgical procedures that eliminate episodes AD include hemorrhoidectomy to treat prolapsing hemorrhoids and shunting procedures to collapse posttraumatic intramedullary cysts.[88]

ORTHOSTATIC HYPOTENSION

Orthostatic hypotension can be a consequence of prolonged bedrest in any individual, but it may be particularly vexing and prominent in individuals with SCI, especially those with tetraplegia or high paraplegia. Orthostatic, or postural, hypotension refers to a fall in blood pressure that results from a change in body position toward the upright. In the person with SCI this usually occurs early in the rehabilitation phase when mobilization out of bed is attempted. The decrease in blood pressure is usually accompanied by an acceleration of the heart rate, dizziness, lightheadedness, loss of vision, or even loss of consciousness. Associated symptoms may include numbness about the face and pallor. Resumption of recumbency generally produces a normalization of blood pressure and symptomatic relief.

The primary event in generating the orthostatic response is the pooling of blood in the paralyzed lower extremities. On sensing the drop in blood pressure, baroreceptor response normally leads to an increase in norepinephrine production and vasoconstriction. In SCI, this response is delayed and inefficient, owing to the inability of the sympathetic nervous system to produce adequate vasoconstriction as a direct result of the cord lesion. The tachycardia represents an attempt to produce a compensatory increase in cardiac output, but this too is inefficient as a result of poor diastolic filling.[27,89]

Treatment of orthostatic hypotension is generally successful with conservative measures. These include use of intermittent compression garments when in bed and use of compression stockings and abdominal binders when out of bed. Adequate hydration is essential as a depleted intravascular volume exacerbates the problem. Gradual progress toward a vertical posture is necessary and reclining wheelchairs and tilt tables are useful. Particular care must be taken in the early morning as this is usually the time of greatest orthostasis.

If conservative measures do not lead to cessation of orthostatic symptoms, sodium chloride may be added in the form of 1-g tablets. This acts to promote volume expansion. Alternatively, mineralocorticoid treatment with fludrocortisone (Florinef) is often very effective and also works to expand the intravesicular volume by salt and water retention. Electrolytes should be monitored closely if this drug is used because hypokalemia may occur. Sympathomimetics, such as ephedrine or pseudoephedrine must be used cautiously by persons with high SCI as they can exacerbate autonomic dysreflexia. Other medications should be evaluated for drugs that can exacerbate the postural hypotension, such as α-blockers. In the chronic phase, orthostatic hypotension has been reported to occur as a consequence of syringomyelia.[90]

RESPIRATORY COMPLICATIONS

Respiratory complications are currently the leading cause of morbidity and mortality in persons with both acute and chronic SCI.[29] All those with tetraplegia and many with paraplegia have some respiratory deficit. While the diaphragm is innervated by high cervical root fibers, other inspiratory and expiratory muscles (especially the abdominal muscles) are affected in lower levels of injury. This decreases the effectiveness of inspiration and the ability to adequately cough making atelectasis more prevalent and the ability to clear secretions more difficult.

In a large prospective multicenter study the incidence of respiratory complications in acute SCI was found to be 67%, most frequently atelectasis, ventilatory failure, and pneumonia.[91] These were more common in persons with high cervical (C1–C4) levels of injury (84%) than in those with lower cervical (C5–C8) (60%) and thoracic (T1–I12) levels (65%). The neurological completeness of the cord lesion, according to the ASIA Impairment scale, was found in this study to have minimal impact on the incidence of respiratory complications.

Prevention of respiratory complications is a major component of SCI care. As noted earlier in this chapter, rehabilitation efforts to improve pulmonary function should be initiated early for all persons with SCI and continued while they remain at risk. These efforts include the use of vital capacity measurements, special beds for position changes, chest percussion, incentive spirometry, inspiratory exercises for strengthening the diaphragm and accessory respiratory muscles, postural drainage, intermittent positive pressure breathing with normal saline or bronchodilator, and elimination of secretions management.[92]

Because respiratory impairment associated with SCI is predominantly a restrictive disorder, the need for oxygen supplementation is limited, except during the acute phase. If oxygen saturations fall, adequate ventilation and secretion management should first be pursued, rather than only increasing the oxygen delivery. Weaning off the ventilator should be attempted as soon as indicated, but options for long-term, ventilator-dependent patients include tracheostomy, noninvasive means of ventilation, and phrenic nerve pacing.[93]

Although respiratory complications are the leading cause of death in those with SCI, the risk decreases with time. Even during the chronic phase of SCI, a home program with monitoring of respiratory status and vital capacity remains important for those with high cord lesions. Risk factors may be decreased when the patient stops smoking, maintains body weight, and receives vaccinations against influenza and pneumonias.

THROMBOEMBOLIC DISEASES

Deep venous thrombosis (DVT) is one of the most common complications of acute SCI and a major cause of morbidity and mortality. The incidence in SCI patients ranges from 47% to 100% depending upon the methods used for assessing the diagnosis.[94,95,96] Clinically evident DVT occurs in roughly 13.8% to 16.3%

of patients, with the incidence slightly higher for patients undergoing surgery.[29,97] The incidence of clinical DVT reported may underestimate the true incidence because the clinical examination is not as helpful in the SCI population as in others at high risk, different tests were used in the various studies, and not all of these studies were not conducted prospectively. The high incidence appears to result from the presence of all three factors of Virchow's triad in the spinal cord patient.[98] This includes venous stasis from muscle paralysis and decreased venous return, hypercoagulability as a result of stimulation of thrombogenic factors following injury, and intimal or vessel wall damage as a result of trauma from the initial injury or afterward.[96]

Clinical features of a DVT include swelling or warmth of the extremity. In the SCI population, some indication of a clot including tenderness to palpation may not be elicited. The differential diagnosis is similar to that of heterotopic ossification (HO) and can coexist with the presence of heterotopic bone. Even if HO is found, this does not rule out a DVT. Because of the potential morbidity and mortality from a DVT, one must have a high index of suspicion and not rely purely on clinical methods to prompt a further investigation.

Although many studies are available to diagnose a DVT, venography is still considered the gold standard, however it is invasive, has the potential for an allergic reaction, and may cause a clot itself. Duplex ultrasonography is an accurate, sensitive, noninvasive test for studying the presence of proximal clots and has gained widespread use.[99] Occasionally, all the veins cannot be examined, and a venogram may still be required. Impedance plethysmography also is used to diagnose proximal clots; however, it is very operator dependent.

The incidence of fatal pulmonary embolism (PE) has been reported to range from 2% to 16% of patients in the first 3 months postinjury. Although there are no characteristic findings of a PE, the most common symptoms include tachypnea, tachycardia, dyspnea, fever, and chest pain. Electrocardiogram (ECG) changes are nonspecific, and most commonly sinus tachycardia is seen. Arterial oxygen saturation may be decreased but is not always abnormal. Pulmonary angiography is the gold standard; however, more frequently ventilation-perfusion (V/Q) lung scanning is performed. A mismatch represents an area of abnormal perfusion with normal ventilation. Although a normal scan rules out an embolus, an abnormal scan does not necessarily indicate its presence.

The use of prophylactic measures to prevent thromboembolic diseases is extremely important. Early initiation is crucial because the highest risk period appears to be during the first 2 weeks following SCI.[94] Rotation beds and external pneumatic compression have been used with some effectiveness.[100] Low-dose subcutaneous heparin (5000 units two or three times per day) decreases the incidence in some studies but was not shown to be effective in others.[30,101,102] Adjusted-dose heparin (partial thromboplastin time [PTT] at 1.5 times control) is considered effective for prophylaxis, but the potential for bleeding is prevalent.[30] Combining pharmacologic and mechanical devices (pneumatic compression boots or electrical stimulation) may be the most effective means of prophylaxis, although electrical stimulation is time consuming and requires more frequent monitoring.[96] Low molecular weight heparin (LMWH) has been shown to be effective for preventing venous thromboembolism, reducing the risk to less than 8%, and is associated with significantly less bleeding than standard heparin.[103,104]

Current recommendations include initiating prophylaxis as soon as possible with a combination of pharmacologic and mechanical means. Pneumatic compression boots are used during the early postinjury period with nurses monitoring the skin every 8 hours.

If their use is delayed for greater than 72 hours, duplex scanning (or other reliable testing) should be obtained before initiating the compression boots. Pharmacologic intervention can include adjusted dose heparin (activated PTT [aPTT] at high normal) with the increased risk of bleeding or a LMWH in which dosage depends on the type used. Newer LMWHs are now becoming available in this country. Prophylaxis should continue for patients at risk for 8 weeks; however, it can be discontinued earlier in motor-incomplete patients and should be continued longer for high-risk patients including high-level, complete tetraplegics and those patients with fractures, obesity, age over 70 years, or a history of thromboembolism.

Once the diagnosis of a DVT is made, prompt treatment with anticoagulation should be initiated to prevent propagation of the thrombosis, pulmonary embolism, and recurrence. Standard treatment is with intravenous heparin adjusting the dose to achieve an aPTT of 1.5 to 2.5 times control. Oral warfarin is then initiated after proper anticoagulation is achieved, and the dosage is adjusted to maintain an international normalized ratio (INR) of 2.0 to 3.0. Treatment with warfarin should continue for 3 to 6 months or longer in patients who have persistent swelling or are at great risk for postphlebitic syndrome.[105,106] Anticoagulation with subcutaneous LMWH has been reported to be effective as the initial treatment of DVT in other patient populations.[107,108] An inferior vena cava filter can be placed if anticoagulation is contraindicated.

SPASTICITY

Spasticity is a syndrome characterized clinically by increased resistance to passive motion, involuntary muscle contractions, and hyperreflexia. The increased resistance is velocity dependent and is unique to upper motor neuron syndromes including SCI.

Spasticity is included as part of the upper motor neuron syndrome. Landau popularized the concept of dividing the upper motor neuron syndrome into positive and negative symptoms.[109] Negative symptoms are deficits in normal functioning caused by CNS injury. Positive symptoms are caused by an increased response of surviving neuron pathways released from control of injured areas of the CNS. Often the negative symptoms are the most disabling to the patient. Positive symptoms such as spasticity, may either be beneficial, or more likely, detrimental. An example of improved function resulting from spasticity would be the ability of a person with SCI to perform stand-pivot transfers by bearing weight on his spastic lower extremities. It is thus important always to keep the upper motor neuron concept of positive and negative symptoms in mind when treating spasticity, as the reduction of spasticity can potentially make the patient less functional.

The *pathophysiology* of spasticity remains unclear. Loss of inhibitory influences on segmental reflexes provides an explanation for increased reflex activity; however, spasticity generally comes on gradually after an initial period of spinal shock. Disinhibition caused by traumatic SCI should cause immediate spasticity according to this theory. Sherrington explained spinal shock as a loss of tonic descending facilitation secondary to injury.[110] Spinal reflexes are then unable to depolarize α motor neurons due to the loss of facilitation. Over time, increased spinal reflex excitability can be attributed to intrinsic changes in the cord. This increased excitability can be caused by denervation supersensitivity, collateral sprouting, or loss of further inhibitory input. Alternatively, spasticity has been theorized to be generated by a hyperexcitable γ efferent system causing discharge of ventral horn cells. The γ system is responsible for altering the discharge of intrafusal fibers and maintaining muscle spindle sensitivity with changing muscle length. Muscle spindles are intrafusal fibers that monitor muscle tension and length. Gamma hyperexcitability as a cause for spasticity has fallen out of favor as new theories focus on changes at the α motor neuron through the intrinsic cord changes described above.[111] As spasticity develops after SCI, associated reflexes such as the cutaneomuscular or flexion withdrawal reflex develop. The clasp knife reflex also is often present in the quadriceps muscle. The clasp knife describes a sudden giving way to passive movement of the lower limb caused by inhibition of antagonistic motor neurons.

EVALUATION

Spasticity is primarily evaluated by the resistance to passive motion of an affected limb. There are several methods that have been developed to quantify spasticity. The Ashworth scale (Box 25-1) and modified Ashworth scale are the most common methods.[112,113] The modified Ashworth scale adds more discrete levels at the lower end of the scale and includes a description of range of motion.

The pendulum test places the patient in a seated position and examines the excursion of the lower limb when dropped from a fully extended position and allowed to swing freely using the knee joint as the pivot. The pendulum test examines the speed, quality of motion, and number of oscillations of the swinging lower limb. The spasm frequency score measures the number of muscle spasms per hour and assigns a numeric score based on this rate as noted in Box 25-2.[114] Gait, transfer, and ADL skills should be assessed to determine the patients function at baseline levels of spasticity. The history should include information about negative symptoms such as decreased endurance and dexterity. Examination should include tests for fine motor control, cutaneomuscular reflexes, and the ability to control any residual motor function. Quantitative scales such as the Ashworth and spasm frequency score are important, but often the patient's subjective reports are equally important as the functional impact of spasticity is difficult to quantify.

BOX 25-1. ASHWORTH SCALE

Grade	Description
1	No increased tone
2	Slight increase in tone, giving a "catch" when the affected part is moved in flexion or extension
3	More marked increased in tone but affected part is easily flexed
4	Considerable increase in tone, passive movement is difficult
5	Affected part is rigid in extension

BOX 25-2. SPASM FREQUENCY SCORE

0 = No spasms
1 = Mild spasm induced by stimulation
2 = Infrequent full spasm occurring less than once per hour
3 = Spasms occurring more than once per hour
4 = Ten or more spasms per hour or continuous contraction

TREATMENT

Although pathologic, spasticity is not a condition that requires treatment in all cases. Many individuals with spasticity choose to live with their level of spasticity, sometimes to the bewilderment of the professional staff members treating them. Treatment of spasticity should generally be undertaken only when the condition causes significant discomfort or interferes with function. Before initiation of therapy, the goals of the intervention should be identified. This identification process then guides the direction of the treatment. The professional staff member must be careful not to impose personal feelings about the patient's spasticity on the decision to treat, especially when the individual has been living with spasticity for long time.

The treatment of spasticity often begins with noninvasive measures. If these are successful, there is no need to seek further treatment; however, if these measures are not, more aggressive treatment is considered. Each step up the therapeutic ladder is taken cautiously with careful consideration of whether the potential reduction of spasticity is worth the potential risks of the intervention.

NONINVASIVE TREATMENT

Physical medicine principles used to inhibit spastic muscle groups of the individual with an SCI include ROM exercises, positioning techniques (bed and wheelchair), orthoses and inhibitive casting, cryotherapy, weight-bearing exercises, electrical stimulation, and biofeedback.

Spastic muscles cause a dynamic imbalance of muscle control in involved extremities. In the upper extremity this results in a tendency toward flexed, adducted, and internally rotated shoulders and flexed elbows (especially in a C5 tetraplegic with unopposed elbow flexion). In the lower extremity, plantar flexion and inversion of the ankle and hip flexion and adduction frequently occurs.

Hypertonicity and muscle imbalance following SCI predisposes patients to fixed muscle shortening and joint capsule tightening with subsequent contracture, pain, and, perhaps, increased disability. There is a high incidence of chronic shoulder pain in persons with tetraplegia when shoulder pain developed early after injury and was associated with spasticity. Absence of ROM exercises within the first 2 weeks after injury led to an increased association.[115] Muscle stretching, particularly steady static stretching to the limits of the ROM of a joint, can result in a reduction of reflex activity that may last for hours after the exercise.[116] Ideally, ROM exercises should be performed once or twice daily on all joints affected by the injury. Education of patients, family members, and other caretakers on proper techniques is essential.

Proper positioning, orthotics, inhibitive casts, and weight-bearing activities are all well-known techniques that can inhibit tone and assist with ROM by promoting prolonged static stretching.[117–120]

Standing on a standing frame or tilt-table can stretch hip and knee flexors and ankle plantar flexors. Pain and loss of ROM in the shoulders in persons with tetraplegia are decreased by placing the arms abducted with elbows extended when in bed.[121] Orthotic management is useful to maintain joint position and limit further deformity and provide prolonged stretch to reduce spasticity while increasing ROM. It includes the use of resting and dynamic splints and the use of serial casting. In the lower extremity, ankle-foot orthotics can control forces leading to spastic equinovarus position and assist in ambulation.

Wheelchair positioning can be crucial in its ability to minimize hypertonicity, particularly in the trunk and neck. For example, increased tone in the trunk can be reduced by slightly tilting the seating unit or wedging the seat.[122]

PHARMACOLOGIC MANAGEMENT

Once conservative measures have failed to satisfactorily control troublesome spasticity, the clinician must decide the most appropriate intervention. Often, this decision is based on whether the spasticity is generalized or regional. Generalized spasticity (e.g., severe flexor spasms of both lower extremities) should be treated with a systemic medication, whereas regional spasticity (e.g., excessive equinovarus tendency at one ankle) is likely to be treated with local injection therapy or bracing. Further, the patient's medical condition must be considered. A person with renal failure has more limited therapeutic options than someone who is healthy because of an increased potential for significant adverse effects of certain antispasticity agents.

THE GABA SYSTEM

Gamma-amino butyric acid (GABA) is believed to be the major inhibitory neurotransmitter in the spinal cord.[123] Medications that augment the quantity or effectiveness of GABA in the cord tend to reduce or normalize muscle tone in persons afflicted with spinal spasticity. Two major GABA receptor subtypes found in the spinal cord are relevant to spasticity management, designated $GABA_A$ and $GABA_B$, respectively.

Baclofen is a structural analog of GABA that exerts its clinical effect by binding to $GABA_B$ receptors. It is often considered the first line pharmacologic intervention in spinal spasticity. Binding of baclofen to $GABA_B$ receptors produces a change in conductance to the cations calcium (Ca^{+2}) and potassium (K^+). It appears that an increased K^+ conductance is responsible for a postsynaptic inhibitory effect of the drug while a decreased Ca^{+2} conductance seems responsible for the presynaptic inhibitory effect. There is an extremely wide dose range for clinical efficacy when given orally. Dosing may begin at 10 to 15 mg/day in divided doses. The dosage should be gradually increased as needed clinically. Although the recommended maximum daily dose is 80 mg, significantly higher oral doses may be both well tolerated and beneficial.[124,125] In general, oral baclofen is well tolerated with the major side effects being fatigue, dizziness, and GI upset. Constipation and diarrhea have been noted, but when occurring in the early phase of SCI, these are more likely related to improper regulation of bowel function. When used in elderly patients or those with renal insufficiency, great care should be taken to avoid changes in mental status, including hallucinations. Spasticity, although uncomfortable, rarely requires immediate control; a slow increase in the dose of baclofen minimizes side effects while allowing for proper dose titration. Dosing is usually in three or four divided daily doses; the half-life is 3.5 hours. Abrupt cessation of the drug should be avoided to reduce the risk of seizures, palpitation, and fever.

Diazepam is the prototypical benzodiazepine used for the treatment of spinal spasticity. Unlike baclofen, diazepam exerts its effect though its binding to the $GABA_A$ receptor.[126] This receptor is composed of a benzodiazepine binding site, a GABA binding site, and a chloride channel. Binding of a benzodiazepine molecule to the receptor complex enhances the affinity of the GABA recognition site for GABA. Binding of GABA to the receptor opens the chloride channel, ultimately resulting in enhanced postsynaptic inhibition and the drugs antispasticity property. Like baclofen, there is a wide dose range for clinical effect. As diazepam and the other benzodiazepines are drugs of potential dependence and abuse, a great deal of concern should be rendered before therapy is instituted with these agents. They are likely to produce lethargy and decreased concentration. Once initiated, dosage increases should be very gradual with close monitoring of the clinical effect to avoid these adverse effects. Therapy with diazepam may begin with as little as 2 mg given at bedtime for nocturnal spasticity with doses up to 60 mg/day not unusual for generalized spasticity. Ketazolam, a long acting benzodiazepine, may simplify benzodiazepine treatment in the future. Although not yet approved for use, it has the advantage of once per day dosing.

THE ADRENERGIC SYSTEM

Two α-2-adrenergic agonists are potentially useful treatments for spinal spasticity. Clonidine, an antihypertensive agent, and tizanidine which received FDA approval in December of 1996, are the prototypical agents in this class. These agents inhibit spasticity at spinal and supraspinal levels by their actions on excitatory interneurons and coeruleospinal pathways, respectively.[127,128] Clonidine, when used orally for spasticity, has modest response rates and may be limited by its hypotensive effect.[129,130] More recently, clonidine became commercially available in a transdermal delivery system that seems to have improved tolerance to the hypotension, though the effectiveness of clonidine as an antispasticity agent remains seemingly modest.[131] Clonidine also may have value when used in combination with other agents such as baclofen.

Tizandine has been demonstrated to be a safe and effective treatment for patients with spinal cord injury and multiple sclerosis.[132,133] Initial dosing of tizandine may begin at 2–4 mg at night and progress gradually upward to maximum individual doses of 36 mg/day in divided doses. As tizanidine is metabolized in the liver, caution should be used by patients with liver disease. The principal side effects include lethargy and dry mouth. Reversible liver function abnormalities have been noted as well as visual hallucinations at the higher dosages. Potentially, tizanidine is a first-line treatment for spinal spasticity, but clinical experience with this agent in North America is very small. In patients with severe spasticity, usage of tizanidine in combination with baclofen or diazepam might be considered; again the clinical experience with this is to be developed in the future.

PERIPHERALLY ACTING AGENTS

Dantrolene sodium differs from the medications discussed previously by virtue of the fact that it gains its myotonolytic properties by acting peripherally, at the level of the muscle. Dantrolene inhibits the release of calcium from the sarcoplasmic reticulum of the muscle cell. This inhibition weakens the calcium dependent excitation-contraction coupling mechanism, which normally produces forceful muscle contraction in skeletal muscle. A significant advantage of dantrolene is that it has virtually no CNS toxicity, making it an attractive agent for use against spasticity in patient with concomitant brain injury. Dantrolene, however, is probably the antispasticity agent most likely to cause muscle weakness and has the potential to cause life-threatening hepatotoxicity. Although the hepatotoxicity is reversible if it is noted early, late identification can prove disastrous. Further, the hepatotoxicity is not a dose-dependent phenomenon. For this reason, dantrolene should not be used in individuals with pre-existing liver disease or in those judged to be unlikely to follow through with frequent blood monitoring of the liver enzymes. Dantrolene also may cause diarrhea. The starting dose of dantrolene is 25 mg 1 to 2 times daily. The dose is then gradually increased until efficacy or evidence of toxicity to a maximum daily dose of 400 mg (100 mg four times daily).

Other medications such as anticonvulsants, phenothiazines, and glycine have all been reported to be potentially useful as antispasticity agents but have been inadequately studied and are currently not widely used in the treatment of spinal spasticity.

Intrathecal Baclofen

The use of intrathecal baclofen has revolutionized the treatment of severe generalized spasticity of spinal cord origin in patients who are unresponsive to oral management and who experience severe side effects from therapeutic dosages. Baclofen is not very lipid soluble and has difficulty crossing the blood-brain barrier. Intrathecal baclofen delivery provides targeted delivery with far greater CSF concentration of drug with far smaller overall doses. Intrathecal baclofen is delivered by a surgically implanted infusion pump placed in a subcutaneous pocket in the abdomen. A catheter is advanced from the pump into the intrathecal space. Dosage adjustments are made by radiotelemetry from a handheld dedicated unit.

Intrathecal baclofen is presently contraindicated in patients with severe autonomic dysreflexia, impaired renal function, during pregnancy and in nursing mothers, children, or patients who suffer from psychotic disorders. Potential patients must also be reliable and able to participate in the care and maintenance of the intrathecal regimen. The pump reservoir needs to be refilled with baclofen at intervals varying with the dosage rate generally every 1 to 3 months. Refill times are calculated and are indicated by a pump low-volume alarm. Refills are easily performed percutaneously through the pump access port.

Patients deemed suitable for treatment of spasticity with intrathecal baclofen are required to undergo a trial dose prior to surgery. A complete evaluation of the patient's Ashworth score, spasm scale, and function is done. The patient then receives a 50 mcg bolus of intrathecal baclofen by lumbar puncture. The patient's vital signs and spasticity are monitored closely over the next 8 hours to evaluate treatment response. If no response is obtained with the 50-mcg bolus, a 75-mcg and, finally, a 100-mcg screening bolus can be tried at 24-hour intervals. It is to be expected that patients react with different response curves to the onset and duration of the bolus dose.

After implantation of the pump, dosing usually begins with twice the screening dose divided over 24 hours. If the screening bolus, however, gives a response lasting more than 12 hours, the screening dose is divided over 24 hours. If no response is evident, the hourly dose can be increased 10% to 20% every 24 hours. Oral baclofen should be tapered off slowly as the intrathecal dose is increased. Response to intrathecal baclofen is very individual. Spinal cord patients have responded to doses as low as 62 mcg/day or as high as 749 mcg/day.[134] Some patients develop a tolerance to intrathecal baclofen therapy and require steadily increasing doses in the first few months of therapy. This need for increased dosage eventually wears off, but a drug holiday may be necessary in rare cases to restore responsiveness. The pump can deliver continuous dosing, periodic boluses, or complex rates throughout the day to accommodate changes in a patient's spasticity. Careful attention must be paid to the patients functional status while titrating intrathecal baclofen doses. Spasms may relent, but the loss of spasticity and increased weakness from baclofen may decrease a patients ability to transfer, stand, or perform activities of daily living. The goal of intrathecal baclofen therapy is to optimize comfort and function, not to decrease Ashworth scores. Studies of intrathecal baclofen usage in spinal spasticity have demonstrated improved functional independence, decreased Ashworth scores, and decreased frequency of spasms.[135,136,137]

Adverse effects of intrathecal baclofen include drowsiness, dizziness, nausea, hypotension, seizures, weakness, and headache. If side effects occur, dosages should be titrated down gently, 10% to 20% per day, to avoid withdrawal. Intrathecal baclofen overdosage is difficult to treat as there is no reliable antidote. The pump should be immediately emptied through the access port, and emergency procedures must be implemented. Mechanical ventilation may be required.

INJECTION THERAPY FOR SPINAL SPASTICITY

Botulinum Toxin

Injections of botulinum toxin intramuscularly offer a new and promising option for the management of spasticity and has recently been added to the treatment armamentarium.

Botulinum toxin is produced by the bacterium *Clostridium botulinum*, which when ingested causes the disease botulism. The toxins themselves are proteins, which have been purified, identified, and differentiated into types A through G based on antigenic characteristics. They bind avidly to receptor sites on the presynaptic nerve terminal in the neuromuscular junction and inhibit the release of acetylcholine resulting in chemical denervation and paralysis. When injected intramuscularly, localized weakness develops without systemic effects.

Type A is the most common serotype found in the United States and is the only form of the toxin approved for clinical use by the FDA. The first clinical use of botulinum toxin was in the 1970s for the treatment of strabismus in primates. By the early 1980s, it had become therapeutically useful for the treatment of strabismus and blepharospasm in humans and since then has been used for ocular dystonias and hemifacial spasm. In the 1990s, botulinum toxin type A has been studied for the treatment of spasticity in patients with cerebral palsy, stroke, multiple sclerosis, traumatic brain injury, and SCI.[138]

The technique involves injecting the toxin into the belly of a selected muscle to weaken that muscle enough to achieve a particular goal. It is not clear that injecting closer to the motor endplate gives a better response than if the muscle belly is injected; therefore, EMG guidance is not required for injection into the motor point but can be helpful when injection of deeper muscles is indicated to confirm localization. The toxin must be diluted with preservative-free saline solution and used within 4 hours. It must be refrigerated until used and the reconstitution must be done gently so as not to disturb the toxin.

The clinical effect depends on many factors, such as the dosage of toxin injected, the size of the muscle to be treated, and the activity of the muscle. The effect becomes clinically evident within 2 to 3 days and may last 2 to 6 months or longer. Although the effect of the toxin on the individual nerve terminal is essentially irreversible, the response slowly subsides with time for reasons that are unclear but may be because of collateral sprouting from nerve terminals and new terminal formation in the injected muscles. Long-term electrophysiologic effects are measurable for more than a year, but there has been no quantifiable cumulative sequelae in most patients.[138]

Botulinum toxin is measured in biologic units. One unit is defined as the median lethal dose (LD_{50}) when injected into the peritoneum of a laboratory mouse. The LD_{50} in primates is approximately 40 u/kg. There are two commercially available products of botulinum toxin type A: DYSPORT, available only in the United Kingdom, and BOTOX, available in the United States. The biologic units are not equivalent in these two products, and when evaluating studies, it is important to know which product is being used so dosages can be compared (1 unit of BOTOX is equivalent to approximately 4 units of DYSPORT). BOTOX is packaged in vials of 100 units each.

Some patients develop resistance to the toxin with repeated injections. This is probably due to an immunologic response in which antibodies develop to the toxin. This can be minimized if doses less than 300 units are given at any one treatment and at no greater than 12-week intervals. Booster injections given weekly or biweekly should be avoided.[138]

The safety of botulinum toxin treatment has not been evaluated in pregnant women or in patients with impaired neuromuscular function; therefore, its use should be avoided in these individuals. The effect may be potentiated by aminoglycoside antibiotic administration and other drugs that interfere with neuromuscular transmission.

Benefits of treatment include the reduction of tone that is localized to a specific group of muscles and, therefore, can be tailored to that particular patient. Effects are dose dependent. If too much weakness results, strength will gradually return. There are no systemic side effects, and other treatments can be used in conjunction with botulinum toxin.

In the SCI population, botulinum toxin has been used to treat detrusor-sphincter dyssynergia by injecting toxin into the external sphincter with improvements in the amounts of postvoid residual urine and the urethral pressure profile and EMG evidence of sphincter denervation. The effects lasted 50 to 60 days.[139–142]

Studies on limb spasticity in the SCI population are in progress, but there are no available data to date. There is no reason to believe, however, that botulinum toxin in SCI would not be as equally efficacious as in other patients with limb spasticity. The patient with an incomplete injury may need treatment for spasticity that is localized to a specific muscle group, but systemic therapy is not indicated.

Successful treatment of spasticity depends on careful patient selection and proper drug administration and dosage. As with treatment of spasticity, all goals may include an increase in ROM, decrease in pain, prevention of contracture, better cosmesis and hygiene, and improvement in balance and gait. Ultimately, what is desired is an improvement in function. This can be difficult to achieve when there is an imbalance between flexor and extensor tone for agonist and antagonist functions. If the balance can be restored, however, by weakening one muscle group, the opposing muscle can function more optimally. For instance, a patient with an incomplete injury and an unsteady gait because of spasticity of the gastrocnemius may respond to an injection of botulinum toxin with decreased tone and subsequent ability to recruit his ankle dorsiflexors, leading to a more efficient gait.

Future research with botulinum toxin includes combination therapies, appropriate dosing, and long-term effects.

Phenol

Phenol has been used as a neurolytic agent in human beings since 1926.[143] As a treatment of spasticity, phenol has been injected intrathecally, epidurally, and at the level of the neural foramen.[144] Certainly, however, it is used most extensively today to perform peripheral nerve or motor point blocks. The antispasticity effect of phenols is caused by nonselective destruction of nerve fibers. The degree of destruction is related to the dilution and quantity of phenol injected and the diluent used. Phenol, like BOTOX, is a treatment for regional spasticity. Its effect is temporary, though the effect can last more than 6 months. When used to perform peripheral nerve blocks, painful paresthesias are a not uncommon side effect.[145] When used to block motor points, the painful paresthesias are avoided; however, the clinical effect of the treatment is lessened and is, therefore, likely to produce benefit only in mild to moderate spasticity. Technically, when injecting phenol into a muscle, selection of motor points is important; therefore, localization with electromyographic (EMG) guidance or via neuromuscular stimulation is required.

SURGICAL TREATMENTS

With the advent of new oral medications, intrathecal baclofen, and botulinum toxin, destructive surgical procedures should be rarely, if ever, used. As progress is made in the area of neurologic restoration, permanent destructive procedures should be avoided in all but the most desperate cases in which other treatment options have been exhausted. Examples of techniques used previously include surgical neurectomy, rhizotomy, and myelotomy.[146]

OSTEOPOROSIS

Following an SCI, a marked calcium resorption and associated hypercalciuria occurs resulting in osteoporosis in all bones in the paralyzed extremities.[147,148,149] The degree of bone loss increases the risk of lower extremity fractures.[149,150,151] Using dual photon absorptometry (DPA), bone loss in the lower extremities following complete lesions is rapid with approximately 22% of the bone depleted 3 months after injury.[152] An additional 5% is lost between the third and fourth months, and at 14 months postinjury approximately one third of the bone has been lost. Bone loss subsequently slows. The bone loss after SCI appears to follow a selective pattern, with the most significant loss occurring from the hips, with the lumbar spine relatively preserved.[153,154]

Using dual energy radiograph (x-ray) absorptometry (DEXA), Garland and colleagues found mean bone mineral density (BMD) in patients with SCI and fracture to be significantly lower than in those with no fractures; however, both groups were below the fracture threshold of 1.0 g/cm^2.[152] Compared with able-bodied controls, the fracture group's mean BMD was 49% of normal. The greater the mobility of the patient, the less bone loss they have.[155] BeDell and coworkers using DEXA found values from the greater trochanter, Ward's triangle, and femoral necks of SCI patients to be 71%, 82%, and 79% of ambulatory individuals, respectively, with age and gender match controls. There was no difference in lumbar spine (L2–L4) bone density levels between the groups.

A number of interventions have been studied to minimize osteoporosis. Functional electrical stimulation (FES) may be beneficial in reducing the rate of bone loss; however, this intervention has not been found to reduce osteoporosis after it has developed in persons with chronic SCI.[149,154,156] The FES cycling has, however, been shown to produce a decrease in the rate of bone loss in persons with acute SCI, and this effect remained even after the FES exercise was discontinued.[157] Standing and ambulation may decrease hypercalciuria, but such activities have not been shown to prevent or reduce osteoporosis, although early performance of such activities may be helpful.[158,159,160]

Pharmacologic agents, including calcitonin, bisphosphonates, and recombinant human growth hormone, have been studied, but none of these have yet been shown to be effective in reducing osteoporosis in persons with SCI.[161]

LOWER EXTREMITY FRACTURES

The incidence of lower extremity fractures in persons with chronic SCI has been reported to be between 1.5% and 6%.[151,162–166] The true incidence, however, may be higher, because not all fractures are clinically recognized. Most of such fractures may be considered pathologic because of the demineralized state of the bones.

The most common site of fracture after SCI is the femur.[151,163–168] Fractures are more common in persons with paraplegia and in those with neurologically complete injuries. The most common reported cause is a fall during transfer, but fractures also may occur during ROM exercises and ADL or without any known cause. The diagnosis of these fractures may be difficult especially in the absence of pain. The presenting symptoms may be a low-grade fever, malaise, and a swollen limb. The search for other causes should be undertaken, but a bony deformity, localized swelling, hematoma, and crepitus suggest a fractured limb. A plain radiograph gives a more definitive diagnosis. Hospitalization is usually not required and may be indicated for those with severe swelling, with uncertain diagnosis, and those in need of surgery.

The main treatment goal is to restore prefacture functional capability, minimize interference with the persons daily routine, minimize the risk of complications, and allow for proper bone healing and satisfactory alignment.[151,166,169]

Lower extremity fractures in ambulatory persons with SCI are treated similar to those occurring in able-bodied persons, with the goal of maintaining normal leg length and alignment.[166,169] In persons with SCI who are not expected to ambulate, normal femoral length and angular alignment is not the primary goal and some degree of shortening and angulation is acceptable but rotational deformity is not. Most fractures in persons with SCI are treated nonoperatively (conservatively) with soft, well-padded splints and frequent skin inspections.[151,166] The padded splint can simply be made of a blanket or pillow wrapped around the fracture site and fixed with adhesive tape, elastic bandage, or stockinette, but splints made of hard materials must be liberally padded. The majority of these fractures heal well, often with rapid union and exuberant callus formation often within 3 to 4 weeks.[162,164,166] Weight-bearing activities, such as tilt table, standing, and stand-pivot transfers, however, should be postponed for a longer period. The patient does not need to remain bed bound and should be permitted to be mobile in the wheelchair within a few days, with the legs flexed at hips and knees and feet flat on the footrest, which maintains good functional positioning. Methods commonly used for able bodied patients for fracture management, that is, surgery, casting, and external fixation, are not indicated for the person with SCI due to the complications. Circumferential plaster casts and skeletal traction may cause problems in the anesthetic limbs.[169,170,171] Surgical interventions for femoral and distal femoral fractures are associated with a high complication rate because of poor bone quality and high risk of osteomyelitis.[151,162,164,165,170,172] Open reduction is, therefore, only rarely necessary. Nonunion of fractures is rare but may occur in 2% to 10%, which is not clinically significant in wheelchair users.[162,164,168,170,173]

Surgical interventions may be indicated when nonsurgical methods do not control rotational deformity of proximal femur fractures, when severe muscle spasm is present when splints are too bulky and interfere with function, when vascular supply is compromised, and when leg shortening and angulation result in unacceptable function or cosmesis.[164,165,166,168,169] Femoral neck and subtrochanteric fractures are probably the most difficult to manage, and occasionally internal fixation may be considered, if a minimal device such as an intramedullary rod can be used.[166] Those with femoral neck fractures can usually maintain prefracture mobility and may be managed without lower extremity immobilization, because splinting this body segment is difficult. Patients with intertrochanteric fractures can be seated in a wheelchair with their feet flat on the footrest and a pillow between the thighs. Femoral shaft and all other distal lower extremity fractures, including tibial, ankle, and foot fractures, are best treated with well-padded or soft splints. Upper limb fractures should be treated in the same fashion as those occurring in able bodied persons, but the clinician must consider the impact of the fracture on functional activities, such as ability to perform transfers, pressure relief, wheelchair propulsion, and ADL.

HETEROTOPIC OSSIFICATION

Heterotopic ossification (HO), ectopic bone within the connective tissue, occurs in 16% to 53% of persons with SCI.[174] Fortunately most HO is an incidental finding on radiograph and not clinically significant.[175,176] Approximately 20% of HO, however, results in significant limitations of joint ROM, interfering with ADL, and 3% to 5% develop severe restrictions or ankylosis of the joint.[177,178]

Heterotopic ossification only occurs below the level of the neurologic lesion in persons with SCI, unless there are other causative factors, such as head injury or burns. The incidence of HO is higher in persons with neurologically complete injury, spasticity, and pressure sores.[179] Most HO occurs 1 to 4 months after SCI, although HO has been reported to develop several years after injury. The most common location of HO is at the anterior aspect of the hip followed by the medial aspect of the knee. The shoulders and elbows may occasionally be affected in persons with high-level tetraplegia. Mature HO is pathologically similar to a fracture callus formation and forms in the connective tissue between the muscle planes but not within the muscle itself.

The cause of HO is still poorly understood. A yet unknown factor may induce a metaplasia of multipotential connective tissue, that is mesenchymal cells, to chondroblasts and osteoblasts.[175,180] Direct trauma does not seem to be a major factor. The presence of a fracture or pressure ulcer can increase the risk of HO formation, however, aggressive ROM has not been shown to predispose persons with SCI to HO.[181]

The early clinical features of HO include swelling, warmth, and fever. In the lower extremities, the differential diagnoses include deep vein thrombosis, hematoma, cellulitis, septic arthritis, fracture, or tumor. After the initial phase the swelling becomes more firm and localized. Occasionally, the early inflammatory phase is not clinically detected and the HO occurs with a decrease ROM of the joint. A specific method for early detection includes a triple phase bone scan, but in this test the first two phases are the most sensitive.[182,183] Alkaline phosphatase levels becomes elevated early but is less specific. Plain radiographs are helpful for detection of HO 7 to 10 days after the initial symptoms develop but do not reveal the process during the earliest phase. HO may result in the development of pressure sores caused by bony pressure or by a change in sitting posture secondary to the extra bone. Risk of DVT may be increased, and peripheral nerve entrapment may occur.[184,185]

Once HO is detected, an aggressive joint ROM exercise program should be initiated. Administration of disodium etidronate may be effective in limiting the extent of the ossification with a dose of 20 mg/kg given daily for 2 weeks, followed by 10 mg/kg for 10 additional weeks, although treatment for a longer period of time has been suggested.[186] The prophylactic use of disodium etidronate has been advocated and shown to be effective in the prevention of HO.[187]

When HO severely limits ROM and impairs function, wedge resection surgery is indicated. Before the surgery the heterotopic bone should be mature to prevent recurrence. The best method to ascertain maturity is through serial bone scans with the appearance of normal bone.[182,187] A normal radiograph and alkaline phosphatase levels are not reliable markers for full bone maturity. Disodium etidronate should be used to prevent recurrence of HO following surgery although its efficacy has not been proved.[175,187] The use of radiation therapy and NSAIDS have not been studied adequately in persons with SCI following surgery for HO.

PAIN

Pain in persons with SCI is a complex and frequently poorly understood clinical complaint with numerous causes. Different categories of SCI pain have been described, but fundamentally two main categories may be identified.[188–192]

1. *Nociceptive pain* caused by a variety of noxious stimuli to the normally innervated body parts, ordinarily above or at the level of the cord injury
2. *Neurogenic pain* related to injury to the nerves roots, cauda equina, and spinal cord

The reported prevalence of SCI pain depends on its perceived severity and the level of the cord injury, but it does not depend on the exact pathology of the cord injury, that is, cord contusion or transection or on the severity of the neurologic lesion as judged by the ASIA Impairment Scale or the ASIA Motor Score.[193,194,195] Thus the prevalence of severe SCI pain has been reported to be 10% to 15% in persons with tetraplegia, 25% in those with thoracic paraplegia, and 42% to 51% in those with lesions of the cauda equina.[190,196–201] The perception of pain and its severity is influenced by numerous factors but in particular by depression and adjustment disorders.[199,201–205]

A physician who treats patients with pain must be thoroughly familiar with the neuroanatomy and neurophysiology of normal pain perception and how this is changed by injury and disease. For in-depth review, the reader is referred to the extensive literature that exists on the subject.[206–210] The literature describes in detail the primary, secondary, and tertiary afferent neurons, the "Gait Control" theory, the influence of different organic chemicals on the nervous systems, such as, substance P, serotonin, norepinephrine, histamine, prostaglandin, bradykinin, potassium ions, and endogenous opiates.[211]

CATEGORIES OF SPINAL CORD INJURY PAIN

Besides categorizing pain in persons with SCI as either nociceptive or neurogenic, it may be helpful clinically to classify such pain according to its area as perceived by the patient, that is above the spinal cord lesion, at the level of the cord lesion, below the cord lesion, or in viscera.

Pain above the level of spinal cord injury in the normally innervated body parts may be caused by a multitude of noxious stimuli, both acute and chronic, as a result of trauma or disease. Of particular significance to persons with SCI is the high incidence of shoulder pain in persons with acute tetraplegia and different forms of chronic or recurrent upper extremity pain related to excessive use of the upper extremities and spine during the performance of self-care activities and wheelchair propulsion.[212] The latter form may variably be caused by myofascial disorders, nerve entrapment syndromes, and premature development of degenerative conditions in the musculoskeletal system.[213–217] Shoulder pain in acute tetraplegia has been found to occur both unilaterally (75%) and bilaterally (61%).[212] Particularly at risk are persons more than 50 years of age, those who do not receive early ROM exercises for the shoulder, those who are improperly positioned in bed, those who have associated injuries to the shoulder, upper extremity, or chest, and those who have weakness of shoulder girdle muscles for whatever reasons. Consequently, those individuals who are older and have higher cervical cord lesions are mostly at risk. Early ROM exercises are effective in preventing such pain and helpful in its treatment.

Neurogenic pain also may occur above the level of the cord lesion and may be generated by entrapment of nerve roots or peripheral nerves or by expanding posttraumatic cystic myelopathy. *Carpal tunnel syndrome* has been reported to occur frequently in wheelchair users with paraplegia, and a 46% incidence of the syndrome has been reported in wheelchair athletes who had electrodiagnostic studies done.[218,219,220] This high incidence may be related to repetitive extrinsic pressure over the carpal tunnel and frequent wrist extension posturing.[213] *Ulnar neuropathy* at the elbow is the second most common nerve entrapment syndrome found in wheelchair athletes and has a reported incidence of 19.4%.[220] Treatment of these nerve entrapments depends on their severity, but in general nonsurgical treatment is initially provided and surgical decompression only considered when this fails.

Reflex sympathetic dystrophy (RSD) may occur unilaterally or bilaterally in the upper extremities of many persons with SCI but primarily in those who have tetraplegia.[221–225] It also may occur infrequently in the upper limbs of those with paraplegia, and it has even been described in the lower extremities. The diagnosis of RSD depends on specific diagnostic criteria.[227] The treatment is usually nonsurgical with physical modalities, analgesic, and antiinflammatory medications and, occasionally, by stellate ganglion block.

Pain perceived to be at the level of the neurologic lesion may be either nociceptive or neurogenic in origin. *Nociceptive* pain is caused by acute or chronic pathological processes affecting the normally or partially innervated tissues within or adjacent to the spine, such as, trauma, spinal instability, degenerative joint disease, infections, or even tumors. Such pain is usually localized to the injured part of the spine and is aggravated by physical activity and prolonged sitting but is often relieved by lying down or by external spinal support. Detailed diagnostic evaluation is required for such pain and if a specific cause is identified, appropriate intervention is required, for example, surgery or antibiotics. When no specific cause is found, such pain is often felt to be myofascial in origin and would then best be treated with nonnarcotic analgesics, spinal support, physical modalities, and back exercises.

Pain of *neurogenic* origin may be described as either radicular or segmental. *Radicular pain* is caused by partial or total damage to one or more nerve roots at the level of the cord injury, that is, by contusion, laceration, compression, traction, or scar formation. Often the dorsal root ganglion is affected resulting in impaired sensation in the corresponding dermatome. Clinically, radicular pain is distributed along the respective dermatome and is variably described as tingling, stabbing, burning, aching, or as a feeling of tightness. Proximal nerve blocks may often produce sufficient pain relief.

Segmental pain is believed to be caused by damage of the gray matter of the dorsal horn of the spinal cord, resulting in hyperactivity of its nociceptor cells.[191,228,229,230] Clinically, segmental pain tends to be bilateral and distributed through one or more adjacent dermatomes. Often the distribution is wider in neurologically incomplete lesions than in those with complete lesions. The terms used by the patient to describe segmental pain are similar to those describing radicular pain. "End-zone pain" represents a form of segmental pain in which there is a combination of hypersensitivity or hyperalgesia with up to three dermatomes at the border of normal and absent sensation.[198,231] During the acute phase of SCI, such pain may preceed some segmental neurologic improvement, but occasionally it may become chronic. Dysesthesia of the hands, referred to by football players as "stingers" and by physicians as "burning hands" syndrome, most likely represents another form of segmental pain, which luckily is usually transient in nature.[232] However, it is often associated with a narrow cervical spinal canal, which makes a careful diagnostic evaluation necessary. A much more difficult clinical problem is the intense hand pain that is often experienced by individuals with neurologically incomplete tetraplegia, such as the central cervical cord syndrome. This condition may often mimic or be associated with reflex sympathetic dystrophy. This so-called "cauda equina pain" is caused by damage of the cauda equina with or without injury to the conus medullaris. It is clearly neurogenic in origin and may be considered to be either radicular, segmental, or both. Clinically, it affects primarily the sacral dermatomes, usually in a symmetric fashion, that is the buttocks, genitals, anus, and feet, and is most often described as being burning or tingling in nature.

Pain perceived as originating below the NLI is usually neurogenic in origin but occasionally nociceptive. When of nociceptive origin, the sensory neural pathways stem from an organ with anatomical location below the spinal lesion, but its peripheral sensory nerves enter the CNS above the lesion, for example, nociceptive pain originating in the trapezius muscle, which anatomically extends to the sixth thoracic vertebra but receives nerve supply from the eleventh cranial nerve, the latissimus dorsi muscle, which anatomically extends to the lumbar spine but receives innervation from the sixth and seventh cervical nerve roots, and the diaphragm, which receives innervation from the third, fourth, and fifth cervical nerve roots. The most common form of pain below the level of the cord injury is a special form of neurogenic pain, which usually is referred to as deafferentation central pain (DCP), although less specific terms for such pain have also been used, for example, central pain, dysesthesia, and phantom pain. The DCP may be defined as a diffuse and nondermatomal pain with unpleasant sensations below the level of the neurologic lesion, which are unaffected by any noxious stimuli.[192] Unfortunately, DCP is both the type of SCI pain that is most common and the one that is most refractive to treatment. Clinically, it may be described as burning, tingling, electric, and a numbing or aching sensation in different sensate body parts, unilaterally or bilaterally. It is usually continuous, except when the person is asleep.[233] The exact origin of DCP is not fully understood, but it is generally believed to rise in the segments of the spinal cord at or just above the site of injury, a view which is supported by the documented beneficial effects of surgical procedures on the dorsal root entry zone at these levels.[228,229,234,235,236] A late onset of DCP occurs with formation of posttraumatic cystic myelopathy or tethering of the cord. Spinal cord injury and sensory deafferentation results in changes of different chemical substances that may be important in pain perception, such as substance P, catecholamines, and endogenous opiates, but it is unclear exactly how these chemicals influence DCP.

Pain in viscera, that is, pain perceived to be within the abdomen or pelvis of persons with SCI is a difficult diagnostic challenge as it is often clinically hard to distinguish between a nociceptive and a neurogenic origin of such pain. Persons with high-level SCI cannot reliably perceive nociceptive abdominal pain and, therefore, other symptoms and signs must be checked or observed for diagnostic clues, such as, nausea, vomiting, and autonomic dysreflexia. It should be recognized, however, that most, if not all, persons with SCI may have some abdominal sensation, and, as a general rule, the lower the cord lesion, the more likely is the pain to be nociceptive rather than neurogenic in origin. Thus it has been reported that persons with cord lesions below T7 can localize abdominal pain earlier and with more accuracy than those with higher lesion.[237] The innervation of the pleura and the peritoneum is normally segmental and correlates roughly with sensation on the skin of the trunk. Sensation from abdominal viscera, however, is nonsegmental and tends to be poorly localized, even in able bodied persons. Almost all persons with tetraplegia, who are able to breathe without mechanical ventilation, retain diaphragmatic sensation, which may be adequate to indicate a subdiaphragmatic pathology by nociceptive means. It is not known if the vagus nerve contains sensory nerve fibers, but if present, such fibers may convey nociceptive pain. When of neurogenic origin, visceral pain may be radicular, segmental, or DCP, although distinguishing between these pain types would be very difficult for the clinician.

Management of pain in persons with SCI is often a difficult and frustrating experience, both for the physician and the patient, but by no means a hopeless endeavor.[192] Every effort should be made to establish an accurate diagnosis, to distinguish nociceptive from neurogenic pain, and to assess all factors that influence the pain perception. Unfortunately, specific cause can rarely be found for neurogenic pain, other than confirming the presence of damaged nervous tissue. Treatment, therefore, tends to be nonspecific, often by trial and error, and seldom results in complete elimination of the pain. However, physicians have long recognized that the intensity of such pain and degree of suffering varies and is influenced by activity level, distraction, depression, adjustment to disability, physical health, and different chemicals.[192] By properly addressing these factors, coping with the pain can be made easier. A specific treatment plan must be created and this must ensure, that no harm be done, that the patient and the family be fully educated about the nature of the pain and treatment options, that the patient actively participates and is involved in the decision making, that the aim should be to improve quality of life, and that every effort be made to obtain maximum pain relief. Multiple interventions should not be initiated simultaneously, but rather implemented one by one over a period to time during which progress is observed by discussion of various activities that are indicative of quality of life rather than by frequent questions regarding the pain itself.

MEDICATIONS

Nociceptive pain usually responds well to a variety of analgesics and muscle relaxants, but these drugs usually have no effect on neurogenic pain. Unfortunately, other medications also have limited effect on neurogenic pain, although frequently prescribed. Such medications should be prescribed by the same physician, administered on a regular basis rather than "as needed," and their effects should be monitored by direct and regular physician contact. The most common groups of medications prescribed for neurogenic pain are discussed below.

Anticonvulsive agents, such as phenytoin, carbamazipine, gabapentin, and divalproex sodium, are commonly prescribed with variable effect. Additionally, minor tranquilizers with some anticonvulsant effect, such as diazepam and clonazepam, have been prescribed also with very limited success.[233]

Psychotropic drugs with antidepressant effect have been used for a long time to treat neurogenic pain including pain of spinal cord origin.[238,239] The most commonly prescribed drugs in these categories are the various tricyclic agents, such as amitriptyline, imipramine, doxepin, and desipramine, but with highly variably success rate. More recently, physicians have used the newer antidepressant agents, such as fluoxetine, paroxetine and setroline, but knowledge on their efficiency for SCI pain is even more limited.

Narcotic drugs (opioids) are still the most effective pain suppressants, but they should be used only after adequate trial with nonnarcotic medications because their use may lead to tolerance, dependence, addiction, and abuse. Intrathecal infusion of morphine by implanted pump has been reported to reduce SCI pain.[233]

Other medications that have been used for neurogenic pain include antihistamines, α-adrenergic antagonists, and local anesthetic agents ordinarily with limited effect.[240,241,242]

ELECTRICAL STIMULATION AND NERVE BLOCKS

Electrical stimulation by different approaches has been used for treatment of pain with different results, including transcutaneous electrical nerve stimulation (TENS)[233,243] electrical stimulation of specific brain regions[244] high-frequency epidural electrical stimulation of the dorsal columns of the spinal cord[245,246] and functional electrical stimulation (FES).[247,248] Peripheral nerve blocks with local anesthetics, phenol or concentrated alcohol, may be effective for various forms of nociceptive pain, and for radicular pain, but is generally ineffective for segmental pain and DCP.

PSYCHOLOGIC TREATMENT

Psychologic treatment by conversational therapy is generally not effective in the management of SCI pain unless it is associated with profound depression or psychotic conditions. Avoiding to imply that the pain may be psychogenic in origin, every effort should be made by the physician to reduce depression and improve the adjustment to the disability. Temporary or partial pain relief may occasionally be obtained by self-hypnosis, relaxation training, meditation, Yoga, biofeedback, or interaction with other persons with SCI pain.[192]

SURGICAL TREATMENT

Surgical treatment may be considered in the management of pain in persons with SCI but primarily when the pain is nociceptive in origin and specific indications exist, for example, spinal instability requiring surgical fusion or pressure on a nerve root requiring decompression. Few persons with SCI and pain of neurogenic origin predictably benefit from surgical interventions. One indication for early surgical operation for neurogenic pain may be an expanding posttraumatic cystic myelopathy in need of shunting. Most surgical procedures for DCP done in the past have been destructive in nature, consisting of ablation or interruption of specific parts of the nervous system.[249] True to their principles of "first, do no harm," most surgeons are hesitant to do further damage to the already traumatized spinal cord. Surgical procedures that have been attempted in the past for neurogenic SCI pain, but now largely abandoned, include lumbar sympathectomy, dorsal root rhizotomy, cordotomy with tractectomy, cordectomy, commissurotomy, stereotactic brain surgery, cingulotomy, and frontal lobotomy.[192] The most common interruptive neurosurgical procedure still done for neurogenic SCI pain is the dorsal root entry zone (DREZ) microcoagulation procedure, which involves a five-level laminectomy, i.e., at the level of injury, two levels above, two levels below, exposing the cord by opening of the dura, sometimes recording abnormal electrical activity within the DREZ, and creating microthermal lesions in the DREZ through special needle electrodes inserted 1 mm apart for the length of the exposed cord.[228,229,230,234,236] The efficacy of this procedure is variable, but results are generally better for segmental pain than for DCP.[234,236] Success rate may be improved by proper selection of patients, accurate placement of microcoagulating electrodes on both sides of the cord, and application of sufficient heat.[234]

MUSCULOSKELETAL CONDITIONS

Musculoskeletal conditions in both acute and chronic SCI are a frequent cause of pain and can be a major contributing factor. Some degree of chronic pain of musculoskeletal origin has been reported in upper extremities of persons with SCI and the complaints of pain become more common as the time postinjury increases.[250,251,252] While persons with paraplegia have a slightly higher prevalence of upper extremity pain, it is reportedly less disabling.

The shoulder is the most frequently reported painful joint with a incidence of 30% to 51%.[250–255] The most common causes of shoulder pain include impingement syndrome from overuse or degenerative joint disease, rotator cuff tear, rotator cuff or bicipital tendinitis, subacromial bursitis, capsulitis, osteoarthritis, myofascial pain syndrome, disuse, and cervical radiculopathy.[251,253,254] Other causes in persons with SCI include muscle imbalance, spasticity, joint contractures, HO, and the presence of a posttraumatic syrinx. The specific cause of shoulder pain in most persons with SCI probably results from a combination of factors and is individually different, but it is widely believed that weight bearing and overuse are the most common causes.[250–255] In the able bodied population, the upper limb is primarily designed for prehensile activities, but in persons with SCI the upper limb becomes a weight-bearing structure, used for most functional activities, such as wheelchair transfers, push-ups for pressure reliefs, and wheelchair propulsion.

The therapeutic approach to shoulder pain in persons with chronic SCI is similar to that in able-bodied persons, bearing in mind special potential causes for those with SCI, for example syringomyelia and heterotopic ossification. A complete physical examination should include assessment of joint ROM, flexibility, strength, sensation, provocative tests for specific abnormalities, and functional assessment. Radiologic tests of the cervical spine or shoulder and electrodiagnostic studies should only be carried out if the diagnosis is unclear or to rule out a specific abnormality.

Treatment of overuse shoulder syndromes should be focused on decreasing the acute pain, addressing the secondary disability caused by the pain, treating the specific condition, and preventing recurrence. Relief of the acute pain usually is accomplished by pharmacologic intervention (NSAIDS, acetaminophen, muscle relaxants), rest, and physical modalities. Injection of local anesthetics or steroids into the subacromial bursa or appropriate space may be helpful. Unlike able-bodied individuals, it is difficult for persons with SCI to completely rest a painful upper limb joint because of its major role in functional activities. During episodes of acute pain, however, a persons with SCI must strive to decrease stresses imposed on the painful joint by using compensatory techniques, such as using a transfer board rather than performing lateral transfers, getting assistance when performing weight shifts, and using a powered wheelchair. At times, however, complete rest may be required. Once pain has subsided, the emphasis of treatment is focused on protecting the shoulder joint and preventing further symptoms. The main objective is to obtain a balance in strength and flexibility of the musculature surrounding the shoulder. Often overlooked for a well-balanced shoulder is maintenance of proper posture and correcting or improving the functional techniques and assistive equipment. One should limit overhead activities (including the use of a trapeze on a bed) and unnecessary upper limb weight bearing.

Significant pain occurs in the other upper limb joints in persons with both paraplegia and tetraplegia.[213] Carpal tunnel syndrome (CTS) symptoms have been reported in as many as two thirds of persons with SCI, and the incidence rises with time after injury.[213,218,219,251,256,257] Pressures within the carpal tunnel at rest in paraplegics have not been shown to be increased, but during functional activities these pressures are greatly elevated, a significant finding in persons who use their hands and wrists repetitively.[218,219,258] Electrodiagnostic studies have shown the presence of CTS in 41% to 63% of persons with SCI.[218,219,256] Compression of the ulnar nerve at the wrist or elbow occurs less frequently than CTS, but is also the result of repetitive trauma in the course of propelling a wheelchair or performing transfers.

The treatment consists of some form of rest, which may be difficult to enforce in persons who use the hands for all functional activities. Splinting of the hands and wrists, especially at night, and steroid injections into the carpal tunnel may be helpful. Techniques of transfers, pressure relief, and wheelchair propulsion should be modified to decrease pressure on the nerves, and excessive flexion or extension of the wrist should be avoided. The use of padded gloves when propelling the wheelchair may protect the hands and wrists. If no relief is obtained, a surgical release may be required. The postoperative limitation of activities must be carefully weighed against the long-term benefits of the procedure.

With advancing age, persons with SCI either lose function or have to modify their equipment to reduce pain. Since most upper limb musculoskeletal problems are due to chronic overuse, it is vital that proper exercise and shoulder protection techniques be learned early during acute rehabilitation and reinforced frequently thereafter. The phrase "no pain, no gain," should be replaced by "conserve it to preserve it" for this group of individuals.

JOINT CONTRACTURES

Joint contractures are common in persons with SCI. In rare cases, joint contractures can improve function, but usually they interfere with nursing care, ADL, and functional mobility and may lead to pain, neuropathy, and development of pressure sores.

Loss of joint ROM and soft tissue mobility frequently develops during prolonged immobilization. On the molecular level, the fixed stiffness of the tissues has been shown to be caused by collagen cross-linking that occurs when soft tissues are not mobilized for sustained periods.[259] The immobilization may be due to prolonged casting, bracing, pain, swelling, or an unbalanced pull from spastic muscle. Contractures occur more quickly if the joint is surrounded by edema. The person with SCI is especially at risk because of the frequently encountered combination of weakness, spasticity, dependent edema, and prolonged bedrest resulting in a loss of motion in any joint and direction.

In rare instances, facilitation of a joint contracture is encouraged to enhance function. Persons with high cervical cord injuries (C4–C6) and decreased grip strength are often taught to avoid passive finger extension and are fitted with wrist-hand orthoses and mitts that result in a shortening of the finger flexor muscles. The subsequent tightening can allow them to use "tenodesis" action, that is, the motion of wrist extension and/or forearm supination to achieve grasp. Many are instructed to avoid excessive stretching of the lumbar and cervical paraspinal musculature to secure good posture. Tight lumbar muscles can allow for increased stability and balance during long and short sitting period, thus improving independence during wheelchair management and mobility, grooming and feeding, during transfers, and during ambulation in which hypermobile trunk can be detrimental. "Selective shortening" of the lower cervical paraspinal musculature often allows for better posture and head control with less active muscle contraction. In cases other than those discussed above, the development of contracture and loss of passive joint motion is unwanted.

Joint contractures are best prevented. Passive ROM and stretching exercises should be performed daily and initiated as early as possible following SCI. Proper positioning of the trunk and extremities when in bed and in the wheelchair is essential for maintaining soft tissue and joint mobility. Relaxation techniques, soft tissue massage, and biofeedback may be used to decrease the activation of the spastic muscles. This is complimented by manual facilitation and strengthening of the weaker muscle groups.

Once joint contracture has developed, a number of therapeutic approaches may be employed. A slow prolonged stretching of the joint, pretreated with pain medication or deep-heating modalities is often effective. Static and dynamic orthoses are used to hold joints at or near their end range position to increase ROM. Static-progressive orthoses, such as static splints which allow adjustments in joint position in relatively small increments, and serial casting are other options for reducing contracture.

Because spasticity plays a large role in the development of joint contractures and prevents completing full ROM, treating the spasticity is very important. Treatment options for spasticity are discussed in an earlier section of this chapter. In addition to pharmacologic intervention, the use of nerve or motor point blocks with a local anesthetic to ascertain the exact role spasticity plays in the loss of ROM is important, by differentiating spasticity from soft tissue contracture. Serial casting is also extremely helpful, as it may decrease spasticity and improve ROM limitations. Because of diminished sensation, the cast should be well padded, especially around bony prominences. Each cast is applied for a few days and can be preceded by a local nerve block to obtain the fullest stretch. The cast can be bivalved to monitor the skin if needed. If there is great risk of skin breakdown, dynamic splints or progressive-static splints may be better, because they can be easily removed.

Despite all attempts, severe joint contractures may be refractory to nonsurgical treatment, and occasionally operative procedures, such as tenotomy, tendon lengthening, myotomy, and neurectomy, may have to be performed especially if results improve hygiene, ease nursing care, prevent skin breakdown, and increase function.

PRESSURE ULCERS

Pressure ulcers, also known as bed sores or decubitus ulcers, are some of the most difficult problems facing persons with SCI. These ulcers impair quality of life by activity restriction and increase the need for medical and nursing care, often by hospitalization or surgery. In acute SCI, more than one third of patients develop such pressure ulcers.[2]

PATHOPHYSIOLOGY

Pressure ulcers are caused by pressure-induced ischemia when vascular structures are compressed between bony prominences and external surfaces. Biomechanical factors related to pressure ulcer development include the magnitude and duration of force application, repetition of force application, and the presence of shearing forces.[260,261,262]

Persons with SCI have many major secondary factors that predispose them to the development of pressure ulcers, including paralysis, loss of sensation, incontinence of urine and stool, spasticity, joint contracture, edema, anemia, and poor nutrition.

COMMON LOCATIONS

Common locations of pressure ulcers include the sacrum, ischial tuberosities, heels, and trochanters. The sacrum is the most common site of ulceration during acute SCI because of prolonged lying in a supine position. Heel ulcers are likely to arise from this position as well, whereas ischial ulcers generally occur later during the course of SCI when the person is sitting without adequate pressure relief. Trochanteric ulcers about the hip usually occur from side lying. Other sites of pressure ulcers that are less commonly seen include the scapulae, often during wearing of a halo vest, the genitals, often related to appliances, such as indwelling or external catheters, and the occiput. All bony prominences, however, must be considered as potential sources of pressure ulceration but especially those below the level of injury.

CLASSIFICATION

Several classifications systems for pressure ulcers exist, each of which describes the pressure ulcers on the basis of depth and extent of tissue damage with higher numbers indicating deeper ulcers.[263,264,265] Because treatment often is based on the depth of the ulcer, all clinicians involved in the treatment should be using the same classification system.

PREVENTION

The surest method of pressure ulcer prevention is proper education of the patient and caregivers. This involves identifying the person at risk and adopting appropriate preventive protocols to avoid prolonged pressure to susceptible areas. In the immediate postinjury period, the person with SCI is confined to bed until hemodynamic and spinal stability is achieved. At this time, pressure-relieving mattresses are very helpful. No mattress, however, can prevent ulcers; therefore, frequent and regular repositioning of the patient and careful skin inspection is necessary. Bed position is best changed every 2 hours and pillows and wedges are strategically placed to maintain patient comfort and provide support. Ankle positioning orthotics provide cushioning to the malleoli and a relief for the heel while preventing plantar flexion contractures. Appropriate bowel and bladder management programs are instituted as early as possible to avoid incontinence and skin maceration. Nutrition instruction is provided to minimize the metabolic effects of the early catabolic state.

Once the rehabilitation phase begins, emphasis is placed on mobility. As more and more time is spent out of bed, the risk of developing ischial pressure ulcers related to sitting in a wheelchair increases. Provision of an appropriate wheelchair is vital as a poorly fitting wheelchair increases risk of ulcer development. Cushion and seat selection is important in maintaining an even pelvis to provide equal pressure distribution in the ischial region. As soon as sitting is begun, a technique must be taught to relieve pressure. If the individual cannot independently perform the pressure relieving maneuver, a caregiver should be trained and the staff should be alerted, but the individual should eventually take responsibility for directing the pressure relieving maneuver. Specific maneuvers include tilting the wheelchair backward, leaning forward to the side, and performing a push up. The maneuver should be performed every 20 minutes. Clothing should be inspected for appropriate fit, especially compression stockings, which can cause pressure ulcers when applied carelessly with bunching of the elastic material.

TREATMENT

Once an ulcer has developed, the treatment depends primarily on depth and degree of tissue involvement. For incipient sores, which appear as erythematous areas over a bony prominence, no specific skin care is needed, although this warning sign should be addressed by more vigilant positioning or a change in equipment. This is also true of a superficial ulcer confined to the skin, providing the exposed tissue is healthy and viable. With proper nutrition and pressure relief, these ulcers usually heal well.

Once the ulcer has penetrated the skin, more aggressive topical therapy is required. Most important is proper wound debridement of devitalized tissue to create a healthy, clean base. Some form of dressing should then be applied. The list of products that promote wound healing is long and largely unproved. An array of gels, pastes, enzymes, biocclusive dressings, and growth factors have been touted and advertised. Whether or not any of these products are superior to normal saline wet-to-dry dressings remains unproved. The advice here is to use whatever product one believes in as long as it does not take the place of regular inspection, pressure relief, and mechanical debridement of necrotic material.

Once the ulcer has reached sufficient depth to expose muscle or bone, or when the ulcer communicates with a joint or body cavity, such as the rectum, the treatment is usually surgical. At this stage, a major activity restriction may be required, for example, prohibiting wheelchair use if the deep ulcer involves the ischial tuberosity. Before undergoing surgical reconstruction, the situation producing the ulcer should be addressed and, if possible, rectified, for example, a wheelchair should be replaced if it does not accommodate a pelvic obliquity and results in uneven ischial weight bearing. Surgical treatment is usually preceded by a bowel preparation to avoid evacuation in the early postoperative period. A Foley catheter is placed. The usual procedure of choice is a myocutaneous rotational flap using local tissue. Free flaps may be required if insufficient local tissue is available. At the time of surgical correction, cultures are sent for the identification of bacterial pathogens that guide the choice of postoperative antibiotics. Following surgery, the patient is positioned to remove all pressure from the repaired segment. Range of motion to involved joints is avoided and spasticity is controlled as aggressively as possible. A low residue diet is prescribed and antidiarrheal agents are frequently used to avoid fecal soilage. Once sutures and drains are removed, the individual gradually resumes activity that allows contact between the flap and external surfaces.

POSTTRAUMATIC CYSTIC MYELOPATHY (SYRINGOMYELIA)

A syrinx is a fluid-filled cavity within the spinal cord that can be a disabling complication of SCI. The incidence of posttraumatic syringomyelia (PTS) was reported to occur in 0.3% to 3.2% of persons with SCI, but since the introduction of MRI, a higher incidence 12% to 22% has been reported.[266–271] Any person with SCI may develop this condition regardless of level of cord injury, neurologic severity, or initial management.[272] A syrinx may develop at any time, as early as 2 months or as late as decades after SCI. It is the most common cause of progressive myelopathy in persons with SCI and is particularly devastating as it may cause weakness or sensory loss after a patient has stabilized after the injury.

The definitive pathogenesis is unknown. A cavity seems to form at the injury site, to be followed later by enlargement and extension above or below the lesion. The cavity is usually initiated at the level of injury in the gray matter of the cord between the dorsal horns and posterior columns, which is a relatively avascular zone between the dorsal and ventral arterial supply.[272] Extension of the cyst then may occur by transmission of the pressure pulses within the epidural veins caused by activities such as coughing, sneezing, straining, or exercises.

The most common presenting symptom of PTS is pain, usually described as a dull ache and is usually increased by straining. The pain is usually located at the site of the original cord injury or may radiate to the neck or upper limbs. The next most common symptom is an ascending sensory level, which may be unilateral, bilateral, or intermittent in nature. Touch sensation is less often affected than pinprick due to the location of the syrinx.[274] Motor weakness is the third most common symptom of PTS, but this rarely occurs in isolation from other symptoms.[272,275] The earliest sign of a syrinx may be the loss of deep tendon reflexes.[267,276] Other symptoms of PTS include hyperhidrosis above and/or below the level of the lesion, change in tone and spasticity (increase or decrease), hypertension, neuropathic joints, change of bladder evacuation, orthostasis, and Horners' syndrome.[90,272,277] With progression of a high cervical syrinx, one may see symptoms of diaphragmatic paralysis and cranial nerve involvement including sensory loss in the trigeminal nerve distribution. Symptoms may be worse in the sitting position because of the gravitational forces on the lower part of the cyst.[278]

Clinical examination and CT with and without myelography were at one time the most common ways of diagnosing PTS, but MRI is now the diagnostic tool of choice. The presence of a spinal cord cyst on MRI does not, however, constitute a clinically significant syrinx and may not be the cause of symptoms because cysts at the level of trauma on routine MRI scanning have been reported in 32 of 63 (51%) patients who were either asymptomatic or tolerating symptoms, none of whom presented with ascending myelopathy.[279] The syrinx may extend over several vertebral segments. No definitive correlation between the size of the syrinx and the severity of the deficits has been noted, although a recent report revealed a positive correlation between the syrinx length and neurologic deterioration.[275] Electrophysiologic studies may be of some value in diagnosing and monitoring of the syrinx.[280]

The natural progression of PTS is not clear. The neurologic status may remain unchanged or slowly progress.[275] Nonprogressive asymptomatic PTS may be treated conservatively by pain control and avoiding straining. Serial clinical examinations and MRI scanning would be advisable. Surgical treatment is only recommended for progressive neurologic deterioration or severe pain. Surgical treatment involves drainage of the cavity and placement of a shunt to the subarachnoid space or peritoneal cavity. Favorable results have been reported following surgery, but the shunt occasionally gets blocked with recurrence of the syrinx. A number of shunt procedures have been described, however, no one procedure has been clearly shown to be superior to others. Relief of pain postoperatively and improvement of motor weakness is usually found, but sensory recovery is not usually as favorable.[274,281] There is good correlation with reduction of the size of the syrinx on postoperative MRI and the result of the surgical treatment.[282] A complete resolution of the syrinx is not, however, necessary for a good clinical outcome.

In summary, there is need for increased awareness with a high index of suspicion for PTS. It represents a treatable cause of pain and should be included in the differential diagnosis of neck and shoulder pain.[283] Early diagnosis can minimize the potentially devastating effects of PTS.

LONG-TERM SURVIVAL AND AGING IN SPINAL CORD INJURY

Spinal cord injury is not fatal if well managed. During the past 25 years, acute and long-term survival rates for persons with SCI have improved dramatically.[284] Despite this improvement, life expectancy still remains below normal.[285] During the first year after injury, the mortality rates are higher than during later years, particularly for more severely injured patients. The most significant prognostic factors related to survival include the severity of injury; that is, the neurologic level and degree of neurologic completeness by ASIA grades impairment scale, age of the patient at the time of injury, and ventilator dependency.[284] Survival rates for persons with SCI who only have sensory sparing or minimal motor function, are more similar to those with neurologically complete lesions than to those with significant motor function below the level of injury. In addition, there is a notable difference in survival rate in persons with SCI for each neurologic level.[285] The older the patient, the poorer the prognosis for survival for all severities of injury.

In the past, renal failure and other urinary tract complications were the leading cause of death in persons with SCI. Because of research efforts leading to changes in clinical care, renal failure as a cause of death has decreased significantly. The current leading cause of death is pneumonia (16.3%) in persons of all ages, neurologic levels, and lengths of time since injury. Nonschemic heart disease (12.2%) is the second leading cause of death with ischemic heart disease ranking sixth (6.5%). Other high-ranking causes of death include septicemia (8.7%), pulmonary emboli (8.1%), and suicide (5.7%).[284] Suicide is the second leading cause of death among persons in younger age groups, the second leading cause of death for persons with paraplegia, and the third leading cause of death between the first and fifth postinjury years. Interestingly, suicide is rare among patients with high-level tetraplegia.[284] Diseases of the urinary tract (3.5%), digestive system (4.8%), and cancer (5.15%) are the next most common causes of death. Overall, cancer mortality rates do not appear to be increased among persons with SCI.

Detailed life expectancies have been reported for all age groups by level of injury.[284] These data, however, are not adequate to individually estimate a persons long-term survival, because the effects of gender, race, genetics, comorbidities, psychologic factors, social support, and quality of care must be taken into account. The data, however, does point to the importance of good care and prevention in improving life expectancy and long-term outcomes, because pulmonary diseases represent 24.4% and suicide 5.7% of deaths. The decrease in renal disorders as a cause of death, shows that when adequate resources, research, and energy are adequate to treat specific medical complications of SCI, such as kidney disease, great strides can be made in improving the quality of care and overall morbidity and mortality.

Along with improved life expectancy, the goals of SCI patients have changed from survival in a sedentary lifestyle in an institutional setting, to maximal activity and independence within the community setting. The process of aging with a SCI may be accompanied by progressive physiologic decline, increasing impairment, disability, handicap, and cost of care.[286] Almost all organ systems are affected by aging. As persons with

SCI age, a premature decline in functional activities can be predicted at an earlier point in life than that of able-bodied individuals of a similar age. As a result, care needs increase prematurely with aging, which have a significant impact on the person with SCI, the family caregivers, and society.[286]

The impairments of aging correspond to the traditional priorities of SCI rehabilitation—skin, bowel, and bladder. Pressure sores are among the most frequent problems of SCI and can be the most costly and disabling. Surface and structural changes of the skin increase its susceptibility to breakdown and infection. Bowel problems include more frequent complaints of constipation, incontinence, bloating, and spastic bowel. This may be due to decreased fecal water content or impairment of other colonic factors. In the general population and in persons with SCI, the incidence of colorectal cancer increases dramatically with age. Fecal occult blood testing is still the most widely used method for colorectal cancer screening; however, this method is not sufficient because approximately three quarters of SCI individuals report some rectal bleeding.

Chronic, recurrent UTIs requiring frequent treatment may continue to occur in the years after SCI. Risk factors contributing to this include age-related changes in the immune system, prostatism, and menopause. When treating UTIs in the aging individual, one should take into account the proper dosages of the antibiotics, the susceptibility to produce adverse effects, and interaction with other medications.

Significant findings in the aging person with SCI included feeling of fatigue, elevated blood pressure, and decreasing functional independence measure (FIM) scores.[287] Pain of neurologic or musculoskeletal origin, including degenerative conditions of the shoulder and overuse injuries, weakness, spasticity, and postural problems in wheelchairs also are seen. Upper and lower extremity joint pain increases significantly with years postinjury from 29.3% at 5 years to 55.2% at 15 years.[287] As previously mentioned, musculoskeletal conditions rank high among indicators when quality of life is considered. With aging, there is an increased incidence of atherosclerosis, hypertension, and obesity. There is a decline in the maximal obtainable heart rate and a decline in maximal physical work capacity. The most significant disability associated with aging relates to functional declines in wheelchair mobility, ambulation, and self-care skills. Treatment options for responding to such changes include skills training, prescribing new or modifying current assistive equipment, using assistance from others, altering priorities for customary activities, and changing attitudes. Appropriate timing and adjustment to this transition is critical to the long-term preservation of function. Because even the most minor functional loss can create profound secondary disability, it is crucial to follow these patients closely to help prepare for and prevent such declines.

One of the greatest threats to maintaining an active lifestyle lies in the area of personal care assistance. Individuals who have relied on a family member for care face substantial difficulties when the family member becomes less capable of providing care because of their own aging. The death of a spouse has implications beyond that of the tragedy for a nondisabled individual. The need for new and additional assistance with decline in function may add considerable emotional stress and financial costs.

A number of studies show that most persons with SCI require additional assistance to maintain their activity level 20 years postinjury[286,287,288,289] and that costs for a patient whose combined age and years postinjury are more than 50 were two times greater than those whose age plus years postinjury were less than 50.[286–289]

Regular follow-up by spinal cord specialists over the life of the patient with SCI cannot be overemphasized. Numerous specific medical, physical, emotional, and home-care needs require the particular knowledge of an SCI specialist. Prevention, detection, timely therapeutic intervention, and modifications to prevent complications must be continued for the lifetime of the individual. If not, the health care system will be more costly for dealing with increased morbidity on an emergency basis rather than for more routine care and prevention.

REFERENCES

1. Guttmann L: *Spinal cord injuries. Comprehensive management and research,* Oxford, 1973, Blackwell Scientific Publications.
2. Stover SL, DeLisa JA, Whiteneck GG, editors: *Spinal cord injury: clinical outcomes from the model systems,* Gaithersburg, MD, 1995, Aspen.
3. Stover SL, et al: System benefits. In Stover SL, DeLisa JA, Whiteneck GG, editors: In *Spinal cord injury: clinical outcomes from the model systems,* Gaithersburg, MD, 1995, Aspen.
4. Seelman KD: Foreword. In Stover SL, DeLisa JA, Whiteneck GG, editors: *Spinal cord injury: clinical outcomes from the model systems,* Gaithersburg, 1995, Aspen.
5. Cales RH, Trunkey ED: Preventable trauma deaths: a review of trauma care systems development, *JAMA* 254:1059–1063, 1985.
6. Lowe DK, et al: Patterns of death, complications and errors in the management of motor vehicle accident victims: implications for a regional system of trauma care, *J Trauma* 23:503–509, 1983.

7. West JG, Trunkey ED, Lim RC: Systems of trauma care: a study of two countries, *Arch Surg* 114:455–460, 1979.
8. Ragnarsson KT, Thomas JP, Zasler ND: Model systems of care for individuals with traumatic brain injury, *J Head Trauma Rehab* 8:1–11, 1993.
9. Englander J, et al: Implementing and evaluating injury prevention programs in the traumatic brain injury model systems of care, *J Head Trauma Rehab* 8:101–113, 1993.
10. Kraus JF, et al: Incidence of traumatic spinal cord lesions, *J Chronic Dis* 28:471–492, 1975.
11. Bracken MB, Freeman DH, Hellenbrand K: Incidence of acute traumatic hospitalized spinal cord injury in the United States, 1970–1977, *Am J Epidemiol* 113:615–622, 1981.
12. Ergas Z: Spinal cord injury in the United States: a statistical update, *Cent Nerv Sys Trauma* 2:19–30, 1985.
13. Fine PR, et al: Spinal cord injury: an epidemiologic perspective, *Paraplegia* 17:237–250, 1979.
14. Clifton GL: Spinal cord injury in the Houston-Galveston area, *Tex Med* 79:55–57, 1983.
15. Go BK, DeVivo MJ, Richards JS: The epidemiology of spinal cord injury. In Stover SL, Whiteneck GG, editors: *Spinal cord injury: clinical outcomes from the model systems,* Gaithersberg, Maryland, 1995, Aspen Publishers.
16. Kalsbek WD, et al: The National Head and Spinal Cord Injury Survey: major findings, *J Neurosurg Suppl* S19–S31, 1980.
17. Kurtzke JF: Epidemiology of spinal cord injury, *Exp Neurol* 48:163–236, 1975.
18. DeVivo MJ, et al: Prevalence of spinal cord injury: a re-estimation employing life table techniques, *Arch Neurol* 37:707–708.
19. Harvey C, et al: New estimates of traumatic SCI prevalence: a survey based approach, *Paraplegia* 28:537–544, 1990.
20. Gibson CJ: Overview of spinal cord injury, *Phys Med Rehab Clin N Am* 3:699–709, 1992.
21. Michaelis LS: International inquiry on neurological terminology and prognosis in paraplegia and tetraplegia, *Paraplegia* 7:1–5, 1969.
22. Ditunno JF Jr, et al: The international standards booklet and functional classification of spinal cord injury, *Paraplegia* 32:70–80, 1992.
23. The American Spinal Injury Association, 2020 Peachtree Road, NW, Atlanta, Georgia 30309.
24. Frankel HL, et al: The value of postural reduction in the initial management of closed injuries of the spine with paraplegia and tetraplegia, *Paraplegia* 7:179–192, 1969.
25. World Health Organization: *International classification of impairment disabilities and handicaps: a manual of classification relating to the consequences of disease,* Geneva, 1980, World Health Organization.
26. *Guide for the use of the uniform data set for rehabilitation;* Buffalo, State University of New York at Buffalo.
27. Staas WE, et al: Rehabilitation of the spinal cord injured patient. In DeLisa JA, editor: *Rehabilitation medicine: principles and practice,* Philadelphia, 1993, JB Lippincott.
28. Bracken MB, et al: A randomized controlled trial of methylprednisolone onalaxin in the treatment of acute spinal cord injury, *N Engl J Med* 322:1405–1411, 1990.
29. Ragnarsson KT, et al: Management of pulmonary, cardiovascular, and metabolic conditions after spinal cord injury. In Stover SL, DeLisa JA, Whiteneck GG, editors: *Spinal cord injury: clinical outcomes from the model systems,* Gaithersburg, 1995, Aspen.
30. Green D, et al: Fixed vs. adjusted dose heparin in the prophylaxis of thromboembolism in spinal cord injury, *JAMA* 260:1255–1258, 1988.
31. Green D, Lee MY, Lim AC: Prevention of thromboembolism after spinal cord injury using low molecular weight heparin, *Ann Intern Med* 113:571–574, 1990.
32. Geerts WH, et al: A perspective study of venous thromboembolism after major trauma, *N Engl J Med* 331:1601–1606, 1994.
33. Geerts WH, et al: A comparison of low-dose heparin with low-molecular-weight heparin as prophylaxis against venous thromboembolism after major trauma, *N Engl J Med* 335:701–707, 1996.
34. Herzog JA: Deep vein thrombosis in the rehabilitation client, *Rehab Nurs* 17:196–198, 1992.
35. Hirsh J: Oral anticoagulant drugs, *N Engl J Med* 324:1865–1875, 1991.
36. Cardenas DD, et al: Management of gastrointestinal genitourinary and sexual function. In Stover SL, DeLisa JA, Whiteneck GG, editors: *Spinal cord injury: clinical outcome from the model systems,* Gaithersburg, 1995, Aspen.
37. Yarkony GM, Heineman AW: Pressure ulcers. In Stover SL, DeLisa JA, Whiteneck GG, editors: *Spinal cord injury: clinical outcomes from the model systems,* Gaithersburg, 1995, Aspen.
38. Yarkony GM, Bass LM, Keenan V, Meyer PR: Contractures complicating spinal cord injury, incidence and comparison between spinal cord center and general hospital acute care, *Paraplegia* 23:265–271, 1985.
39. Sypert GW: External spinal orthotics. *Neurosurgery* 20:642–649, 1987.
40. Axelsson P, Johnsson R, Stromqvist B: Effect of lumbar orthosis on intervertebral mobility determined by roentgen stereo photo grammetric analysis, *Spine* 7:678–681, 1992.
41. Axelsson P, Johnsson R, Stromqvist B: Lumbar orthoses with unilateral hip immobilization. Effect on intervertebral immobility determined by roentgen stereo photo grammetric analysis, *Spine* 18:876–879, 1993.
42. Marino RJ, et al: Superiority of motor level over single neurological level of categorizing tetraplegia, *Paraplegia* 33:510–513, 1995.

43. Coughlan JK, et al: Lower extremity bracing in paraplegia—a follow up study, *Paraplegia* 18:25–32, 1980.
44. Mickelberg R, Reid S. Spinal cord lesions and lower extremity bracing: an overview and follow-up study, *Paraplegia* 19:379–385, 1981.
45. Bradley WE: Innervation of the male urinary bladder, *Urol Clin North Am* 5(2):279–293, 1978.
46. Barrett DM: Electromyography: the practical approach. In Barrett DM, Weir AJ, editors: *Controversies in neurourology,* New York, 1984, Churchill Livingston.
47. Khanna OP: Cystometry: water. In Barrett DM, Weir AJ, editors: *Controversies in neurourology,* New York, 1984, Churchill Livingston.
48. Barkin M, et al: The urologic care of the spinal cord injury patients, *J Urol* 129:335–339, 1983.
49. King RB, et al: Clean and sterile intermittent catheterization methods in hospitalized patients with spinal cord injury, *Arch Phys Med Rehab* 73:798–802, 1992.
50. Maynard FM, Glass J: Management of the neuropathic bladder by clean intermittent catheterization: 5 year outcomes, *Paraplegia* 25:106–110, 1987.
51. Lammertse DP, et al: The relative risk of bladder cancer associated with indwelling catheters. Paper presented at American Paraplegic Society 42nd Annual Conference, Las Vegas, Sept 3, 1996.
52. Chancellor MB, Erhard MJ, Rivas DA: Clinical effect of alpha-1 antagonism by terozosin on external and internal urinary sphincter function, *J Am Paraplegia Soc* 16(4):207–214, 1993.
53. Perkash I: Efficacy and safety of terozosin to improve voiding in spinal cord injury patients, *J Spinal Cord Med* 18(4):236–239, 1995.
54. Dykstra DD, Sidi AA: Treatment of detrusor-sphincter dyssynergia with botulinum-A toxin: a double blind study, *Arch Phys Med Rehab* 91:24–26, 1990.
55. Schellhammer PF, Haskler RH, Bunts RC: External sphincterotomy: an evaluation of 150 patients with neurogenic bladder, *J Urol* 110:199–202, 1993.
56. Chancellor MB, et al: Management of sphincter dyssynergia using the sphincter stent prosthesis in chronically catheterized SCI men, *J Spinal Cord Med* 18(2):88–93, 1995.
57. Chancellor MB, et al: Prospective comparison of external sphincter balloon dilation and prosthesis placement with external sphincterotomy in spinal cord injured men, *Arch Phys Med Rehab* 75:297–305, 1994.
58. Linder A, Leach GE, Raz S: Augmentation cystoplasty in the management of neurogenic bladder disease and urinary incontinence, *J Urol* 135:969–971, 1986.
59. Sidi AA, et al: Augmentation enterocystoplasty for the management of voiding dysfunction of spinal cord injury patients, *J Urol* 143:83–85, 1990.
60. Chao R, et al: Bladder neck closure with continent augmentation or suprapubic catheter in patients with neurogenic bladders, *J Am Paraplegia Soc* 16(1):18–22, 1992.
61. Neal DE: Autoagumentation in the management of detrusor hyper-reflexia. Paper presented at American Paraplegic Society 42nd Annual Conference, Las Vegas, Sept 4, 1996.
62. Neumayer L, et al: The acutely affected abdomen in paraplegic spinal cord injury patients, *Ann Surg* 212:561, 1990.
63. Apstein M, Dalecki-Chipperfield K: Spinal cord injury as a risk factor for gallstone disease, *Gastroenterology* 92:966, 1987.
64. Stone J, et al: Chronic gastrointestinal problems in spinal cord injury patients: a prospective analysis, *Am J Gastroenterol* 85:1114–1119, 1990.
65. Glickman S, Kamm MA: Bowel dysfunction in spinal cord injury patients, *Lancet* 347:1651–53, 1996.
66. Kurnick NB: Autonomic hyperreflexia and its control in patients with spinal cord lesions, *Ann Intern Med* 44:678–86, 1956.
67. Lindsay R, et al: Incidence and clinical features of autonomic dysreflexia in patients with spinal cord injury, *Paraplegia*: 18:285–92, 1980.
68. Juler GL, Eltorai IM: The acute abdomen in spinal cord injury patients, *Paraplegia* 23:118–23, 1985.
69. Lee, BY, et al: Autonomic dysreflexia revisited, *J Spinal Cord Med* 18:75–87, 1995.
70. Kurnick NB: Autonomic hyperreflexia and its control in patients with spinal cord lesions, *Ann Intern Med* 44:678–86, 1956.
71. Kewolramani LS: Autonomic dysreflexia in traumatic myelopathy, *Am J Phys Med* 54:1–21, 1980.
72. Eltorai I, et al: Fatal cerebral hemorrhage due to autonomic dysreflexia in a tetraplegic patients. Case reports and review, *Paraplegia* 30:355–360, 1992.
73. Brown BT, Carrion HM, Politano VA: Guanethidine sulfate in the prevention of autonomic hyperreflexia, *J Urol* 122:55–57, 1979.
74. Abouleish E: Hypertension in a paraplegic parturient, *Anesthesia* 53:348–349, 1980.
75. Kewalramani LS: Autonomic dysreflexia in traumatic myelopathy, *Am J Phys Med* 54:1–21, 1980.
76. Pryor J: Autonomic hyperreflexia, *N Engl J Med* 285:860, 1971.
77. Fromst GP: Atrial fibrillation associated with autonomic dysreflexia in patients with tetraplegia, *Arch Phys Med Rehabil* 72:592–594, 1991.
78. Guttmann L, Frankel HL, Paeslack V: Cardiac irregularities during labor in paraplegic women, *Paraplegic* 8:144–151, 1965.
79. Frankel YC, Mathias CJ, Spalding JM: Mechanisms of reflex cardiac arrest in tetraplegic patients, *Lancet* 2:1183–1185, 1975.
80. Wayne EM, Vukov JG: Eye findings in autonomic hyperflexia, *Ann Optholmol* 9:41–42, 1977.
81. Guttman FL, Whitteridge D: Effects of bladder distention on autonomic mechanisms after spinal cord injuries, *Brain* 70:361–404, 1947.
82. Dunn KL: Autonomic dysreflexia: a nursing challenge

in the care of patients with spinal cord injury, *J Cardiovasc Nurs* 5:57–64, 1991.

83. Gerber JG, Nies AS: Antihypertensive agents and the drug therapy of hypertension. In Gibmon AG, et al: editors: *The pharmacologic basis of therapeutics,* ed 8. New York, 1994, Pergamon Press.
84. Krum H, et al: A study of the alpha-1 adrenoreceptor blocker prazosin in the prophylactic management of autonomic dysreflexia in high spinal cord injury patients, *Clin Auto Res* 2:83–88, 1992.
85. Trap CS, Bennett CJ: Autonomic dysreflexia and its urological implications: a review, *J Urol* 146:141–146, 1991.
86. Linden R, Liffler EJ, Kedia KR: A comparison of the efficacy of an alpha-1 adrenergic blocker and a slow calcium channel blocker in the control of autonomic dysreflexia, *Paraplegia* 23:34–38, 1985.
87. Riccobone AR: Long term follow-up of sphincterotomy in the treatment of autonomic dysreflexia, *Neurourol Urodynamic* 14:43–46, 1995.
88. Hrez DA, Gregerson M, Pearl L: Rehabilitation neurosurgery, *Neurosurgery* 18:311–315, 1986.
89. Halar E, Bell K: Contracture and other deleterious effects of immobility. In Delisa JA, et al, editors: *Rehabilitation medicine principles and practice,* ed 2 Philadelphia, 1988, JB Lippincott.
90. Maynard FM: Post traumatic cystic myelopathy in motor incomplete quadriplegia presenting as progressive orthostasis, *Arch Phys Med Rehab* 65:30–32, 1984.
91. Jackson A, Groomes TE: Incidence of respiratory complications following spinal cord injury, *Arch Phys Med Rehab,* 75:270–275, 1994.
92. Bach JR: Avoiding pulmonary morbidity and mortality for patients with paralytic or restrictive pulmonary syndromes, *Phys Med Rehab Clin North Am* 7(2):423–443, 1996.
93. Bach JR: New approaches in the rehabilitation of the traumatic high level quadraplegic, *Am J Phys Med Rehab* 70(1):13–19, 1991.
94. Merli G, et al: Deep vein thrombosis in acute spinal cord injured patients, *Arch Phys Med Rehab* 69:661–664, 1988.
95. Todd J, et al: Deep venous thrombosis in acute spinal cord injury: comparison of 125 I fibrinogen leg scanning, impedance plethysmography and venography, *Paraplegia* 14:50–57, 1976.
96. Merli G, et al: Etiology, incidence, and prevention of deep vein thrombosis in acute spinal cord injury, *Arch Phys Med Rehab* 74:199–205, 1993.
97. Weingarden SI. Deep venous thrombosis in spinal cord injury: overview of the problem, *Chest* 102(suppl):636S–639S, 1992.
98. Virchow R: Neuer Fall Von Todlichen Embolie Der Lungenarterie, *Arch Pathol Anat* 10:225–228, 1856.
99. White J, et al: Diagnosis of deep vein thrombosis using duplex ultrasound, *Ann Intern Med* 11:1297–1304, 1989.
100. Yarkony GM, Chen D. Rehabilitation of patients with spinal cord injuries. In Braddom RL, editor: *Physical medicine and rehabilitation,* Philadelphia, 1996, WB Saunders.
101. Kulkarni JR, et al: Prophylactic low dose heparin anticoagulant therapy in patients with spinal cord injuries: a retrospective study, *Paraplegia* 30:169–172, 1992.
102. Frisbie J, Sasahara A: Low dose heparin prophylaxis for DVT in spinal cord injured patients: a controlled study, *Paraplegia* 19:343–346, 1981.
103. Green D: Prophylaxis of thromboembolism in spinal cord injured patients, *Chest* 102:(suppl) 649S–651S, 1992.
104. Green D, et al: Prevention of thromboembolism in spinal cord injury: role of low molecular weight heparin, *Arch Phys Med Rehab* 75:290–292, 1994.
105. Merli G: Management of deep venous thrombosis in spinal cord injury, *Chest* 102:652S–657S, 1992.
106. Lim AC, Roth EJ, Green D: Lower limb paralysis: its effect on the recanalization of deep vein thrombosis, *Arch Phys Med Rehab* 73:331–333, 1992.
107. Levine M, et al: A comparison of low molecular weight heparin administered primarily at home with unfractioned heparin administered in the hospital for proximal deep vein thrombosis, *N Engl J Med* 334:677–681, 1996.
108. Koopman MMW, et al: Treatment of venous thrombosis with intravenous unfractionated heparin administered in the hospital as compared with subcutaneous, low-molecular weight heparin administered at home, *N Engl J Med* 334:682–687, 1996.
109. Landau WM: Spasticity: What is it? What is it not? In Feldman RG, Young RR, Koella QP, editors: *Spasticity: disordered motor control,* Chicago, 1980, Year Book Medical.
110. Delisa JA: *Rehabilitation medicine principles and practice,* ed 2, Philadelphia, 1993, JB Lippincott.
111. Gordon J: Receptors in muscle and their role in motor control. In Downey J, et al editors: *The physiological basis of rehabilitation medicine,* ed 2, Boston 1994, Butterworth-Heinemann.
112. Brar SP, et al: Evaluation of treatment protocols on minimal to moderate spasticity in multiple sclerosis, *Arch Phys Med Rehab* 72:185–189, 1991.
113. Bohannon RW, Smith MB: Interrater reliability of a modified Ashworth Scale of Muscle Spasticity, *Phys Ther* 67:206–207, 1987.
114. Priebe MM, et al: Assessment of spasticity in spinal cord injury with a multidimensional problem, *Arch Phys Med Rehab* 77:713–716, 1996.
115. Nance, PW: A comparison of clonidine, cyproheptadine and baclofen in spastic spinal cord injured patients, *J Am Para Soc* 17:151–157, 1994.
116. Scott JA, Donovan WH: The prevention of shoulder pain and contracture in the acute tetraplegic patient, *Paraplegia* 19(5):313–319, 1981.
117. Odeen I: Reduction of muscular hypertonous by long-term muscle stretch, *Scand J Rehab Med* 13:93–99, 1981.

118. Yarkony GM, editor: *Spinal cord injury: medical management and rehabilitation.* Procedure manual. Rehabilitation Institute of Chicago, Gaithersburg, 1994, Aspen.
119. Hill JP, editor: *Spinal cord injury. A guide to functional outcomes in occupational therapy. Procedure manual. Rehabilitation Institute of Chicago,* Rockville, 1986, Aspen.
120. Delisa JA, et al, editors: *Rehabilitation medicine principles and practice,* Philadelphia, 1988, JB Lippincott.
121. Kottke FJ, Lehman JF, editors: *Krusen's handbook of physical medicine and rehabilitation,* ed 4, Philadelphia, 1990, WB Saunders.
122. Falk AB, et al: *Positioning for function. Wheelchairs and other assistive technologies,* Valhalla, 1990, Valhalla Rehabilitation Publications.
123. Noth J: Trends in the athophysiology and pharmacotherapy of spasticity, *J Neurol* 238:131–139, 1991.
124. Bianchine JR: Drugs for Parkinson's disease, spasticity and acute muscle spasms. In Goodman LS, et al: editors: *The pharmacological basis of therapeutics,* ed 7, New York, 1995, MacMillian Publishing.
125. Kirkland LR: Baclofen dosage: a suggestion (letter), *Arch Phys Med Rehab* 65:214, 1985.
126. Bormann J: Electrophysiology of GABA A and GABA B receptor subtypes, *Trends Neurol Sci* 11:112–116, 1985.
127. Coward DM: Pharmacology and mechanism of action of tizanidine (Sirdalud). In Emre M, Benicke R, editors: *Spasticity: the current state of research and treatment.* Cornforth, 1989, Pasthenon.
128. Coward DM: Tizandine: neuropharmacology and mechanism of action, *Neurology* 44:(supp 19):S6–S11, 1994.
129. Maynard FM: Early clinical experience with clonidine in spinal spasticity, *Paraplegia* 24:175–82, 1986.
130. Donovan WM, et al: Clonidine-effect on spasticity: a clinical trial, *Arch Phys Med Rehab* 69:193–519, 1988.
131. Weingarden SI, Belen JG: Clonidine transdermal system for treatment of spasticity in spinal cord injury, *Arch Phys Med Rehabil* 73:876–877, 1992.
132. Nance PW, et al, and the North American Tizanidine Study Group: Efficacy and safety of Tizanidine in the treatment of spasticity in patients with spinal cord injury, *Neurology* 44(Suppl 9) 544–552, 1994.
133. Smith C, et al, US Tizanidine Study Group: Tizanidine treatment of spasticity caused by multiple sclerosis: results of a double blind, placebo-controlled trial, *Neurology* 44(Suppl 9):534–543, 1994.
134. Penn RD, et al: Intrathecal baclofen in severe spinal spasticity, *N Engl J Med* 320:1517–1521, 1989.
135. Azouui P, et al: Intrathecal baclofen in severe spinal spasticity, *N Engl J Med* 320:1517–1521, 1989.
136. Penn R: Intrathecal baclofen for spasticity of spinal orgin: seven years of experience, *J Neurosurg* 77:236–240, 1992.
137. Abel NA, Smith RA: Intrathecal spinal spasticity, *Arch Phys Med Rehab* 75:54–58, 1994.
138. O'Brien C, et al: Botulinum toxin. A clinical monograph. Proceeding of the 12th World Congress of International Federation of Physical Medicine and Rehabilitation, Sidney, 1995, Littleton, CO, 1995, Postgraduate Institute for Medicine.
139. Dykstra DD, Sidi AA: Treatment of detrusor-sphincter dyssynergia with botulinum-A toxin: a double-blind study, *Arch Phys Med Rehab* 71(1):24–26, 1990.
140. Dykstra DD, et al: Effects of botulinum A-toxin on detrusor-sphincter dyssynergia in spinal cord injury patients, *J Urol* 139(5):919–922, 1988.
141. Schurch B, et al: Botulinum-A toxin as a treatment of detrusor-sphincter dyssynergia: a prospective study in 24 spinal cord injury patients, *J Urol* 155(3):1023–1029, 1996.
142. Schurch B, et al: Effects of botulinum-A toxin on the periurethral striated sphincter of the neurogenic bladder. Preliminary study, *J Urol (Paris)* 97(7):375–380, 1990.
143. Doppler K: Die Sympathikodiaphtherise (chemische sympathikusavischoltung) an der arteria femoralis, *Med Klin* 22:1954–1956, 1926.
144. Wood KM: The use of phenol as a neurolytic agent: a review, *Pain* 5:205–229, 1978.
145. Moritz V: Phenol block of peripheral nerves, *Scand J Rehab Med* 5:160–163, 1973.
146. Katz RT: Management of spasticity, *Am J Phys Med Rehab* 88:108–116, 1988.
147. Garland DE, et al: Osteoporosis after spinal cord injury, *J Orthop Res* 10:371–378, 1992.
148. Chantraine A: Actual concept of osteoporosis in paraplegia, *Paraplegia* 16:51–58, 1978.
149. Hangartner TN, et al: Tibial bone density loss in spinal cord injured patients: effects of FES exercise, *J Rehab Res Dev* 31:50–61, 1994.
150. Ingram RR, et al: Lower limb fractures in the chronic spinal cord injured patient, *Paraplegia* 27:133–139, 1989.
151. Ragnarsson KT, Sell GH: Lower extremity fractures after spinal cord injury: a retrospective study, *Arch Phys Med Rehab* 62:418–423, 1981.
152. Garland DE, et al: Cone mineral density about the knee in SCl patients with pathological fractures, *Contemp Ortho* 26:375–379, 1993.
153. Leslie WD, Nance PW: Dissociated hip and spine demineralization: a specific finding in spinal cord injury, *Arch Phys Med Rehab* 74:960–964, 1993.
154. BeDell KK, et al: Effects of functional electrical stimulation-induced lower extremity cycling on bone density of spinal cord–injured patients, *Am J Phys Med Rehab* 75:29–34, 1996.
155. Saltzstein RJ, Hardin S, Hastings J: Osteoporosis in spinal cord injury: using an index of mobility and its relationship to bone density, *J Am Para Soc* 15:232–234, 1992.
156. Leeds EM, et al: Bone mineral density after bicycle ergometry training, *Arch Phys Med Rehab* 71:207–279, 1990.
157. Jackson RD, Mysiw WJ: Intermittent compressive forces, not muscle contraction, can reduce neurogenic

osteoporosis. Proceedings of the 76th annual meeting of the Endocrine Society, Anaheim, June 15–18, 1994.

158. Kaplan PE, et al: Reduction of hypercalciuria in tetraplegia after weight bearing and strengthening exercises, *Paraplegia* 19:289–293, 1981.
159. Kunkel CF, et al: Effect of standing on spasticity, contracture, and osteoporosis in paralyzed males, *Arch Phys Med Rehab* 74:73–78, 1993.
160. Miniare P. Immobilization osteoporosis: review, *Clin Rheumatol* 8:95–103, 1989.
161. Elias A, Gwinup G. Immobilization osteoporosis in paraplegia, *Am Para Soc* 15:163–170, 1992.
162. Comarr AE, Hutchinson RH, Bors E: Extremity fracture in patients with spinal cord injuries, *Am J Surg* 103:732–739, 1962.
163. Eichenholtz SN: Management of long bone fractures in paraplegic patients, *J Bone Joint Surg* 47A:299–310, 1963.
164. Freehafer AA, Mast WA: Lower extremity fractures in patients with spinal cord injury, *J Bone Joint Surg* 46A:683–694, 1965.
165. Freehafer AA, Hazel CM, Becker CL: Lower extremity fractures in patients with spinal cord injury, *Paraplegia* 19:367–372, 1981.
166. Freehafer AA: Limb fractures in spinal cord injury, *Arch Phys Med Rehab* 76:823–827, 1995.
167. Ingram RR, Suman RK, Freeman PA: Lower limb fractures in the chronic spinal cord injured patient, *Paraplegia* 27:133–139, 1989.
168. Notthee WM: A review of long bone fractures in patients with spinal cord injuries, *Clin Orthop* 155:65–70, 1981.
169. McMaster WC, Stauffer ES: Management of long bone fractures in the spinal cord injured patient, *Clin Orthop* 112:44–52, 1975.
170. Baird R, Kreitenberg A, Eltorai I: External fixation of femoral shaft fractures in spinal cord injury patients, *Paraplegia* 24:183–190, 1986.
171. Azaria M, Anner A, Ohry A: Long bone fractures in spinal cord injured patients, *Orthop Rev* 12:69–75, 1993.
172. Michaelis LS: *Orthopedic surgery of the limbs in paraplegia,* Berlin, 1964, Springer-Verlag.
173. Finerman GA, Stover SL: Heterotopic ossification following hip replacement or spinal cord injury: two clinical studies with EHDP, *Metab Bone Dis Relat Res* 3:337–342, 1981.
174. Stover SL, Niemann KM, Tulloss JR: Experience with surgical resection of heterotopic bone in spinal cord injury patients, *Clin Orthop* 363:71–77, 1991.
175. Wharton GE, Morgan DH: Ankylosis in the paralyzed patient, *J Bone Joint Surg* 52:105–112, 1970.
176. Maynard FM, et al: Management of Neuromusculoskeletal Systems. In Stover SL, DeLisa JA, Whiteneck GG, editors: *Spinal cord injury clinical outcomes fundamental systems,* Gaithersburg, 1995, Aspen.
177. Wharton GE, Garland DE: Clinical observations on fractures and heterotopic ossification in the spinal cord and traumatic brain injured populations, *Clin Orthop* 233:86–101, 1988.
178. Lal S, et al: Risk factors for heterotopic ossification in spinal cord injury, *Arch Phys Med Rehab* 70:387–390, 1989.
179. Chantraine A, Minaire P: Para-osteoarthropathies, *Scand J Rehab Med* 13:31–37, 1981.
180. Stover SL, Hataway CJ, Zeiger HE: Heterotopic ossification in spinal cord injury patients, *Arch Phys Med Rehab* 56:199–204, 1975.
181. Freed JH, et al: The use of the three phase bone scan in the early diagnosis of heterotopic ossification and in the evaluation of Didronel therapy, *Paraplegia* 20:208–216, 1982.
182. Ozel JA, Rudd TG: Heterotopic bone formation: clinical, laboratory and imaging correlation, *J Nucl Med* 26:125–132, 1985.
183. Haselkorn J, Britell CW, Cardenas DD: Diagnostic imagery of heterotopic ossification with coexistent deep venous thrombosis in flaccid paraplegia, *Arch Phys Med Rehab* 72:227–229, 1991.
184. Brooke MM, et al: Heterotopic ossification and peripheral nerve entrapment: early diagnosis and excision, *Arch Phys Med Rehab* 72:425–429, 1991.
185. Garland DE, et al: Diphosphonate treatment for heterotopic ossification in spinal cord injury patients, *Clin Orthop* 176:197–200, 1983.
186. Stover SL, Hahn HR, Miller JM: Disodium etidronate in the prevention of heterotopic ossification following spinal cord injury (preliminary report), *Paraplegia* 14:146–156, 1976.
187. Burke DC, Woodard JM: Phantom sensations in spinal paralysis. In Vinkin PJ, Bruyn GW, editors: *Handbook of clinical neurology,* Amsterdam, 1976, North Holland Publishing.
188. Donovan WH, et al: Neurophysiological approaches to chronic pain following spinal cord injury, *Paraplegia* 20:135–146, 1982.
189. Britell CW, Mariano AJ: Chronic pain in spinal cord injury, *Phys Med Rehab* 5:71–82, 1991.
190. Woolsey RM: Pain in spinal cord disorders. In Young RE, Woolsey RM, editors: *Diagnosis and management of disorders of the spinal cord,* Philadelphia, 1995, WB Saunders.
191. Ragnarsson KT: Management of pain in persons with spinal cord injury, *J Spinal Cord Med* 20:186–199, 1997.
192. Melzack R, Loeser JD: Phantom body in pain in paraplegics: evidence for central "pattern generating mechanism" for pain, *Pain* 4:195–210, 1978.
193. Ditunno JF Jr, et al: The international standards booklet for neurological and functional classification of spinal cord injury, *Paraplegia* 32:70–80, 1994.
194. American Spinal Injury Association: *International standards for neurological and functional classification of spinal cord injury,* Chicago, 1992, The Association.

195. Cohen MJ, et al: Comparing chronic pain from spinal cord injury to chronic pain of other origins, *Pain* 35:57–63, 1988.
196. Davidoff G, et al: Function-limiting dysesthetic pain syndrome among traumatic spinal cord injury patients: a cross sectional study, *Pain* 29:39–48, 1987.
197. Rose M, et al: Pain following spinal cord injury: results from a postal survey, *Pain* 34:101–102, 1988.
198. Mariano AJ: Chronic pain and spinal cord injury, *Clin J Pain* 8:87–92, 1992.
199. Richards JS: Chronic pain in spinal cord injury: review and comment, *Clin J Pain* 8:119–122, 1992.
200. Cairns DM, Adkins RH, Scott MD: Pain and depression in acute traumatic spinal cord injury: origins of chronic problematic pain, *Arch Phys Med Rehab* 77:329–335, 1996.
201. Nepomuceno C, et al: Pain in patients with spinal cord injury, *Arch Phys Med Rehab* 60:605–609, 1979.
202. Richards JS, et al: Psychosocial aspects of chronic pain in spinal cord injury, *Pain* 8:355–366, 1980.
203. Elliott T, Harkins SW: Psychosocial concomitants of persistent pain among persons with spinal cord injuries, *J Neurorehab* 1:7–16, 1991.
204. Summers JD, et al: Psychosocial factors in chronic spinal cord injury, *Pain* 47:183–189, 1991.
205. Clark WC: Pain and suffering. In Downy JA, et al, editors: *The physiological basis of rehabilitation medicine,* ed 2, Boston, 1994, Butterworth-Heinemann.
206. Price D: *Psychological and neural mechanisms for pain,* New York, 1988, Raven Press.
207. Fields HL: *Pain,* New York, 1987, McGraw Hill.
208. Fields HS: *Pain syndromes in neurology,* London, 1990, Butterworth.
209. Bonica JJ: Anatomic and physiological basis of nociception and pain. In Bonica JJ, editor: *The management of pain,* vol 1, ed 2, Philadelphia, 1990, Lee and Febiger.
210. Melzack R, Wall PD: Pain mechanisms: a new theory, *Science* 150:971–979, 1965.
211. Waring WP, Maynard FM: Shoulder pain in acute traumatic quadriplegia, *Paraplegia* 29:37–42, 1991.
212. Apple DF, Cody R, Allen A: Overuse syndrome of the upper limb in people with spinal cord injury. In Apple DF Jr, editor: *Physical fitness: a guide for individuals with spinal cord injury,* Baltimore, 1996, Department of Veterans Affairs.
213. Ferrara MS, Davis RW: Injuries to elite wheelchair athletes, *Paraplegia* 28:335–341, 1990.
214. Taylor D, Williams T: Sports injuries in athletes with disabilities: wheelchair racing, *Paraplegia* 33:296–299, 1995.
215. Dozono K, et al: Peripheral neuropathies in the upper extremities of paraplegic wheelchair marathon racers, *Paraplegia* 33:208–211, 1995.
216. Burnham RS, Steadward RD: Upper extremity peripheral nerve entrapments among wheelchair athletes: prevalence, location and risk factors, *Arch Phys Med Rehab* 75:519–524, 1994.
217. Aljure J, et al: Carpal tunnel syndrome in paraplegia patients, *Paraplegia* 23:182–186, 1985.
218. Gellman H, et al: Carpal tunnel syndrome in paraplegia patients. *J Bone Joint Surg* 70A:517–519, 1988.
219. Burnham RS, Steadward RD: Upper extremity peripheral nerve entrapments among wheelchair athletes, prevalence, location and risk factors, *Arch Phys Med Rehab* 75:519–524, 1994.
220. Gellman H, et al: Reflex sympathetic dystrophy in cervical spinal cord injury patients, *Clin Orthop* 233:126–131, 1988.
221. Cremer SA, Maynard F, Davidoff G: The reflex sympathetic dystrophy syndromes associated with traumatic myelopathy: report of five cases, *Pain* 37:187–192, 1989.
222. Philip PA, Philip M, Monga TN: Reflex sympathetic dystrophy in central cord syndrome: case report and review of the literature, *Paraplegia* 28:48–54, 1990.
223. Weinapel SF: Reflex sympathetic dystrophy following traumatic myelopathy, *Pain* 18:345–349, 1984.
224. Gallien P, et al: The reflex sympathetic dystrophy syndrome in patients who have had a spinal cord injury, *Paraplegia* 33:715–720, 1995.
225. Aisen PS, Aisen ML: Shoulder hand syndrome in cervical spinal cord injury, *Paraplegia* 32:588–592, 1994.
226. Kozin F, et al: The reflex sympathetic dystrophy syndrome (RSDS) III. Scintigraphic studies, further evidence of the therapeutic efficacy of systemic corticosteroids and proposed diagnostic criteria, *Am J Med* 70:23–30, 1981.
227. Nashold BS, Bullitt D: Dorsal root entry zone lesions to control central pain in paraplegics, *J Neurosurg* 55:414–419, 1981.
228. Nashold BS, Ostdahl RN: Dorsal root entry zone lesions for pain relief, *J Neurosurg* 51:59–66, 1979.
229. Nashold BS Jr, Alexander E: Neurosurgical treatment of deafferentation pain. In Tollison CD, editor: *Handbook of chronic pain management,* Baltimore, 1989, William & Wilkins.
230. Tunks E: Pain in spinal cord injured patients. In Bloch RF, Bashbaum M, editor: *Management of spinal cord injuries.* Baltimore, 1986, Williams & Wilkins.
231. Maroon JC: "Burning hands" in football spinal cord injuries, *JAMA* 238:2049–2051, 1977.
232. Fenollosa P, et al: Chronic pain in the spinal cord injured: statistical approach and pharmacological treatment, *Paraplegia* 31:722–729, 1993.
233. Edgar RE, et al: Computer assisted DREZ microcoagulation: post-traumatic spinal deafferentation pain, *J Spinal Disord* 6:48–56, 1993.
234. Hyndman OR: Lissauer's tract section. A contribution to chordotomy for the relief of pain (preliminary report), *J Inter Coll Surg* 5:294–400, 1942.
235. Friedman AH, Nashold BS: DREZ lesions for relief of pain related to spinal cord injury, *J Neurosurg* 65:465–469, 1986.
236. Charney KJ, Juler GL, Comarr AE: General surgery

problems in patients with spinal cord injuries, *Arch Surg* 110:1083–1088, 1975.

237. Mersky H, Hester RA: The treatment of chronic pain with psychotropic drugs, *Postgrad Med J* 48:594–598, 1972.
238. Max MB, et al: Effects of desipramine, amitriptyline and fluoxetine on pain in diabetic neuropathy, *N Engl J Med* 326:1250–1256, 1992.
239. Rumore MM, Schlichtin DA: Clinical efficacy of antihistamines as analgesics, *Pain* 25:7–22, 1986.
240. Ghostine SY, et al: Phenoxybenzamine in the treatment of causalgia. Report of forty cases, *J Neurosurg* 60:1263–1268, 1984.
241. Loubser PG, Donovan WH: Diagnostic spinal anesthesia in chronic spinal cord injury pain, *Paraplegia* 29:25–36, 1991.
242. Davis R, Lentini R: Transcutaneous nerve stimulation for treatment of pain in patients with spinal cord injury, *Surg Neurol* 4:100–101, 1975.
243. Richardson DE, Akil H: pain reduction by electrical stimulation in man, *J Neurosurg* 47:178–183, 1977.
244. Krainick JU, Phoden U: Dorsal column stimulation. In PD Wall, R Melzack, editors: *Textbook of pain*, Edinburgh, 1989, Churchill Livingstone.
245. Illis LS, Sedgwick EM, Tallis RC: Spinal cord stimulation in multiple sclerosis: clinical results. *J Neurol Neurosurg Psych* 43:1–14, 1980.
246. Twist DJ, et al: Neuroendocrine changes during functional electrical stimulation, *Am J Phys Med Rehab* 71:156–162, 1992.
247. Sipski ML, DeLisa JA, Schweer S: Functional electrical stimulation bicycle ergometry: patient perceptions, *Am J Phys Med Rehab* 68:147–149, 1989.
248. Guttman L: *Spinal cord injuries. Comprehensive management and research,* ed 2, Oxford, 1976, Blackwell Scientific.
249. Edgar RE, et al: Computer assisted DREZ microcoagulation: post-traumatic spinal deafferentation pain, *J Spinal Disord* 6:48–56, 1993.
250. Subbarao JV, Klopfstein J, Turpin R: Prevalence and impact of wrist and shoulder pain in patients with spinal cord injury, *J Spinal Cord Med* 18:9–13, 1995.
251. Sie IH, et al: Upper extremity pain in the post rehabilitation spinal cord injured patients. *Arch Phys Med Rehabil* 73:44–48, 1992.
252. Gellman H, Sie I, Waters RL: Late complications of the weight bearing extremity in the paraplegic patient, *Clin Orthop* 233:132–135, 1988.
253. Bayley JC, Couchran TP, Sledge CB: The weight bearing shoulder. The impingement syndrome in paraplegics, *J Bone Joint Surg* 69A:676–678, 1987.
254. Nichols PJ, Norman PA, Ennis J: Wheelchair users shoulder? Shoulder pain in patients with spinal cord lesions, *Scand J Rehab Med* 11:29–32, 1979.
255. Wylie EJ, Chakera TM: Degenerative joint abnormalities in patients with paraplegia of duration greater than 20 years, *Paraplegia* 26:101–106, 1988.
256. Davidoff G, Werner R, Waring W: Compressive mono neuropathies of the upper extremity in chronic paraplegia, *Paraplegia* 29:17–24, 1991.
257. Tun CG, Upton J: The paraplegic hand: electrodiagnostic studies and clinical findings, *J Hand Surg* 5:716–719, 1988.
258. Gelberman RH, et al: The carpal syndrome, *J Bone Joint Surg* 63A:680–683, 1981.
259. Botte MJ, Abrams RA, Bodine-Fowler SC: Treatment of acquired muscle spasticity using phenol peripheral nerve blocks, *Orthopedics* 18:151–159, 1995.
260. Kosiak M: Etiology and pathology of ischemic ulcers, *Arch Phys Med Rehab* 40:62–69, 1959.
261. Brand PW: Pressure sores. In Kened RM, Cowden JM, Scales JT, editors: *Bed sore biomechanics,* London, 1976, Macmillan.
262. Bennett L, et al: Skin stress and blood flow in sitting paraplegic patients, *Arch Phys Med Rehab* 65:196–190, 1984.
263. Shea JP: Pressure sore classification and management, *Clin Orthop* 112:89–100, 1975.
264. National Pressure Ulcer Advisory Panel: Pressure ulcer prevalence, cost and risk assessment: Concensus development conference statement, *Decubitus* 2:24, 1989.
265. Yarkony G, et al: Classification of pressure ulcers, *Arch Dermatol* 126:1218–1219, 1990.
266. Umbach I, Halpern A: Review article: postspinal cord injury syringomyelia, *Paraplegia* 29:219–221, 1991.
267. Dworkin GE, Stass W: Post-traumatic syringomyelia, *Arch Phys Med Rehab* 66:329–331, 1985.
268. Williams B: Post traumatic syringomyelia In HL Frankel, editor: *Handbook of clinical neurology*; vol 17, Amsterdam, 1992, Elsever Science Publishers.
269. Sett P, Crockard HA: The value of MRI and the follow-up management of spinal injury, *Paraplegia* 29:396–410, 1991.
270. Frisbie JH, Aguilera EJ: Chronic pain after spinal cord injury; an expedient diagnostic approach, *Paraplegia* 28:460–465, 1990.
271. Hussey RW, et al: Prospective study of the occurrence rate of post-traumatic cystic degeneration of the spinal cord utilizing MRI, *J Am Para Soc* 13:1–20, 1990, Abstract 41, 35th Annual Conference of the American Paraplegic Society.
272. Biyani A, Masri WS: Post traumatic syringomyelia: a review of literature; *Paraplegia* 32:723–731, 1994.
273. McDonald RI, Findlay JM, Tator CH: Microcytic spinal cord degeneration causing post traumatic myelopathy, *J Neurosurg* 68:466–471, 1988.
274. Rossier AB, et al: Post traumatic syringomyelia, incidence, clinical presentation, electro physiologic studies, syrinx protein and results of conservative and operative treatment, *Brain* 108:439–461, 1995.
275. Schurch B, Wichmann W, Rossier AB: Post traumatic syringomyelia: a prospective study of 449 patients with spinal cord injury, *J Neurol Neurosurg Psych* 60:61–67, 1996.

276. Watson N: Ascending cystic degeneration of the cord after spinal cord injury, *Paraplegia* 19:89–95, 1981.
277. Ben Zur PH: Intermittent Horners syndrome: recurrent, alternate Horners syndrome in cervical cord injury, *Ann Ophthalmol* 7:955–962, 1975.
278. Quencer RM, Gleen BA, Eismont FJ: Post traumatic spinal cord cysts; clinical features and characterization with metrizamide computed tomography, *Radiology* 146:415–423, 1983.
279. Backe HA, et al: Post traumatic spinal cord cysts evaluated by magnetic resonance imaging, *Paraplegia* 29:607–612, 1991.
280. Dyro FM, Rossier AB: Electrodiagnostic abnormalities in 15 patients with post traumatic syringomyelia. Pre and post operative procedures, *Paraplegia* 23:233–242, 1985.
281. Davis CHG, Symon L: Mechanisms and treatment of post traumatic syringomyelia, *Br J Neurosurg* 3:669–674, 1989.
282. Grant R, et al: MRI measurement of the syrinx size before and after operation, *J Neurol Neurosurg Psych* 50:1685–1687, 1987.
283. Cole M, et al: Post traumatic syringomyelia late occurrence of distant pain after spinal injury, *J Neuro Rehab* 6:201–202, 1992.
284. DeVivo MJ, Stover SL: Long term survival and causes of death in spinal cord injury. In Stover SL, DeLisa JL, Whiteneck GG, editors: *Spinal cord injury: clinical outcomes from the model systems,* Gaithersburg, 1995, Aspen.
285. DeVivo MJ, Stover SL, Black KJ: Prognostic factors for twelve year survival after spinal cord injury, *Arch Phys Med Rehab* 73:156–162, 1992.
286. Menter RR, et al: Impairment, disability, handicap and medical expenses of persons aging with spinal cord injury, *Paraplegia* 29:613–619, 1991.
287. Mentor RR, Hudson LM: Effects of age at injury and the aging process. In Stover SL, DeLisa JA, Whiteneck GG, editors: *Spinal cord injury: clinical outcomes from the models systems,* Gaithersburg, 1995, Aspen.
288. Menter RR. Aging with a spinal cord injury, *Phys Med Rehab Med Clin North Am* 3:879–891, 1992.
289. Whiteneck GG, et al: *Aging with spinal cord injury,* New York, 1993, Demos.

26

CONCEPTS AND ISSUES OF SPINE DEVICE DEVELOPMENT AND REGULATION

James T. Robertson
Deborah Hyatt

HISTORICAL OVERVIEW

As in any field of medicine, our knowledge of the spine and spinal treatments can be traced back to ancient times. The following historical summary relies on Wiltse's brief but comprehensive 1991 history of spinal disorders and treatments.[1]

The history of spinal treatments began with the ancient Greeks. Approximately 1300 BC, Hippocrates developed a traction table for reduction of fractures and fracture-dislocations. Before 200 AD, the Greek physician Galen had described and named lordosis, kyphosis, and scoliosis, and he had attempted to correct these abnormalities. In the seventh century, Paul of Aegina used splints to reduce fractures and performed the first laminectomies. Unfortunately, much of the knowledge and skills of these and other ancient physicians was lost during the "Dark Ages" that followed the collapse of the Roman Empire. Centuries would pass before our understanding of spinal disorders and traumas would rise to the same level.

During the Renaissance, Versalius and Paré defined the study of anatomy, and Paré recognized cord compression as a cause of paraplegia. The term *orthopedics* was coined by Nicholas Andry (1658–1742), who published the first book on the musculoskeletal system. The first orthopedic hospital was established at about the same time, accompanied by the wide distribution of orthopedic literature. Laminectomies also were performed and were widely and hotly debated. The use of aseptic techniques, anesthesia, and radiographs were all established in the 1800s.

At that time, scoliosis and other deformities were treated with exercise, bracing or casts, and distraction in a bed or frame. Spinal fusion was first described in 1911 by Albee and Hibbs, and Hibbs originated a technique to treat tuberculosis of the spine and scoliosis.[2,3] Myelography was developed through the 1920s and 1930s. In the 1930s and 1940s fusion as a treatment for scoliosis fell temporarily into disfavor; later improvements in pre- and postoperative care, bracing, and casting restored the technique to a respectable status. The Scoliosis Research Society was established in 1966.

Cervical fusion was developed by Gallie in the late 1930s and advanced by William Rogers in the 1940s.[4,5] An anterior approach for combined discectomy and fusion and for multiple-level fusion was developed in the 1950s.[6,7] These advances continued through the 1960s, with Robinson and Southwick using rods wired to the facets and Hodgson promulgating the anterior technique, which he employed in wedge osteotomy for congenital kyphosis.[8,9]

Internal fixation of the lumbar spine can be traced back to 1887, when B. F. Wilkins performed an internal reduction and fixation of the posterior lumbar on a newborn.[10] The procedure was rarely performed over the next several decades for lack of a suitably strong, inert metal. In the 1930s, Charles Venable used implants made of a cobalt-chromium-molybdenum alloy, Vitallium.[11,12] Vitallium, which is biocompatible, could be left in vitro long enough to complete bone healing. Venable's success paved the way for later advances in biomaterials research, including the use of stainless steel, titanium, and tantalum, and the recent developments of methylmethacrylate, other plastics, and ceramics.

Modern techniques for internal lumbar fixation date back to the 1940s when King recommended using screws through the facets.[13] The first reported use of inserting screws directly into the pedicle was described in 1959.[14] Dwyer combined anterior disk excision, screw insertion, and fixed-cable compression in 1969.[15] In the 1960s and 1970s, Harrington combined cast correction and meticulous fusion and developed new spinal instrumentation for use in the treatment of scoliosis.[16,17] In the 1970s and 1980s, Roy-Camille and several colleagues published their work using plate systems, rod systems, and pedicle screws, separately and in combination.[18,19] Magerl also performed pedicle screw fixation, inserting Schanz screws into the pedicles percutaneously or internally and using a variety of external and internal fixators.[20] Diagnostic magnetic resonance imaging (MRI) and somatosensory evoked potentials for intraoperative spinal cord monitoring were both developed in the 1970s. In 1982, Luque reported on his system of sublaminar wires and posterior rods to treat scoliosis, a method that allowed segmental stabilization without large postoperative casts.[21] In 1984, Cotrel and Dubousset presented the first rotating scoliosis-correcting system, using screws, rods, cross connectors, and hooks.[22]

Many more internal fixation devices have been developed through the 1980s and 1990s, including plates and plating systems designed for use on the anterior and lateral aspects of vertebral bodies.

Looking back over the history of spinal medicine, we can certainly appreciate the decades and centuries of study and effort that have led to so many recent advances. We can certainly celebrate the past 50 years of progress, during which modern spinal devices were developed and refined. We should also keep in mind, however, that many of today's devices are founded on the same, essentially unchanged, concepts that drove the achievements of King, Harrington, and others. As exciting as the past few decades have been, it is even more exciting to recognize that spinal surgery is still in a pioneering age. There are many advances yet to come, and surgeons and their patients will continue to benefit as new surgical techniques and devices are developed.

THE CONTEMPORARY PRODUCT DEVELOPMENT PROCESS

Product development involves far more than simply product design and testing. For companies in the surgical device arena, it also requires extensive communications and contact with surgeons and other healthcare professionals, intense research and development (R&D) efforts, and an awareness of the many forces at work in the U.S. and global medical device markets. In this section, we focus on the first two of these aspects, and present an overview of the steps involved in bringing a surgical device successfully to market.

PRODUCT DEVELOPMENT IN RESPONSE TO AN IDENTIFIED NEED

For companies in the surgical device arena, the first step in product development typically occurs when a surgeon describes for an engineer a surgical situation that could be improved, or patient need that could be met, by the development of a new product. Thus, medical product development springs from a surgical/engineering perspective in which a product is developed to meet an existing, identified need. This differs from the development of consumer products in which a need for the product is more often "created" through marketing strategies. The surgical/engineering perspective also differs from the exploratory focus, which generates advances in fields such as toxicology, microbiology, chemistry, and physics.[23]

To identify patient needs and produce problem-solving devices, surgical device manufacturers stay in close contact with their primary customers—surgeons. Top executives, managers, engineers, R&D personnel, and sales and marketing teams attend surgical meetings, read the literature, observe in the operating room, participate in in-service training programs, conduct focus groups, and pursue other avenues of communication with surgeons. Among the issues that manufacturers seek to address through surgeons are the need for a range of device sizes, surgical risk factors, new surgical approaches and techniques, and, of course, surgeon preferences. Individual surgeons or researchers also may serve as catalysts in the development of particular products. For example, Sofamor Danek's developmental work on anterior plating systems that culminated in the ZPlate-ATL anterior fixation system was supported by Dr. Zdeblick at the University of Wisconsin, following identification of the need for a product that could address the growing trend toward anterior internal fixation of the thoracic and thoracolumbar spine when anterior stabilization is required for a patient.[24]

After identification of a need, surgical product development proceeds using a surgical/engineering approach: the objectives of the proposed device are defined by surgeons for engineers, and the design criteria (e.g., expected implant size range, compression-distraction capability, and the need for a low-profile design) are established by engineers in consultation with surgeons. The aim is to determine the necessary product attributes and how to combine them to achieve an optimum solution. Prototypes are then developed and informally evaluated by the company and by surgeons working with cadavers or simulated bones. If a prototype proves viable, it is repeatedly modified and reevaluated in a cyclic process in which the company and surgeon "fine tune" the design.

TYPICAL STEPS IN THE PRODUCT DEVELOPMENT "PATHWAY"

As shown in the "pathway" chart (Fig. 26-1), several key steps may take place during development of a device system. The following outline is meant only to illustrate the general shape and flow of this process, not to establish any particular activities or a certain order of events as being essential. Certainly, more, fewer, or different steps may occur depending on the company and type of product under development.

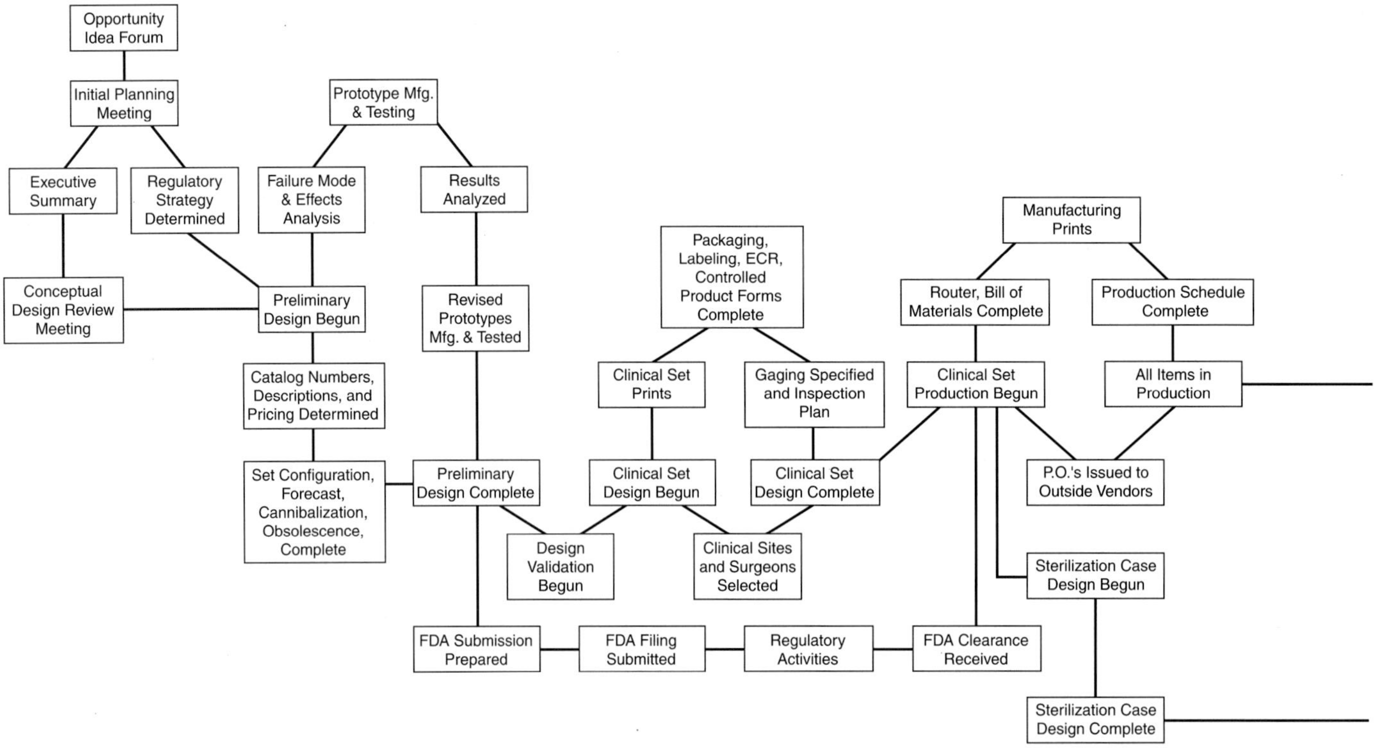

FIGURE 26-1

Typical product development "pathway."

- First, after a surgeon describes a surgical situation or patient need that may be improved, a review meeting is held to assess current solutions, new design criteria, and possible improved solutions. A target solution is described, and potential advantages and disadvantages of the proposed product are discussed, with surgeon and engineer input.
- Upon reaching consensus, an initial planning meeting is held, during which the remainder of the pathway is plotted by the surgeon and the responsible development and business representatives. The team addresses general business issues, reviews the design concept, and proposes a development strategy.
- A failure mode and effects analysis (FMEA) is performed. The FMEA identifies the potential ways in which the product might fail and assigns a severity rating to each potential failure mode. This procedure not only addresses alterations in product design that may be needed to prevent a specific failure mode but also identifies the kinds of testing and quality control necessary to provide maximum product performance and safety.
- At the same time, planning and early preparation of initial documentation for submission to the U.S. Food and Drug Administration (FDA) also begin. The FDA documentation proceeds as noted in the time line at the bottom of Figure 26-1, with the goal of achieving clearance at approximately the time that the company is prepared to go into production. (For more information on this process, see the following section, Testing and Regulatory Guidelines and Requirements.)
- Prototype manufacture begins. As stated before, the prototype is revised and reviewed by surgeons until the preliminary design is considered complete. An initial set of components is then manufactured.
- During manufacture of the first full set of components and instruments, product packaging and labeling is completed, and quality control standards are established. Surgeon experience and input is critical to ensure that the product meets all of the defined objectives.
- During evaluation, additional design adjustments may be made based on surgeon assessment and feedback.
- Marketing programs are completed, along with production and inspection schedules, and the system is readied for release.

COMPUTER-AIDED TECHNOLOGIES USED IN PRODUCT DEVELOPMENT

Today, the device design and production is extraordinarily sophisticated, thanks in part to modern

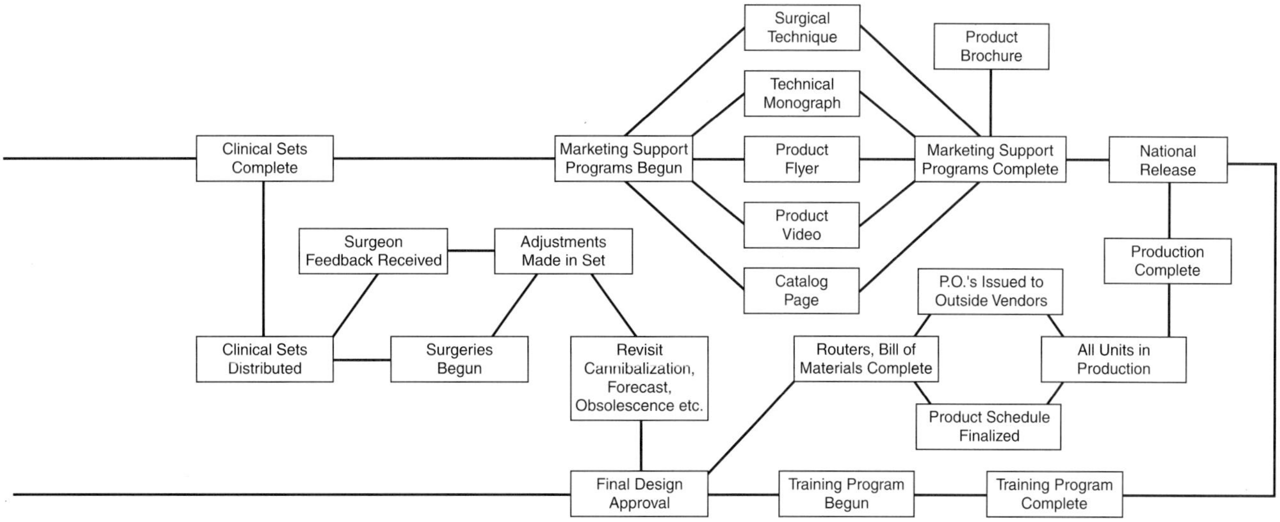

FIGURE 26-1

Continued

technology. Companies now often use computer-assisted design (CAD), manufacture (CAM), and engineering (CAE) programs and technologies, which provide nearly instantaneous and virtually unlimited options.

The CAD systems, for example, offers three-dimensional design capabilities in even the earliest concept stages, saving time and money over traditional hard-prototype production. Using this technology, designers can employ structural analysis, identify shortcomings in relation to performance parameters, and test "what if" scenarios to determine how design changes will affect product performance. Once a computer-generated design appears on-target other computer systems, such as Rapid prototype equipment, can interface with the CAD program to generate plastic prototypes for evaluation, mold-making, and casting.

The CAM and CAE systems are used in much the same way through development and production of not only the various prototypes but also of the clinical sets and, eventually, the final marketable product.

TESTING AND U.S. REGULATORY GUIDELINES AND REQUIREMENTS

U.S. FOOD AND DRUG ADMINISTRATION REGULATIONS

As Figure 26-1 shows, preparation of documents for submission to the FDA is integral to device marketing. Clearance by the FDA is required for interstate sale of any implantable device, but there is much confusion about the role of the FDA and how the FDA regulates devices. It is important to first understand the agency's background and the laws under which it operates. This summary of FDA history and regulations, and the following examination of Good Laboratory Practices (GLP) and Good Manufacturing Practices (GMP), FDA spinal device testing requirements, and voluntary standards followed by U.S. manufacturers, rely largely on the 1993 writings of Melkerson, Yahiro, and Mishra, and on separate 1989 articles authored by Callahan and by Buckman.[25,26,27]

The U.S. FDA was created in 1906, under the Food and Drug Act. The first device regulations were enacted in 1938 when the FDA was given the responsibility of regulating misbranded and adulterated devices.[28] The FDA's role and authority were broadened by the Medical Device (MD) Amendments of 1976, which gave the FDA comprehensive regulatory powers over medical devices and provided much of the current definition of device. The MD Amendments are also important because devices that were on the market before enactment of the Amendments on May 28, 1976 are regulated as "preamendments" devices, while those created after that date are regulated as "new" devices. The Safe Medical Devices Act (SMDA) of 1990 is equally important because it expanded the FDA's regulatory powers. Additional amendments in 1992 further expanded the definition of *device* and the FDA's authority (Box 1).[29]

510 (k), PREMARKET APPROVAL, AND INVESTIGATIONAL DEVICE EXEMPTION PROCESSES

There are, essentially, three routes by which implantable devices may be cleared for interstate shipping for clinical testing or for interstate sale by the FDA. These processes—510 (k), Premarket Approval (PMA), and Investigational Device Exemption

(IDE)—all make different statements about the FDA's acceptance of a device's credentials. (Box 2)

- Premarket notification, or 510(k) clearance, means that a device can be marketed as "substantially equivalent" (SE) to a device that was already on the market prior to enactment of the Medical Device Amendments or has already met the SE standard.[30] To be considered SE, the proposed device must be substantially equivalent in design, materials, and intended use to the predicate device.[31] Alternatively, if the new device is intended for the same use, but is not technologically equivalent, the manufacturer must be able to demonstrate that the new device is as safe and effective as the predicate device. Testing of a 510(k)-cleared device may include nonclinical laboratory or clinical testing. 510(k) clearance does not mean, and is not meant to imply, that the device has undergone clinical testing.

Box 1. Medical Device Definition From the Medical Device Amendments of 1976

Definition: *Medical device* is defined as "any instrument, apparatus, implement, machine, contrivance, implant, in vitro reagent, or other similar or related article, including any component, part, accessory, which is:

- recognized in the official National Formulary, or the *United States Pharmacopeia*, or any supplement to them;
- intended for use in the diagnosis of disease or other conditions, or in the cure, mitigation, treatment, or prevention of disease, in man or other animals; or
- intended to affect the structure or any function of the body of man or other animals; and
- does not achieve any of its principle purposes through chemical action within or on the body of man or other animals and which is not dependent upon being metabolized for the achievement of any of its principal intended purposes.

Good Manufacturing, Laboratory Practices, and Testing Standards

Good Manufacturing Practices (GMP), developed by the FDA, provide guidelines by which a manufacturer's quality controls may be evaluated; therefore, the FDA requires compliance with these standards. As part of the application for an IDE and PMA, the manufacturer must fully describe the company's procedures and processes related to the production, packing, and storage of its products.[33]

Similarly, Good Laboratory Practices (GLP), promulgated by the FDA, have been adopted for use by many manufacturers. Generally speaking, these voluntary standards concern laboratory testing and manufacturing of a wide range of consumer products, not just medical devices. Some sections of the standards,

Box 2 Overview of Routes to FDA Clearance or Approval of Surgical Devices

- Premarket Notification, 510(k). Clears "substantially equivalent" devices for interstate sale in the U.S. Does not necessarily require or imply clinical testing.
- Premarket Approval, PMA. Approves devices for interstate sale in the U.S., following FDA acceptance of device's safety and effectiveness. Requires rigorous testing, including clinical trials.
- Investigational Device Exemption, IDE. Allows interstate shipping and clinical testing. Required for virtually all devices subject to PMA approval and even for some devices that are subject to 510(k).
- Premarket Approval (PMA) is for all devices that the FDA determines are not substantially equivalent. The PMA process requires scientific testing and proof of the device's safety and effectiveness. It is interesting to note that a device may require a PMA for certain sought-after indications and, at the same time, may be allowed on the market through the 510(k) process for other indications, provided that a substantially equivalent predicate device exists for the latter indications. In one instance, for example, total hip replacement implants that had not yet demonstrated sufficient bone/implant ingrowth for noncemented use were cleared for cemented application, based on their substantial equivalence to predicate, cemented devices.
- The Investigational Device Exemption (IDE) allows interstate shipping and clinical testing of a device so that the manufacturer can collect clinical data. All devices that undergo clinical testing in the United States must have, or must be determined to be exempt from, an IDE. Federal regulations describe the information needed in an IDE application. Once the IDE is approved, clinical trials begin. The testing schedule allows a specified number of cases to be treated at a specified number of sites. Adherence to the investigational protocol requires that unanticipated adverse reactions be reported immediately to the FDA.[32] Ultimately, if the device is determined to present an unreasonable risk to the human subjects involved in the trial, the investigation must be terminated.

however, are of particular importance to surgical device manufacturers.

One such section of the GLP is the one pertaining to the proper preparation and maintenance of the written study protocol, which addresses why and how each test is to be conducted. If aims or conditions change during the course of the testing, the protocol must be revised, those revisions noted, and the reasons for the changes in the protocol fully explained. Another key section of the GLP concerns the characterization and handling of test and control articles (the device, system, or material under study). This section requires that the physical characteristics of the article—its strength, purity, composition, and identification—be established and documented for each batch of tested and control products. Obviously, this helps to ensure the validity of the product performance in testing. Perhaps the most pertinent section of the GLP is the one related to record-keeping and reports. The standard requires a full final report, which may be proceeded by interim reports. The final report should include complete information on the testing entities, identify and explain all changes in the protocol that occurred, and—most importantly—fully disclose all data resulting from the tests and all conclusions drawn from that data.

CURRENT PRODUCT TESTING STANDARDS FOLLOWED BY U.S. SPINAL DEVICE MANUFACTURERS

U.S. TESTING STANDARDS

There are a number of testing standards that the FDA requires for spinal fixation devices. These tests are used primarily to mechanically evaluate spinal systems to support either (1) a claim of substantial equivalence for products submitted to the 510(k) process, or (2) the preclinical characterization of implants that require an IDE and subsequent PMA. Recommended tests include strength testing to determine the point of ultimate failure of a device, fatigue testing to determine the device's endurance limits, and stability testing to measure the nondestructive rigidity of the product. The FDA encourages manufacturers to perform preclinical testing, when possible, on the entire spinal construct.[26]

The FDA's emphasis on testing "for failure," so to speak, works hand in hand with the goal of spinal manufacturers to provide product safety and effectiveness. Companies often design and enact many product tests, including those that the FDA frequently requests, as part of the product development FMEA. To clarify the changeable nature of this process, one must understand that although certain tests are common, there is no single, "absolute" way to test for any particular product characteristic. Rather, the manufacturer develops tests and testing methods, which are specific to the product, taking into account its intended use and the characteristics that the product must display for successful performance in a human subject. Thus, a company may fully and adequately test a product, in keeping with the FDA's testing requirements and recommendations, without necessarily following an exact testing schedule or agenda. Rather than undermining the validity of product testing, the nature of this process supports and underscores efforts by surgical device manufacturers to establish the safety and effectiveness of their products.

Many spinal manufacturers use the standards issued by a number of national associations. These organizations include the American Society of Testing and Materials (ASTM), the Association for the Advancement of Medical Instrumentation (AAMI), and the American National Standards Institute (ANSI). Among these standards are, for example, ASTM's Provisional Standard (PS) 5-94, which addresses issues of "construct" and "interconnection" performance in lumbar and anterior systems.

INTERNATIONAL TESTING STANDARDS

International organizations are also establishing testing, quality control, and manufacturing standards. The primary entity is the International Standards Organization (ISO). The ISO issues standards in three major areas—product, testing, and quality systems—which are denoted as ISO 9002, 9003, and 9004, respectively. Generally, "ISO 9001" is used to refer to these standards in toto.

Under the European Union's (EU) Medical Device Directive, which becomes fully effective for devices in June, 1998, manufacturers wishing to sell medical devices in the EU will be required to comply with ISO 9000 standards and attain "CE mark certification." In fact, achievement of CE mark certification will, in 1998, be imperative for companies wishing to market their products in the EU, as noncertified products will face a trade barrier.

One must keep in mind the innovative and evolving nature of today's surgical device manufacturing industry. As noted before, most of the current products have been available for less than a decade. As new designs and materials are developed, and as the global demand for quality medical products increases, the establishment of valid, quantifiable testing methods and product standards will continue to be of great interest and concern to spinal device manufacturers.

FDA REGULATION IMPACT ON SPINE SURGEONS AND PATIENTS

The complex, time-consuming, and often bureaucratic process of achieving 510(k) clearance of PMA approval of a medical device can have a significant effect on spine surgeons and their patients. The reasons for this can range from confusion over the surgeon's role in selecting devices for treatment, to delayed or reduced product availability, to surgical changes that have occurred in response to what is considered a constraining regulatory environment. The following discussion of these issues relies largely on the Wilkerson Group's 1995 report to the Health Industry Manufacturer's Association, Buckman, and Callahan.[23,26,27]

Environment Created by FDA Regulations

There is no question that FDA regulations have had a significant impact on the healthcare industry. The following summary addresses a number of associated issues, including misconceptions about the agency, and describes a number of effects that the current regulatory environment has had on product development in recent years.

Misconceptions About the FDA

There are a number of common misconceptions about the role of the FDA and the scope of its authority. Perhaps the most common one is that all legally marketed devices have been cleared by the FDA as being safe and effective for their labeled, intended use. Technically, this is true for PMA-cleared devices, but these account for only a small fraction of the legally marketed orthopedic devices on the market today. The vast majority of devices have been cleared through the 510(k) process, in which the FDA makes no general statement about the device, other than that it meets the criteria of substantial equivalence.

A second common misconception is that any device on the U.S. market has been cleared by the FDA. A device, however, may be investigational or may have been custom-produced to meet a specific surgeon's needs in a specific case.

Finally, it is commonly thought that the FDA regulates the actions of individual physicians. In point of fact, the U.S. FDA does not regulate the choice, method, or manner by which any physician treats any patient, provided that the treatment is not part of an IDE study. The FDA's sole responsibility regarding medical devices is to ensure their proper entry into the market, and the agency concerns itself only with the manufacturer's role in this process. Although a physician may lawfully use a drug or device "off label," that is, in a dosage or manner other than labeled, it is not clear whether such off-label use or other regulatory status must be disclosed by the physician to the patient.

The Medical Device Package Insert

A package insert is usually included with every cleared medical device sold in the United States. The wording and inclusion of the package insert, which discloses the product's intended use, indications and contraindications, potential adverse reactions, and the like, are closely scrutinized by the FDA. Because, however, the agency does not regulate physicians or interfere in any way with treatment decisions, many surgeons feel free to, and do, use products in nonlabeled ways. One example would be the noncemented application of a hip or knee replacement system that is labeled for cemented use only. Another example, more familiar to the spine surgeon, is the use of available bone plate or screw systems for pedicle fixation, again in an off-label use of the product. Surgeons are using these legally marketed systems in unlabeled ways to provide what has been documented to be the best patient treatment in individual cases.

This emphasis on providing the best care underlies the understood "standard of care" by which physicians operate. Standard of care means, in the simplest terms, common adherence to accepted medical practices, which are believed to offer the best outcome for the patient. By its nature, this concept can lead to off-label use, because the physician's treatment decisions are based on the needs of the patient, not on whether or not a particular device is labeled for a particular use.

PRODUCT AVAILABILITY

Perhaps the single greatest effect that FDA regulation has on spine surgeons and their patients is that manufacturers now face long delays in bringing new products to market. There are a number of factors that have slowed FDA response time in recent years, but the Wilkerson Group attributes longer review times largely to the agency's increasing focus on issues of product efficacy and clinical use, in addition to the traditional emphasis on product safety.[23] The Group's 1995 report bluntly states that the FDA now demands more rigorous product testing than ever before, with a resulting slowdown in response time for PMAs and 510(K) s, forcing manufacturers to work within an ever-more complicated, time-consuming, and costly regulatory environment.

The nominal FDA response time to submitted IDEs, 510(k)s and PMAs is 30 days, 90 days, and 180 days, respectively. In point of fact, however, the typical clearance time for a 510(k) was more than 7 months in 1994, a threefold increase over the 1989 average. The problem is not that the FDA is failing to respond to the submitted 510(k) within the allotted timeframe, but that the agency's response is often largely a request for more information. This essentially "restarts the clock" on the process. Obviously, repeated requests for additional information can greatly slow down what was originally a well-defined process. The same may be held to be true when a company attempts to receive IDE or PMA approval.

Lengthening clearance and approval processes and concerns over the regulatory process itself and product/company liability issues have affected manufacturers and the medical device market in a number of ways (as, again, documented by the Wilkerson Group):[23]

- Research and development costs have increased, sometimes to prohibitive levels. This is particularly true in the case of younger, smaller companies, many of which are involved in innovative and cutting-edge product development. Such products often cannot meet substantially equivalent standards for 510(k) clearance, and must be proceed through the (already) more rigorous and more costly PMA process. Prohibitive costs also can keep larger, established companies from developing new designs and materials, particularly if the product has a limited application and cannot be marketed to a broad enough customer base.

  Companies are less likely to expand on or improve their existing product line. The FDA may require a modified product to again complete the clearance or approval process. As might be expected, this is particularly true if the device is to be constructed of a new material, or if its intended use is to be expanded. The device may no longer meet the substantially equivalent threshold, which requires the company to work through the IDE and PMA processes.

  Some companies have moved their research and development and manufacturing operations overseas, where regulatory compliance is perhaps more straightforward and efficient. Thus, new products and technologies are introduced into foreign markets, rather than to U.S. surgeons. These products may or may not ever receive FDA clearance, and U.S. surgeons may or may not ever gain access to the devices. Obviously, this reduces treatment options in the United States to the detriment of patients in this country. The movement to produce and sell products overseas also can affect the U.S. economy as high-tech jobs and facilities are lost and money is invested and spent elsewhere. Other companies have elected to acquire facilities and companies already operating in foreign countries, thus increasing their presence in the global market and potentially opening the way for quicker worldwide distribution of their devices, without the resulting loss of jobs and funds.
- Development and introduction of innovative new surgical techniques and technologies has slowed. This prevents surgeons from learning and taking advantage of the latest medical treatments and can even force the surgeon to fall back on an existing treatment that is not likely to provide an acceptable outcome. Obviously, this is to the detriment of both the surgeon and patient.
- Managed-care operators and other private healthcare payers are increasingly pressuring surgeons to forego the use of innovative or newer treatments to contain initial costs.[35]
- The flow of venture capital into the medical devices arena has decreased because of concern over costs. Academic medical centers and research-oriented universities have been affected, as well, by loss of research dollars.
- Concern over product liability and related litigation has forced some companies to abandon work on innovative new products, to divest themselves of potentially risky business, or even to quit the medical devices arena altogether. This applies not only to manufacturers of surgical devices but also to companies that are closely allied to them. For example, some producers of raw materials who traditionally supplied medical device manufacturers have withdrawn from the market. (For example, Teflon material is no longer available to the medical industry.)[36] When this occurs, manufacturers are forced to seek, sometimes unsuccessfully, other suppliers.[37]

WHAT SURGEONS SHOULD DO

As noted throughout the previous discussion, use of a surgical device is entirely up to the discretion of the surgeon, but there are several underlying considerations that each physician should take into account when considering use of a surgical device or when performing in an investigational capacity.

- If involved in a clinical investigation, the surgeon must abide by the investigational protocol and IDE regulations. This is critical, as adherence to the protocol and regulations are closely scrutinized by the FDA, and deviation can create delays or even prevent the product from receiving market clearance. Proper patient follow-up is also critical, as a failure to do so greatly decreases the data available from the trial and its usefulness in attaining approval.[38]
- If considering use of an unfamiliar product, the surgeon should take care to study its testing, performance, and failure data closely. Only the surgeon can determine if a particular device is appropriate for use in a particular case.
- If considering use of a familiar or unfamiliar product for off-label use, again, the surgeon should closely consider available product use information before making a final determination.

TODAY'S DEVICES FOR SPINAL SURGERY

Despite, or perhaps because of, the "pioneering" aspects of the spinal device industry, a number of innovative new products are available to the surgeon.[39,40]

- Rod-and-screw systems often are used for lumbar or thoracic spinal fixation. They may be implanted by a posterior or anterior surgical approach, depending on product design and intended use. One such product offered currently on the market is the GDLH posterior spinal system used for posterior application only.[41]
- The GDLH® system uses a single-level laminar claw to enable hook fixation; the tapered hook shoes reduce intrusion into the canal space. The top-loading, top-tightening connectors provide procedural flexibility, while the threaded hook posts enable incremental segmental correction. The posts may be sheared off at connector level to ensure a low profile.[47] (Figure 26-2)
- Plate-and-screw systems may be used for fixation of the cervical, thoracic, or lumbar spine. Current device systems include the Orion anterior cervical plate system, the ZPlate-Thoracic anterior fixation system, and the ZPlate-ATL anterior fixation system, which is intended for thoracic or lumbar use.
- The Orion system offers plate lengths from 25 mm to 110 mm, a range of screwwidths, and variable screw lengths. Additionally, the Orion plate features a premachined lordotic curve for a more anatomic fit. The slotted center opening in the plate allows optional screw placement. Finally, the independent locking mechanism for the endplate screws is designed to reduce micromotion and the risk of screw back-out (Fig. 26-3).[43,44]
- The ZPlate-Thoracic and ZPlate-ATL systems are technically plate and screw devices, but they also offer many of the benefits of rod and screw systems, because of the combination of holes and slots in the plates themselves. This allows easier distraction and compression of the bone graft, using fewer components. The ATL plate is 25 mm wide, with a 1.5-inch radius of curvature, whereas the Thoracic plate is a narrower 22 mm, to fit the smaller bodies of the thoracic spine, and features a premachined kyphotic curve for a more anatomic fit. Both systems include bolts and screws in a variety of lengths for greater surgical flexibility. (Figs. 26-4 and 26-5).[45,46]
- Cable systems are used for cervical fusion. One such product is the Atlas cable system.
- The Atlas system includes three different cables, offered in titanium and stainless steel, and several components and instruments—the cable tensioner, provisional crimper, and integral bar crimp—which are part of the product. The system

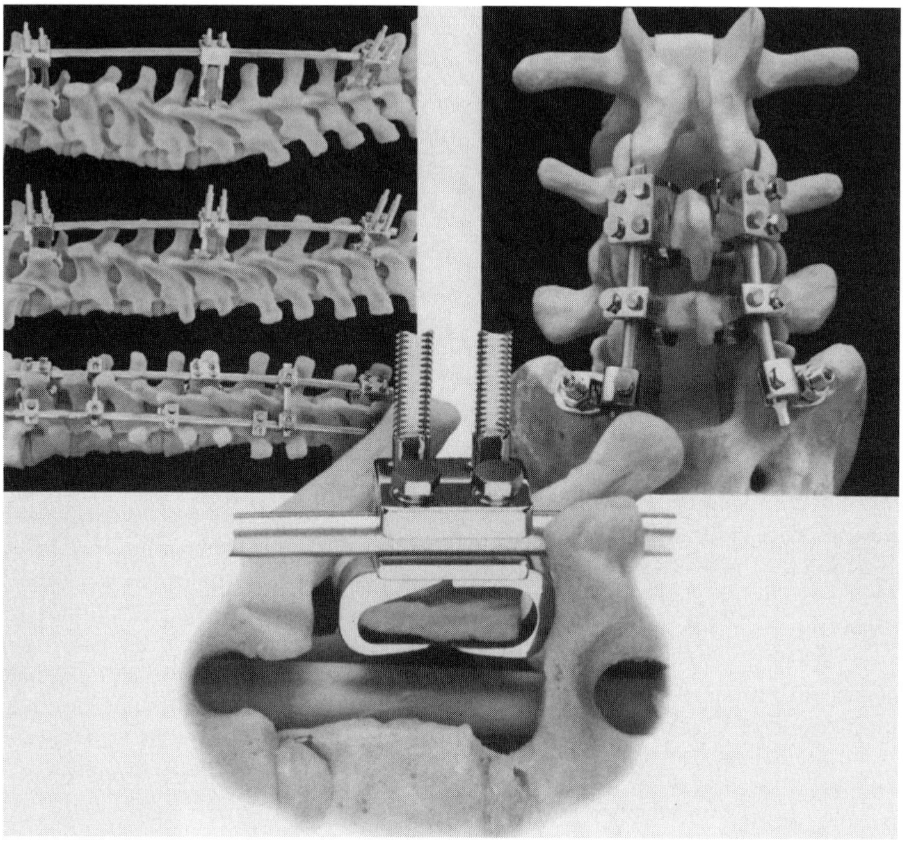

Figure 26-2

GDLH posterior spinal system. (Photo © 1994 Sofamor Danek.)

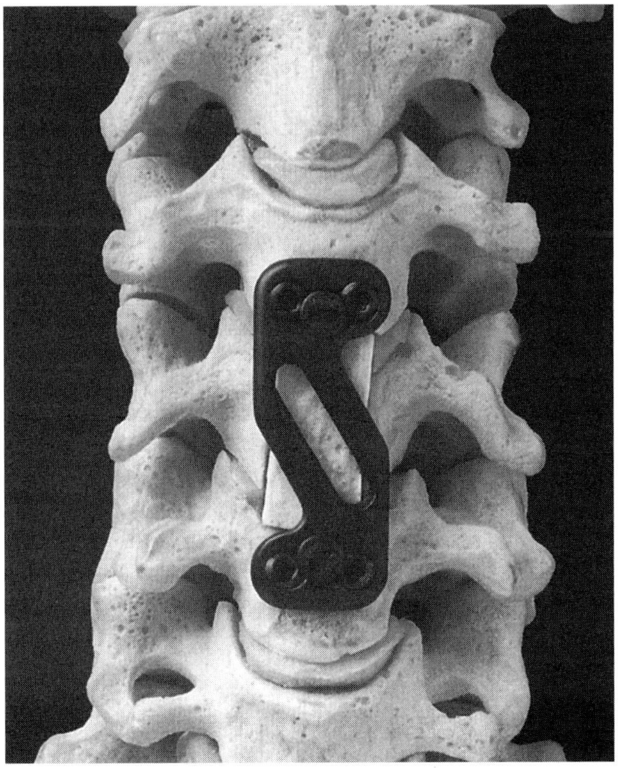

FIGURE 26-3

ORION anterior cervical plate system. (Photo © 1994 Sofamor Danek.)

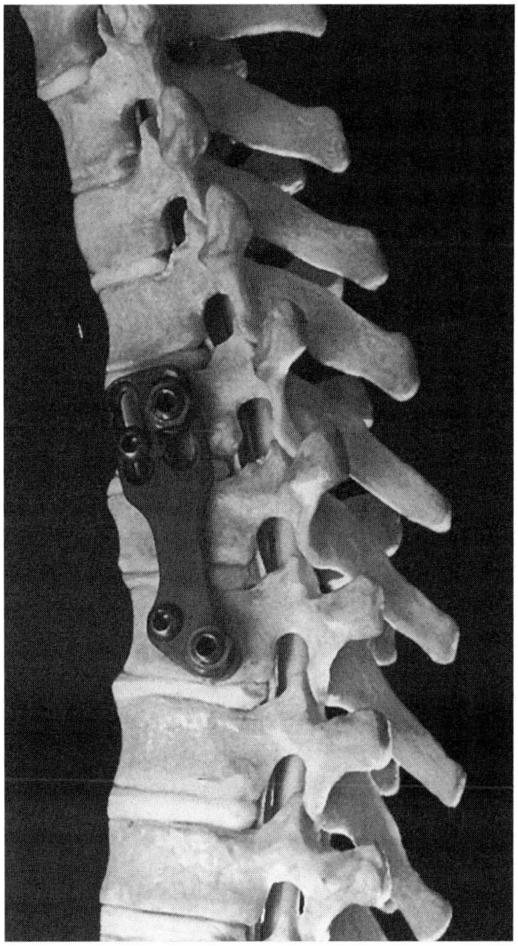

FIGURE 26-4

ZPlate-Thoracic anterior fixation system. (Photo © 1995 Sofamor Danek.)

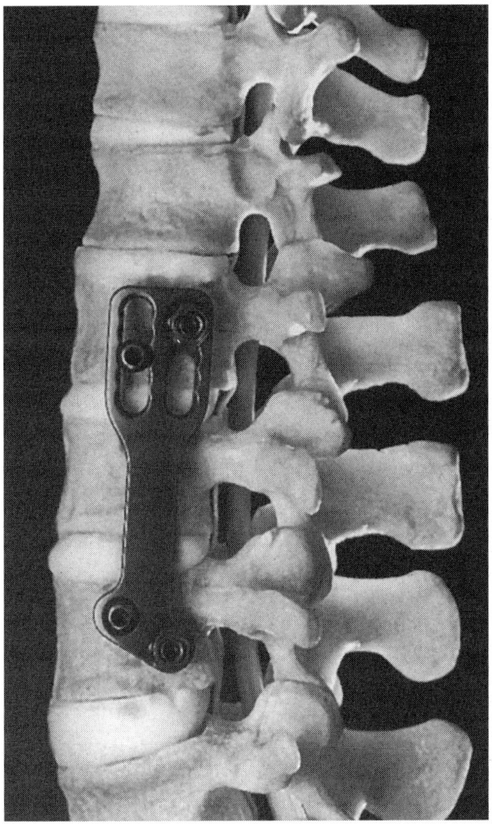

FIGURE 26-5

ZPlate-ATL anterior fixation system. (Photo © 1995 Sofamor Danek.)

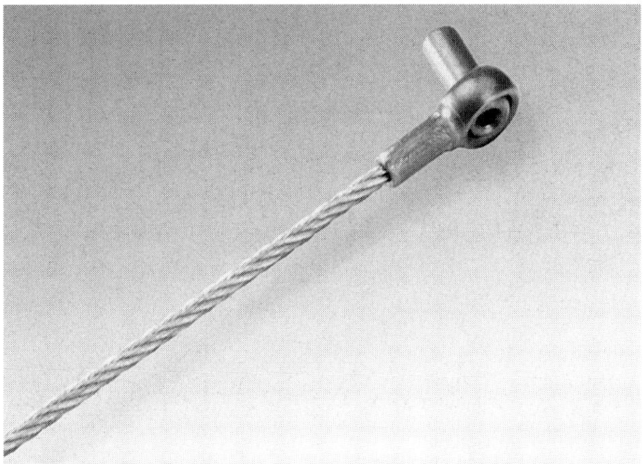

FIGURE 26-6

ALTAS cable system. (Photo © 1994 Sofamor Danek.)

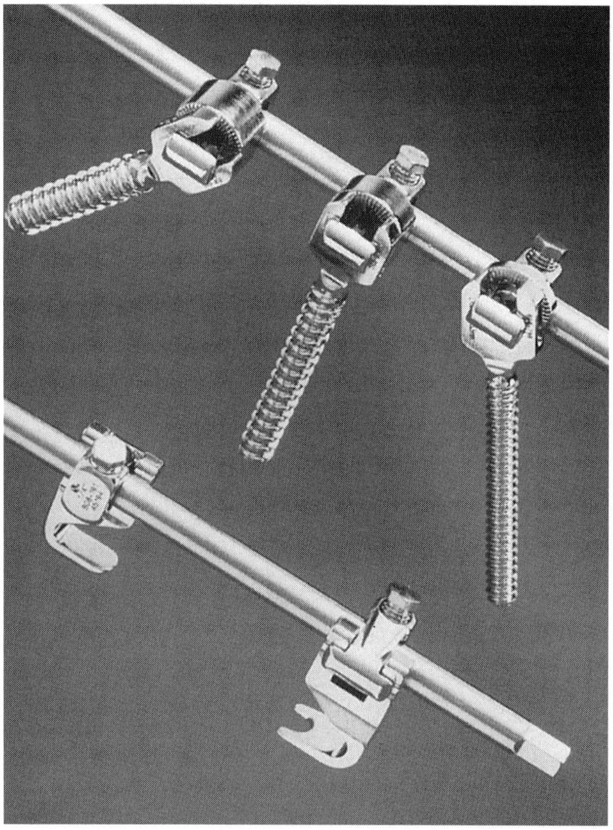

FIGURE 26-7

TSRH spinal system. (Photo © 1995 Sofamor Danek.)

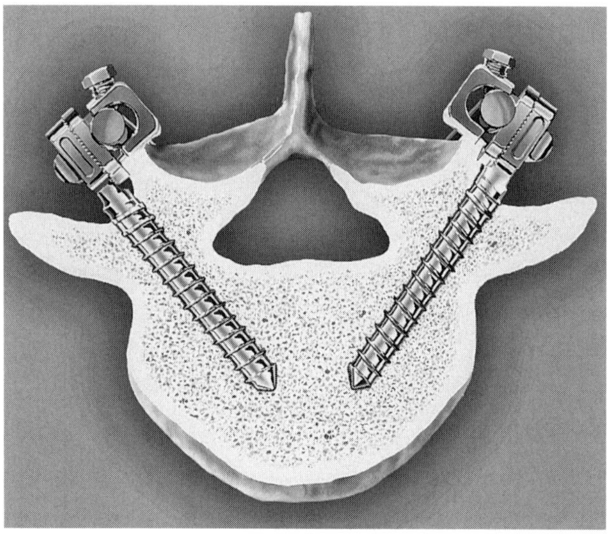

FIGURE 26-8

TSRH spinal system. (Photo © 1995 Sofamor Danek.)

is designed for surgical flexibility, strength, and control (Fig. 26-6).[47]

- Universal systems provide flexibility in addressing a wide range of spinal conditions. The TSRH® spinal system is one such offering.[48]
- The TSRH system may be used to treat deformities, degenerative conditions or trauma, or for anterior spinal fixation procedures. The system offers a variety of specialized components and component-instruments sets, including TSRH® top tightening components. The TSRH spinal system is also indicated for severe grades III and IV spondylisthesis at the L5-S1 joint (Figs. 26-7 and 26-8).[49,50,51]

FUTURE DEVICES FOR SPINAL SURGERY

Perhaps even more exciting than the development of new implant designs is the burgeoning field of biotechnology in which many spinal manufacturers are now participating. Anticipated biotechnologic advances, including biologic products and new biomaterials, are expected to provide tremendous opportunities for improvement in the treatment of spinal disorders well into the next century.

One exciting new biomaterial is Hedrocel, porous tantalum. This proprietary material has potential for broad applications in the treatment of certain spinal disorders, most notably in the manufacture of interbody fusion devices. Hedrocel material consists, essentially, of approximately 80% tantalum and 20% air. Its unique, open-pore structure was developed to provide an enhanced medium for bone growth. Not only does Hedrocel material offer the exceptional biocompatibility of tantalum, but it also can be manufactured to match more closely the modulus of elasticity of bone. Undoubtedly, the development of Hedrocel material and other new biomaterials offers significant hope for continuing advances in spinal devices and treatments.

Another exciting product that may be "just over the horizon" is a bone morphogenetic protein (BMP) delivery system. The hope is that a BMP delivery system may one day replace the need for bone grafts by helping the patient's body to regenerate bone where needed. The history of study into BMPs actually dates back to the 1960s when animal research demonstrated that demineralized bone matrix could generate the formation of ectopic bone. More recent research has resulted in the successful isolation, identification, and reproduction of a number of BMPs. Currently, companies are focusing their research on the development of an appropriate carrier that can deliver an optimum dose of the protein to the site where bone regrowth is needed.[53] Obviously, this venture holds great promise for improved treatment of spinal disorders and trauma.

As companies continue to research and develop new devices, biomaterials, and biologic products for spinal reconstruction, new surgical treatments and techniques will surely be developed. Just as certainly, surgeons will continue to apply the knowledge and skills that have been accumulated and passed down through the ages. And today's practitioners will, in turn, pass on their knowledge and skills to the next generation of spinal surgeons in the hope of benefiting them and their patients.

REFERENCES AND NOTES

1. Wiltse LL: The history of spinal disorders. In Frymoyer JW, editor: *The adult spine: principles and practice,* New York, 1991, Raven Press.
2. Albee FH: Transplantation of a portion of the tibia into the spine for Pott's disease, *JAMA* 57:885, 1911.
3. Hibbs RA: An operation for progressive spinal deformities, *NY Med J* 93:1013, 1911.
4. Gallie WE: Skeletal traction in treatment of fractures and dislocations of the cervical spine, *Ann Surg* 106:770–776, 1937.
5. Rogers WA: Treatment of fracture-dislocation of the cervical spine, *J Bone Joint Surg* 24:245–258, 1942.
6. Robinson RA, Smith GW: Anterolateral cervical disc removal and interbody fusion for cervical disc syndrome, *Bull John Hopkins Hosp* 96:233, 1955.
7. Bailey RW, Badgley CE: Stabilization of the cervical spine by anterior fusion, *J Bone Joint Surg* 42A:565–594, 1960.
8. Robinson RA, Southwick WO: Indications and techniques for early stabilization of the neck in some fracture dislocations of the cervical spine, *S Med J* 53:565–579, 1960.
9. Hodgson AR, Stock FE: Anterior spine fusion for treatment of tuberculosis of the spine, *J Bone Joint Surg* 42A:295–310, 1960.
10. Wilkins BF: Separation of the vertebrae with protrusion of hernia between the same-operation-cure, *St Louis Med Surg J* 54:340–341, 1888.
11. Venable CS, Stuck WG: Electrolysis controlling factor in the use of metals in treating fractures, *JAMA* 3(1):349, 1939.
12. Vitallium is a registered trademark of Howmedica, Inc.
13. King D: Internal fixation for lumbosacral fusion, *J Bone Joint Surg* 30A:560–565, 1948.
14. Boucher HH: A method of spinal fusion, *J Bone Joint Surg* 41B:248–259, 1959.
15. Dwyer AF, Newton NC, Sherwood AA: An anterior approach to scoliosis. A preliminary report, *Clin Orthop* 62:192–202, 1969.
16. Harrington, PR: Treatment of scoliosis: correction and internal fixation by spine instrumentation, *J Bone Joint Surg* 44A:591–610, 1962.
17. Harrington, PR: Technical details in relation to the successful use of instrumentation in scoliosis, *Orthop Clin North Am* 3(1):49–67, 1972.
18. Roy-Camille R, Roy-Camille M, Demeulenaere C: Osteosynthesis of dorsal, lumbar, and lumbosacral spine with metallic plates screwed into vertebral pedicles and articular apophyses, *Presse Med* 78:1447–1448, 1970.
19. Roy-Camille R, Saillant G, Mazel C: Internal fixation of the lumbar spine with pedicle screw plating, *Clin Orthop* 203:7–17, 1986.
20. Magerl F: *External skeletal fixation of the lower thoracic and upper lumbar spine: current concepts of external fixation of fractures,* Berlin, 1982, Springer Verlag.
21. Luque G: The anatomic basis and development of segmental spinal instrumentation, *Spine* 7:256–259, 1982.
22. Cotrel Y, Dubousset J: The use of pedicle screws and universal instrumentation for spinal fixation. Paper presented at the AO Trauma Course, Davos, Switzerland, December, 1985.
23. *Report in brief: forces reshaping the performance and contribution of the U.S. medical device industry.* Prepared for the Health Industry Manufacturers Association, The Wilkerson Group, Inc., 1995.
24. Dr. Thomas A. Zdeblick, Associate Professor of Orthopaedic Surgery, University of Wisconsin.
25. Melkerson MN, Yahiro MA, Mishra NK: Regulatory perspective for orthopedic devices. In Morrey BF, editor: *Biological, material, and mechanical considerations of joint replacement,* New York, 1993, Raven Press.
26. Callahan TJ: The process of FDA approval of a spinal implant: governmental perspective, *J Spinal Disord* 2(4):288–291, 1989.
27. Buckman, PM: Spine instrumentation and the FDA: what spine surgeons should know, *J Spinal Disord* 2(4):292–295, 1989.
28. Adulterated devices are defined under Section 501 of the Medical Device Amendments as being unsafe, defective, filthy, manufactured under unsanitary conditions, etc.
29. It is important to note that the U.S. Food and Drug Administration regulates under a number of laws, in addition to those noted above. These laws include the Federal Food, Drug, and Cosmetic Act, the Fair Packaging and Labeling Act, the Radiation Control for Health and Safety Act, and certain sections of the Public Health Service Act related to control of communicable diseases and biology products for human use.
30. Named after the applicable section of the Medical Device Amendments.
31. As Buckman stresses, the predicate device has to have

been in commercial distribution for the same intended use as the proposed device. If not, 510(k) clearance of the proposed device is not possible, and the manufacturer must proceed with the more rigorous and complex PMA process. For example, even though the use of screws in the pedicle can be documented as early as 1959, the FDA believes that except for a limited indication no fixation system intended for this specific purpose was ever commercially distributed prior to enactment of the MD Amendments. This has proven a major stumbling block in recent years to manufacturers working on pedicle screw systems, as only the PMA process was open to them; 510 (k) clearance was simply not an option.

32. Manufacturers are required to report any device-related malfunctions, serious injuries and deaths to the FDA by the Medical Device Reporting regulation, 21 Code of Federal Regulations (CFR) Part 803.
33. 21 Code of Federal Regulations (CFR) Part 812.20, Ch. 1, April 1, 1994 edition.
34. Deleted in pages.
35. In the early 1990s, delays in determining Medicare coverage of investigational devices caused cancellation of a number of clinical trials. The issue was settled in September, 1995, and Medicare now reimburses for the majority of investigational devices, and even for off-label use, if it is deemed by the patient's physician to be a medical necessity.
36. Teflon is a registered trademark of DuPont.
37. As stated above, the characteristics of a device include the material from which it is constructed, and the specifics of that material in terms of its purity, chemical composition, strength, etc. If the exact same material cannot be purchased through another supplier, and the device must be constructed of a "different" material, the manufacturer may be required to resubmit the product to the 510 (k) or PMA process. For this reason, the loss of material suppliers can affect a company's ability to keep even previously reviewed devices on the market.
38. Per Callahan, a minimum of 85% patient follow-up is desirable in an orthopedic clinical trial. Naturally, confidentiality of all patient records is maintained; only summary results are ever released by the FDA.
39. Several of the products referenced here are intended for pedicle screw use, but only in patients (a) having severe spondylolisthesis {grades 3 and 4} of the L5-S1 vertebral joint, (b) receiving fusion using autogenous bone graft only, (c) having the device fixed or attached to the lumbar and sacral spine {L3 and below}, and (d) having the device removed after the development of a solid spinal fusion mass. The FDA also stipulated that the labeling for this use bear the following warning statements:

WARNINGS

- When used as a pedicle screw system, this device system is intended only for grade 3 or 4 spondylolisthesis at the fifth lumbar–first sacral (L5-S1) vertebral joint.
- The screws of this device system are not intended for insertion into the pedicles to facilitate spinal fusions above the L5-S1 vertebral joint.
- Benefit of spinal fusions utilizing any pedicle screw fixation system has not been adequately established in patients with stable spines.
- Potential risks identified with the use of this device system, which may require additional surgery, include: device component fracture, loss of fixation, nonunion, fracture of the vertebra, neurological injury, and vascular or visceral injury.

See Warnings, Precautions, and Potential Adverse Events sections of the product's package insert for a complete list of potential risks.

40. Many of the products described herein are covered in whole or in part by U.S. patents or patents pending.
41. This product is named after the Hospital Dr. German Diaz Lombardo in Mexico City, Mexico.
42. *GDLH posterior spinal system,* 1994, Sofamore Danek.
43. *ORION anterior cervical plate system . . . the answer to cervical plate fixation,* 1995, Sofamore Danek.
44. Lowery GL: *ORION anterior cervical plate system surgical technique,* 1995, Sofamor Danek.
45. *Raising the standard . . . a little higher,* 1995, Sofamor Danek.
46. Zdeblick, TA: *ZPLATE-ATL anterior fixation systems surgical technique,* 1995, Sofamor Danek.
47. *ATLAS cable system: Evolution of the cable system for spinal applications,* 1995, Sofamor Danek.
48. This product is named after the Texas Scottish Rite Hospital for Children in Dallas, Texas.
49. *TSRH spinal system: Continuing the evolution of universal spinal instrumentation,* 1994, Sofamor Danek.
50. *TSRH spinal system: TSRH top tightening,* 1993, Sofamor Danek.
51. Simmons EH, Simmons ED Jr, Markowitz HD: *TSRH pedicle screw spinal system: severe spondylisthesis of L5-S1 grade 3 and 4 surgical technique,* 1995, Sofamor Danek.
52. Hedrocel is a registered trademark of Implex Corp. Hedrocel material is produced by Implex Corporation and is proprietary to Sofamor Danek for use of the material in spinal applications.
53. Medical Data International: Carriers for bone-growth factors, *Inside Surgery* III (5-6): 1995.

INDEX

A

Abdominal injuries, spinal surgeon evaluation of, 37
Abdominal pain, spinal cord injury, 398
Abdominal viscera, penetrating spinal trauma and, 300
Acceleration-deceleration injuries: *see also* Motor vehicle accidents
  airbags and, 98-99
  cervical symptoms after, 97
  clinical presentation of, 98-100
  diagnosis and treatment of, 101-102
  disk annular injury, 100
  esophageal hemorrhage and, 100
  headache and, 99
  long-term outcome after, 102-103
  longus colli muscle tears, 100
  normal anatomy and, 96
  soft tissue injuries to spine from, 96
  temporomandibular joint injuries, 100
Acute care after spinal injury, 3, 366
Adamkiewicz, artery of, 6
Adrenergic system, spinal spasticity and, 392
Aging and spinal cord injury, 360, 404-405
Airbags, acceleration-deceleration injuries and, 98-99
Alkaline phosphatase, 283
American Spinal Injury Association, neurologic level of injury classification, 2
Anastomotic network, in spinal canal, 6
Anatomy
  of coccyx, 239
  of sacrum, 235-236
  of spine, 6
Anesthesia
  cervical spine injury and, 148
  hypotensive, 195
  spinal trauma and, 35
Annulus, lacerated, 64
Antibiotic treatment
  prophylactic, after thoracic spine surgery, 194
  spinal cord injury and, 350
Anticonvulsive agents, 399
Antidepressant medications, 399
Aorta
  anterior thoracolumbar junction and, 23
  arterial circulation to spine and, 6
  penetrating spinal trauma and, 300
Apophyses, development of, 6
Arachnoiditis, penetrating spinal trauma and, 306
Arcuate ligament, anterior thoracolumbar junction and, 23
Arterial circulation, from posterior spinal branches, 6
Artery: *see* specific type
Ashworth scale, 390
Athletic competitions, emergency care and, 33
Atlantoaxial subluxation
  rheumatoid arthritis and, 108
  rotatory, in children, 257
Atlantooccipital joint
  fracture of, 40
  injuries, pediatric, 247
  subluxation of, 40
Atlas
  development of, 242
  injuries/fractures of, 137, 156-158
    classification of, 157
    diagnosis of, 156
    surgical management of, 158
    treatment of, 157
  rotary fixation in, 45
Atlas-dens interval, radiographic measurement of, 105
Attendant care, 3
Autonomic dysreflexia, 385-387
  clinical presentation of, 386
  etiology of, 386
  management of, 387
  pathophysiology of, 386
  spinal cord injury and, 358
Axial compression, to craniovertebral junction, 42
Axial loading injuries, 173-179
  diagnosis of, 173
  surgical management of, 173-176
  treatment of, 173
Axis
  development of, 242
  fractures of, 138
  rotary fixation in, 45
  traumatic spondylolisthesis of, 161-165

B

Baclofen
  intrathecal, 393
  spinal spasticity and, 391
Ballistics, penetrating spinal trauma and, 298
Batson's plexus, anterior surgical approach to cervical spine and, 9
Bedboard
  emergency care and, 34
  pressure sores and, 34
Biomechanics
  C1-C2 articulation and, 149
  lower cervical spine and, 150
  of cervical spine fixation, 149
  of odontoid fractures, 150
Bladder dysfunction
  neurogenic, 382
    management of, 383

Bladder dysfunction—con't
neurogenic—con't
pharmacologic management of, 384
surgical management of, 384
spinal cord injury and, 355-356
Bladder, neuroanatomy of, 382
Blood loss, during surgery, 194-195
Blood supply, to spine, 6
Body cast, 187
Bone grafts
osseous healing and, 287
surgical complications of, 279-280
Bone metabolism, pseudarthrosis and, 293
Bone morphogenetic protein delivery system, 424
Bone scintigraphy, pseudarthrosis diagnosis, 294
Botulinum toxin, for spinal spasticity, 393
Bowel function, spinal cord injury and, 356
Bowel injuries, 37
Brace: *see also* Orthoses
poster, 135
Brachiocephalic artery, anterior approach to thoracic spine and, 17
Bradycardia, quadriplegia and, 134
Brain injury
acceleration-deceleration, 96
neurologic assessment and, 34
Bullet wounds: *see* Gunshot wounds
Burst fractures
deformity after, 316
of thoracolumbar junction, 203, 206
traction for, 377

C

C1-C2 articulation, biomechanics of, 149
C1-C2, articular processes injuries, 61
C1-C4, Frankel grade A, B, C and, 3
C2 pedicle screw placement, 1567
C5-C9, Frankel grade A, B, C and, 3
C7, avulsion fracture of, 71
Callus formation, fracture healing and, 283
Calvarium, acceleration-deceleration injury and, 96
Cardiac dysrhythmia, after spinal cord injury, 374
Cardiopulmonary arrest, after spinal cord injury, 374
Cardiorespiratory resuscitation, after spinal cord injury, 350
Carotid sheath, anterior surgical approach to cervical spine and, 9
Carpal tunnel syndrome, 397
Cartilage cells, 6
Cauda equina syndrome, emergency surgery and, 37
Cautery, during costotransversectomy, 21
Cellular debris, fracture healing and, 283
Central cord hemorrhage, 83
Central cord syndrome, 71
cervical instability in children and, 107
recovery after, 351
Cerebrospinal fluid, acceleration-deceleration injury and, 96
Cervical collars, 376
Cervical fusion, posterior, 170
Cervical instability, 97
anatomic considerations in, 144
assessment and determination of, 144-145
childhood disorders at risk for, 106-107
classification of, 145-146
CT assessment of, 145
Glasgow Coma Scale and, 145
immobilization and, 134
in children
central cervical cord syndrome and, 107
Ehlers-Danlos syndrome and, 107
Grisel's syndrome and, 106
Klippel-Feil syndrome and, 107
Lesch-Nyhan syndrome, 107
mucopolysaccharidoses and, 107
odontoid hypoplasia and, 107
os odontoideum and, 107
Rubinstein-Taybi syndrome and, 107
trisomy 21 and, 106
upper respiratory infections and, 106
MRI assessment of, 145
nonsurgical management of, 134-143
operative vs. nonoperative management, 146-147
outcome studies, 146-147
radiographic assessment of, 145
radiologic evaluation of, 105
subaxial, assessment of, 145
surgical management of, 144-184
trauma classification, 146
Cervical manipulation, spinal cord injury and, 108
Cervical spine
compressive flexion injuries, 138
development of, 242
distractive flexion injury, 140
fractures/dislocations of, vertebral artery injury and, 148
Frankel classification and, 3
instability of: *see* Cervical instability
lower
anterior surgical approach to, 9
fractures/dislocations of, 138
injuries to, 62-63
posterior, surgical approach to, 13
radiography of, 39
realignment of, 35
stability of, 135
surgical approaches to
posterior, 13
retropharyngeal, 11
transoral, 11
trauma classification, 146
upper, anterior surgical approaches to, 11
vertebral arteries in, 6
vertical compression fractures of, 140
Cervical spine fixation biomechanics, 149-153
anterior instrumentation and, 150
C1-C2 articulation and, 149
occipital-cervical junction, 149
posterior instrumentation and, 151
Cervical spine injuries/trauma
anesthetic considerations in, 148
immobilization, pediatric patients, 244-245

in elderly, 311
lower, 165-172
in children, 258
surgical complications of, 276-278
surgical management of, upper, 153-165
surgical treatment of, children, 261-263
Cervicothoracic junction, fusion of, 170
Cervicothoracic spine, surgical approaches to
anterior cervicothoracic junction, 17
transsternal, 17
Chance fractures, 79
of lumbar spine, 217
Charcot arthropathy, 317
Chest tube, pneumothorax prevention and, 20
Children
atlantoaxial rotatory subluxation in, 257
atlantooccipital injuries, 247
battered
intraocular bleeding and, 261
spinal injuries in, 258-261
subdural hematoma and, 261
whiplash shaken baby syndrome and, 258
cervical instability in, 105-107
central cervical cord syndrome and, 107
Ehlers-Danlos syndrome and, 107
Grisel's syndrome and, 106
Klippel-Feil syndrome and, 107
Lesch-Nyhan syndrome, 107
mucopolysaccharidoses and, 107
odontoid hypoplasia and, 107
os odontoideum and, 107
Rubinstein-Taybi syndrome and, 107
trisomy 21 and, 106
upper respiratory infections and, 106
cervical spine injuries in, surgical treatment of, 261-263
halo fixation in, 261
hangman's fractures in, 252
odontoid fractures in, 251
rotary fixation in, 45
slipped vertebral apophysis, 269
spinal cord injury
after minor trauma and, 105
long-term sequelae of, 272
without radiographic abnormality, 256
spinal development, 242-243
spinal embryology, 242-243
spinal fractures/injuries, 250-251
diagnosis and management of, 241-275
immobilization and transport, 244-245
incidence and demography of, 241
Jefferson, 250-251
spinal pathoanatomy and, 243-244
spondylolysis, 81
spondylosis of C2 in, 252
thoracolumbar spine injuries in, 263-271
compression fractures, 266
flexion-distraction, 266
fracture dislocations, 266
traumatic spondylolysis in, 270
vertebral anomalies/trauma, 254-256
Chondroblasts, fracture healing and, 283
Circulation
arterial, of spine, 6
venous, of spine, 6
Circulatory injuries, spinal surgeon evaluation of, 37
Clay-shovelers' fracture, 71
Cobb elevators, 20
Coccydynia
diagnosis of, 239-239
falls and, 239
treatment of, 240
Coccygeal pain
evaluation of, 239
treatment of, 240
Coccyx
anatomy of, 239
fractures of, 235-240
pressure sores and, 34
Comminuted fractures, fracture healing and, 288
Complications: *see* Surgical complications
Compression fractures
adolescent kyphosis and, 75
deformity after, 316
of C1, radiography of, 43
of thoracolumbar spine, 203, 206
in children, 266
Scheuermann's disease and, 75
vertical, 140
Computed tomography
acceleration-deceleration injuries, 101
C1-C2 articular process injuries, 62
cervical instability assessment, 145
craniooccipital facets anatomy, 41
dens fractures, 46
disk herniation and, 91
distraction-flexion injuries, 63-67
hyperextension fractures of lumbar spine, 79-81
intraspinal epidural hematoma and, 36
Jefferson fracture, 43
late deformity after spinal trauma, 321
pediatric spinal injury, 245
penetrating spinal trauma, 87-88, 300-303
pseudarthrosis diagnosis, 294
sacral fractures, 236
SCI after minor trauma, 105
spinal
injury evaluation, 35, 39, 82
technique of, 40
spondylolysis, 81
stress fractures, 82
thin section, spinal anatomy and, 39
upper thoracic spine fractures, 187
Concussion, 33
Corticosteroids, 34
Costotransversectomy, 21, 23, 193
Craniocervical region
burst fractures of, 67
clay-shovelers' fracture and, 71
compression injuries of, 67-70
distraction injuries to, 63
distraction-flexion injuries of, 63-67
flexion injuries in, 63-67

Craniocervical region—con't
fractures of, 61-75
hyperextension injuries, 70-73
Cranio-occipital facets, 41
Craniovertebral junction
axial compression of, 42
dislocation of, 40
embryology of, 56
Cranium, dural sinuses in, 6
Crus, anterior thoracolumbar junction and, 23

D

Dean's injury sequelae, 101
Decompression
after spinal cord injury, 332-335
historical results of, 332
anterior cervical, complications of, 148
anterior, axial loading injuries and, 173-176
epidural hematoma and, 36
penetrating spinal trauma and, 303-305
surgical, timing of, 147-148
upper thoracic spine fractures, 188
Deep venous thrombosis
after spinal cord injury, 134
multisystem injuries and, 37
spinal cord injury and, 388
Deformities after spinal trauma, 315-330
burst fractures and, 316
Charcot arthropathy and, 317
classification of, 322
complications, 327
compression fractures and, 316
computed tomography evaluation of, 321
kyphosis and, 316
operative treatment of, 324-329
pathomechanics of, 315-319
patient evaluation, 319-322
seat belt injuries and, 317
treatment of, 322-324
Degenerative disk disease, 88
Denis classification system for spinal fractures, 201
Dens
fractures of, 46
Jefferson fracture and, 43
pseudarthrosis, os odontoideum and, 53
subluxation of, 56
Diaphragmatic pleura, anterior approach to thoracolumbar junction and, 21
Disability, 371
Disk avulsion, 98
Disk herniation
incidence in general population, 91
trauma and, 88
with unstable spinal injuries, 165
Diskography, pseudarthrosis diagnosis, 294
Dissection
during costotransversectomy, 21
pulse identification and, 10
subperiosteal, 19
Distraction injuries of craniocervical region, 63
Distraction-flexion injuries, 63-67, 140
Down syndrome: *see* Trisomy 21
Dural sinuses, 6
Dural tears
after spinal trauma, 335-339
clinical presentation of, 335
etiology of, 335
repair techniques, 336
during thoracic spine surgery, 195

E

Ecchymosis, long-bone fractures and, 35
Economic impact of spinal cord injury, 2
Edema
long-bone fractures and, 35
traction and, 36
Ehlers-Danlos syndrome, 107
Elbows, pressure sores and, 34
Elderly
spinal injuries in, 310-314
cervical, 311
epidemiology of, 311
lumbar, 312
management of, 310
thoracic, 312
traumatic spinal cord injury in, 313
Electrical stimulation, fracture healing and, 286
Electroencephalogram, evoked potentials and, 120
Electromyography
motor root monitoring and, 130
spinal cord monitoring and, 130
Embryology, 6
of spine, 242-243
Emergency care
athletic competitions and, 33
bedboard and, 34
decompression for intraspinal epidural hematoma, 36
musculoskeletal examination and, 35
of spine trauma, 33
pressure sores and, 34
spinal cord injury, corticosteroids and, 34
spinal stabilization, 36
spinal surgery, 36
cauda equina syndrome and, 37
epidural hematoma and, 37
Emergency department, triage in, 33
Emergency medical services, 3
spinal cord injury and, 366
Endochondral ossification, fracture healing and, 284
Endothelial cell-derived growth factor, 283
Environmental modifications, 3
Epidermal growth factor, fracture healing and, 283
Epidural hematoma, intraspinal, decompression and, 36
Epidural veins, anterior surgical approach to cervical spine and, 9
Equipment needs
after spinal cord injury, 380
for tetraplegics, 380
Equipment, durable, 3
Erector spinae muscles, during costotransversectomy, 21

Esophageal hemorrhage, acceleration-deceleration injuries and, 100
Esophageal hiatus, anterior thoracolumbar junction and, 23
Esophagus
  anterior surgical approach to cervical spine and, 9
  position of, 10
Evaluation, severity of SCI, 2
Evoked potentials
  electrophysiologic basis of, 120-121
  monitoring
    during spine surgery, 119
    general principles of, 121-122
    waveform generation and nomenclature, 123-125
  motor, 119, 126-131
    spinal cord stimulation and, 128
  somatosensory, 119
    intraoperative monitoring of, 122
  wake-up test and, 125
Extremities
  peripheral fractures in, 35
  ranging of, 37

F

Facet dislocation
  bilateral, 171-172
  unilateral, 171
Facet dislocation/subluxation, intervertebral disk injury and, 64
Falls
  coccydynia and, 239
  spinal cord injury after, 2, 105
Fetus, spinal development, 6
Fever, multisystem injuries and, 37
Fibroblasts, fracture healing and, 283
Finochietto rib retractors, 19
Fistula, traumatic, penetrating spinal trauma, 306
Fixation
  internal, fracture healing and, 286-287
  rotary, 45
Flat-back syndrome, 214
Flexion injuries
  compressive, 138
  of craniocervical region, 63-67
Flexion-distraction injuries
  of thoracolumbar junction, 207
  of thoracolumbar spine, in children, 263
Food and Drug Administration, surgical device regulation, 417-419
Foraminotomy, 178
Fracture dislocation
  of thoracolumbar junction, 207
  of thoracolumbar spine, children, 266
Fracture healing, 283
  cellular debris and, 283
  complications of, 288
  electrical stimulation and, 286
  fibroblasts and, 283
  inflammatory phase of, 283
  internal fixation and, 286-287
  lymphocytes and, 283
  macrophages and, 283
  mediators of, 285-286
  mesenchymal cells and, 283
  modeling phase, 284
  necrotic tissue and, 283
  osteoblasts and, 283
  polymorphonuclear cells and, 283
  rapid acceleration process and, 285
  remodeling and, 284
  reparative phase, 283
Fracture pattern, lumbar spine, 215
Fractures: *see also* specific type
  comminuted, fracture healing and, 288
  long-bone, 35
  peripheral, of extremities, 34
  spinal: *see* Spinal fractures
Frankel Neurologic Classification, spinal cord injury costs and, 3
Functional assessment, after spinal cord injury, 368-372, 371-372
Functional outcomes, after spinal cord injury, 379
Fusion
  axial loading injuries and, 173-176
  nonsteroidal antiinflammatory medications and, 293
  osteoconduction and, 291
  osteoinduction and, 291
  process of, 291

G

Gamma-amino butyric acid, spinal spasticity and, 391
Gangliosides, spinal trauma and, 332
Gastrointestinal disturbances, 375, 385
GDLH system, 422
Gestation, spinal development during, 6
Glasgow Coma Scale, 145
Gliosis, intrinsic, 84
Glycosphingolipids, 332
Grafts: *see* Bone grafts
Grisel's syndrome, 106
Gunshot wounds
  bullet removal and, 304
  characteristics of, 298
  emergency care and, 33
  lead toxicity and, 305
  patient evaluation, 300-303
  spinal cord injury resulting from, 2, 188-189
    costs of, 3
  velocity effects on tissue damage, 188
  wound ballistics, 298

H

Halo device, 135
Halo fixation, in children, 261
Halo vest management, 146
Handicap, 371
Hangman's fractures, 56-61
  immobilization and, 138

Hangman's fractures—con't
  pediatric, 252
  traction for, 377
Head trauma, physical examinations and, 35
Headache, acceleration-deceleration injuries and, 99
Health care expenditures
  of spinal cord injury, 3
  public concern, 1
Health maintenance organization
  spending reductions and, 1
  spinal cord injury and, 1
Heart disease, spinal cord injury and, 404
Heart, anterior approach to thoracolumbar junction and, 21
Hedrocel, 424
Hematoma, drain placement for prevention of, 11
Herniation, acute nuclear, 64
Heterotopic ossification, spinal cord injury and, 359, 396-397
HMO: *see* Health maintenance organization
Hyperextension fractures/injuries, 70-73, 176-179
  diagnosis of, 101-102, 176-177
  of lumbar spine, 79-81
  surgical management of, 178-179
  treatment of, 101-102, 177
Hyperflexion injury, 168-170
  diagnosis of, 168
  surgical management of, 170
  treatment of, 168
Hyperreflexia, spinal cord injury and, 358
Hypoperfusion, traction and, 36
Hypotension, multisystem injuries and, 37

I

Iatrogenic injuries, to vertebral artery, 148
Immobilization
  after spinal injury, 135
    children, 244-245
  cervical instability and, 134
  fracture of atlas and, 137
  fracture of axis and, 138
  halo device and, 135
  lower cervical fractures/dislocations and, 138
  odontoid fractures and, 137
  Philadelphia collar and, 135
  poster brace and, 135
  types of, 135-136
Impairment, 371
Infection
  bladder, 356
  fracture healing and, 288
  penetrating spinal trauma and, 305
  pharyngeal wound, 11
  pressure sores and, 34
  retropharyngeal approach to cervical spine and, 12
  urinary tract, 384
Inferior vena cava
  anterior thoracolumbar junction and, 23
  penetrating spinal trauma and, 300
Intercostal artery
  during costotransversectomy, 21
  ligation of, 6
  spinal circulation and, 6
Intercostal muscles, anterior approach to thoracic spine and, 19
Intercostal nerve
  anterior approach to thoracic spine and, 19
  during costotransversectomy, 21
Intercostal vein, anterior thoracolumbar junction and, 23
Interleukin 1, fracture healing and, 283
Internal fixation, 286-287
Internal iliac arteries, 6
Interspinous fixation, 170
Intervertebral disk
  cervical spine radiograph, 10
  excision of, 11
  facet dislocation/subluxation and, 64
Intoxication, neurologic assessment and, 34
Intraabdominal injury, penetrating spinal trauma and, 300
Intramedullary hemorrhage, MRI appearance of, 82
Irrigation during transoral approach to cervical spine, 11

J

Jefferson fractures
  dens and, 43
  pediatric, 250-251
  radiograph of, 43
  traction for, 377
Jewett and Taylor braces, 187
Joint capsular injury, 100
Joint contractures, 401-402

K

Kidney
  dysfunction, spinal cord injury and, 382
  penetrating spinal trauma and, 300
Klippel-Feil syndrome, 255
  cervical instability in children and, 107
Kyphosis
  adolescent, compression fracture and, 75
  after spinal fracture, 316
  pressure sores and, 34

L

Laminectomy, 178, 303
Larynx, anterior surgical approach to cervical spine and, 9
Lateral mass plates, 170
Lead toxicity, gunshot wounds and, 305
Lesch-Nyhan syndrome, cervical instability in children and, 107
Life support, emergency care and, 34
Ligation of intercostal artery, 6
Liver injuries, 37
Longitudinal ligament, posterior, ossification of, 108
Longus colli muscle, subperiosteal reflection of, 10

Lower extremity fractures, spinal cord injury and, 395
Lumbar artery, spinal circulation and, 6
Lumbar lordosis, 117
Lumbar spine
  deformities, 214
    after spinal trauma and, 325
  development of, 242
  flat-back syndrome and, 214
  flexion injuries of, 75-79
  Frankel classification and, 3
  lumbar arteries in, 6
  radiography of, 39
  spondylolysis of, 81-82
  surgical approaches to
    anterior, 25
    anterior lumbosacral, 27
    paraspinal, 31
    retroperitoneal, 25, 27
    transperitoneal, 25
    Wiltse, 31
  wedge compression fracture of, 75-79
Lumbar spine fractures/injuries, 214-232
  classification of, 217-220
  diagnosis of, 214-215
  fracture pattern of, 215
  hyperextension, 79-81
  in elderly, 312
  load-sharing classification system, 220
  neurologic status and, 215
  nonoperative treatment of, complications of, 225
  operative treatment of, 225-232
    anterior vs. posterior surgery, 226-232
    considerations for, 222
    indications for, 225-226
  operative vs. nonoperative treatment of, 220-225
    neurologic factors, 220-225
  osteoporotic, 215-216
    treatment of, 225
  stress, 81-82
  surgical complications of, 279
  treatment of, 215-220
Lumbocostal arch, anterior approach to thoracolumbar junction and, 23
Lumbocostal trigone, anterior thoracolumbar junction and, 23
Lumbosacral spine, surgical approaches to
  anterior, 27
  posterior, 29
Lymphocytes, fracture healing and, 283

M

Macrophages, fracture healing and, 283
Magnetic resonance imaging
  acceleration-deceleration injuries, 101
  central cord syndrome and, 71
  cervical instability assessment, 145
  compression injuries of craniocervical region, 67
  disk herniation and, 91
  distraction injuries craniocervical region, 64
  hyperextension injuries, 71
  intramedullary hemorrhage and, 82
  Jefferson fracture, 43
  pediatric spinal injury, 245
  penetrating wounds of spine and, 87-88
  progressive posttraumatic myelomalacic myelopathy, 84
  sacral fractures, 236-237
  spinal cord injury
    after minor trauma, 105
    diagnosis, 82-87
  spinal cord swelling, 82
  spinal injury, 331
    diagnosis, 39
    evaluation, 35
    technique of, 40
  wedge compression fracture of lumbar spine, 77
  wedge deformity and, 75
Mayfield horseshoe, 117
McAfee classification system, 201
Median raphe, posterior approach to cervical spine and, 13
Medical devices: *see also* Spinal devices; Surgical devices
  FDA regulations and, 420
  package inserts, 420
  product availability, 420
Medico-legal claims
  disk herniation and, 88-91
  spinal injury and, 88-91
Meningitis, transoral approach to cervical spine and, 11
Mentation problems, acceleration-deceleration injuries and, 99
Mesenchymal cells, 283
Methylprednisolone, 34
Microscope, operative, during transoral approach to cervical spine, 11
Minerva orthosis, 376-377
Motor function, spinal cord and, 2
Motor vehicle accidents: *see also* Acceleration-deceleration injuries
  emergency care and, 33
  hangman's fractures and, 61
  long-term outcome after, 102-103
  mechanism of trauma, 97-98
  prevention of, 2
  soft tissue injuries to spine and, 96
  spinal cord injury and, 2
  whiplash and, incidence rates, 97
MRI: *see* Magnetic resonance imaging
Multisystem injury, 33
Muscle necrosis, 34
Musculoskeletal conditions, spinal cord injury and, 400-401
Musculoskeletal examination, 35
Myelography
  intraspinal epidural hematoma and, 36
  sacral fractures, 237
  spinal cord injury diagnosis, 82
Myelopathy
  posttraumatic cystic, 359, 403-404
  progressive posttraumatic myelomalacic, 84
Myotome, 369

N

Narcotic drugs, 399
Nasotracheal tube, 12
National Spinal Cord Injury Model System Database, 1
  SCI epidemiology and, 1
Neck, numbness/neuroma of, 13
Necrosis
  muscle, 34
  skin, 34
Necrotic tissue, fracture healing and, 283
Neural compromise, 77
Neural structure injury, 82-87
Neurologic assessment
  after spinal cord injury, 135, 368-372
  brain injury and, 34
  intoxication and, 34
  penetrating spinal trauma and, 300
  sacral fractures and, 237
Neurologic category, 2
Neurologic compression, surgical decompression and, 147-148
Neurologic compromise, intraoperative, prevention of, 195
Neurologic condition
  changes in, 35
  noncontiguous fractures and, 35
Neurologic deterioration
  emergency spinal surgery and, 36
  intraspinal epidural hematoma and, 36
  penetrating spinal trauma and, 305
Neurologic injury, prevention of, 37
Neurologic level of injury, 2, 369
Neurologic recovery, 2
Neurophysiologic monitoring, during spine surgery, 119-133
  requirements for, 119
Neuropraxia, upper extremity, 117
Neurosurgical procedures, 331-344
Nonsteroidal antiinflammatory medications, pseudarthrosis and, 293
Notochord forms, 6

O

Occipital condyle
  compression of, 42
  fracture of, diagnosing, 41
Occipital-cervical junction, biomechanics of, 149
Occipitoatlantal injury, 136
Occipitocervical dissociation, 153
  classification and treatment of, 153
  diagnosis of, 153
  surgical management of, 154
Occipitocervical screw-plate fixation, 154
Occipital condyle fractures, 153
Odontoid fractures, 137, 159-161
  biomechanics of, 150
  classification of, 159
  diagnosis of, 159
  in children, 251
  operative vs. nonoperative management, 146
  surgical management of, 160
  traction for, 377
  treatment of, 160
Odontoid hypoplasia, 107
Opioids, 399
Orion system, 422
Oropharynx, preparation for surgery of, 11
Orthopedic Trauma Association, cervical spine trauma classification, 146
Orthoses
  cervical, 376-377
  cervical-thoracic, 376-377
  Minerva, 376-377
  spinal, 376-379
  thoracolumbosacral, 377
Orthostatic hypotension, spinal cord injury and, 387-388
Os odontoideum, 53
  cervical instability in children and, 107
  dens pseudarthrosis and, 53
Osseous healing
  bone grafts and, 287
  complications of, 288
  electrical stimulation and, 286
  in spinal injuries, 283-290
  spinal fusion and, 287
Ossific nuclei, 6
Osteoarthritis, spinal cord injury and, 108
Osteoblasts
  fracture healing and, 283
  spinal fracture and, 283
Osteoconduction, 291
Osteoinduction, 291
Osteoporosis
  lumbar spine fractures and, 215-216
  spinal cord injury and, 395
  wedge deformity and, 75
Osteoprogenitor cells, 284

P

Pain
  categories of, 397
  electronic stimulation for, 399
  functional electrical stimulation, 399
  in viscera, 398
  medications for, 399
  neurogenic, 397
  nociceptive, 398
  of neurogenic origin, 398
  penetrating spinal trauma and, 305
  psychologic treatment for, 399
  radicular, 398
  segmental, 398
  spinal cord injury and, 397-400
  surgical treatment for, 400
Pancreas, injuries to, 37
Paraparesis, 369
Paraplegia, 369

- complete, 2
- incidence of, 2
- incomplete, 2

Paraspinal muscles, during costotransversectomy, 21
Paresis, flaccid, 37
Pars, fracture of, 81
Pathoanatomy of spine, 243-244
Patient positioning
- during spinal surgery, 111-118
  - lateral decubitus position, 113-116
  - prone position, 113
  - supine position, 112-113
- surgical management of spinal trauma, 111-118

Patients, surgical devices and, FDA regulation impact on, 419-420
Pedicle development, 6
Penetrating spinal trauma, 87-88, 298-309
- arachnoiditis and, 306
- complications of, 305-306
- decompression and, 303-305
- epidemiology of, 298
- infection and, 305
- injury characteristics, 298
- lead toxicity and, 305
- neurologic deterioration and, 305
- neurologic injury and, 302
- neurologic recovery after, 302
- pain and, 305
- patient evaluation, 300-303
- spinal stability and, 302
- surgical complications and, 281
- surgical evaluation, 303-305
- syrinx and, 306
- traumatic fistula and, 306
- wound ballistics, 298

Perforators, spinal blood supply and, 6
Pericardium, 21
Pharyngeal wound infection, 11
Phenol, for spinal spasticity, 394
Philadelphia collar, 135
Phrenic nerves, anterior approach to thoracolumbar junction and, 21
Physical therapy, 102
Platelet-derived growth factor, 283
Pneumothorax, 20
Polymorphonuclear cells, 283
Poster brace, 135
Pressure sores, 402
- classification of, 402
- common locations of, 402
- emergency care and, 34
- pathophysiology of, 402
- prevention of, 402
- treatment of, 403

Pretracheal fascia, 10
Prevention of spinal cord injury, 4
Prevertebral fascia, blunt dissection of, 10
Prevertebral fat line, displacement of, 69
Productivity loss, 4
Progressive posttraumatic myelomalacic myelopathy, 84
Proteinases, 283
Pseudarthrosis, 291-297
- causation of, 293
- classification of, 292
- clinical significance of, 292
- definition of, 291
- dens, 53
- diagnosis of, 293
- histology of, 291
- incidence of, 295
- osteoconduction and, 291
- osteoinduction and, 291
- prevention of, 296
- surgical diagnosis of, 294
- treatment of, 295

Psoas major, 23
Psoas minor, 23
Psychotropic drugs, 399
Pulmonary embolism, multisystem injuries and, 37
Pyelonephritis, spinal cord injury and, 355

Q

Quadratus lumborum, anterior thoracolumbar junction and, 23
Quadriparesis, 369
Quadriplegia, 369
- bradycardia and, 134

R

Radicular arteries, 6
Radicular problems, evaluation of, 102
Radiography
- acceleration-deceleration injuries, 101
- ankylosing spondylitis, 107-108
- atlas-dens interval measurement, 105
- cervical instability assessment, 145
- cervical spine stability assessment, 135
- Chance fracture and, 79
- craniovertebral junction, 56
  - dislocation of, 40
- distraction-flexion injuries, 63-67
- during traction, 36
- hangman's fractures, 61
- Jefferson fracture, 43
- lateral cervical spine, 10
- lateral compression fracture of C1, 43
- os odontoideum and, 53
- patient transferring and, 111
- prevertebral fat line displacement, 69
- pseudarthrosis diagnosis, 294
- rotary subluxation, 45
- sacral fractures, 236
- spinal injury
  - diagnosis, 39
  - pediatric, 245
- spinal instability and, 35
- thoracolumbar injuries and, 73
- thoracolumbar spine fractures, 200

Radiography—con't
  torticollis and, 45
  upper cervical instability, in children, 105
  upper thoracic spine fractures, 187
Radiologist, spinal surgeon and, 39
Rapid acceleration process, 285
Reflex sympathetic dystrophy, 397
Rehabilitation, 3
  after spinal cord injury, 350, 365-413, 379
    comprehensive, 367
    model systems of care, 366
  after thoracic spine fractures, 194
Rehospitalization, 3
Respiratory complications
  infections, cervical instability in children and, 106
  insufficiency, after spinal cord injury, 374
  of spinal cord injury, 388
Retraction, during transoral approach to cervical spine, 11
Retractors
  blunt, 10
  Finochietto rib, 19
  McGarver, 11
  rib spreading, 19
Rheumatoid arthritis, 108
Ribs, anterior thoracolumbar junction and, 23
Ring curettes, 20
Risser jacket, 187
Rotary fixation, 45
  diagnosis of, 46
Rotary subluxation, 45
Rubinstein-Taybi syndrome, cervical instability in children and, 107

S

Sacral fractures, 235-240
  classification of, 237-238
  computed tomography of, 236
  imaging of, 236-237
  MRI of, 236-237
  myelography of, 237
  neurologic evaluation of, 237
  neurologic injuries and, 237
  occult insufficiency, 238
  radiography of, 236
  tomography of, 236
  treatment of, 238-239
Sacral spine
  Frankel classification and, 3
  sacral artery in, 6
Sacrum, anatomy of, 235-236
Scalp, numbness/neuroma of, 13
Scapulae, pressure sores and, 34
Scheuermann's disease, 75
Schmorl's node type lesions, 75
SCI: *see* Spinal cord injury
Scintigraphy, pseudarthrosis diagnosis, 294
Sclerotomes development, 6
Seat belt fractures/injuries, 77
  deformity after, 317
Segmental artery, 6
Sensory level, 369
Sexual functioning, 360
Shoulder harnesses, 98
Skeletal injury classifications, 145
Skin necrosis, 34
Smith-Robinson extension, 190
Smoking, pseudarthrosis and, 293
Soft tissue trauma: *see* Whiplash
Somite development, 6
Spasticity, 389-393
  adrenergic system and, 392
  evaluation of, 390
  GABA system and, 391
  injection therapy for, 393
    botulinum toxin, 393
    phenol and, 394
  intrathecal baclofen and, 393
  peripherally acting agents and, 392
  pharmacologic management of, 391
  spinal cord injury and, 356
  surgical treatment for, 395
  treatment of, 391
Spinal anatomy, acceleration-deceleration injury and, 96
Spinal cord
  function, Glasgow Coma Scale and, 145
  reaction to traumatic injury, 345-349
  stimulation of, motor evoked potentials and, 128
  swelling, MRI appearance of, 82
Spinal cord injury
  acute care after, 366
  acute management of, 373-376
  acute phase case, 352
  after minor trauma, 105-110
    in adults, 107-109
    in children, 105
    misdiagnosis of, 105
  aging and, 360, 404-405
  autonomic dysreflexia and, 358, 385-387
    clinical presentation of, 386
    etiology of, 386
    management of, 387
    pathophysiology of, 386
  bowel function and, 356
  cardiac dysrhythmia and, 374
  cardiopulmonary arrest and, 374
  causes of, 2
  cervical manipulation and, 108
  cervical, surgical complications of, 276-278
  Charcot arthropathy after, 317
  children, long-term sequelae of, 272
  chronic phase of, 354
  clinical syndrome of, 370-371
  closed management of, 347
  corticosteroids and, 34
  costs of, 1, 2
  decompression after, 332-335
    historical results of, 332
  decubitus ulceration and, 355
  deep venous thrombosis and, 134, 388
  economic impact of, 2
  elderly patients with, 310
  emergency medical services, 366

epidemiology of, 1, 367
etiology of, 368
evaluation of, 2
extremity complications and, 359
falls and, 2
Frankel Neurologic Classification and, 3
functional assessment of, 368-372, 371-372
functional outcomes after, 379
future implications, 4
gangliosides and, 332
gastrointestinal problems and, 375, 385
gunshot wounds and, 2, 188-189
health care expenditures and, 1
heterotopic ossification and, 359, 396-397
history of, 345
immobilization after, 135
in adults, 107-109
in children, without radiographic abnormality, 256
incidence of, 1
incomplete, syndromes of, 145
indirect costs of, 4
initial treatment of, 134
joint contractures and, 401-402
kidney dysfunction and, 382
long-term survival after, 404-405
lower extremity fractures and, 395
medical complications after, 373
methylprednisolone and, 34
mobility loss in, 37
motor vehicle accidents and, 2
MRI diagnosis of, 82-87
multisystem involvement and, 37
muscle function loss in, 37
musculoskeletal conditions associated with, 400-401
neurogenic bladder dysfunction, 382
  management of, 383
  pharmacologic management of, 384
  surgical management of, 384
neurologic assessment, 135, 368-372
neurologic level of injury, 2
neurologic recovery after, 352
occipitoatlantal injury and, 136
orthopedic vs. neurosurgical management of, 345
orthoses and, 376-379
orthostatic hypotension and, 387-388
osseous healing in, 283-290
osteoporosis and, 395
pain and: *see under* Pain
pathophysiology of, 346
penetrating spinal trauma and, 303-305
posttraumatic cystic myelopathy and, 359, 403-404
pressure sores and, 402-403
prevention of, 1, 367
psoriatic spondylitis and, 108
quality of life and, 1
recovery and functional outcome after, 350-362
rehabilitation after, 365-413, 379
respiratory complications and, 388
respiratory insufficiency during, 374
rheumatoid arthritis and, 108
scope of, 1
secondary problems associated with, 355-362
severity of, 2
sexual function and, 360
spasticity and, 356, 389-393
  evaluation of, 390
  pharmacologic management of, 391
  treatment of, 391
surgical intervention, 347-349
  timing of, 147-148
syringomyelia and, 403-404
thromboembolic disease and, 388
traumatic, in elderly, 313
trends in, 1
urinary tract complications, 384
urologic dysfunction after, 375
urologic problems and, 355-356
violence and, 2

Spinal cord monitoring
  dermatomal somatosensory evoked potentials and, 130
  electromyography and, 130
  intraoperative, 119-133
    somatosensory evoked potentials and, 121
    techniques of, 121-131
  segmental neurophysiologic, 129-131

Spinal devices, current product testing, 419

Spinal fractures/injuries: *see also* Spinal cord injury
  acceleration-deceleration injuries and, 98
  anatomic derangement, 39
  anesthesia and, 35
  computed tomography evaluation of, 35
  computed tomography of, 40
  costs of, 1
  dural tears and, 335-339
    clinical presentation of, 335
    etiology of, 335
  emergency management of, 33
  emergency surgery in, 36
  epidemiology of, 1, 331-332
  functional outcome after, 350-362
  imaging of, 39
  in elderly, 310-314
    epidemiology of, 311
  late deformity after, 315-330
    burst fractures and, 316
    Charcot arthropathy and, 317
    classification of, 322
    complications, 327
    compression fractures and, 316
    kyphosis and, 316
    lumbar spine, 325
    operative treatment of, 324-329
    pathomechanics of, 315-319
    patient evaluation, 319-322
    seat belt injuries and, 317
    thoracic spine, 325
    treatment of, 322-324
  magnetic resonance imaging of, 40
  medical-legal claims of, 88-91
  MRI evaluation of, 35
  neurosurgical procedures, 331-344
  noncontiguous, 35
  osseous healing in, 283-290
  osteoblasts and, 283

Spinal fractures/injuries—con't
  patient positioning in, 111-118
  pediatric, 250-251
    atlantooccipital injuries and, 247
    diagnosis and management, 241-275
    evaluation of, 245
    incidence and demography, 241
    pseudosubluxation and, 247
    radiology of, 245
  penetrating: *see* Penetrating spinal trauma
  physical examination and, 35
  posttraumatic syringomyelia and, 339
    diagnosis of, 339
    incidence of, 339
    management of, 339-340
    pathophysiology of, 339
  pseudarthrosis and, 291-297
    classification of, 292
    clinical significance of, 292
  radiographic evaluation of, 35
  recovery after, 350-362
  surgical approaches for: *see* Surgical approaches/techniques
  surgical complications in, 276-282
  treatment of, historical overview, 414-415
Spinal fusion, osseous healing and, 287
Spinal instability
  evaluating, 35
  patient transfers and, 117
Spinal manipulation, cord injury after, 105
Spinal stability
  penetrating spinal trauma and, 302
  thoracolumbar junction fractures and, 200
Spinal stabilization, emergency, 36
Spinal surgeon
  evaluation for spinal fracture, 34
  FDA regulation impact on, 419-420
  interaction with treatment team, 33
  radiologist and, 39
Spinal surgery: *see also* Surgical approaches/techniques
  blood loss during, 194-195
  complications of: *see* Surgical complications
  devices for, 421-424
    future, 424-425
  dural injury during, 195
  flexion-distraction injury and, 65
  general preparation for, 276
  historical perspective, 199
  intraoperative neurologic compromise prevention, 195
  neurophysiologic monitoring during, 119-133
  patient positioning during, 111-118
    complications of, 116-117
    lateral decubitus position, 113-116
    prone position, 113
    supine position, 112-113
  patient transfer and, 111-112
  penetrating spinal trauma, bullet/blade removal, 304
  timing of, 147-148
Spinal treatments, historical overview, 414-415
Spine: *see also* specific sections
  anatomy of, 6
  arterial circulation to, 6, 7
  circulation of, 6
  development of, 6, 242-243
    ossification, 242
  during life-saving intervention, 33
  embryology of, 6, 242-243
  emergency technicians and, 33
  immobilization of, 34
  pathoanatomy of, 243-244
  penetrating wounds of, 87-88
  soft tissue injury: *see* Whiplash
  surgical approaches to, 6
  venous circulation to, 6
Spinous processes, 13
Spondylitic spurs, 69
Spondylitis
  ankylosing, 107-108
  psoriatic, 108
Spondylolisthesis
  spondylolytic, 81
  traumatic, of axis, 161-165
Spondylolysis, traumatic, in children, 270
Spondylosis of C2, pediatric, 252
Stab wounds, 300
  blade removal and, 304
  characteristics of, 298
  patient evaluation, 300-303
Stabilization: *see* Spinal stabilization
Sternocleidomastoid muscle, anterior surgical approach to cervical spine and, 9
Stomach injuries, 37
Strap muscles, anterior surgical approach to cervical spine and, 9
Stress fractures, spondylolysis and, 81
Stress ulceration, corticosteroids and, 34
Subaxial spine
  anterior cervical approach to, 9
  stability of, assessment, 145
Subluxation
  atlantoaxial rotatory, in children, 257
  rotary, 45
Supraspinous ligament, clay-shovelers' fracture and, 71
Surgeon: *see* Spinal surgeon
Surgical approaches/techniques, 6: *see also* Spinal surgery
  anterior cervical approach to subaxial spine, 9
  atlas injuries, 158
  axial loading injuries, 173-176
  cervical spine
    anterior cervical approach to subaxial spine, 9
    in children, 261-263
    lower, 9
    posterior, 13
    upper
      anterior approach to, 11
      anterior retropharyngeal, 11
      anterior transoral, 11
      transoral approach to, 11
  cervicothoracic spine
    anterior cervicothoracic junction approach to, 17
    transsternal approach to, 17
    transthoracic approach to, 17
  foraminotomy, 178
  hyperextension injuries, 178-179

hyperflexion injuries, 170
laminectomy, 178
lumbar spine
anterior, 25
fractures of, 215-232
paraspinal, 31
retroperitoneal, 25
transperitoneal, 25
Wiltse, 31
lumbosacral spine
anterior, 27
posterior, 29
odontoid fractures, 160
thoracic spine
anterior approach to, 17
anterior thoracolumbar junction approach to, 21
costotransversectomy approach to, 21
posterior, 25
transthoracic approach to, 17
upper
fractures of, 187-188
with spinal canal compromise, 190-194
vertebral fractures of, 185-198
thoracolumbar spine, anterior, 24
Surgical complications
anterior cervical decompression, 148
avoidance of, 280
cervical injury treatment, 276-278
diagnostic quality and, 280-281
dural injury, 280
during transoral approach to cervical spine
meningitis, 11
pharyngeal wound infections, 11
grafts and, 279-280
lumbar spine surgery, 279
patient positioning and, 116-117
penetrating trauma and, 281
recognition and avoidance of, 276-282
retropharyngeal approach to cervical spine and, 12
spinal trauma and, 276-282
thoracic spine injury, 278-279
Surgical devices
current product testing, 419
currently available, 421-424
future, 424-425
international testing standards, 419
manufacturing, laboratory practices and testing, 418-419
premarket approval, 417
product availability, 420
product development process, 415-417
testing and regulatory guidelines and requirements, 417-419
Swelling, long-bone fractures and, 35
Sympathetic trunk, anterior thoracolumbar junction and, 23
Syringomyelia, 339-342, 403-404
diagnosis of, 339-340
incidence of, 339
management of, 339-340
pathophysiology of, 339
Syrinx, penetrating spinal trauma and, 306

T

T1-S5, Frankel grade A, B, C and, 3
TED hose, 37
Temporomandibular joint, acceleration-deceleration injuries and, 100
Teratogenic effects, 6
Tetraparesis, 369
Tetraplegia, 369
complete, 2
incidence of, 2
incomplete, 2
Tetraplegic, equipment needs for, 380
Thoracic corsets, 187
Thoracic pedicle screw placement, 170
Thoracic spine
anatomy of, 185
bony disruption of, 73
deformity after spinal trauma and, 324
development of, 242
disk herniation without fracture, 73
flexion-compression trauma to, 73
flexion-rotation injuries to, 73
Frankel classification and, 3
intercostal arteries in, 6
radiography of, 39
surgical approaches to
anterior thoracolumbar junction, 21
costotransversectomy, 21
costransversectomy approach to, 23
posterior, 25
trauma to, 73
vertebral fractures of, 185-198
Thoracic spine fractures/injuries
in elderly, 312
surgical complications, 278-279
upper
blood loss during surgery, 194-195
diagnostic imaging of, 186-187
gunshot wounds and, 188
orthoses for, 187
postoperative management of, 194
preoperative evaluation of, 186-187
surgical decision-making, 187-188
surgical management of, 190-194
treatment of, 187
Thoracolumbar instability, determination of, 203
Thoracolumbar junction
anterior approach to, 21
deformity after spinal trauma and, 324
distraction-extension injuries of, 208
flexion-distraction injuries of, 207
fracture dislocation of, 207
fractures/injuries of, 73-75
burst, 206
classification of, 73, 200
compression, 206
in children, 263-271
management of, 199-208
nonoperative treatment of, 203-206
operative treatment of, 206-213
radiographic analysis of, 200

Thoracolumbar junction—con't
  fractures/injuries of—con't
    spinal stability and, 200
  surgical approach to, 23
  surgical approaches, anterior, 24
Thoracolumbosacral orthoses, 377
Thromboembolic disease
  spinal cord injury and, 388
  support hose, 37
Thrombophlebitis, deep vein, 134
Tissue damage, projectiles and, 188
Tomography of sacral fractures, 236
Tongue deviation, 42
Torticollis, radiography and, 45
Trachea, anterior surgical approach to cervical spine and, 9
Tracheotomy, airway reestablishment and, 11
Traction
  C-arm during, 36
  cervical, 377
  cervical spine realignment and, 35
  edema and, 36
  hypoperfusion and, 36
  radiograph during, 36
  sedation/analgesia and, 35
Transcutaneous electrical nerve stimulation, whiplash and, 102
Transforming growth factor, 283
Trapezius, 13
Trauma
  "fine-toothed comb" examination, 35
  basic treatment for, 34
  disk herniation and, 91
  head: *see* Head trauma
  life support and, 34
  minor, spinal cord injury after, 105-110
  musculoskeletal examination and, 35
  patients, emergency technicians and, 33
Trisomy 21
  cervical instability in children and, 106
  vertebral anomalies and, 255
Trochanters, pressure sores and, 34
TSRH system, 424

U

Ulnar neuropathy, 117, 397
Urinary tract
  complications of
    infections, 384
    stones, 385
  evaluation of, 383
Urologic dysfunction, after spinal cord injury, 375
Urologic injuries, spinal surgeon evaluation of, 37

V

Venous circulation, of spine, 6
Vertebrae, wedge deformity of, 75
Vertebral alignment, radiography and, 39
Vertebral anomalies/trauma, in children, 254-256
Vertebral apophysis, slipped, in children, 269
Vertebral artery
  anatomic variability of, 11
  injury, 148
  spinal circulation and, 6
Vertebral body
  development of, 6
  mechanical failure of, 317
  of thoracic spine, 185
Vertebral column, function of, 39
Vertebral foramen, 185
Vertebral fractures, 70
  of upper thoracic spine, 185-198
Vertebral vein system, 7
Violence
  gunshot wounds, 2
  increase in rate of, 2
  spinal cord injury and, 2

W

Wage losses, 4
Wedge deformity, 75
Whiplash, 96
  diagnosing, 102
  epileptiform activity after, 98
  incidence of, 97
  long-term outcome after, 102-103
  physical therapy program, 102
  transcutaneous electrical nerve stimulation and, 102
  treatment of, 102
Whiplash shaken baby syndrome, 258
  intraocular bleeding and, 261
  subdural hematoma and, 261
Wiltse approach to lumbar spine, 31
Wound closure, during costotransversectomy, 21
Wound infection, during transoral approach to cervical spine, 11

Z

Zygapophyseal trauma, 10